Clinical Pocket Companion for

Maternal-Child Nursing Care

Optimizing Outcomes for Mothers, Children, and Families

D0827384

Clinical Pocket Companion for

Maternal-Child Nursing Care

Optimizing Outcomes for Mothers, Children, and Families

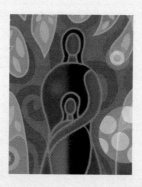

Susan L. Ward, PhD, RN
Professor of Nursing
Nebraska Methodist College
Omaha, Nebraska

Shelton M. Hisley, PhD, RNC, WHNP-BC
Assistant Professor of Nursing (Retired)
University of North Carolina at Wilmington
Wilmington, North Carolina

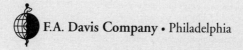

F.A. Davis Company • Philadelphia

F.A. Davis Company
1915 Arch Street
Philadelphia, PA 19103
www.fadavis.com

Printed in the United States of America

Last digit indicates print number: 10 9 8 7 6 5 4 3 2 1

Publisher, Nursing: Lisa B. Deitch
Developmental Editor: Shirley Kuhn
Director of Content Development: Darlene D. Pedersen
Senior Project Editor: Padraic J. Maroney
Manager of Art and Design: Carolyn O'Brien

As new scientific information becomes available through basic and clinical research,
recommended treatments and drug therapies undergo changes. The author(s) and
publisher have done everything possible to make this book accurate, up to date, and
in accord with accepted standards at the time of publication. The author(s), editors,
and publisher are not responsible for errors or omissions or for consequences from
application of the book, and make no warranty, expressed or implied, in regard to the
contents of the book. Any practice described in this book should be applied by the
reader in accordance with professional standards of care used in regard to the unique
circumstances that may apply in each situation. The reader is advised always to check
product information (package inserts) for changes and new information regarding
dose and contraindications before administering any drug. Caution is especially urged
when using new or infrequently ordered drugs.

Library of Congress Cataloging-in-Publication Data

Ward, Susan L.
  Clinical pocket companion for Maternal-child nursing care : optimizing outcomes
for mothers, children, and families / Susan L. Ward, Shelton M. Hisley.
    p. ; cm.
  Companion for Maternal-child nursing care : optimizing outcomes for mothers,
children, and families / Susan L. Ward, Shelton M. Hisley. Philadelphia : F.A. Davis,
c2009.
  Includes bibliographical references and index.
  ISBN-13: 978-0-8036-1855-8
  ISBN-10: 0-8036-1855-7
  1. Maternity nursing—Handbooks, manuals, etc. 2. Pediatric nursing—Handbooks,
    manuals, etc. I. Hisley, Shelton M. II. Ward, Susan L. Maternal-child nursing care.
    III. Title. [DNLM: 1. Maternal-Child Nursing—methods—Handbooks. 2. Cultural
    Diversity—Handbooks. 3. Evidence-Based Nursing—methods—Handbooks.
    4. Holistic Nursing—methods—Handbooks. WY 49 W263c 2010]
  RG951.W369 2010
  618.2'0231—dc22   2009022384

We dedicate the Clinical Pocket Companion to the nurses, students, and faculty who use this book as they provide holistic and culturally sensitive nursing care to mothers, children, and families.

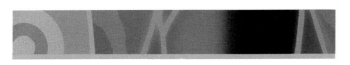

preface

The *Clinical Pocket Companion for Maternal-Child Nursing Care: Optimizing Outcomes for Mothers, Children, and Families* is a handy, concise resource that provides the essential elements for safe, effective nursing practice in maternal and child health. This versatile clinical aid can be beneficial to students and practicing nurses alike. Use it to supplement and reinforce information provided in the parent text during the clinical portion of the course. It also makes a great study guide. As a maternal-child health nurse, you will find it a convenient resource to retrieve important information quickly in a variety of patient settings. Presented in an easy-to-use format, this must-have tool for clinical practice offers students and practicing professional nurses an opportunity to ensure that the care they provide to mothers, children, and families is safe, timely, evidence-based, and culturally sensitive.

The clinical pocket companion is comprised of 32 chapters and is organized in a format that parallels the parent text. The first 14 chapters address ante-, intra-, and post-partal care of the childbearing woman; the final 18 chapters center on the care of infants, children and adolescents.

Pertinent information needed for safe clinical practice is condensed and summarized in a format to facilitate easy retrieval and quick reference. Illustrations enhance and clarify the major concepts presented. Special features focus on the themes of caring, sensitivity, empowerment, holism, spirituality, health promotion, complementary care, and safety.

Each chapter in this clinical pocket companion is organized into the following features:

- Key Terms - Definitions to enhance understanding of key concepts of care
- Focused Assessment - Essential elements of the nursing assessment for specific maternal-child conditions
- Clinical Alerts – Help you to recognize emergent or critical situations
- Diagnostic Tests – Various tests necessary for specific conditions

- Medications – Crucial information about commonly prescribed medications and herbal agents
- Nursing Procedures – Step-by-step instructions to ensure proper technique and positive outcomes
- Ethnocultural Considerations – Emphasize culturally-sensitive care in the clinical setting
- Teaching the Family – Clear teaching guidelines for parents to care for themselves, their infants, and children
- Additional Information for the Clinical Setting – Essential information to facilitate the delivery of safe, effective care in specific circumstances
- Resources – To direct you to various Internet and other sources for additional information

The *Clinical Pocket Companion for Maternal-Child Nursing Care: Optimizing Outcomes for Mothers, Children, and Families* is an easy-to-follow resource designed to help guide your every-day care of patients in the clinical setting. Use it to help you perform an appropriate assessment; formulate a nursing care plan; recognize abnormal findings; teach the mother, child, and family; interpret diagnostic and laboratory data; and provide safe, effective, culturally-sensitive care.

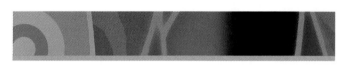

contributors

Deborah Bambini, PhD, WHNP-BC, CNE
Assistant Professor
Grand Valley State University
Grand Rapids, Michigan

Linda Nicholson Grinstead, PhD, RN, CPN, CNE
Professor
Grand Valley State University
Grand Rapids, Michigan

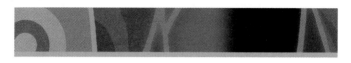

acknowledgments

We thank the editors and production staff of the F.A. Davis Company for their expertise and guidance, especially:

- Lisa Deitch, Publisher, Nursing
- Shirley Kuhn, Special Projects Editor
- Darlene D. Pedersen, Director of Content Development
- Padraic Maroney, Senior Project Editor
- Sam Rondinelli, Assistant Director of Production
- David Orzechowski, Managing Editor
- Julia Reukauf, Marketing Specialist

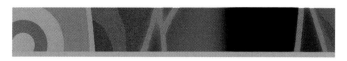

table of contents

chapter **1**　**Caring for Women, Families, and Children in Contemporary Society**　**1**

Infants and Children: Focused Assessment　2
Teaching the Family　2
Ethnocultural Considerations　6
Adolescents: Focused Assessment　6
Teaching the Family　7
Adult Health: Focused Assessment　7
Diagnostic Tests　10
Medications　10
Ethnocultural Considerations　11
Teaching the Family　11
Additional Information for the Clinical Setting　14

chapter **2**　**Reproductive Anatomy and Physiology**　**17**

Focused Assessment　18
Female Reproductive System　18
Male Reproductive System　23

chapter **3**　**Human Sexuality and Fertility**　**25**

Focused Assessment　26
Diagnostic Tests　26
Medications　28
Teaching the Family　28
Ethnocultural Considerations　34
Teaching the Family　38
Additional Information for the Clinical Setting　39

chapter **4**　**Conception and Development of the Embryo and Fetus**　**41**

Focused Assessment　42
Medications　45
Ethnocultural Considerations　47
Teaching the Family　47
Additional Information for the Clinical Setting　50
Resources　50

chapter **5**   **Physiological and Psychosocial Changes During Pregnancy**   **51**

Focused Assessment   52
Diagnostic Tests   56
Ethnocultural Considerations   57
Teaching the Family   58
Psychosocial Adaptations in Pregnancy   59
Additional Information for the Clinical Setting   60
Clinical Alert   61

chapter **6**   **The Prenatal Assessment**   **63**

Focused Assessment   65
Medications   73
Ethnocultural Considerations   75
Teaching the Family   75
Additional Information for the Clinical Setting   75

chapter **7**   **Promoting a Healthy Pregnancy**   **78**

Focused Assessment   78
Diagnostic Tests   79
Medications   81
Ethnocultural Considerations   81
Teaching the Family   82
Resources   87

chapter **8**   **Caring for the Woman Experiencing Complications During Pregnancy**   **89**

Bleeding During Pregnancy: Focused Assessment   91
Clinical Alerts   92
Diagnostic Tests   94
Ethnocultural Considerations   94
Teaching the Family   95
Hypertensive Complications in Pregnancy: Focused Assessment   96
Clinical Alerts   97
Medications   99
Teaching the Family   103
Additional Information for the Clinical Setting   104
Endocrine Complications in Pregnancy: Focused Assessment   105
Clinical Alert   107
Diagnostic Tests   107
Medications   108

Ethnocultural Considerations 108
Teaching the Family 108
Additional Information for the Clinical Setting 109
Infections that May Adversely Affect Pregnancy:
Focused Assessment 110
Diagnostic Tests 120
Medications 120
Special Conditions and Circumstances that May Adversely
Affect Pregnancy 121
Focused Assessment 123
Clinical Alerts 124
Diagnostic Tests 124
Medications 129
Ethnocultural Considerations 132
Additional Information for the Clinical Setting 133
Resources 134

chapter **9**　**The Process of Labor and Birth**　**136**

Focused Assessment 138
Promoting Effective Pushing 156
Clinical Alerts 157
Medications 157
Ethnocultural Considerations 159
Teaching the Family 159
Additional Information for the Clinical Setting 159
Resources 160

chapter **10**　**Promoting Patient Comfort During Labor and Birth**　**161**

Focused Assessment 163
Clinical Alerts 164
Medications 166
Ethnocultural Considerations 171
Teaching the Family 172
Additional Information for the Clinical Setting 172
Resources 174

chapter **11**　**Caring for the Woman Experiencing Complications During Labor and Birth**　**175**

Focused Assessment 177
Clinical Alerts 181
Medications 181
Ethnocultural Considerations 183

Teaching the Family   184
Additional Information for the Clinical Setting   185

chapter **12**   **Caring for the Postpartal Woman
                   and Her Family**   **202**

Focused Assessment   203
Assessment and Care of the Perineum   207
Promotion of Infant Nourishment   209
Clinical Alerts   210
Medications   210
Ethnocultural Considerations   215
Teaching the Family   216
Additional Information for the Clinical Setting   219
Resources   221

chapter **13**   **Caring for the Woman Experiencing
                   Complications During the Postpartal
                   Period**   **222**

Focused Assessment   223
Clinical Alerts   226
Diagnostic Tests   241
Medications   242
Teaching the Family   246
Additional Information for the Clinical Setting   248
Resources   249

chapter **14**   **Physiological Transition of the Newborn**   **251**

Focused Assessment   252
Clinical Alert   261
Diagnostic Tests   261
Medications   263
Ethnocultural Considerations   264
Additional Information for the Clinical Setting   264

chapter **15**   **Caring for the Normal Newborn**   **266**

Focused Assessment   268
Clinical Alerts   282
Diagnostic Tests   283
Medications   284
Ethnocultural Considerations   287
Teaching the Family   287
Additional Information for the Clinical Setting   290
Resources   291

chapter **16**   **Caring for the Newborn at Risk**   **293**

Focused Assessment   293
Clinical Alerts   301
Diagnostic Tests   301
Medications   303
Ethnocultural Considerations   305
Teaching the Family   305
Additional Information for the Clinical Setting   306
Resources   312

chapter **17**   **Caring for the Developing Child**   **314**

Focused Assessment   314
Clinical Alerts   315
Ethnocultural Considerations   316
Teaching the Family   316
Additional Information for the Clinical Setting   318
Resources   323

chapter **18**   **Caring for the Child in the Hospital
and in the Community**   **324**

Focused Assessment   324
Clinical Alerts   347
Diagnostic Tests   349
Medications   353
Ethnocultural Considerations   358
Teaching the Family   359
Additional Information for the Clinical Setting   362
Resources   370

chapter **19**   **Caring for the Family Across Care Settings**   **372**

Focused Assessment   372
Clinical Alert   374
Teaching the Family   374
Additional Information for the Clinical Setting   375
Resources   380

chapter **20**   **Caring for the Child with a Psychosocial
or Cognitive Condition**   **381**

Focused Assessment   381
Clinical Alerts   385
Medications   387

Ethnocultural Considerations   389
Teaching the Family   389
Additional Information for the Clinical Setting   391
Resources   394

chapter **21**   **Caring for the Child with a Respiratory
Condition**   **396**

Focused Assessment   396
Clinical Alerts   398
Diagnostic Tests   400
Medications   403
Ethnocultural Considerations   406
Teaching the Family   407
Additional Information for the Clinical Setting   412
Resources   415

chapter **22**   **Caring for the Child with a Gastrointestinal
Condition**   **416**

Focused Assessment   417
Clinical Alerts   418
Diagnostic Tests   420
Medications   424
Ethnocultural Considerations   425
Teaching the Family   426
Additional Information for the Clinical Setting   428
Resources   432

chapter **23**   **Caring for the Child with an Immunological
or Infectious Condition**   **434**

Focused Assessment   435
Clinical Alerts   436
Diagnostic Tests   438
Medications   439
Teaching the Family   446
Additional Information for the Clinical Setting   448
Resources   452

chapter **24**   **Caring for the Child with a Cardiovascular
Condition**   **453**

Focused Assessment   454
Clinical Alerts   456
Diagnostic Tests   458
Medications   460

Ethnocultural Considerations   461
Teaching the Family   462
Additional Information for the Clinical Setting   463
Resources   477

chapter **25** **Caring for the Child with an Endocrinological or Metabolic Condition**   **479**

Focused Assessment   479
Clinical Alerts   482
Diagnostic Tests   483
Medications   486
Ethnocultural Considerations   488
Teaching the Family   489
Additional Information for the Clinical Setting   495
Resources   498

chapter **26** **Caring for the Child with a Neurological or Sensory Condition**   **499**

Focused Assessment   500
Clinical Alerts   505
Diagnostic Tests   507
Medications   507
Ethnocultural Considerations   511
Teaching the Family   512
Additional Information for the Clinical Setting   513
Resources   521

chapter **27** **Caring for the Child with a Musculoskeletal Condition**   **525**

Focused Assessment   525
Clinical Alerts   531
Diagnostic Tests   533
Medications   536
Ethnocultural Considerations   538
Teaching the Family   539
Additional Information for the Clinical Setting   539
Resources   546

chapter **28** **Caring for the Child with an Integumentary Condition**   **547**

Focused Assessment   548
Clinical Alerts   552
Diagnostic Tests   554

Medications   555
Ethnocultural Considerations   559
Teaching the Family   559
Additional Information for the Clinical Setting   563
Resources   571

chapter **29**   **Caring for the Child with a Renal,
Urinary Tract, or Reproductive Condition   574**

Focused Assessment   574
Clinical Alerts   580
Diagnostic Tests   583
Medications   591
Ethnocultural Considerations   596
Teaching the Family   597
Additional Information for the Clinical Setting   599
Resources   607

chapter **30**   **Caring for the Child with a Hematological
Condition   610**

Focused Assessment   611
Clinical Alerts   614
Diagnostic Tests   618
Medications   624
Ethnocultural Considerations   625
Teaching the Family   626
Additional Information for the Clinical Setting   630
Resources   639

chapter **31**   **Caring for the Child with Cancer   640**

Focused Assessment   640
Clinical Alerts   643
Diagnostic Tests   646
Medications   653
Ethnocultural Considerations   659
Teaching the Family   659
Additional Information for the Clinical Setting   661
Resources   669

chapter **32**   **Caring for the Child with a Chronic
Condition or the Dying Child   671**

Focused Assessment   672
Clinical Alerts   676
Medications   677

Ethnocultural Considerations   677
Teaching the Family   678
Additional Information for the Clinical Setting   678
Resources   689

Photo and Illustration Credits   **691**

Index   **698**

Caring for Women, Families, and Children in Contemporary Society

KEY TERMS

climacteric – Transitional time in a woman's life marked by declining ovarian function and decreased hormone production

dysmenorrhea – Painful menstruation that interferes with daily activities

dysplasia – Abnormal development of tissues or organs

endometriosis – Benign disorder of the reproductive tract characterized by the presence and growth of endometrial tissue outside of the uterus.

hyperprolactinemia – Excessive secretion of prolactin

leiomyoma – Fibroid, a benign smooth muscle uterine tumor

menopause – Permanent cessation of menstrual periods; can only be dated with certainty 1 year after menstruation ceases

mittelschmerz – Abdominal pain in the region of an ovary during ovulation; usually occurs midway through the menstrual cycle

perimenopause – Period of transition of changing ovarian activity before menopause and through the first few years of amenorrhea

prostaglandins – Chemical mediators produced by the tissues and found in many parts of the body; play an important role in menstrual cramps

Infants and Children

FOCUSED ASSESSMENT

Recommended Immunization Schedule for Children

Vaccine ▼ Age ►	Birth	1 month	2 months	4 months	6 months	12 months	15 months	18 months	19–23 months	2–3 years	4–6 years
Hepatitis B[1]	Hep B	Hep B		see footnote 1		Hep B					
Rotavirus[2]			Rota	Rota	Rota						
Diphtheria, Tetanus, Pertussis[3]			DTaP	DTaP	DTaP	see footnote 3	DTaP				DTaP
Haemophilus influenzae type b[4]			Hib	Hib	Hib[4]	Hib					
Pneumococcal[5]			PCV	PCV	PCV	PCV				PPV	
Inactivated Poliovirus			IPV	IPV		IPV					IPV
Influenza[6]						Influenza (Yearly)					
Measles, Mumps, Rubella[7]						MMR					MMR
Varicella[8]						Varicella					Varicella
Hepatitis A[9]						HepA (2 doses)				HepA Series	
Meningococcal[10]										MCV4	

Range of recommended ages [   ]   Certain high-risk groups [   ]

Source: Centers for Disease Control and Prevention (2008).

TEACHING THE FAMILY

Nutrition

Guidelines for Infant Feeding	
Infant/Child Age	**Feeding Guidelines**
Birth–1 Month	Breast every 2–3 hours Bottle every 3–4 hours 2–3 oz. per feeding
2–4 Months	Breast or bottle every 3–4 hours 3–4 oz. per feeding
4–6 Months	Breast or bottle 4–6 times per day 4–5 oz. per feeding
6–8 Months	Iron-fortified rice cereal Breast or bottle 4 times per day 6–8 oz. per feeding

Infant/Child Age	Feeding Guidelines
8–10 Months	Finger foods Chopped or mashed foods Sippy cup with formula, breast milk, juice or water Breast or bottle 4 times per day 6–8 oz. per feeding
10–12 Months	Self-feeds with fingers and spoon Most table foods Breast or bottle 4 times per day 6–8 oz. per feeding

Introducing Solid Foods to Infants

Tips for Introducing Solid Foods to Infants
- The infant displays readiness at approximately 6 months of age.
- Assess for developmental cues: ability to sit well with support; disappearance of the extrusion reflex.
- Begin with iron-fortified rice cereal.
- Add vegetables, then fruits.
- Introduce one food at a time; wait 3 to 5 days between new foods.
- Introduce food before formula or breastfeeding; follow each solid food meal with breast milk or formula.

Alert: If the infant is not growing or gaining weight, or if he is unable to suck or swallow or shows any sign of an allergic reaction, promptly seek help from the primary health care provider, nearby clinic, or emergency room.

Additional Information
- Avoid salt, sugar, and additives.
- **Never** prop bottles, put food in bottles, or mix food with formula (choking hazard).
- Offer only small bites of food to prevent choking; when feeding, pay close attention to the infant.

(American Academy of Pediatrics, 2005)

Dental Care

Guidelines for Parents
- Teething typically begins between 4 and 7 months.
- It is normal for an infant to have any number of teeth ranging from no teeth to 8 or more teeth by the first birthday.

- Most children have all 20 primary teeth by the third birthday.
- Signs of teething:
  - Drooling, irritability, desire to chew on objects, crying episodes, disrupted sleep, change in eating patterns
- Interventions for teething discomfort:
  - Give infant a cool wet washcloth to chew on.
  - Place teething rings in the refrigerator for a few minutes before applying.
  - Rub gums with a clean finger.
- Take the infant to the dentist within 6 months of the eruption of the first tooth.
- Cleanse the gums with a damp washcloth or soft toothbrush.
- Do not use toothpaste until the child reaches age 2.

Sleep and Rest

Sleep Requirements			
Age	Hours of Sleep	Additional Naps	Tips
Newborn	15–20	—	"Back to sleep": Always place infant on back for sleep
3 Months	15	—	Put infant to bed drowsy but awake so that he learns to fall asleep on his own.
6 Months	9–14	Two 2-hour naps	
1 Year	9–14	May decrease slightly	
Toddler/ Preschool	14	Usually one nap for 1.5–3 hours	Bedtime resistance often appears. Utilize bedtime rituals.
School Age	10–12 +/–	—	

Prevent Plagiocephaly

- Infant skulls are soft and flexible during the first year of life as the skull enlarges to accommodate the growing brain. During this time, the infant skull can become misshapen or deformed by external pressure. This condition is rarely life threatening, but can cause permanent facial and skull deformities, or in severe cases, the child's vision can be affected.

- Constant pressure on one area of the infant's head can flatten or reshape it. Proper positioning during sleep and waking periods spent in car seats and infant chairs often require the infant to spend considerable time on his back.
- Place the infant on the stomach to play for several times each day. When the infant is very young, place a rolled towel or blanket under his arms for support. This intervention removes pressure from the skull and facilitates the development of strong neck and arm muscles needed for sitting and crawling.
- Place the infant on his side during awake times.
- Alternate the direction the infant faces in the bassinette or crib during sleep times. If the infant's crib is positioned against a wall, alternate the end of the bed where the infant's head is placed to allow her to look out toward the room instead of the less stimulating wall.
- Seek medical advice if a flattened area on the baby's skull does not improve with positioning changes; a customized helmet may be necessary.

Promoting Safety for Infants and Children

Review with parents:

- Car seat guidelines
- Household smoke and carbon monoxide detectors; fire extinguishers
- Storage of medications and cleaning supplies: Install child-safety latches.
- Crib safety: Ensure that bars are less than 2 3/8 inches apart; mattress fits snugly; free from sharp edges and toxic paint.
- Hazards of microwave ovens: Never use to warm infant bottles or food.
- Use of pacifiers: Never place around infant's neck or attach to clothing.
- Proper use of highchairs, strollers, swings, playpens; avoid walkers.
- Infant care basics:
  - Keep one hand on the infant when on a changing table or other high surface.
  - At bath time, test water temperature with wrist, keep both hands on infant.
- Use safety gates at all stairways.

ETHNOCULTURAL CONSIDERATIONS

Infant Feeding

Culture plays an important role in infant feeding. For many new immigrants and members of ethnic minorities, the traditions of their homeland, the consumption of traditional foods, and maintaining traditional food preparations provide comfort in an environment that is new *and* unknown, and is a way of sustaining cultural identity. Some cultural practices include breastfeeding on demand and early introduction of solid foods, whereas others feel that exposure of the breast is indecent and therefore decreases the mother's comfort with breastfeeding. It is imperative for nurses to recognize biases that the Western view of health and nutrition is the only appropriate method to feeding an infant. Nurses need to evaluate the effect of the cultural practices objectively and intervene only if the mother or infant is at risk for harm.

Adolescents

FOCUSED ASSESSMENT

Components of Health Promotion Screening

Screening should include (Michigan Quality Improvement Consortium, 2005a):

- Height, weight, and body mass index (BMI)
- Risk evaluation and counseling:
  - Nutrition, obesity, physical activity, dental health, tobacco use, immunizations, human immunodeficiency virus (HIV) prevention, sexually transmitted diseases prevention and sexual health, sexual abuse, preconception counseling for all women of childbearing age, medication use, and sun exposure
- Safety:
  - Intimate partner violence, seat belt use, use of helmets, firearm safety, and use of smoke and carbon monoxide detectors in the home
- Behavior assessment:
  - Depression, suicide threats, alcohol and drug use, anxiety, stress reduction, risk-taking behaviors and coping skills
  - Consideration of developmental tasks

- Piaget: Thought becomes more abstract
- Erikson: Role experimentation; peer influence
- Freud: Puberty and development of sexuality

TEACHING THE FAMILY

Safety

Discuss the following topics:

- Decision making
- Strategies for conflict resolution
- Reproductive health safety
- Risk-taking behaviors (substance use and abuse, violence, tattooing, body piercing)
- Signs of depression, suicide, eating disorders
- Injury prevention (seatbelt, helmet, other protective wear for sports)

Health Promotion

- Adequate calcium and vitamin D intake
- Adequate sleep, rest, and exercise
- Preparation for the first gynecological visit (ages 13–15); pelvic examination by age 21 or 3 years after the initiation of sexual activity

Adult Health

FOCUSED ASSESSMENT

Preventive Screening Recommendations			
Service	19–39 Years	40–64 Years	65 + Years
Aspirin Prophylaxis	Discuss with women post-menopause, men older than 40 years, and younger individuals at increased risk for coronary heart disease.		
Breast Cancer Screening		Annual mammogram for women with risk factors; every 1–2 years for women 50 to 64 years of age with no risk factors	Annual mammogram for women with risk factors; every 1–2 years for women 65 and older with no risk factors *(continued)*

Preventive Screening Recommendations (Continued)

Service	19–39 Years	40–64 Years	65 + Years
Cervical Cancer Screening	First Pap smear at age 21 or 3 years after first sexual intercourse, whichever is earlier; every 3 years after 3 consecutive normal results	Every 3 years after 3 consecutive normal results	Pap smear with new sexual partner
Chlamydia and Gonorrhea Screening	All sexually active females, including asymptomatic women age 25 years and younger		
Colon Cancer Screening	All persons 50–79 years of age		
Hypertension Screening	Blood pressure screening every 2 years if <120/80 mm Hg; annual blood pressure screening if 120–139/80–89 mm Hg		
Influenza Vaccine	Annually between October and March for individuals age 50 years and older, those with chronic illnesses, members of the health care team, and others at high risk		
Pneumococcal Vaccine	Immunize individuals at high risk once; re-immunize once after 5 years if at risk for losing immunity.		Immunize at age 65 if not done previously; re-immunize once if first vaccination received >5 years ago and before age 65.
Problem Drinking Screening	Screen for problem drinking among all adults and provide brief counseling.		
Tobacco Cessation Counseling	Assess all adults for tobacco use and provide ongoing cessation services for those who smoke or are at risk for smoking relapse.		
Total Cholesterol and HDL Cholesterol Screening	Fasting fractionated lipid screening for men older than age 34 every 5 years	Fasting fractionated lipid screening for men older than age 34 and for women older than age 44 every 5 years	
Vision Screening			Asymptomatic elderly adults

Sources: American College of Obstetricians and Gynecologists (2007); U.S. Preventive Services Task Force (2007); Institute for Clinical Systems Improvement (2005).

Breast Cancer Risk Factors

- Defects in breast cancer gene 1 (*BRCA1*) or breast cancer gene 2 (*BRCA2*)
- Gender: 100 times more likely to occur in females than in males
- Age: Increasing age, with 50% appearing by age 50
- Personal history of breast cancer in at least one breast
- Family history of breast cancer
- Exposure to radiation
- Excess weight
- Exposure to estrogen: Early onset of menarche, late menopause, or use of hormonal therapy
- Race: Caucasians more likely to develop breast cancer than Hispanics or African Americans
- Smoking
- Exposure to carcinogens
- Excessive use of alcohol
- Diagnosis of precancerous breast changes
- Increased breast density revealed on mammography

(American Cancer Society [ACS], 2006)

Osteoporosis Risk Factors

- Older age, due to decreased estrogen after menopause
- Slender build and small frame
- Low body weight (< 70 kg [150 lbs.])
- Shortened exposure to estrogen, through late menarche or early menopause
- Family history of osteoporosis
- Smoking
- Decreased physical activity or sedentary lifestyle
- Excessive caffeine or alcohol use
- Low calcium and vitamin D intake
- Southeast Asian and Caucasian ethnicity
- Use of corticosteroids, commonly used to treat chronic respiratory disorders and arthritis

DIAGNOSTIC TESTS

Cholesterol and Lipid Screening

Guidelines for Interpreting Lipid Screening Results	
Total Cholesterol	
Below 200 mg/dL:	Desirable
240 mg/dL and above:	High, increased risk of cardiac disease
LDL Cholesterol	
Below 100 mg/dL:	Desirable; target goal for those with cardiac disease or multiple risk factors
100–129 mg/dL:	Elevated; target goal for those with two or more risk factors
130–160 mg/dL:	Borderline high; target goal for those with zero to one risk factor
Above 160 mg/dL:	Significantly elevated
HDL Cholesterol	
Below 40 mg/dL:	Adds a risk factor for cardiac disease
60 mg/dL and above:	Desirable
Triglycerides	
Below 150 mg/dL:	Desirable
200 mg/dL and above:	High

Source: Veterans Health Administration, Department of Defense (2006).

MEDICATIONS

Herbal Remedies for Anxiety and Depression

Herbal remedies for anxiety and depression include kava kava, passionflower, valerian root, gotu kola, and St. John's wort. Although these herbs are believed to reduce anxiety, stress, and muscle tension, the nurse should provide education on the potential side effects of these substances, which include gastrointestinal discomforts, nausea, and dizziness.

ETHNOCULTURAL CONSIDERATIONS

Breast Cancer Screening

There are notable differences in breast cancer screening practices among women of different ethnic backgrounds. Although African American women are at a lower risk for developing breast cancer than Caucasian women are, they are more likely to die from breast cancer due to late diagnosis. According to Husaini et al. (2001), African American women are more likely to have mammogram screening if they are older, married, have a higher level of education, and believe that early detection could lead to a cure. A positive family history of breast cancer and church affiliation have no influence on the incidence of detection.

Asian American and Pacific Islander women have very low rates of breast cancer screening. Factors responsible for the low screening rates include lack of health insurance, low income, and lack of a primary care provider (Kagawa-Singer & Pourat, 2000).

Breast cancer causes a significant number of deaths in Filipino women. In a study by Wu and Bancroft (2006), researchers found that women were more likely to follow recommended screenings if there was support from physicians and family members and if they had insurance. The presence of physical symptoms, family history of breast cancer, and health literacy promote adherence to recommendations.

TEACHING THE FAMILY

Breast Self-Examination (BSE)

1. Visually inspect the breasts in front of a mirror. Assess for color, contour, shape, and size. Assess for dimpling or puckering of the skin; change in nipple direction; and redness, rash, or swelling

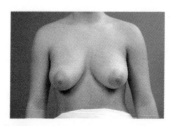

2. Repeat the first step with the arms slightly raised above the head.

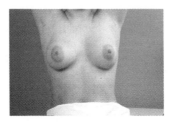

3. Inspect and palpate the nipple. Gently squeeze the nipple between the thumb and forefinger, looking for discharge. Many women, especially those who have had children, are able to express some discharge by squeezing the nipples. Discharge that is of concern is most often spontaneous (ACS, 2007).

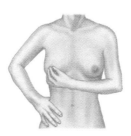

4. Palpate the breast and axillae. Recline on the bed and place a pillow under each shoulder during palpation. Use the left hand to palpate the right breast and the right hand to palpate the left breast. Using the finger pads of the three middle fingers, palpate the entire surface of the breast. Use overlapping dime-sized circular motions and apply three different levels of pressure: light pressure is best to feel the tissue closest to the skin; medium pressure is best to feel a little deeper; and firm pressure is used to feel the tissue closest to the chest and ribs.

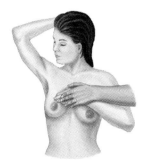

5. Move around the breast in an up-and-down pattern, checking the entire breast area until only the ribs are felt.
6. Repeat the entire technique on the other breast (ACS, 2007).

How to Recognize and Cope with Fibrocystic Changes in the Breast

- Palpable thickening in breast tissue, associated with cyclic tenderness, pain
- Common, benign, usually appear during second and third decades of life
- Treat by relieving symptoms (e.g., analgesics, nonsteroidal anti-inflammatory drugs such as ibuprofen), diuretics, use of support bra, avoidance of tobacco and alcohol, application of heat to breasts.

How to Perform Testicular Self-Examination

1. Examine the testicles, one at a time. One should be slightly larger than the other (usually the right one).
2. Feel for lumps and bumps along the front and sides.
3. Using both hands, place your thumbs over the top of each testicle and your index fingers and middle fingers underneath the testicle. Gently roll the testicle, using slight pressure, between your fingers.

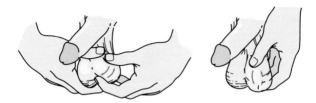

4. The epididymis, which carries the sperm, can be felt at the top of the back part of each testicle. It should feel soft and rope-like and be slightly tender to pressure. This is a normal finding.

5. Notify your physician if you notice any swelling, lumps, pains, or changes in color or size of either testicle (The Nemours Foundation, 2007).

ADDITIONAL INFORMATION FOR THE CLINICAL SETTING

Speaking with an Adolescent About Losing Weight

- Discussions about weight loss can be a sensitive issue for many overweight patients, especially during adolescence. Body weight has a dramatic effect on the development of self-image and self-esteem.
- Begin the conversation with expressions of respect that are sensitive to cultural differences related to food choices and eating patterns. Regardless of whether or not the patient is ready to begin a weight control program, she may still benefit from talking openly about healthy eating and exercise.
- Begin with a simple question to determine if the patient is willing to talk about the issue: *"Cindy, can we talk about your weight? What are your thoughts about your weight right now?"* *"What kind of help would you like from me regarding your weight?"*
- Avoid the use of words that may make patients feel uncomfortable, such as "obese," "obesity," "fat," and "excess fat."
- To determine the degree of readiness to engage in weight control, additional questions can be asked: *"What are your goals concerning your weight?"*

Health Promotion Counseling for Perimenopausal Women

Counsel perimenopausal women about:

- Healthy lifestyle strategies: Smoking cessation, consuming a variety of foods low in saturated fat and cholesterol, limiting salt and alcohol intake, maintaining a healthy weight, and being physically active
- Prevention of osteoporosis: Consuming foods rich in vitamin D and calcium, obtaining moderate exposure to sunlight, engaging in weight-bearing exercises; smoking cessation; and limiting alcohol intake
- Treatment of menopausal symptoms: Alternative therapies; antidepressants; stress reduction; avoidance of spicy foods, alcohol, and caffeine; getting adequate sleep; being physically active; use of selective estrogen receptor modulators (SERMs) for severe symptoms only

Empowering Women to Cope with Symptoms of Menopause

Dietary supplements and herbal therapies have long provided women with alternative treatments to alleviate some of the symptoms associated with menopause (e.g., soy, vitamins, probiotics, and herbs such as black cohosh). Research evidence does not support the ideas that they are efficacious in minimizing menopausal symptoms (Nedrow et al., 2006).

Complementary therapies that are currently being studied for their benefit in diminishing menopausal symptoms include:

- Mind–body therapy
- Energy therapy: Electromagnetic forces, life-force energy
- Manipulative and body-based therapy: Chiropractic, osteopathy, massage
- Traditional Chinese medicine

While there is no current evidence to support their effectiveness in minimizing the symptoms of menopause, these complementary methods are considered to be much safer than herbal and vitamin therapies.

Health Promotion for Older Adults

- Exercise and activity: Improve strength, endurance, flexibility, and balance

- Cognitive functioning
  - Stress management
  - Coping strategies
  - Medical management of physical illnesses
  - Healthy lifestyle choices: good nutrition, moderation of alcohol, elimination of tobacco use
- Functional assessment
- Immunizations
  - Influenza
  - Pneumococcus

REFERENCES

American Academy of Pediatrics. (2005). Policy statement: Breastfeeding and the use of human milk. *Pediatrics, 115*(2), 496–506.

American Cancer Society (ACS). (2006). What are the risk factors for breast cancer? Retrieved from http://www.cancer.org/docroot/CRI/content/CRI_2_4_2X_What_are_the_risk_factors_for_breast_cancer_5.asp?sitearea= (Accessed October 29, 2008).

American Cancer Society (ACS). (2007). How to perform a breast self-exam. Retrieved from http://www.cancer.org/docroot/CRI/content/CRI-2-6x-How-to-perform-a-breast-self-exam-5.asp (Accessed March 4, 2008).

American College of Obstetricians and Gynecologists. (2007). *Women's health care: a resource manual* (3rd ed.). Washington, DC: Author.

Husaini, B.A., Sherkat, D.E., Bragg, R., Levine R., Emerson, J.S., Mentes, C.M., et al. (2001). Predictors of breast cancer screening in a panel study of African American women. *Women and Health, 34*(3), 35–51.

Institute for Clinical Systems Improvement (ICSI). (2005, October). *Preventive services in adults*. Bloomington, MN: Author.

Kagawa-Singer, M., & Pourat, N. (2000). Asian American and Pacific Islander breast and cervical carcinoma screening rates and healthy people 2000 objectives. *Cancer, 89*(3), 696–705.

Michigan Quality Improvement Consortium. (2005a, July). *Adult preventive services (ages 18–49)*. Southfield, MI: Author.

Nedrow, A., Miller, J., Walker, M., Nygren, P., Huffman, L.H., & Nelson, H.D. (2006). Complementary and alternative therapies for the management of menopause-related symptoms: A systematic evidence review. *Archives of Internal Medicine, 166*(14), 1453–1465.

Nield, L.S., & Kamat, D.M. (2006). Odd skull shapes: Heads up on diagnosis and therapy, *Consultant for Pediatricians, 5*(11), 701–709.

The Nemours Foundation. (2007). How to perform a testicular self-examination. Retrieved from http://www.kidshealth.org/teen/sexual_health/guys/tse.html (Accessed March 14, 2008).

Veterans Health Administration, Department of Defense. (2006). *VHA/DoD clinical practice guideline for the management of dyslipidemia in primary care*. Washington, DC: Author.

Wu, T.Y., & Bancroft, J. (2006). Filipino American women's perceptions and experiences with breast cancer screening. *Oncology Nursing Forum, 33*(4), E71–E78.

Reproductive Anatomy and Physiology

KEY TERMS

adrenarche – Changes that occur at puberty as a result of increased secretion of adrenocortical hormones

ferning – Palm leaf or arborization pattern found on microscopic examination of a sample of certain fluids such as cervical mucus and amniotic fluid

gonad – Sex gland that produces hormone (ovary and testis)

graafian follicle – Mature ovarian cyst that contains the nearly mature ovum (oocyte); on rupture of the follicle, it is discharged from the ovary (ovulation); the corpus luteum develops within the ruptured graafian follicle

gravid – Pregnant

menarche – The first menstrual period

oocyte – Incompletely developed ovum

oogenesis – Process of oocyte development that results in maturation of human ova

puberty – Biological time frame between childhood and adulthood; during this time the reproductive organs mature and the individual becomes functionally capable of reproduction

sex chromosome – Chromosome associated with the determination of sex: X (female); Y (male)

spinnbarkheit – The formation of a stretchable thread of cervical mucus; occurs at the time of ovulation due to the influence of estrogen

thelarche – Beginning of breast development

FOCUSED ASSESSMENT

Assessment of the reproductive system should start with a general health assessment:

- Chief complaint
- Associated/alleviating factors
- Past medical history
- Family health history
- Social history
- Timeline of development of the secondary sexual characteristics

Female Body Changes Associated with Puberty				
Type of Body Change	**Body Change**	**Definition**	**Average Age Initiated**	**Average Age Completed**
Growth Spurt	Adolescent growth spurt	Height increase 2.4–4.3 inches (6–11 cm) in 1 year	10	11.8
Secondary	Thelarche	Breast budding	9.8	14.6
	Adrenarche	↑ adrenal androgen secretion → axillary and pubic hair	10.5	
Primary	Menarche	First menstrual period	12.8	

FEMALE REPRODUCTIVE SYSTEM

External Structures

Include mons pubis, labia majora, labia minora, clitoris, vestibule of the vagina, urethral (urinary) meatus, Skene's glands, Bartholin's glands, vaginal introitus, hymen, and perineum (Fig. 2-1).

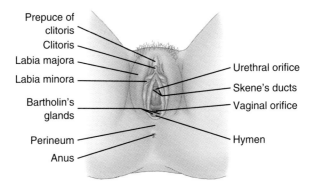

Figure 2-1 Female external genitalia.

The Pelvic Floor
- Muscles include the levator ani and coccygeus.
  o Provide support for internal pelvic structures.

Internal Structures

Include the ovaries, fallopian tubes, uterus, adjacent structures (adnexa), and vagina (Figs. 2-2 and 2-3).

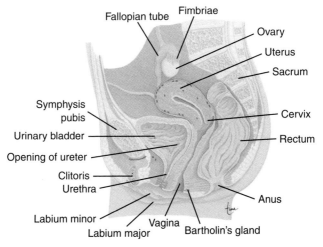

Figure 2-2 Midsagittal view of the female reproductive system.

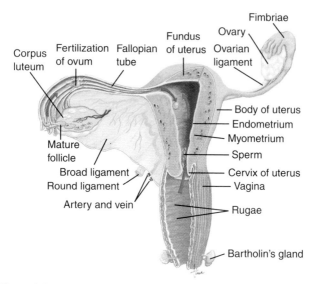

Figure 2-3 The female reproductive system shown in anterior view.

Uterine Anatomy
- Corpus: Upper two thirds of uterine body
- Isthmus: Slight constriction midway between the corpus and the cervix
- Cervix: Lower, narrow end of the uterus, opens into the vagina

Uterine Support Structures
Include the broad, round, cardinal, pubocervical, and uterosacral ligaments (support upper and middle portions of the uterus); and pelvic floor muscles (support lower portion of the uterus).

Bony Pelvis (Fig. 2-4)
- Composed of sacrum, coccyx, and two innominate (hip) bones.
- Includes the "false pelvis" and the "true pelvis."
- True pelvis is divided into inlet, midpelvis, outlet.

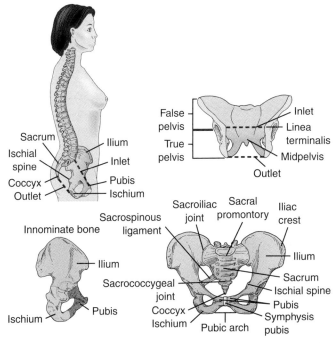

Figure 2-4 The female bony pelvis.

The Breasts

- Considered accessory organs of the reproductive system.
- Consist of glandular, fibrous, and adipose tissue suspended by Cooper's ligaments.
- Primary function is infant nourishment.
- Lactation is triggered by prolactin.
- Parts include nipples, areolae, and Montgomery tubercles.

The Menstrual Cycle and Reproduction

The menstrual cycle is hormonally mediated through events in the hypothalamus, anterior pituitary gland, and ovaries (Fig. 2-5). Interrelationships exist among the levels of hormone secretion, development of the ovarian follicles, and changes in the uterine endometrium (Fig. 2-6).

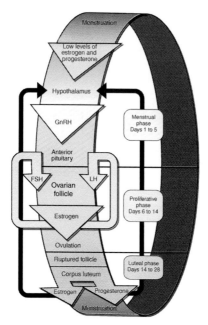

Figure 2-5 Hormonal feedback mechanisms that regulate the female menstrual cycle.

Body Changes Related to the Menstrual Cycle and Ovulation
- Cervical mucus
  - Increased amount: Watery, clear
  - Increased elasticity (spinnbarkheit)
  - Increased ferning
- Physiological changes
  - Increased basal body temperature
  - Mittelschmerz

Natural Cessation of Menses
- Climacteric phase: Decline in ovarian function and loss of estrogen and progesterone production
- Perimenopausal phase: Precedes menopause; characterized by physical/psychological changes related to estrogen depletion
- Menopause (last menstrual period)
- Postmenopausal phase: Time after menopause; estrogen produced by the adrenal glands

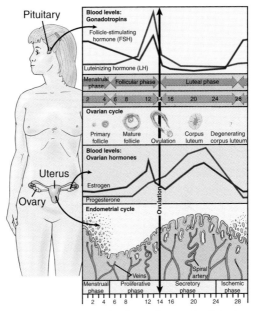

Figure 2-6 The female reproductive cycle. Levels of the hormones secreted from the anterior pituitary are shown relative to one another and throughout the cycle. Changes in the ovarian follicle are depicted. The relative thickness of the endometrium is also shown.

MALE REPRODUCTIVE SYSTEM

External Structures

Consist of the perineum, penis, and scrotum (Fig. 2-7).

Internal Structures

Include the testes, epididymis, ducts (vas deferens, ejaculatory duct), urethra, spermatic cords, and accessory glands (seminal vesicles, prostate, bulbourethral glands and urethral glands).

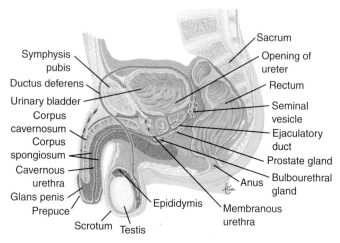

Figure 2-7 The male reproductive system shown in a midsagittal section through the pelvic cavity.

Hormonal Influence

Testosterone is the dominant male hormone.

- At puberty, stimulates enlargement of testes and accessory organs
- Prompts development of the secondary sex characteristics and a linear growth spurt

Human Sexuality and Fertility

KEY TERMS

abortion – Termination of pregnancy before the fetus reaches a viable age, usually less than 20 weeks of gestation or when the fetus weighs less than 500 grams

elective a. Voluntary termination of a pregnancy for other than medical reasons

therapeutic a. Abortion performed when the pregnancy endangers the mother's mental or physical health or when the fetus has a known condition that is incompatible with life

abstinence – Refraining from vaginal intercourse

basal body temperature (BBT) – Lowest body temperature taken immediately on awakening and before arising

bilateral tubal ligation (BTL) – Method of female sterilization in which both fallopian tubes are blocked to prevent conception

contraception – Prevention of conception

dyspareunia – Pain with sexual intercourse

hysterosalpingography – Radiography of the uterus and fallopian tubes after injection of a radiopaque iodine-based dye

infertility – Inability to achieve pregnancy during a year or more of unprotected intercourse

intrauterine device (IUD) – Small plastic device that is inserted into the uterus and left in place for an extended period of time to prevent implantation of a fertilized ovum

menorrhagia – Menstrual bleeding that is excessive in number of days or amount of blood

sterility – Absolute factor prevents reproduction

theoretical effectiveness – Effectiveness in a laboratory setting

toxic shock syndrome (TSS) – Severe, acute disease most often caused by *Staphylococcus aureus*; has also been associated with the use of high-absorbency tampons during menstruation but may complicate any staphylococcal infection

user effectiveness – Number of women who will become pregnant within 1 year of typical use (includes user error)

vasectomy – Male sterilization that involves ligation or the removal of a segment of the vas deferens

zygote – Fertilized ovum that results from the union of an ovum and a sperm

FOCUSED ASSESSMENT

Components of a Reproductive Health History

- General health history: Chronic health problems, tobacco, alcohol and other substance use, medications, herbal supplements
- Menstrual history: Age at onset, frequency, duration, flow, presence of dysmenorrhea or breast tenderness
- Obstetric history: Outcomes of past pregnancies; plans for future pregnancies
- Sexual history and risk assessment: Previous sexually transmitted infections (STIs), dyspareunia, postcoital bleeding, frequency of intercourse (is it consensual?), number of past sexual partners, current partner(s), gender, sexual practices, use of protective devices
- Past contraceptive use: Any difficulties with specific methods

DIAGNOSTIC TESTS

Common Diagnostic Methods Used in the Evaluation of Female Infertility	
Type/Name of Test	**Role of the Nurse**
Prediction of Ovulation Identifies the LH surge (24–36 hours before ovulation) and absence of ovulation. Tests include basal body	Teach the couple how the information helps to determine timing of intercourse to coincide with ovulation. Instruct the woman about recording the BBT and

Type/Name of Test	Role of the Nurse
temperature (BBT), commercial ovulation predictor kits, and assessment of cervical mucus.	assessing the cervical mucus; reinforce directions for using commercial ovulation predictor kits.
Postcoital Test (PCT); Huhner Test Assessment of the quality and quantity of cervical mucus and sperm function at the time of ovulation	Instruct the patient to arrange to come in to the office 6–12 hours after intercourse for evaluation of the cervical mucus.
Ultrasound Examination To evaluate structure of the pelvic organs, identify maturing ovarian follicles and the timing of ovulation	Reassure the patient that sonography uses sound waves, not radiation, to evaluate the pelvic structures. The examination may be conducted transabdominally or transvaginally and specific instructions are given, depending on method.
Hysterosalpingography Radiopaque dye is injected through the cervix, into the uterus and tubes. Evaluates structural integrity of the uterus and tubes.	May experience cramping, referred shoulder pain. Use nonsteroidal anti-inflammatory drugs (NSAIDs) as needed for pain. Report heavy cramping, bleeding, fever or malodorous discharge.
Tests of Endocrine Function Used to evaluate the hypothalamus, pituitary gland and ovaries. Levels of follicle-stimulating hormone (FSH), luteinizing hormone (LH), estrogen, and progesterone are assessed.	Timing of blood tests is very important for accurate interpretation of the results. Explain that FSH and LH stimulate ovulation; and estrogen and progesterone make the endometrium receptive for implantation of the fertilized ovum.
Endometrial Biopsy Involves the removal of a sample of the endometrium with a small pipette attached to suction. Provides information about the effects of progesterone (produced by the corpus luteum after ovulation) on the endometrium.	Teach the patient about the purpose and appropriate timing of the test: it should be performed not earlier than 10–12 days after ovulation (2–3 days before menstruation is expected). Cramping, pelvic discomfort, and vaginal spotting may occur; a mild analgesic (e.g., ibuprofen) may be used to alleviate the discomfort.
Hysteroscopy and Laparoscopy Endoscopic exam of the interior of the uterus and the pelvic organs under general anesthesia. Hysteroscopy may be performed without general anesthesia in the office. Abnormalities such as polyps, myomata (fibroid tumors), and endometrial adhesions are identified.	Explain the purpose of the test and other procedures that may be done at the same time. When general anesthesia is to be used, the patient should take nothing by mouth for several hours before the planned procedure. Advise her that since carbon dioxide gas will be instilled into the abdomen to enhance organ visibility, she may experience postoperative cramping and referred shoulder pain, which can be relieved with a mild analgesic.

Basic Infertility Evaluation and Workup	
Female	**Male**
CBC	Semen analysis: Sperm count should be:
Urinalysis	Volume of 2–6 mL of semen
Pap smear and wet mount	
Serology	>20 million sperm per 1 mL of semen
Luteinizing-hormone-surge	>50% forward moving sperm
ovulation predictor kit	>30% normal sperm
FSH cycle day 3 if >35 years old	
Rh factor, blood grouping	<1 million WBCs/mL of semen
Hysterosalpingography (to reveal	
uterine or tubal obstruction or	
abnormalities)	

MEDICATIONS

Counseling About Medications that Decrease the Effectiveness of Oral Contraceptives

- Take a thorough history.
- Use of certain medications (e.g., Rifadin, Rimactane), isoniazid, barbiturates, and griseofulvin (Fulvicin-U/F, Gris-PEG, Grifulvin V) can decrease effectiveness of oral contraceptives and higher doses of estrogen must be used.
- Vomiting and diarrhea affect the absorption of oral contraceptives; thus patients who experience these symptoms should use a backup method such as condoms.
- Interactions with certain drugs such as acetaminophen, anticoagulants, and some anticonvulsants (e.g., phenytoin sodium, carbamazepine, primidone, topiramate) may reduce the efficacy of oral contraceptives.

TEACHING THE FAMILY

Contraception

Topics to discuss with the patient:

- Use and satisfaction with previous methods
- Lifestyle, ability to manage chosen method
- Indications, contraindications, side effects, efficacy
- Reinforce that no method is 100% effective except abstinence.

Methods of Contraception

Medication-Free Contraception

Method	Description	Teaching
Natural Family Planning (NFP)	Identify fertile time and avoid intercourse during that time.	The only method acceptable to the Roman Catholic Church
Fertility Awareness Methods (FAM)	Identify fertile time and use abstinence or other contraceptive method during that time. Utilizes assessment of BBT, cervical mucus changes, abdominal bloating, and mittelschmerz.	Both NFP and FAM require patients who are very aware of the subtle changes during cycles and who have regular, predictable cycles. Both partners must be motivated to use the method successfully. Stress or illness can affect the timing of the cycle. User effectiveness: 75%
Coitus Interruptus	Withdrawal	Ejaculation may occur before full withdrawal. User effectiveness: 71%
Lactational Amenorrhea Method (LAM)	Breastfeeding	Can be effective if breastfeeding exclusively. Some lactating mothers ovulate without menstruating. If exclusively breastfeeding, infant younger than 6 months of age, and no menses since childbirth, user effectiveness approaches 98%.
Abstinence	Refrain from intercourse.	Requires commitment and self-control. User effectiveness: 100%

Barrier Methods of Contraception

With all barrier methods, wash hands before and after use.

Method	Description	Teaching
Diaphragm	Rubber/latex dome-shaped barrier inserted into vagina to cover cervix **CONTRAINDICATIONS:** Latex allergy, predisposition to urinary tract infections (UTIs)	Use spermicide in center and around edges. Place up to 6 hours before intercourse **Must** leave in place 6–24 hours after intercourse. Wash with warm, soapy water. Inspect for holes and tears. *(continued)*

Barrier Methods of Contraception (Continued)

Method	Description	Teaching
		Re-fit with 20% weight change or pregnancy. Provides no protection against STIs. Side effects: UTI, irritation from spermicide User effectiveness: 84%
Cervical Cap	Thimble-shaped latex device fits firmly around cervix **CONTRAINDICATIONS:** History of toxic shock syndrome (TSS), pelvic inflammatory disease (PID), cervical disease, latex allergy	Use spermicide in the cap before placement. Requires dexterity. Provides no protection against STIs. Side effects: Cervical irritation, allergic reaction User effectiveness: 74%
Male Condoms	Placed over erect penis before ANY genital, oral, or anal contact **CONTRAINDICATIONS:** Latex allergy (polyurethane and natural membrane condoms are available but offer no protection against HIV and STIs).	Penis must be erect for placement. Leave space at tip as reservoir. Remove while still erect, grasping at the base and avoiding spillage. Avoid using condoms with the spermicide nonoxynol-9. Side effects: Allergic reaction User effectiveness: 85%
Female Condoms	Polyurethane vaginal sheath with a ring at each end	More expensive than male condom Not latex, so safe for latex allergies Also use spermicides User effectiveness: 75%–82%
Spermicides	Gels, creams, films, and suppositories inserted into vagina to kill sperm before they can ascend **CONTRAINDICATIONS:** Cervicitis	Suppositories and films require 15 minutes to become effective. Provides no protection against STIs. Side effects: Allergic reaction, topical irritation User effectiveness: 71%
Contraceptive Sponge	Round, disposable polyurethane device permeated with spermicide (nonoxynol-9) that fits over cervix	Moisten thoroughly with tap water. Provides protection for up to 24 hours. Must remain in vagina at least 6 hours after intercourse. Provides no protection against STIs. User effectiveness: 84%–87%

Hormonal Methods of Contraception

Combined Hormonal Methods

All combination hormonal contraceptives have both estrogen and progestin, which, in combination, decrease FSH and LH. Progestins also thicken cervical mucus to prevent sperm penetration.

Method	Description	Teaching
Oral Contraceptive Pills (OCPs)	Many different formulations including 21/7 pattern (21 days of hormones, 7 days off); 24/4 pattern; and continuous **CONTRAINDICATIONS:** *Absolute* – smoking and >35 years of age; moderate to severe hypertension (BP 160/100); undiagnosed uterine bleeding; diabetes >20 years duration or with vascular changes; history of pulmonary embolism or deep venous thrombosis (DVT); ischemic heart disease or stroke; severe migraine headaches; known/suspected breast cancer; impaired liver function; pregnancy; major immobilizing surgery within the past month; cholecystitis *Relative:* Hypertension; migraine headaches; epilepsy; obstructive jaundice in pregnancy; gallbladder disease; surgery with prolonged immobilization; sickle cell disease	Must take at the same time every day. Use backup method during first week. Provide no protection against STIs Medications that may interfere: Rifampin, isoniazid, barbiturates, griseofulvin, certain anticonvulsants, anticoagulants, acetaminophen Report ACHES: **A**bdominal pain **C**hest pain **H**eadaches **E**ye problems **S**evere leg pain Side effects: Amenorrhea, nausea, bloating, spotting, breast tenderness, headaches during first 3 months User effectiveness: 95%
Transdermal Patch	Same contraindications as for OCPs	Apply to abdomen, buttock, upper outer arm, upper torso once a week for 3 weeks, then 1 week off for withdrawal bleeding. Rotate sites. Side effects: Same as for OCPs *(continued)*

Combined Hormonal Methods (Continued)

Method	Description	Teaching
		In addition: Local irritation User effectiveness: 99%
Vaginal Ring	Same contraindications as for OCPs	Side effects: Same as for OCPs; also vaginal irritation, infection User effectiveness: 98%

Contain only progesterone, which provides contraception by thickening the cervical mucus to prevent sperm penetration and inhibits implantation. The injections and implant also suppress ovulation.

Pills	"Mini pill" Ovulation may occur. **CONTRAINDICATIONS:** Hepatitis; cancer; colitis	Timing of dosage is very important! Side effects: Irregular menses User effectiveness: 92% May be used while breastfeeding No protection against STIs
Injections	Medroxyprogesterone 150 mg IM deltoid or gluteal or 104 mg SQ abdomen or anterior thigh Also suppresses ovulation. Give first injection within 5 days of menses.	Side effects: Irregular bleeding; amenorrhea; weight gain; depression; headache; breast tenderness User effectiveness: 98%–99% No protection against STIs Must return to office/clinic every 3 months for injection
Implant	Subdermal implant inserted on inner side of upper arm. Suppresses ovulation. Implanon is effective for 3 years.	Side effects: Irregular bleeding; amenorrhea; emotional lability; weight gain; headache; depression; dysmenorrhea; acne User effectiveness: Approaches 100% No protection against STIs

Other

Emergency Postcoital Contraception	"Morning after pill": Estrogen + progestin or progestin-only Take first dose within 72 hours of coitus and second dose 12 hours later.	Side effects: Nausea and vomiting Effectiveness: Estrogen + progestin = 89% of those who would have become pregnant; Progestin only = 95% Provides no protection against STIs.
Intrauterine device (IUD)	Small plastic device inserted into the uterus	Insert during menses.

Other

	Exact mechanism not known but causes sterile inflammatory response that results in a spermicidal intrauterine environment ParaGard (contains copper wire): Replace every 10 years. Mirena (contains progestin): Replace every 5 years; may produce amenorrhea. **CONTRAINDICATIONS:** Pregnancy; current STI; abnormal vaginal bleeding; cancer of genital tract; uterine anomalies or fibroid tumor; allergy to IUD components	Teach the patient to check for presence of "strings" after menses. Side effects: With ParaGard: Menorrhagia; dysmenorrhea. With Mirena: Decreased dysmenorrhea; decreased menorrhagia; amenorrhea Effectiveness: 98%–99% Provides no protection against STIs. Teach **PAINS** warning signs: **P**eriod late **A**bdominal pain, dyspareunia **I**nfection exposure or vaginal discharge **N**ot feeling well, fever/chills **S**tring missing, shorter, or longer
Sterilization	Permanent and irreversible Women: Bilateral tubal ligation (BTL); microinserts Men: Vasectomy	Outpatient or after childbirth (inpatient) Effectiveness: 96.3%–99% Office procedure (microinserts) Not considered complete until 2 negative semen analyses are obtained after procedure. Effectiveness: 99%
Clinical Pregnancy Termination	Elective: Performed at the woman's request Therapeutic: Performed for health reasons Vacuum aspiration: Most commonly used surgical method up to 12 weeks' gestation Dilation and evacuation: Second-trimester procedure	Potential complications: Bleeding, infection Reinforce need for follow-up care. Administer Rh$_o$ (D) immune globulin if indicated (i.e., non sensitized Rh$_o$ D-negative woman). Provide psychosocial support Teach about side effects associated with medications used with medical abortion: Nausea, vomiting, cramping.

(continued)

Combined Hormonal Methods (Continued)	
Other	
Medical termination: Can be performed for up to 63 days of gestation. Antimetabolites (e.g., methotrexate), abortifacients (e.g., mifepristone) and medications that induce uterine contractions (e.g., misoprostol) are used.	Teach about signs of complications: Fever 104°F (40°C), abdominal pain, prolonged or heavy bleeding, foul vaginal discharge, no menses within 6 weeks. Teach about contraception.

ETHNOCULTURAL CONSIDERATIONS

Obtaining a Sexual History for Infertility Care

Culturally influenced practices and taboos may create feelings of discomfort for couples when asked specific details of their intimate lives during the infertility care interview. Nurses must be sensitive to these issues and aware of cultural variations. For example, Orthodox Jewish law forbids a couple from engaging in sexual intercourse for 7 days after the menstrual period. This tenet can create an infertility problem if ovulation occurs during the early days after menstruation.

Drugs that Adversely Affect the Female Reproductive System		
Drug Class	**Drug**	**Possible Adverse Reactions**
Androgens	Danazol	Vaginitis, with itching, dryness, burning, or bleeding; amenorrhea
	Fluoxymesterone, methyltestosterone, testosterone	Amenorrhea and other menstrual irregularities; virilization, including clitoral enlargement
Antidepressants	Tricyclic antidepressants	Changed libido, menstrual irregularity
	Selective serotonin reuptake inhibitors	Decreased libido, anorgasmia
Antihypertensives	Clonidine, reserpine	Decreased libido
	Methyldopa	Decreased libido, amenorrhea

Drug Class	Drug	Possible Adverse Reactions
Antipsychotics	Chlorpromazine, perphenazine, prochlorperazine, thioridazine, trifluoperazine, haloperidol	Inhibition of ovulation (chlorpromazine only), menstrual irregularities, amenorrhea, change in libido
Beta Blockers	Atenolol, labetalol hydrochloride, nadolol, propanolol hydrochloride, metoprolol	Decreased libido
Cardiac Glycosides	Digoxin	Changes in cellular layer of vaginal walls in postmenopausal women
Corticosteroids	Dexamethasone, hydrocortisone, prednisone	Amenorrhea and menstrual irregularities
Cytotoxics	Busulfan	Amenorrhea with menopausal symptoms in premenopausal women, ovarian suppression, ovarian fibrosis and atrophy
	Chlorambucil	Amenorrhea
	Cyclophosphamide	Gonadal suppression (possibly irreversible), amenorrhea, ovarian fibrosis
	Methotrexate	Menstrual dysfunction, infertility
	Tamoxifen	Vaginal discharge or bleeding, menstrual irregularities, pruritus vulvae (intense itching of the female external genitalia)
	Thiotepa	Amenorrhea
Estrogens	Conjugated estrogens, esterified estrogens, estradiol, estrone, ethinyl estradiol	Altered menstrual flow, dysmenorrhea, amenorrhea, cervical erosion or abnormal secretions enlargement of uterine fibromas, vaginal candidiasis
	Dienestrol	Vaginal discharge, uterine bleeding with excessive use
Progestins	Medroxyprogesterone acetate, norethindrone, norgestrel, progesterone	Breakthrough bleeding, dysmenorrhea, amenorrhea, cervical erosion, and abnormal secretions

(continued)

Drugs that Adversely Affect the Female Reproductive System (Continued)

Drug Class	Drug	Possible Adverse Reactions
Thyroid Hormones	Levothyroxine sodium thyroid USP, and others	Menstrual irregularities with excessive doses
Miscellaneous	Lithium carbonate	Decreased libido
	L-Tryptophan	Decreased libido
	Spironolactone	Menstrual irregularities, amenorrhea, possible polycystic ovarian syndrome

Source: Dillon, P.M. (2007). *Nursing health assessment. Clinical pocket guide.* Philadelphia: F.A. Davis, pp. 234–235

Selected Medications Used in the Treatment of Infertility

Medication	Actions	Nursing Considerations and Side Effects
Clomiphene Citrate (Clomid)	An antiestrogen that binds with estrogen receptors to trigger FSH and LH release	Contraindicated with hepatic impairment. Patients may experience ovarian enlargement, vasomotor flushes, abdominal distention, nausea and vomiting, breast tenderness, blurred vision, headache, pelvic pain, abnormal uterine bleeding. May cause multiple ovulation.
Bromocriptine Mesylate (Parlodel)	Reduces elevated prolactin secretion by the anterior pituitary, which improves gonadotropin-releasing hormone secretion and normalizes follicle-stimulating hormone and luteinizing hormone release. Ovulation is restored and increased progesterone by the corpus luteum supports early pregnancy.	Patients may experience nausea and vomiting, headache, dizziness, orthostatic hypotension, blurred vision, diarrhea, metallic taste, dry mouth, urticaria, rash.

Medication	Actions	Nursing Considerations and Side Effects
Gonadotropin-releasing Hormone (GnRH) Agonists (GONADORELIN; GOSERELIN [ZOLADEX], LEUPROLIDE [LUPRON], NAFARELIN [SYNAREL])	Stimulates release of pituitary FSH and LH in patients with deficient hypothalamic GnRH secretion. FSH and LH stimulate ovulation (female) and testosterone and spermatogenesis (male).	Advise patients of potential side effects: Headache, depression, nasal irritation (Synarel), vaginal dryness, breast swelling and tenderness, hot flashes, vaginal spotting, decreased libido, and impotence.
GnRH Antagonists (CETRORELIX [CETROTIDE], GANIRELIX [ANTAGON], ABARELIX [PLENAXIS], HISTRELIN [SUPPRELIN])	Reduces the extent of endometriosis; used with medications that stimulate ovulation by suppressing LH and FSH.	Patients are closely monitored for ovarian hyperstimulation (ascites with or without pain, pleural effusion, ruptured ovarian cysts, multiple births), headache, nausea.
Human Chorionic Gonadotropin (hCG) (PROFASI HP, PREGNYL, CHOREX)	Used after failure to respond to therapy with clomiphene citrate; induces ovulation; used in conjunction with gonadotropins (FSH and LH [Pergonal], [Repronex], [Humegon]); ovulation usually occurs within 18 hours. Also stimulates production of progesterone by the corpus luteum.	When used with menotropins, risk for ovarian hyperstimulation, and arterial thromboembolism; other side effects include headache, irritability, restlessness, and depression.
Progesterone (IM, Intravaginal)	Provides luteal phase support—prepares the endometrial lining to promote implantation of the embryo.	Common side effects include nausea, weight gain, and fluid retention.

TEACHING THE FAMILY

Herbs to Avoid When Attempting to Achieve Pregnancy	
Category	**Herb**
Anthraquinone Laxatives	Aloe
	Buckthorn
	Cascara sagrada
	Docks
	Meadow saffron
	Senna
Uterine Stimulants	American mandrake
	Black cohosh
	Blue cohosh
	Bloodroot
	Calamus
	Cayenne
	Fennel
	Feverfew
	Flax seed
	Goldenseal
	Lady's mantle
	Licorice
	Make fern
	Sage
	Tansy
	Thuja
	Thyme
	Wild cherry
	Wormwood
	Mayapple
	Mistletoe
	Passion flower
	Pennyroyal
	Periwinkle
	Poke root
	Rhubarb
Alkaloids/Bitter Principles	Barberry
	Bloodroot
	Celandine
	Cinchona
	Ephedra
	Goldenseal

ADDITIONAL INFORMATION FOR THE CLINICAL SETTING

Advanced Reproductive Technologies (ART)

Treatment	Procedure	Indications for Use/Special Considerations	Complications
In Vitro Fertilization (IVF)	Administration of medications to induce ovulation. Oocytes are harvested and mixed with prepared sperm in a culture dish to form embryos. Three or four embryos are placed into the hormonally prepared uterus.	Tubal blockage or damage, endometriosis, cervical mucus abnormalities, male/female immunological infertility, cervical factors, infertility of unknown etiology.	Failure Multiple pregnancy
Intrauterine Insemination (IUI)	Retrieved and prepared sperm are placed into the uterus at the time of natural or induced ovulation.	Seminal deficiencies (e.g., oligospermia [low sperm count]), cervical factors (e.g., inhospitable mucus, stenosis), unexplained infertility	Failure Multiple pregnancy
Gamete Intrafallopian Transfer (GIFT)	Oocytes and sperm are placed in the fallopian tube.	Requires at least one functioning fallopian tube.	Failure Tubal pregnancy Multiple pregnancy
Zygote Intrafallopian Transfer (ZIFT) **Tubal Embryo Transfer (TET)**	After in vitro fertilization, zygotes are placed in one fallopian tube. Placement occurs at the embryo stage.	Requires at least one functioning fallopian tube.	Failure Tubal pregnancy Multiple pregnancy
Intracytoplasmic Sperm Injection (ICSI)	Micromanipulation process for an individual sperm cell which is injected directly into an ovum (in the laboratory)	Absence of the vas deferens; severe male factor (e.g., oligospermia, poor sperm quality)	Failure

(continued)

Advanced Reproductive Technologies (ART) (Continued)

Treatment	Procedure	Indications for Use/Special Considerations	Complications
Cryopreservation	Freezing method	Permits storage of sperm or ovarian tissue or embryos that result from IVF for the future.	Failure

REFERENCE

Dillon, P.M. (2007). *Nursing health assessment. Clinical pocket guide.* Philadelphia: F.A. Davis.

Conception and Development of the Embryo and Fetus

KEY TERMS

amnion – The innermost of the two fetal membranes that form the sac and contain the fetus and the fluid that surrounds it in utero

chorion – Fetal membrane closest to the intrauterine wall; gives rise to the placenta and continues as the outer membrane that surrounds the amnion

chorionic villi – Vascular projections from the chorion, which will form the fetal portion of the placenta

chromosome – A linear strand within the cell nucleus that carries genes; composed of DNA and proteins

dizygotic – Originating from two zygotes (i.e., fraternal twins)

embryo – Conceptus from the fourth day after fertilization until approximately the eighth gestational week

fetus – The developing human, in utero, after completion of the eighth gestational week, until birth

genetics – The study of single genes and their effects

gestation – The period of intrauterine fetal development from conception to birth

karyotype – Photomicrograph of the chromosomes of a single cell; the chromosomes are then arranged in numerical order

monozygotic – Originating from a single fertilized ovum (i.e., identical twins)

mutation – Spontaneous, permanent change in the normal gene structure

neural tube defect – A group of congenital structural disorders that result from a failure of the embryonic neural tube to close during development (i.e., cranial fusion disorders: anencephaly, encephalocele; spinal fusion disorders: spina bifida, meningomyelocele, meningocele)

teratogen – Substance that adversely affects normal cellular development in the embryo/fetus

trisomy – Condition in which a chromosome breaks and all or a part of the chromosome is transferred to a different part of the same chromosome or to a different chromosome. Most common trisomies in live newborns: trisomy 18 (Edward syndrome); trisomy 21 (Down syndrome); trisomy 13 (Patau syndrome)

FOCUSED ASSESSMENT

The first prenatal visit should include a careful history to determine factors that may affect the pregnancy:

- Cultural: Health practices and values
- Psychological: Feelings about the pregnancy, preparation, social support, stressors, future plans
- Physical: Past health history, current health issues, menstrual/ovulatory history, structural abnormalities, medications, substance use, tobacco
- Environmental: Exposure to toxins in the home or work place, second-hand smoke, stress

Embryonic and Fetal Growth and Development

Weeks	Weight	Length (crown to rump)	Characteristics	Implications
2 weeks	?	2 mm	Blastocyst implanted in uterus	Adequate secretion of progesterone by corpus luteum crucial to maintain endometrium
4 weeks	0.4 g	4 mm	Embryo is curved, tail prominent. Upper limb buds and otic pits present. Heart prominence evident.	Central nervous system (CNS), organ, and tissue development begins and vulnerable to teratogens.

Weeks	Weight	Length (crown to rump)	Characteristics	Implications
				Folic acid supplement is important.
8 weeks	2 g	3 cm	Head rounded with human characteristics. Unable to determine sex. Intestines still present in umbilical cord. Ovaries and testes distinguishable.	Ends embryonic period and begins fetal period. Organ systems and neuromuscular development remain vulnerable.
12 weeks	19 g	8 cm	Has a human appearance, with disproportionately large head. Eyes fused. Skin pink and delicate. Upper limbs almost reached final length. Intestines in the stomach. Sex distinguishable externally.	Fetus becomes more resistant to damage from teratogens. Able to auscultate heart tones with Doppler ultrasound stethoscope.
16 weeks	100 g	13.5 cm	Scalp hair appears. External ears present. Lower limbs well developed. Arm to leg ratio proportionate. Fetus active.	Maternal serum alpha-fetoprotein (MSAFP) reliable until 22 weeks.
20 weeks	300 g	18.5 cm	Head and body hair (lanugo) present. Vernix covers skin. Quickening felt by the woman.	Ultrasound examination often performed to detect growth abnormalities.
24 weeks	600 g	23 cm	Skin reddish and wrinkled. Some subcutaneous fat present. Some respiratory-like movements. Fingernails present. Lean body.	Fetus now viable.

(Continued)

Embryonic and Fetal Growth and Development (Continued)

Weeks	Weight	Length (crown to rump)	Characteristics	Implications
28 weeks	1100 g	27 cm	Eyes open with eyelashes present. Much hair present. Skin slightly wrinkled; more fat now present.	Gestational diabetes, related to maternal insulin resistance and fetal growth, becomes detectable by glucose tolerance test.
32 weeks	1800 g	31 cm	Skin is smooth. Increase in weight gain more than length. Toenails present. Testes descending.	
36 weeks	2200 g	34 cm	Skin pale, body plump. Body lanugo almost gone. Able to flex arm and form grasp. Umbilicus in center of body. Testes in inguinal canal, scrotum small with few rugae. Some sole creases present.	
40 weeks	3200+ g	40 cm	Skin smooth and pink. Lanugo on upper back and shoulders. Ear lobes formed and firm. Chest prominent and breasts often protrude slightly. Testes with well defined rugae. Labia majora well developed. Creases cover soles of feet.	

MEDICATIONS

Organogenesis occurs from approximately the second until the eighth week of gestation. During this time, the embryo is extremely vulnerable to teratogens.

Teratogen Exposure During Organogenesis	
Teratogen	**Effect**
Fat-soluble Vitamins: Vitamin A Vitamin D deficiency Vitamin E: High doses	Both high and low doses can cause malformations: CNS, microtia, clefts (fissure or elongated opening). Poor fetal growth, neonatal hypocalcemia, rickets, poor tooth enamel May increase risk for bleeding problems.
Alcohol	One of the most potent teratogens known. Safe threshold not established. Associated with fetal alcohol spectrum disorder (FASD) which includes neurological and physical changes.
Tobacco	Small for gestational age (SGA), cleft lip, impaired infant neurobehavior, decreased babbling in infants
Caffeine	Half-life triples during pregnancy. Readily crosses the placenta. CNS stimulant, causing maternal tachycardia and hypertension and affects fetal heart rate and movement; may be associated with preterm labor and intrauterine growth restriction (IUGR) although no clear causation exists.
Cocaine and Crack	Vasoconstriction of uterine vessels Associated with spontaneous abortion, abruptio placentae, stillbirth, IUGR, fetal distress, meconium staining, preterm birth Altered neurological and behavior patterns, neonatal strokes and seizures, congenital genitourinary and limb malformations, intestinal atresia, and heart defects
Opiates	Maternal: Spontaneous abortion, premature rupture of the membranes, preterm labor, increased incidence of STIs, hepatitis, malnutrition Fetal: Death, IUGR, prenatal asphyxia, prematurity, intellectual impairment, neonatal infection
Sedatives	Maternal: Lethargy, drowsiness, CNS depression. Infant: Neonatal withdrawal syndrome, seizures, delayed lung maturity

(continued)

Teratogen Exposure During Organogenesis (Continued)

Teratogen	Effect
Amphetamines	Maternal: Malnutrition, tachycardia, withdrawal symptoms Fetus: IUGR, prematurity, cardiac anomalies, cleft palate, placental abruption Infant: Hypoglycemia, sweating, poor visual tracking, lethargy and difficulty feeding
Marijuana	Maternal: Anemia, low weight gain Fetus: IUGR Infant: Hyperirritability, tremors, photosensitivity, adverse effects on cognitive and language development
Radiation (high levels)	Damage to chromosomes and embryonic cells, stunted fetal growth, mental retardation, deformities, abnormal brain function, cancer that develops later in life
Lead	Spontaneous abortion, fetal anomalies (hemangiomas, lymphangiomas, hydrocele, minor skin abnormalities, undescended testes), preterm birth

FDA Pregnancy Categories

Category	Interpretation
A	Adequate, well-controlled studies in pregnant women have not shown an increased risk of fetal abnormalities.
B	Animal studies have revealed no evidence of harm to the fetus; however, there are no adequate and well-controlled studies in pregnant women. **or** Animal studies have shown an adverse effect, but adequate and well-controlled studies in pregnant women have failed to demonstrate a risk to the fetus.
C	Animal studies have shown an adverse effect and there are no adequate and well-controlled studies in pregnant women. **or** No animal studies have been conducted and there are no adequate and well-controlled studies in pregnant women.
D	Studies (adequate well-controlled or observational) in pregnant women have demonstrated a risk to the fetus. However, the benefits of therapy may outweigh the potential risk. For example, the drug may be acceptable if needed in a life-threatening situation or serious disease for which safer drugs cannot be used or are ineffective.

Category	Interpretation
X	Studies, adequate well-controlled or observational, in animals or pregnant women have demonstrated positive evidence of fetal abnormalities. The use of the product is contraindicated in women who are or may become pregnant.

ETHNOCULTURAL CONSIDERATIONS

Racial and Ethnic Groups with Increased Risk for Diseases Caused by Recessive Genes	
Racial/Ethnic Group	**Disease**
African, Mediterranean, Caribbean, Latin American, or Middle Eastern descent	Hemoglobin gene mutations are more common in persons from these areas. African Americans have an increased incidence of sickle cell anemia. Southeast Asians have a greater likelihood of carrying hemoglobin E, an abnormal hemoglobin.
Mediterranean or Asian origin	These individuals have a higher risk for the hereditary anemia thalassemia.
Jewish ancestry	Individuals with Jewish ancestry have an increased risk for diseases associated with inborn errors of metabolism caused by different enzyme deficiencies (e.g., Tay–Sachs, Canavan, and Gaucher).
Caucasian or northern European descent	The most common disorder found among this population is cystic fibrosis.

TEACHING THE FAMILY

Empowering Through Education

- Teach all women of childbearing age who are capable of becoming pregnant to consume 0.4 mg of folic acid daily to reduce the incidence of neural tube defects.
- Include prenatal screening for maternal drug/substance use as a component of care for all pregnant women.
- Provide pregnant women with information on normal fetal growth and development.
- Display fetal growth charts in visible areas and discuss developmental landmarks throughout gestation to enhance the patient's and family's understanding.

- When appropriate, assemble a team composed of nutritionists, social workers, and home health workers to ensure healthy fetal growth and development.
- Include fathers and other support persons in prenatal education to help optimize the outcome.

TORCH Infections

TORCH infections are a group of maternal infectious diseases that cause harm to the embryo or fetus, especially during the first 12 weeks of gestation when developmental anomalies may occur (Box 4-1). TORCH is an acronym for *t*oxoplasmosis, *o*ther (e.g., hepatitis, syphilis), *r*ubella, *c*ytomegalovirus, and *h*erpes simplex.

Box 4-1 TORCH Infections

Toxoplasmosis

- Associated with consumption of infested, undercooked meat and poor hand washing after handling cat litter.
- If mother acquires toxoplasmosis after conception and passes it to the fetus via the placenta, fetal infection occurs.
- Most infants are asymptomatic at birth, but develop symptoms later.

Maternal Effects: Flu-like symptoms in the acute phase.
Fetal/Neonatal Effects: Miscarriage likely in early pregnancy. In neonates, CNS lesions can result in hydrocephaly, microcephaly, chronic retinitis, and seizures; retinochoroiditis may appear in adolescence or adulthood.

Other Infections

- Most commonly includes the hepatitis virus.
- Hepatitis A virus spread by droplets or hands, transmission rare but can occur.
- Hepatitis B virus can be transmitted via placenta, but transmission usually occurs when the infant is exposed to blood and genital secretions during labor and birth.

Maternal Effects: Fever, malaise, nausea, abdominal discomfort; may be associated with liver failure
Fetal/Neonatal Effects: Preterm birth, hepatitis infection, intrauterine death

Rubella (German measles)

- Spread by respiratory droplets.
- Obtain signed consent prior to administration of vaccine.

- Vaccine may be safely given to breastfeeding mothers.
- Instruct patients not to become pregnant for 1 month after receiving the immunization.

Maternal Effects: Fever, rash, mild lymphedema

Fetal/Neonatal Effects: Miscarriage, IUGR, cataracts, congenital anomalies, hepatosplenomegaly, hyperbilirubinemia, mental retardation, and death. Other symptoms may develop later. Infants born with congenital rubella are contagious and should be isolated.

Cytomegalovirus (CMV)

- Spread by respiratory droplets, semen, cervical and vaginal secretions, breast milk, placental tissue, urine, feces, and banked blood (nearly 50% of adults in the United States have antibodies for this virus).

Maternal Effects: Asymptomatic illness, cervical discharge, and mononucleosis-like syndrome

Fetal/Neonatal Effects: Fetal death or severe generalized disease with hemolytic anemia and jaundice, hydrocephaly or microcephaly, pneumonitis, hepatosplenomegaly, mental retardation, cerebral palsy, deafness; blood, brain, and liver are most often affected.

Herpes Simplex Virus (HSV)

- HSV II is sexually transmitted.
- Infant usually infected during exposure to lesion in birth canal, most at risk during a primary infection in the mother (50% born vaginally will develop some form of herpes; 60% will die; half of survivors develop problems).

Maternal Effects: Blisters, rash, fever, malaise, nausea, and headache

Fetal/Neonatal Effects: Miscarriage, preterm birth, stillbirth; transplacental infection is rare but can cause skin lesions, IUGR, mental retardation, microcephaly, seizures, and coma.

Communicating with the Family When a Fetal Anomaly Has Been Identified

- When prenatal testing identifies a fetus with a congenital anomaly, families are faced with a flood of emotions and difficult decisions. The nurse plays an important role in providing support and education regarding options available to these couples. A nonjudgmental and caring attitude is vital at this difficult and vulnerable time.

Therapeutic communication is enhanced when the nurse uses statements such as:

- "It's normal to have fear, grief, or even be angry."
- "It's normal to have concerns about your ability to have a normal baby."

- "I am here to answer your questions and listen to your concerns. If I don't know the answers. I will either find and share them or arrange for a colleague to meet with you.

The nurse should avoid using statements such as:

- "You can always have other children."
- "I know how you feel."
- "At least you don't know the baby yet."

ADDITIONAL INFORMATION FOR THE CLINICAL SETTING

Preterm Birth at Less Than 38 Weeks of Gestation

- Nurses must understand fetal growth and development in order to anticipate specific problems when infants are born prematurely.
- An infant born at 28 weeks of gestation has significantly different needs from an infant born at 38 weeks of gestation.

Understanding Abnormalities in Sex Chromosomes

Turner syndrome (monosomy X)

- Most common sex chromosome deviation in females
- Characterized by chromosomal constitution of 45X
- Affected females usually exhibit juvenile external genitalia, undeveloped ovaries, short stature, webbing of the neck, impaired intelligence.

Klinefelter syndrome (trisomy XXY)

- Most common sex chromosome deviation in males
- The extra X chromosome results in poorly developed male secondary sexual characteristics, small testes, infertility, and possible impaired intelligence.

RESOURCES

http://www.ornl.gov/sci/techresources/Human_Genome/publicat/tko/01_foreword.html

http://www.healthypeople.gov/Publications

http://www.nichd.nih.gov/health/topics/preconception_care.cfm

Physiological and Psychosocial Changes During Pregnancy

KEY TERMS

angioma – Tiny, bluish end-arterioles occurring on the neck, thorax, face, and arms; often appear during the second to fifth month of pregnancy and disappear after birth

Chadwick's sign – Bluish purple coloration of the vaginal mucous membrane caused by increased vascularity; visible from approximately the fourth week of pregnancy; a probable sign of pregnancy

chloasma – Increased pigmentation over the cheeks, hairline, brow, and nose of the pregnant woman and in some women taking oral contraceptives; also called the "mask of pregnancy" or "melasma gravidarum"

colostrum – Breast fluid that may be secreted from the second trimester of pregnancy onward; most evident in the first 2 to 3 days after birth and before the onset of true lactation

decidua – The endometrium or lining of the uterus during pregnancy; it is shed after giving birth

diastasis recti abdominis – Separation of the two rectus muscles along the median line of the abdominal wall

epulis gravidarum – Benign red, raised nodules of the gingiva seen in pregnant women

Goodell sign – Softening of the tip of the cervix; a probable sign of pregnancy

leukorrhea – Whitish-yellow discharge from the cervical canal or the vagina; may be normal physiologically or caused by vaginal/endocervical pathology such as infection

linea alba – White line of connective tissue in the middle of the abdomen that extends from the sternum to the mons pubis

linea nigra – Line of darker pigmentation seen in some women during the latter part of pregnancy; appears on middle of the abdomen and extends from the umbilicus to the mons pubis

mean arterial pressure (MAP) – Average of the systolic and the diastolic blood pressures

Montgomery tubercles (glands) – Small, nodular sebaceous glands on and around the areola that provide lubrication for the nipple tissue

operculum – Plug of mucus that fills the cervical canal to protect a pregnancy from outside pathogens

palmar erythema – Rash occurring on the surface of the palms, sometimes seen during pregnancy

pruritis gravidarum – Severe itching during pregnancy

ptyalism – Excessive production of saliva

striae gravidarum – "Stretch marks"—reddish lines on the breasts, abdomen, and thighs caused by stretching of the skin during pregnancy

supine hypotension syndrome (vena caval syndrome) – Fall in blood pressure caused by decreased venous return when the gravid uterus presses on the ascending vena cava when the woman is lying flat on her back; symptoms include dizziness, diaphoresis, nausea and pallor

FOCUSED ASSESSMENT

Physiological Adaptations in Pregnancy

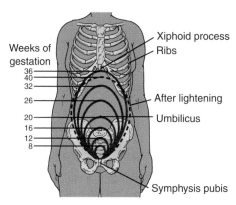

Figure 5-1 Pattern of uterine growth during pregnancy.

Hormones in Pregnancy		
Hormone	**Action**	**Effect**
Estrogen	Hyperplasia and hypertrophy	Breast tissue enlargement, uterine enlargement, enhanced uterine contractility
Progesterone	Smooth muscle relaxant, vasodilation, inhibits prolactin and oxytocin actions until needed	Slows gastrointestinal (GI) tract to increase absorption of nutrients, relaxes uterus to prevent labor until ready.
Prolactin	Increases 10-fold.	Responsible for initial lactation.
Oxytocin	Causes uterine contractions, stimulates milk ejection.	Labor, "let down" reflex
Prostaglandins	Increase response of the myometrium to the effects of oxytocin.	May contribute to onset of labor, softening of the cervix. Decreased levels may contribute to hypertension and preeclampsia.
Relaxin	Produced by the placenta, softens ligaments.	Lumbar lordosis, change in the center of gravity

Summary of Physiological Adaptations in Pregnancy

Organ/System	Change	Effect
Uterus	Hyperplasia and hypertrophy, hyperemia	Weight increases from 70 g to 1100 g.
Cervix	Hyperemia	Chadwick's sign, operculum, leukorrhea
Vagina and vulva	Hyperemia, elevated glycogen levels, decreased pH	Leukorrhea, increased risk of *Candida albicans*
Ovaries	Luteinizing hormone (LH) causes corpus luteum to produce progesterone for 6–7 weeks.	Corpus luteal cyst may enlarge to golf-ball size, then resolves.
Breasts	Estrogen and progesterone stimulate changes in tissue and mammary gland action.	Early: Enlargement, fullness, tingling, increased sensitivity. Montgomery tubercles enlarge and secrete lubricant, striae develop; colostrum is formed.
Integumentary System	Estrogen, progesterone, melanocyte-stimulating hormones increase. Increased adrenal steroid levels cause connective tissue changes.	Photosensitivity, chloasma, linea nigra, palmar erythema, angiomas Connective tissue becomes fragile, causing striae.
Neurological System	Unclear	Changes in attention span, concentration, memory, sleep pattern changes
Cardiovascular System	Changes in vascular permeability and vasodilation, relaxation of vascular resistance	Carpal tunnel syndrome, syncope, orthostatic hypotension, vasodilation; allows improved heat dispersion and increases risk for varicose veins, hemorrhoids.
Heart	Hypertrophy, displacement from growing fetus	Exaggerated first and third sounds, systolic murmur
Blood Volume	Increased by 40%–45%	Murmur
Iron	Increased need due to additional oxygen demands	"Physiological anemia of pregnancy" or "pseudoanemia" (normal hemodilution effect related to the plasma volume increase that exceeds the increase in erythrocytes)

Organ/System	Change	Effect
Clotting Factors	Fibrinogen volume increases by 50%.	Increased sedimentation rate, increased factors VII, VIII, IX, and X, leading to a hypercoagulable state
Cardiac Output	Increases by 30%–50%.	Pulse increases, blood pressure drops in second trimester, then returns to normal after 20 weeks; supine hypotension syndrome.
Immune System	Depressed leukocyte function	Increased susceptibility to infection
Respiratory System	Tidal volume increases 30%–40%; estrogen causes hypertrophy and hyperplasia of lung tissue; progesterone causes relaxation of bronchi, bronchioles, alveoli.	Increased oxygen consumption and vital capacity, decreased diaphragmatic movement and increased lateral chest wall movement to compensate for changes
Eyes, Ears, Nose, Throat	Eyes: Corneal thickening, fluid retention, decreased intraocular pressure. Nose: Increased mucus production Throat: Hyperemia	Blurred vision Rhinitis of pregnancy, epistaxis Difficulty swallowing
GI Tract	Increased blood flow, change in mucosa, progesterone slows GI motility, weakens gastroesophageal sphincter, slows bile emptying.	Changes in taste and smell, gingivitis, ptyalism, reflux, pyrosis, nausea/vomiting of pregnancy; hemorrhoids, constipation, pruritis gravidarum
Urinary System	Increased blood flow to kidneys by 30%–50%, pressure on structures by gravid uterus, progesterone relaxes urethra and sphincter musculature	Increased glomerular filtration rate (GFR) and renal tubular reabsorption. Increased excretion, urgency, frequency, nocturia, predisposed to urinary tract infections (UTIs)
Endocrine System		
THYROID	Increased blood flow, hyperplasia from estrogen, elevated levels of triiodothyronine (T_3) and thyroxine (T_4)	Enlarges up to two times, basal metabolic rate (BMR) increases up to 25%.
PARATHYROID	Hyperplasia from estrogen	Calcium demand increases. *(continued)*

Summary of Physiological Adaptations in Pregnancy (Continued)		
Organ/System	Change	Effect
PANCREAS	Hypertrophy and hyperplasia of insulin-producing beta cells of the islets of Langerhans	Alterations in carbohydrate metabolism
Musculoskeletal System	Hypertrophy of the round ligaments supporting the uterus	"Round ligament pain"
	Abdominal wall weakens. Weight shifts upward and outward.	Diastasis recti
	Symphysis pubis separates, bones of pelvis become loose.	Compensated by lordosis to maintain the center of gravity over the legs. "Pregnancy waddle"

DIAGNOSTIC TESTS

Common Laboratory Values in Pregnancy		
Laboratory Values	Usual Normal Female Value	Normal Value in Pregnancy
Serum Values		
Hemoglobin (Hgb)	11.7–15.5 g/dL	Decreased by 1.5–2 g/dL Lowest point occurs at 30–34 weeks
Hematocrit (Hct)	38%–44%	Decreased by 4–7%, lowest point at 30–34 weeks
Leukocytes	4.5–11.0 × 10³/mm³	Gradual increase of 3.5–10³/mm³
Platelets	150–400 × 10³/mm³	Slight decrease
Amylase	30–110 U/L	Increased by 50–100%
Chemistries		
Albumin	3.4–4.8 g/dL	Early decrease by 1 g/dL
Calcium (total)	8.2–10.2 mg/dL	Gradual decrease of 10%
Chloride	97–107 mEq/L	No significant change
Creatinine	0.5–1.1 mg/dL	Early decrease by 0.3 mg/dL
Fibrinogen	200–400 mg/dL	Progressive increase of 1–2 g/L
Glucose (fasting)	65–99 mg/dL	Gradual decrease of 10%
Potassium	3.5–5.0 mEq/L	Gradual decrease of 0.2–0.3 mEq/L
Protein (total)	6.0–8.0 g/dL	Early decrease of 1 g/dL, then stable

Laboratory Values	Usual Normal Female Value	Normal Value in Pregnancy
Sodium	135–145 mEq/L	Early decrease of 2–4 mEq/L then stable
Urea nitrogen	8–20 mg/dL	Decrease in first trimester by 50%
Uric acid	2.3–6.6 mg/dL	First trimester decrease of 33%, rise at term
Urine Chemistries		
Creatinine	11–20 mg/kg per 24 h	No significant change
Protein	10–140 mg per 24 h	Increased by 250–300 mg/day by the 20th week
Creatinine clearance	75–115 mL/min/ 1.73 m^2	Increased by 40%–50% by the 16th week
Serum Hormones		
Cortisol	8–21 g/dL	Increased by 20 g/dL
Prolactin	3.3–26.7 ng/mL	Gradual increase, 5.3–215.3 ng/mL, peaks at term
T_4 total	5.5–11.0 mcg/dL	5.5–16.0 mcg/dL
T_3 total	70–204 ng/dL	Early sustained increase of up to 50% 116–247 ng/dL (last 4 months of gestation)

Sources: Hacker, Moore, & Gambone (2004); Van Leeuwen, Kranpitz, & Smith, (2006).

ETHNOCULTURAL CONSIDERATIONS

Pregnancy-related Beliefs and Practices

All cultures have beliefs and practices related to the pregnancy and birthing experience. Careful assessment of the patient's beliefs regarding pregnancy and birth is essential to providing culturally sensitive care. The following areas require special attention: the state of pregnancy as a healthy versus a taboo state, nutritional practices such as hot/cold balance, expression of pain during labor, involvement of the father and other family members, over-the-counter remedy or herbal use, and other cultural beliefs.

TEACHING THE FAMILY

Health Education Topics Related to the Physiological Adaptations of Pregnancy			
Topics to Include	**First Trimester**	**Second Trimester**	**Third Trimester**
Physiological Changes of Pregnancy and Related Discomforts	Pain and tingling in breasts Nausea and vomiting (morning sickness) Urinary frequency Fatigue Mood swings	Enlargement of the abdomen Skin pigmentation Striae gravidarum Vascular spiders Constipation Heartburn or gastric reflux Leg cramps Groin pain from round ligament stretching Leukorrhea	Dyspnea Leg and feet cramps Constipation Indigestion, heartburn, gastric reflux Pedal edema Fatigue Vaginal discharge Urinary frequency Braxton Hicks contractions versus true labor
Danger Signs to Report to the Health Care Provider	Vaginal bleeding Abdominal cramping or pain Severe or prolonged vomiting	Vaginal bleeding Burning or painful urination Fever, increased pulse rate Decreased or absent fetal movements Unrelenting nausea and vomiting Abdominal pain or cramping Swelling of face or fingers, headaches, visual disturbances or epigastric pain	Visual disturbances Headache Hand and facial edema Fever Vaginal bleeding Abdominal pain; uterine contractions Premature rupture of the membranes Decreased or absent fetal movements Swelling of face or fingers, headaches, visual disturbances or epigastric pain
General Health Teaching	Schedule of return visits for routine prenatal care General hygiene	Reinforcement and reiteration of previous teaching Comfort measures	Signs and symptoms of labor/preterm labor

Topics to Include	First Trimester	Second Trimester	Third Trimester
	Comfort measures	Anticipatory guidance	When to call the health care provider, when to go to the birthing center or hospital
	Anticipatory guidance	Choices of prenatal education classes	
	Sexual activity and restrictions	Signs and symptoms of preterm labor	Comfort measures
	Physical activities, exercise and rest		Anticipatory guidance
	Nutritional guidance		Reinforcement and reiteration of previous teaching
	Avoidance of alcohol, fetal alcohol effects		Encouragement to attend a labor and birth class
	Effects of smoking, and smoking cessation strategies if indicated.		

Source: Mattson & Smith (2004).

PSYCHOSOCIAL ADAPTATIONS IN PREGNANCY

Health Education Topics Related to the Psychosocial Adaptations to Pregnancy

Topics to Include	First Trimester	Second Trimester	Third Trimester
Psychosocial Changes During Pregnancy	Ambivalence about pregnancy	Active dream and fantasy life	Dislikes being pregnant but loves the child
	Introversion	Concerns with body image	Anxious about childbirth, but sees labor and birth as deliverance
	Passivity and difficulty with decision making	Nesting behaviors	
	Sexual and emotional changes	Sexual behavior adjustment	The couple experiments with various mothering or fathering roles
	Changing self-image	Expanding to a variety of methods of expressing affection and intimacy	Woman is introspective
	Ethical dilemmas of prenatal testing		

Source: Mattson & Smith (2004).

ADDITIONAL INFORMATION FOR THE CLINICAL SETTING

Maternal Tasks of Pregnancy

General Principles	Pregnancy progressively becomes part of the woman's total identity She feels unique because she cannot share her sensory experience with others. Her focus turns inward and she is overly sensitive. She seeks the company of other women and especially pregnant women. Absence of a female support system during pregnancy is a singular index of a high-risk pregnancy.
Acceptance of Pregnancy "Binding-in"	*First trimester.* The woman accepts the idea of pregnancy but not the child. *Second trimester.* With sensation of fetal movement, or "quickening," the woman becomes aware of the child as a separate entity. *Third trimester.* The woman wants the child and is tired of being pregnant.
Acceptance of the Child	*First trimester.* Acceptance of the pregnancy by self and others. *Second trimester.* The family needs to relate to the infant. *Third trimester.* The critical issue is the unconditional acceptance of the child; conditional acceptance may imply rejection by the mother or family members.
Reordering of Relationships, Giving of Self	*First trimester.* Examines what needs to be given up; trade-offs for having the infant May grieve the loss of a carefree life. *Second trimester.* Identifies with the child. *Third trimester.* Has decreased confidence in her ability to become a good mother to her child.
Safe Passage	*First trimester.* Focuses on herself, not on her infant. *Second trimester.* Develops a strong attachment and places great value on her infant. *Third trimester.* Has concern for herself and her infant as a unit, shares a symbiotic relationship. At the seventh month, she is in a state of high vulnerability. She views labor and birth as deliverance and as a hope, not as a threat.

Source: Mattson & Smith (2004).

Developmental Tasks and the Pregnant Adolescent

- Developing a personal value system
- Choosing a vocation or career
- Developing a personal body image and sexuality
- Achieving a stable identity
- Attaining independence from parents

These tasks may be overshadowed by the developmental tasks of pregnancy and create conflicts.

CLINICAL ALERT

Avoiding Supine Hypotension Syndrome

The woman may experience supine hypotension syndrome, or vena caval syndrome (faintness related to bradycardia) if she lies on her back. The pressure from the enlarged uterus exerted on the vena cava decreases the amount of venous return from the lower extremities and causes a marked decrease in blood pressure, with accompanying dizziness, diaphoresis, and pallor (Fig. 5-2). Place the woman on her left side to relieve these symptoms.

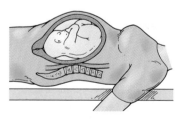

Figure 5-2 Supine hypotension, or vena caval syndrome, may occur if the pregnant woman lies on her back. The weight of the gravid uterus causes compression of the vena cava.

REFERENCES

Hacker, N.F., Moore, J.G., & Gambone, J.C. (2004). *Essentials of obstetrics and gynecology* (4th ed.). Philadelphia: W.B. Saunders.

Mattson, S., & Smith, J.E. (2004). *Core curriculum for maternal-newborn nursing.* St. Louis, MO: W.B. Saunders

Van Leeuwen, A.M., Kranpitz, T.R., & Smith, L. (2006). *Davis's comprehensive handbook of laboratory and diagnostic tests with nursing implications* (2nd ed.). Philadelphia: F.A. Davis.

The Prenatal Assessment

KEY TERMS

alpha-fetoprotein (AFP) – Fetal antigen; elevated levels in amniotic fluid are associated with neural tube defects; decreased levels may indicate an increased risk of having an infant with Down syndrome.

 MSAFP Maternal serum alpha-fetoprotein

amenorrhea – Absence of menses

ballottement – Passive movement of the unengaged fetus

Braxton Hicks sign – Mild, intermittent uterine contractions

Chadwick's sign – Bluish-purple coloration of the vaginal mucous membrane caused by increased vascularity; visible from approximately the fourth week of pregnancy; a probable sign of pregnancy

diethylstilbestrol (DES) – Synthetic estrogen that was once given to women in early pregnancy to prevent miscarriage. In utero exposure to DES is associated with reproductive tract malformations and vaginal cancer in females and increased rates of infertility in males and females

EDB – Estimated date of birth; also called "estimated date of delivery" (EDD); formerly termed the "estimated date of confinement" (EDC)

engagement – Entry of the presenting part into the maternal pelvis. Fetus is not ballottable.

fetal heart rate (FHR) – Beats per minute (bpm) of the fetal heart; normal range is 110–160 bpm

fetal lie – Position of the fetal spine in relation to the maternal spine: longitudinal (the same as the mother); transverse (fetal spine is horizontal across maternal spine); oblique (fetal spine is at some angle between the longitudinal and the transverse lie).

fundus – Dome-shaped upper portion of the uterus between the points of insertion of the fallopian tubes

Goodell sign – Softening of the tip of the cervix; a probable sign of pregnancy

gravidity – Total number of a woman's pregnancies

Hegar sign – Softening of the lower uterine segment; a probable sign of pregnancy

human chorionic gonadotropin (hCG) – Hormone produced by the chorionic villi; the biologic marker in pregnancy tests

Leopold maneuvers – Four maneuvers to assess the lie, presentation and position of the fetus

LMP – Last menstrual period

multigravida – Woman who has been pregnant two or more times

multipara – Woman who has carried two or more pregnancies to viability, whether they ended in live infants or stillbirths

Naegele's rule – Method for calculating the estimated date of birth: LMP + 7 days – 3 months

nulligravida – Woman who has never experienced a pregnancy

nullipara – Woman who has not yet carried a pregnancy to the point of viability

parity – Number of pregnancies carried to the point of viability, regardless of whether the infant or infants were alive or stillborn

Piskacek sign – Uterine asymmetry with a soft prominence on the implantation site; a probable sign of pregnancy

position (of the fetus) – Location of a fixed reference point on the fetal presenting part in relation to a specific quadrant of the maternal pelvis

presentation – Fetal part that enters the pelvic inlet first and leads through the birth canal during labor. If the head is "presenting," terms used are cephalic, vertex. Other presentations are breech and shoulder

primigravida – Woman who is pregnant for the first time

pseudocyesis – "False pregnancy"; condition in which a woman has the usual signs of pregnancy (e.g., abdominal enlargement, weight gain, cessation of menses, morning sickness) but is not pregnant

quickening – Maternal awareness of the sensation of fetal movement, usually occurs around 17 to 20 weeks of gestation

Rh factor – Inherited antigen present on erythrocytes. The individual who has the factor is known as "positive" (Rh+) for the factor; one who does not have the factor is known as Rh negative (Rh–)

Rh immune globulin (RhIg) – Solution of gamma globulin that contains Rh antibodies

FOCUSED ASSESSMENT

First Visit During the First Trimester

- Comprehensive health history
- Medical history (patient and father of the baby [FOB]; include hospitalizations, chronic and acute illnesses, immunizations, family history)
- Reproductive history
- Menstrual history (age at onset of menses [menarche], frequency, duration, flow)
- Risk exposure (diethylstilbestrol [DES], sexually transmitted infections [STIs], sexual practices)
- Obstetric history: Previous pregnancies (losses, births, preterm labor/birth, preeclampsia, gestational diabetes, perception of the childbearing experience)
- Current pregnancy: Last menstrual period (LMP)–was it "normal?"; any concerns; discomforts; establish the estimated date of birth (EDB)
- Social history (education level, work history, environmental exposure to teratogens, substance use, smoking, alcohol use, occupational hazards)
- Sexual history
- History of intimate partner violence (IPV) (assess every patient)
- Cultural practices (health practices, pregnancy practices, parenting practices, social support)
- Psychological assessment (depression, stress level, coping strategies, developmental stage, adjustment to pregnancy)
- Nutritional assessment (dietary recall, dietary restrictions, prenatal vitamins, folic acid, use of herbal or homeopathic remedies)
- Complete physical assessment: Head-to-toe with clinical pelvimetry, uterine size/fundal height measurement (Fig. 6-1), Pap smear, chlamydia and gonorrhea cultures, fetal heart tones (FHT) if >12 weeks of gestation, body mass index (BMI)
- Patient education

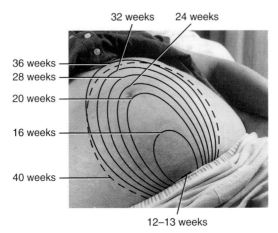

Figure 6-1 Fundal measurement should approximately equal the number of weeks of gestation.

Screening/Diagnostic Tests
- Pap smear
- Chlamydia, gonorrhea
- Complete blood count (CBC: hemoglobin, hematocrit, differential)
- Blood type and rhesus (Rh) factor
- Antibody screen (Kell, Duffy, rubella, varicella, toxoplasmosis, and anti-Rh)
- RDR/VDRL (for syphilis)
- Hepatitis B surface antigen (HbsAB)
- HIV
- Sickle cell screen (women of African, Asian, Middle Eastern descent)
- Urine (protein, ketones, glucose; culture for asymptomatic bacteriuria if indicated)

Assess for Intimate Partner Violence
Developed by the Massachusetts Medical Society (Alpert et al., 1992), "RADAR" is an acronym to guide nurses as they interview patients about relationship violence:

- Routinely screen every patient.
- Ask directly, kindly, and in a nonjudgmental manner.
- Document your findings.
- Assess the patient's safety.
- Review options and provide referrals.

Document Past Pregnancies and Their Outcomes

Pregnancy Classification System	
G	**G**ravida
T	Number of **T**erm pregnancies
P	Number of **P**reterm deliveries
A	Number of **A**bortions, both spontaneous and induced
L	Number of **L**iving children

Assess for Signs of Pregnancy		
Presumptive	**Probable**	**Positive**
Amenorrhea	Abdominal enlargement	Fetal heartbeat
Nausea and vomiting	Hegar sign, Piskacek sign	Visualization of the fetus
Urinary frequency	Goodell sign	Fetal movement palpated by a health care professional
Breast tenderness	Chadwick sign	
Quickening	Braxton Hicks sign	
Skin changes	Positive pregnancy test	
Fatigue	Ballottement	

Calculate the EDB Using Naegele's Rule

Naegele's rule is used to calculate the estimated date of birth (EDB; estimated date of delivery [EDD]).

This calculation is based on the first day of the woman's last normal period.

7 days are added to the LMP and 3 months subtracted and where necessary a year added.

For example, if the woman's LMP was June 8, 2007:

Add 7 days = June 15, 2007

Subtract 3 months = March 15, 2007

Add a year = March 15, 2008   EDB = 3/15/08

(An alternative way is to add 7 days and then add 9 months = year where needed)

Remember to ask the woman about her LMP.
　　　　　　　　Did her period start on the expected date?
　　　　　　　　Was blood loss normal (the same as her usual menstrual blood loss)?
　　　　　　　　Was her period different in any way?

(continued)

Calculate the EDB Using Naegele's Rule (Continued)

Was she using a form of contraception and if so, when was this method discontinued? (Hormonal contraception may delay the return to a normal ovulation pattern).

These questions will help you to determine an accurate date for the woman's last normal menstrual period.

Remember: Some women experience bleeding at the time of implantation, which normally occurs 7 to 9 days after fertilization. Care needs to be taken not to mistakenly use the date of implantation bleeding as the LMP.

Essential Components of Subsequent Prenatal Visits

- Review overall health status (signs/symptoms, discomforts, changes in medications, psychological assessment) and warning signs of pregnancy
- Assess maternal well-being (vital signs, weight, edema, reflexes and clonus if indicated, signs of preterm labor, intimate partner violence)
- Assess fetal well-being (FHTs after week 12) (Fig. 6-2), presence of fetal movements, uterine growth (fundal height measurement), Leopold maneuvers (Figs. 6-3, 6-4, 6-5, and 6-6), and presentation/position (Fig. 6-7)

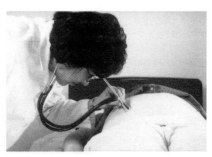

Figure 6-2 Auscultation of the fetal heart tones with a fetoscope.

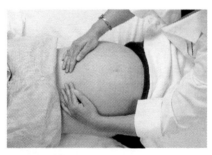

Figure 6-3 First Leopold maneuver.

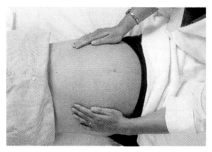

Figure 6-4 Second Leopold maneuver.

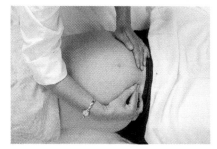

Figure 6-5 Third Leopold maneuver.

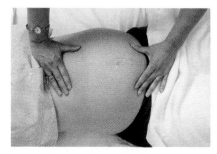

Figure 6-6 Fourth Leopold maneuver.

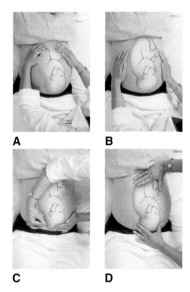

A   **B**

C   **D**

Figure 6-7 Assessing fetal presentation/position.

Assessments Specific to Trimester

First Trimester
Every 4 weeks:

- Evaluate weight, blood pressure (BP), urine for glucose, ketones, and protein, fundal height, fetal heart tones (FHTs).
- Evaluate adjustment to pregnancy, nutritional intake, nausea/vomiting, discomforts.

Second Trimester
Every 4 weeks:

- Evaluate weight (normal gain is 1–2 pounds/week), BP, urine for glucose and protein, fundal height, FHTs, fetal movements, perform Leopold maneuvers.
- Nutrition, AFP testing by 20 weeks, general survey ultrasound at 20 weeks.
- Discuss plans for childbirth and prenatal classes.
- Perform preterm labor (PTL) assessment and reinforce teaching about PTL.

Third Trimester

Every 2 weeks from 28 to 32 weeks until 34 weeks, then weekly:

- Evaluate weight (normal gain is 1–2 pounds/week), BP, urine for glucose and protein, fundal height, FHTs, fetal movements, perform Leopold maneuvers.
- At 24–28 weeks perform screen for gestational diabetes, obtain culture for Group B *Streptococcus*.
- Assess for contractions, readiness for childbirth, social support.

Diagnostic Tests	
Test	**Description**
Ultrasound Examination	Routinely performed by many clinicians during the first trimester to confirm dates and to ensure a singleton gestation – may also be obtained later in the pregnancy.
Prenatal Screening*	MSAFP: Screening for open neural tube defects and Down syndrome. Done around 16 weeks of gestation; if indicated, follow-up may include amniocentesis.
Screening for Gestational Diabetes	Offered around 24–28 weeks of gestation Patient drinks solution containing 50 grams of glucose. Blood is drawn 1 hour later; results should be below 140 mg/dL.
Rh Screening	To check for Rh antibodies; if negative, 300 mcg Rh_o immune globulin (RhoGAM) is administered at 28–32 weeks (nonsensitized Rh[D]-negative women).
Hemoglobin/Hematocrit	Usually repeated mid-pregnancy and then as indicated.
Group B *Streptococcus* Screening	Usually offered at 37 weeks of gestation to determine whether antibiotic coverage is needed during labor.

*See Timetable for Prenatal Diagnosis.

Timetable for Prenatal Diagnosis

Test	Significance
Maternal Serum Alpha-fetoprotein Screening (MSAFP)	Sample of maternal blood obtained between 14 and 16 weeks of pregnancy.
	High levels may be indicative of an open neural tube defect, but may also result from incorrect dates, multiple pregnancy or fetal demise.
	Low levels of serum AFP are associated with Down syndrome. The incidence of Down syndrome increases with maternal age to approximately 1 in 100 at age 40 or older.
Triple Test: AFP, human chorionic gonadotropin (hCG) and unconjugated estriol	Levels of hCG are increased when trisomy 21 (Down syndrome) is present.
	A low level of hCG can indicate trisomy 18. The sensitivity of the AFP test in detecting trisomy 21 is increased by 40%–50% when hCG levels are added.

MEDICATIONS

Effects of Recreational Drug Use in Pregnancy

Name	Street Name	Route	Effect	Pregnancy	Newborn
Methamphetamines **Dextroamphetamine**	Meth Crank Speed Ice	Smoked Snorted Swallowed Injected Inhaled	Stimulant	Spontaneous abortion Prematurity Breastfeeding not recommended	Withdrawal Tremors Poor muscle tone ?↑SIDS
Cocaine	Coke	Inhaled Smoked	Stimulant	Spontaneous abortion Placental abruption Preterm birth Breastfeeding not recommended	Birth defects – abnormalities of brain, skull, face, eyes, heart, limbs, intestines, genitals and urinary tract. Neonatal withdrawal Visual disturbances Delay in cognitive and/or learning ability
Ecstasy (methylenedioxymethamphetamine [MDMA]; compound may contain amphetamines and hallucinogens)	E, Adam, Roll, Bean, X and XTC, Clarity, Essence, Stacy, Lover's Speed, Eve	Pill form usually swallowed Crushed and snorted Injected per rectum (known as 'shafting') Smoked	Stimulant Mood enhancer	Spontaneous abortion Placental abruption Preterm birth	Congenital abnormalities: Cleft palate Low birth weight Rats exposed to ecstasy showed memory and learning deficiencies.

(continued)

Effects of Recreational Drug Use in Pregnancy (Continued)

Name	Street Name	Route	Effect	Pregnancy	Newborn
Marijuana, Cannabis	Pot Weed Grass Mary Jane	Ingested Smoked Snorted Injected	Stimulant Psychedelic Depressant	Intrauterine growth restriction (IUGR) Preterm birth	Possible link to increased incidence of childhood cancers. Withdrawal symptoms. Decrease in verbal ability and memory, plus lower impulse control
Heroin	Boy, brown, china white, dragon, gear, H, horse, junk, skag, smack	Swallowed	Sedative	Spontaneous abortion, IUGR Preterm labor/birth Stillbirth	Neonatal withdrawal syndrome

ETHNOCULTURAL CONSIDERATIONS

Hypertension and Pregnancy

Hypertension is more prevalent in African American and Mexican American cultures, probably due to hereditary factors (Nabel, 2003). It is the most common medical condition affecting pregnancy and may worsen as the pregnancy progresses.

TEACHING THE FAMILY

Strategies to Enhance the Childbearing Year

- Provide education related to stage of pregnancy (i.e., what physical changes to expect or danger signs that need to be reported such as vaginal bleeding or fluid loss, abdominal pain or visual disturbances).
- Encourage attendance in prenatal education classes.
- Encourage tour of facility where patient intends to give birth.
- Educate about care of the newborn (e.g., car seats, male circumcision, immunizations) so that parents can make informed decisions.

ADDITIONAL INFORMATION FOR THE CLINICAL SETTING

Goals that Guide Nursing Care

- To recognize deviations from normal
- To provide individualized, evidence-based care
- To provide culturally appropriate prenatal education designed to meet the patient's learning style and needs
- To empower women to become actively involved in their pregnancy by being informed recipients and shared decision-makers

Procedure 6-1 Obtaining A Mid-Stream Urine Sample

Purpose

A technique for obtaining a clean sample of urine so that it can be examined for bacteria, protein, glucose, and ketones. Findings provide information about the patient's hydration status (e.g., amount, color, specific gravity), infection status (e.g., leukocytes), nutritional status (e.g., ketones), and the status of possible complications such as gestational diabetes (i.e., glucose) or preeclampsia (e.g., protein).

Preparation

1. Complete the information requested on the container label. Include the patient's full name and the date and time of collection of the specimen. If a requisition is needed, note the date and time on the requisition.

2. Explain the procedure to the woman to ensure she understands why a urine sample is requested, the purpose of any tests to be performed, and directions on how to obtain a mid-stream urine sample.

Equipment

- Approved empty sterile container for collection
- Towelette for cleaning in between the labia
- Tissue

Steps

Instruct the patient to do the following:

1. Wash and dry hands thoroughly or use an alcohol-based hand-rub.

2. Remove the container cap and set it on a clean, even surface with the inner surface pointing up. Do not touch the inner surface of the lid or the container.

3. Sit on the toilet seat and separate the labia (vaginal lips) using your nondominant hand. Clean the urogenital area from the front to back with the towelette provided. Wipe for only one stroke and then discard the towelette

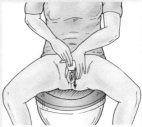

Patient cleansing labia

Procedure 6-1 (Continued)

4. Holding the labia apart, begin to pass urine. Allow the beginning urine to go directly into the toilet.

5. Continue to urinate and hold the container under the urine stream. Avoid touching the inside of the container. Remove the container when it is approximately half full.

6. Carefully replace the cap and secure tightly.

7. Wash your hands again after the specimen collection.

Document the procedure.

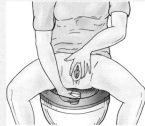

Patient urinating into specimen cup.

Clinical Alert Pregnant women are at an increased risk for developing urinary tract infections, especially if they are diabetic or have gestational diabetes. Urinary tract infections may also predispose to the onset of preterm labor.

Teach the Patient

Teach the patient to recognize common signs of a urinary tract infection:

• Dysuria: Pain (burning sensation) on urination

• Urinary frequency associated with small amounts of urine

• Hematuria: Blood or red blood cells in the urine

REFERENCES

Alpert, E.J., Freud, K.M., Park, C.C., Patel, J.C., & Sovak, M.A. (1992). *Partner violence: How to recognize and treat victims of abuse.* Massachusetts Medical Society, Waltham, MA.

Nabel, E.G. (2003). Cardiovascular disease. *New England Journal of Medicine, 349*(1), 60–72.

Promoting a Healthy Pregnancy

KEY TERMS

anorexia nervosa – Eating disorder marked by weight loss, emaciation, a disturbance in body image, and fear of weight gain

body mass index (BMI) – A method of evaluating the appropriateness of weight for height. Formula for calculating BMI: $BMI = \dfrac{Weight \text{ (in kilograms)}}{Height^2 \text{ (in meters)}}$

bulimia nervosa – Eating disorder marked by recurrent episodes of binge eating, self-induced vomiting and diarrhea, excessive exercise, strict dieting or fasting, and an exaggerated concern about body shape and weight

intrauterine growth restriction (IUGR) – Undergrowth of the fetus; may be due to deficient nutrient supply, intrauterine infection or associated with a congenital malformation

pica – Consumption of non-nutritive substances or food

small for gestational age (SGA) – Inadequate growth for gestational age

FOCUSED ASSESSMENT

At each prenatal visit: update health history, perform physical examination (as indicated) and conduct appropriate laboratory/diagnostic testing (see Chapter 6)

DIAGNOSTIC TESTS

Genetic Screening During Pregnancy

Disorder	Population Affected	Pathology	Pregnancy and Newborn Complications
Sickle Cell Disease	African Americans Persons of Mediterranean descent	Autosomal recessive hemolytic disease. Involves an abnormal substitution of an amino acid in the structure of hemoglobin. Red blood cells assume abnormal, sickle shape in response to triggers, including hypoxia, infection, dehydration. Results in inability to oxygenate tissues. Leads to occlusion and rupture of blood vessels.	Spontaneous abortion Preterm labor Intrauterine growth restriction Stillbirth
Tay-Sachs Disease	Ashkenazi Jews Jewish people from Eastern or Central Europe French-Canadians Cajuns	Both parents must carry and pass on the trait to the child.	Infants appear normal at birth, until about 3 to 6 months of age when the neurological system begins to deteriorate. Death occurs between the ages of 2 and 4 years.
Thalassemia	Greeks Italians Southeast Asians Filipinos	Disorder of hemoglobin synthesis Thalassemia minor: person is heterozygous for the trait; experiences fewer symptoms. Thalassemia major: person is homozygous for the trait; experiences more severe symptoms.	Children appear normal at birth. During the first 2 years, children become pale, lethargic, and develop jaundice. Results in enlarged liver, spleen, and heart. Death results from heart failure and infection. *(continued)*

Genetic Screening During Pregnancy (Continued)

Disorder	Population Affected	Pathology	Pregnancy and Newborn Complications
Hemophilia	Males are affected. Females are carriers.	Mutation in the gene of coagulation factor VIII. Causes a defect in blood clotting. Leads to frequent bleeding episodes and hemorrhage.	Males can have excessive bleeding when circumcised. Increased incidence of intracranial hemorrhage Easy bruising and bleeding with injuries
Glucose-6-Phosphate Dehydrogenase (G6PD) Deficiency	African Americans Seen mostly in males	Causes drug-induced destruction of red blood cells when taking certain medications (e.g., sulfonamides)	Increased incidence of pathological jaundice or hyperbilirubinemia due to destruction of red blood cells
Cystic Fibrosis	Caucasians	Autosomal recessive genetic disorder Causes exocrine gland dysfunction	Results in chronic obstructive lung disease from thick mucus secretions in the lungs Frequent lung infections occur Causes a deficiency in pancreatic enzymes that prevents normal digestion

MEDICATIONS

Ferrous Sulfate (**fer**-us **sul**-fate)

Pregnancy Category B

Indications Prevention/treatment of iron-deficiency anemia

Actions An essential mineral found in hemoglobin, myoglobin, and many enzymes. Prevents iron deficiency.

Therapeutic Effects Prevents/treats iron deficiency.

Pharmacokinetics
Absorption Therapeutically administered PO iron may be 60% absorbed; absorption is an active and passive transport process.

Contraindications and Precautions
Use cautiously in Peptic ulcer, ulcerative colitis; indiscriminate chronic use may lead to iron overload.
Adverse Reactions and Side Effects Constipation, dark stools, diarrhea, epigastric pain, gastrointestinal bleeding

Route and Dosage (mg elemental iron) 100–200 mg/day (2–3 mg/kg per day) in three divided doses

Nursing Implications
1. Assess nutritional status and dietary history to determine possible cause of anemia and need for patient teaching.
2. Assess bowel function for constipation or diarrhea; notify care provider and use appropriate nursing measures if these symptoms occur.

Data from Deglin, J.H., & Vallerand, A.H. (2009). Davis's drug guide for nurses (11th ed.). Philadelphia: F.A. Davis.

ETHNOCULTURAL CONSIDERATIONS

Vitamin D Deficiency

African Americans and other women with dark skin are at the greatest risk for vitamin D deficiency. Women who habitually cover most of their skin with clothing and those who live in northern latitudes with limited exposure to sunlight are also more likely to be deficient in vitamin D.

Anemia During Pregnancy

In the United States, maternal anemia occurs most commonly among adolescents, African American women, and women of lower socioeconomic status.

The Consumption of Non-nutritive Substances

Causes of pica are believed to include nutritional deficiencies, cultural and familial factors, stress, low socioeconomic status, and biochemical disorders. In some cultures, certain non-nutritive food substances are thought to bring health or have positive spiritual effects for those who consume them. Individuals of other cultures believe that the consumption of specific non-nutritive substances plays a role in enhancing fertility or promoting luck within the family.

TEACHING THE FAMILY

Nutrition to Promote a Healthy Pregnancy		
Element	Recommendation During Pregnancy	Comments
Calories	300 kcal/day increase	Focus on healthy eating.
Protein	Moderate increase	Caution regarding undercooked meats, fish high in mercury (shark, swordfish, tilefish, king mackerel).
Water	8–10 8-oz. glasses per day	Four to six glasses should be water; the rest may be other fluids (limit caffeine to <300 mg/day).
Calcium	1000 mg/day	Supplements are important.
Vitamin D	5 mcg	Exposure to sunlight and fortified foods usually adequate. Dark-skinned women are more at risk for deficiency.
Iron	18 mg/day	Starting by 12 weeks of gestation, usually requires supplementation.
Vitamin C	80–85 mg/day	Enhances iron absorption.
Folic Acid	800 mcg/day	Aids in iron absorption; necessary for DNA and RNA production. Deficiency is related to neural tube defects.

Recommended Total Weight Gain During Pregnancy for a Single Birth

Pre-Pregnancy BMI	Recommended Total Weight Gain
Underweight (<19.8)	28–40 lbs.
Normal weight (19.8–26)	25–35 lbs.
Overweight (>26–29)	15–20 lbs.
Obese (>29)	15+ lbs.

Source: National Heart, Lung and Blood Institute (2006).

Iron Supplements

- Teach patients to avoid substances known to decrease iron absorption (bran, tea, coffee, milk, oxylates [found in spinach and Swiss chard], egg yolk) when taking iron supplements.
- Take iron between meals with a beverage other than tea, coffee, or milk.

Vitamin B_{12} Deficiency

- Counsel patients who are vegetarians about the risk for vitamin B_{12} deficiency.
- Associated with the following maternal problems: megaloblastic anemia, glossitis, and neurological deficits
- Infants born to mothers with vitamin B_{12} deficiency are more likely to have megaloblastic anemia and to exhibit neurodevelopmental delays.

Coping with Fatigue

Advise the woman to:

- Get plenty of rest (go to bed earlier, take naps and breaks when possible).
- Cut down on external commitments (e.g., volunteer and social events).
- Eat a healthy, balanced diet; include iron-rich foods and protein; include foods with vitamin C to help with iron absorption.
- Exercise moderately at least 30 minutes each day. Brisk walking is the best exercise for improving alertness and boosting energy levels.

- Avoid food and beverages containing caffeine.
- Drink plenty of fluids.
- Minimize stress.
- Ask for help. One's partner, children, and friends can help, but only if they are aware that help is needed.

Exercise

Advise the woman to:

- Monitor her breathing rate (she should be able to talk comfortably while exercising).
- Protect against overheating.
- Stop when she becomes tired and never exercise to the point of exhaustion.
- Avoid exercises that could cause trauma to the abdomen, rigorous bouncing, arching of the back, or bending beyond 45-degree angle.
- Drink adequate fluids.
- Remember that balance changes as pregnancy progresses.

Complementary Care

- Massage therapy: Increases blood flow to maternal and fetal tissues; enhances relaxation.
- Chiropractic care: Treats lower back pain and headaches related to increased hormone levels.
- Acupuncture and acupressure: Treat many physical ailments during pregnancy without the introduction of medications.
- Relaxation exercises, meditation, and breathing techniques: increase blood flow to maternal and fetal tissues; increase relaxation.
- Light therapy: Enhances mood and treats depression.
- Reflexology: Stimulates nerve pathways to increase blood flow and energy flow to corresponding areas of the body.
- Aromatherapy: Enhances relaxation.

Dealing with Common Discomforts in Pregnancy

Trimester	Common Discomforts	Relief Measures
First	Nausea and vomiting	Consume small, frequent meals, dry crackers. Remain upright after meals. Consider vitamin B_6, acupressure.
	Fatigue	Establish bedtime routine; take naps.
	Urinary frequency and nocturia	Ensure adequate intake; decrease fluid intake 2–3 hours before bedtime. Perform Kegel exercises. Seek help if urine is bloody or if hesitancy or burning during urination is experienced.
	Dyspepsia	Remain upright after eating; consume small, frequent meals; avoid fatty foods and cold liquids.
	Gum hyperplasia and bleeding	Use soft toothbrush and see dentist as recommended.
Second	Dependent edema	Avoid constrictive clothing; elevate legs; use side-lying position when resting.
	Leg varicosities	
	Hyperventilation and shortness of breath	Take slow, steady breaths, raise arms above the head.
	Numbness and tingling of fingers	Wear wrist brace when sleeping.
	Supine hypotensive syndrome	Rest on the side and rise slowly.
	Fatigue	As above
	Urinary frequency	As above
	Dyspepsia	As above
	Flatulence	Avoid gas-forming foods, chewing gum, large meals
	Gum hyperplasia and bleeding	As above
	Leg cramps	Regular exercise, elevate legs, dorsiflex feet, consume adequate calcium and phosphorous
Third	Dependent edema	As above
	Leg varicosities	As above
	Dyspareunia	Try various positions, alternative methods for satisfaction
	Nocturia	As above

(continued)

Dealing with Common Discomforts in Pregnancy (Continued)

Trimester	Common Discomforts	Relief Measures
	Round ligament pain	Warm bath, apply heat, support uterus with pillow or pregnancy girdle
	Supine hypotensive syndrome	As above
All Trimesters	Ptyalism	Small frequent meals, avoid starchy foods, suck on hard candies
	Nasal congestion	Increase fluids, vaporizer, steamy shower
	Back pain	Good body mechanics, physical therapy
	Leukorrhea	Panty liner, cotton underwear
	Constipation	Fluids, fiber, exercise
	Insomnia	Sleep hygiene, proper alignment with pillows

Signs and Symptoms of Danger

Trimester	Warning Sign	Possible Complication(s)
	Severe, persistent nausea and vomiting	Hyperemesis gravidarum Hydatidiform mole
First	Abdominal pain and vaginal bleeding	Spontaneous abortion
	Chills, fever, malaise, anorexia	Infection, e.g., UTI
	Headache, vision changes, elevated blood pressure, edema	Preeclampsia
	Increased vaginal secretions	Vaginitis Premature rupture of the membranes
Second	Regular, persistent contractions or backache	Preterm labor
	Decreased fundal height	IUGR
	Increased fundal height (>2 cm/week)	Hydramnios, multiple gestation, fetal macrosomia
	Decreased fetal movement	Fetus in danger from any of the above
Third	The same as found in the second trimester	As above
	Positive glucose challenge test	Gestational diabetes

Trimester	Warning Sign	Possible Complication(s)
	Painless vaginal bleeding	Placenta previa
	Abdominal pain with or without vaginal bleeding	Abruptio placentae

RESOURCES

American College of Obstetricians and Gynecologists (ACOG)

Association of Women's Health, Obstetrical, and Neonatal Nursing (AWHONN)

USDHHS & U.S. Department of Agriculture

The document "Dietary Guidelines for Americans 2005" is an evidence-based resource guide for professionals and consumers that offers strategies for promoting health and reducing the risk for chronic diseases through diet and physical activity. Dietary guidelines, food composition, the food guide pyramid, dietary supplements, and resource lists are included in the guide (USDHHS & U.S. Department of Agriculture [USDA], 2005) (http://www.nal.usda.gov/fnic/).

REFERENCES

Deglin, J.H., & Vallerand, A.H. (2009). *Davis's drug guide for nurses* (11th ed.). Philadelphia. F.A. Davis.

Obesity and Women's Reproductive Health (2006). National Heart, Lung and Blood Institute. Retrieved from http://www.nhlbi.nih.gov/guidelines/ obesity/e_txtbk/ratnl/22111.htm (Accessed December 7, 2008).

Caring for the Woman Experiencing Complications During Pregnancy

KEY TERMS

amniotic infection syndrome – Placental, fetal membrane, and umbilical cord inflammation that occurs after premature rupture of the membranes (PROM)

asymptomatic bacteriuria – Presence of at least 10^5 colony-forming bacteria without symptoms

condylomata acuminata – Genital warts

disseminated intravascular coagulation (DIC) – Hematological disorder characterized by a pathologic form of clotting that is diffuse and consumes large amounts of clotting factors; causes widespread external or internal bleeding or both

ectopic pregnancy – A pregnancy that implants outside of the uterine cavity

erythroblastosis fetalis – Hemolytic disease of the newborn, usually caused by isoimmunization that has resulted from Rh incompatibility or ABO incompatibility

gestational diabetes mellitus (GDM) – Onset of diabetes during pregnancy

glycosylated hemoglobin (Ghb) – Glycohemoglobin (a minor hemoglobin) with glucose attached; Ghb/HbA1c concentration represents the average blood glucose level over the preceding 5 to 6 weeks

Homans' sign – Early sign of deep venous thrombosis in the leg; on dorsiflexion, pain occurs from inflammation of the blood vessel. A negative Homans' sign does not rule out deep vein thrombosis.

hydatidiform mole (molar pregnancy) – Gestational trophoblastic neoplasm, usually results from fertilization of an egg that contains no nucleus

hydramnios (polyhydramnios) – Amniotic fluid in excess of 2.0 liters

hydrops fetalis – Most severe form of fetal hemolytic disorder; may be a sequela to maternal isoimmunization.

isoimmunization – Development of antibodies in a species of animal with antibodies from the same species (e.g., development of anti-Rh antibodies in an Rh-negative mother following exposure to Rh-positive fetal blood)

kernicterus – Bilirubin encephalopathy that involves the deposit of unconjugated bilirubin in brain cells and results in neurological damage or death

ophthalmia neonatorum – Neonatal eye inflammation from *Neisseria gonorrhoeae* that can result in permanent blindness from perforation of the globe of the eye

pregestational diabetes mellitus – Onset of diabetes before pregnancy

premature rupture of the membranes (PROM) – Rupture of the amniotic sac at least 1 hour before the onset of labor at any gestational age

preterm premature rupture of the membranes (PPROM) – Rupture of the membranes before the onset of labor and before 37 completed weeks of gestation

preterm rupture of the membranes – Rupture of the membranes before 37 completed weeks of gestation

salpingectomy – Surgical removal of the fallopian tube

salpingostomy – Surgical opening of a fallopian tube

thyrotoxicosis – Excessive thyroid activity

tocolysis – Use of medications (tocolytics) to inhibit uterine contractions

type 1 diabetes – An absolute insulin deficiency (Expert Committee on the Diagnosis and Classification of Diabetes Mellitus [ECDCDM], 2003)

type 2 diabetes – A combination of insulin resistance and inadequate insulin production (ECDCDM, 2003)

vertical transmission – Transmission of infection occurs antepartally when the virus or bacteria crosses the placenta, intrapartally when it travels (via the bloodstream) from the vagina up into the uterus during labor or following rupture of the membranes, or postpartally through transfer in the breast milk

Bleeding During Pregnancy

FOCUSED ASSESSMENT

The Perinatal Patient at Risk: Causes of Bleeding in Early Pregnancy

Cause	Assessment	Implications	Risk Factors
Implantation	Scant spotting for 1–2 days 1–2 weeks after conception, Painless	Does not affect the pregnancy.	
Abortion: 10%–20% of all pregnancies are "lost."	*Complete*: Complete expulsion of products of conception (POC) before 20 weeks of gestation	Watch for infection, offer counseling.	More than three previous pregnancy losses
	Threatened: Bleeding before 20 weeks of gestation but no cervical dilation	Rest; call if bleeding or cramping increases.	
	Incomplete: Partial expulsion of POC	Dilation and curettage Counseling	
	Inevitable: No expulsion of POC yet but bleeding and dilated cervix	Watch for infection.	
	Missed: Death of embryo or fetus but POC are not expelled		
Ectopic Pregnancy	Abdominal pain, spotting, missed menstrual period	Pregnancy loss, hemorrhage if ruptures, salpingostomy or methotrexate. Counseling	Previous ectopic or other abdominal surgeries, pelvic inflammatory disease (PID), endometriosis
Gestational Trophoblastic Disease	"Molar pregnancy": Bleeding, uterus larger than expected, hyperemesis, preeclampsia, absence of fetal heart tones (FHTs)	Hemorrhage, anemia, shock, choriocarcinoma, not a viable pregnancy Counseling	Maternal age, history of previous molar pregnancy, Clomid

(continued)

The Perinatal Patient at Risk: Causes of Bleeding in Later Pregnancy (Continued)			
Cause	**Assessment**	**Implications**	**Risk Factors**
Placenta Previa (Fig. 8-1) Implantation of placenta near or over the cervix	Painless bleeding in second half of pregnancy *Complete:* Placenta covers entire cervix *Partial:* Placenta covers part of the cervix *Marginal:* Placenta encroaches on cervical margin	Vaginal birth not possible with complete placenta previa. Seek immediate care if **any** bleeding or labor. **No vaginal digital exam**	Prior cesarean birth, multiple gestation, smoking, cocaine use, age >35 years, African or Asian ethnicity
Placental Abruption (abruptio placentae) (Fig. 8-2) Premature separation of a normally implanted placenta	Severe abdominal pain, abnormal contractions, increased uterine tone, fetal compromise, third trimester *Concealed:* Bleeding is confined within the uterine cavity, 20% of cases *Revealed:* Vaginal bleeding present	Fetal mortality in 35% of all placental abruptions Maternal mortality 0.5%–5% Actual blood loss is often more than what is visible	Trauma Cocaine use

CLINICAL ALERTS

Early Identification of Maternal Hemorrhage

- The maternal pulse (tachycardia) and/or fetal heart rate (bradycardia or tachycardia) may be the first indicators of maternal instability.
- Blood pressure is a very poor indicator of blood volume deficit.
- Due to the expanded blood volume that normally occurs during pregnancy, the patient may be asymptomatic and exhibit vital signs that remain within normal parameters despite a large amount of blood loss.

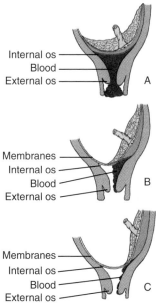

Internal os
Blood
External os
A

Membranes
Internal os
Blood
External os
B

Membranes
Internal os
Blood
External os
C

Figure 8-1 Placenta previa. *A.* Complete. *B.* Partial. *C.* Marginal.

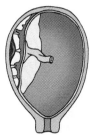
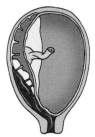
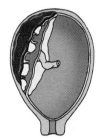

Partial separation
(concealed hemorrhage)

Partial separation
(apparent hemorrhage)

Complete separation
(concealed hemorrhage)

Figure 8-2 Abruptio placentae.

Care for the Patient Experiencing an Abruptio Placentae

- Hospitalization
- Intravenous placement with a large-bore catheter (16-gauge)
- Lab work: Includes complete blood count (CBC), coagulation studies (fibrinogen, prothrombin time [PT],

partial thromboplastin time [PTT], platelet count, fibrin degradation products), type and screen for 4 units of blood, Kleihauer-Betke for Rh-negative patients. A "clot test" may be performed: a red top tube of blood is drawn, set aside, and checked for clotting. If a clot does not form within 6 minutes or if it forms and lyses within 30 minutes, a coagulation defect is probably present and the fibrinogen level is <150 mg/dL.

- If birth is not imminent, possibly betamethasone to promote fetal lung maturity
- RhoGAM if indicated
- Continuous evaluation of intake and output
- Continuous electronic fetal monitoring
- Delivery (cesarean or vaginal birth) may be initiated depending on maternal–fetal status
- Continuous maternal–fetal assessment, with ongoing information and emotional support for the patient and her family

DIAGNOSTIC TESTS

With any incidence of bleeding during pregnancy, the following laboratory tests are commonly performed:

- CBC
- Coagulation studies (fibrinogen, PT, PTT, platelet count, fibrin degradation products)
- Type and screen for blood
- Kleihauer–Betke for Rh-negative patients; Rh(D)-negative patients should receive RhoGAM to prevent isoimmunization
- Ultrasound to assess viability of pregnancy, location of placenta, location of conceptus, and to assess for abruption

ETHNOCULTURAL CONSIDERATIONS

Religious Beliefs and Blood Transfusions

Jehovah's Witness prohibits its members from receiving blood products or their derivatives. When bleeding occurs during pregnancy and blood is deemed necessary to save the woman's and/or fetus' life, a very challenging situation exists. Non-blood products may be given but are not always successful. Sometimes a court order is obtained so that blood can be administered to save the life of the woman and/or fetus. Respect the family's beliefs and support them during this very difficult time when the health of both the woman and her fetus as well as their religious beliefs are being challenged.

TEACHING THE FAMILY

Communicating with the Family Who Has Experienced a Perinatal Loss

Approach the family with compassion and sincerity. Expressions of caring are conveyed in the following statements:

- "I understand this is a very difficult time for you and your family, but I want you to know that I am here and willing to listen if you want to talk. You let me know if and when you are ready."
- "It is normal for you to be sad and you will probably feel like this for some time. Losing a baby, no matter how far along in your pregnancy, is very difficult. I can recommend some support groups if you think you might be interested." (If the patient says she does not want the information at this time, continue with) "Please do not hesitate to call us if you change your mind. We can always give you the information."
- "Does your baby have a name?" (refer to the fetus by name instead of "the fetus")

Hypertensive Complications in Pregnancy

Specific Conditions and Implications

Condition	Definition	Implications
Chronic Hypertension (HTN)	HTN present before pregnancy	At increased risk for preeclampsia
Gestational HTN (transient)	HTN appearing after the 20th week of pregnancy without proteinuria	Resolves by 12 weeks postpartum
Preeclampsia	HTN (BP >140/90 mm Hg) with proteinuria appearing after 20 weeks of gestation	Risk for abruption, intrauterine growth restriction (IUGR), fetal demise, disseminated intravascular coagulation (DIC), renal failure, seizure

(continued)

Specific Conditions and Implications (Continued)		
Condition	Definition	Implications
Hemolysis, Elevated Liver Enzymes, Low Platelets (HELLP syndrome)	A complication of preeclampsia that can manifest at any time during pregnancy and the puerperium	Arteriolar vasospasms lead to hemolysis, and decreased blood flow to the liver, resulting in tissue ischemia and hemorrhagic necrosis (elevated liver enzymes). In response to the endothelial damage caused by the vasospasms, platelets aggregate at the site and a fibrin network is set up, leading to a decrease in the circulating platelets (low platelets).
Eclampsia	The occurrence of a grand mal seizure	Can occur during pregnancy, labor, or within 72 hours after birth

FOCUSED ASSESSMENT

Risk Factors for Preeclampsia

- Primigravida (6–8 times greater risk)
- Age extremes (<17 years and >35 years)
- Diabetes
- Preexisting hypertension
- Multiple gestation (5 times greater risk)
- Fetal hydrops (10 times greater risk)
- Hydatidiform mole (10 times greater risk)
- Preeclampsia in a previous pregnancy
- Family history
- Obesity
- Immunological factors
- Chronic renal disease
- Rh incompatibility
- African American ethnicity
- Pregnancies that result from donor insemination, oocyte donation, embryo donation (American College of Obstetricians and Gynecologists [ACOG], 2002; Sibai, Dekker, & Kupfermine, 2005)

Assessment Guidelines

Cardiovascular System
- Blood pressure, heart sounds, lung sounds
- Edema

- Early signs or symptoms of pulmonary edema (tachycardia or tachypnea)
- Daily weight taken at the same time of the day and on the same scale
- Skin color, temperature, and turgor
- Capillary refill: May indicate decreased perfusion if >3 seconds

Renal System
- Proteinuria: 24-hour urine sample
- Output of at least 30 mL/hr
- Intake/output measurement

Central Nervous System
- Level of consciousness
- Headache, visual disturbances*
- Hyperreflexia
- Clonus

Hepatic System
- Elevated liver enzymes
- Enlarged liver
- Epigastric pain*

Document the presence or absence of these symptoms.

CLINICAL ALERTS

Facilitating Effective CPR for the Pregnant Patient

Instruct the pregnant patient never to lie on her back. Explain that the weight of the baby exerts pressure on the large blood vessels and impedes blood flow back to the heart. If the pregnant patient experiences a cardiac arrest, this information is essential. CPR is not effective if the fetus remains on the large blood vessels. One nurse must take responsibility to displace the uterus to the left while the cardiac compressions are being performed.

Care of the Pregnant Patient Post Seizure

- Do not attempt to shorten or abolish the initial seizure. Attempts to administer anticonvulsants intravenously without secure venous access can lead to phlebitis and venous thrombosis.
- Prevent maternal injury.

- Maintain adequate oxygenation; administer oxygen via face mask at 10 L/min.
- Minimize the risk of aspiration. Position the patient on her side to facilitate drainage. Ensure suction equipment is ready and working.
- Give adequate magnesium sulfate to control seizures. As soon as possible following the seizure, venous access should be secured with a 4- to 6-gram loading bolus of magnesium sulfate given over 15 to 20 minutes. If the patient seizes after the loading dose, another 2-gram bolus may be given intravenously, over 3 to 5 minutes.
- Correct maternal acidemia. Blood gas analysis allows monitoring of oxygenation and pH status. Respiratory acidemia is possible following a seizure.
- Avoid polytherapy. Maternal respiratory depression, respiratory arrest, or cardiopulmonary arrest is more likely in women who receive polytherapy to arrest a seizure. Remember that anticonvulsants are respiratory depressants and may interact.
- Check the fetus(es) (all must be accounted for). Following a seizure there may be loss of FHR variability and bradycardia on the fetal monitoring tracing.
- Check the patient for ruptured membranes, contractions, and cervical dilation.
- Prepare for birth as indicated.
- Support the patient and her family. This is a very frightening event for them and they need reassurance and need to be kept aware of the plan of care and the well being of their baby (Poole, 2004).

Documentation After a Patient Seizure

- Time and length of seizure
- Associated symptoms
- Vital signs including fetal heart assessment
- Presence or absence of uterine contractions
- Any untoward results such as the rupture of membranes or signs of placental abruption
- Medications that were given. Remember to have the physician write or co-sign any verbal orders that were given during the emergency (Poole, 2004)

Accidental Overdose of Magnesium Sulfate Administration Can Pose a Significant Risk to Both Mother and Newborn

Current Recommendations to Prevent Magnesium Sulfate Accidents

- A standardized unit protocol with standing orders that address the initial bolus and maintenance dose to be administered; how the pump should be programmed; the maintenance IV solutions that will be used and the frequency of the maternal–fetal assessment.
- Administer IV magnesium sulfate (including the initial bolus) only through a controlled infusion device with free-flow protection.
- Use universal standardized dose prepackaged magnesium sulfate.
- Have a second nurse check the initial magnesium sulfate IV bag and pump settings (and every magnesium sulfate IV bag that is added and each subsequent rate change).
- Use a 100-mL (4 g) or 150-mL (6 g) IV piggyback (IVPB) for the initial bolus instead of giving a bolus from the main bag with a rate change on the pump.
- Use color-coded tags on the lines as they go into the pumps and into the IV ports.
- Provide 1:1 nursing care for women in labor who are receiving magnesium sulfate.
- When care is transferred to another nurse, have both nurses together at the bedside review the pump settings for both the magnesium sulfate and mainline IV fluids and review written physician orders for magnesium sulfate infusion orders.
- Implement periodic magnesium sulfate overdose drills with airway management and calcium administration with the physician and nurse team members participating together.
- Maintain the calcium antidote in the patient's room in a locked box.

(Simpson & Knox, 2004).

MEDICATIONS

Magnesium Sulfate (mag-**nee**-zhum **sul**-fate)

Pregnancy Category D

Indications Anticonvulsant in severe eclampsia or preeclampsia. Unlabeled use: Preterm labor.

Actions Plays an important role in neurotransmission and muscular excitability

Therapeutic Effects Resolution of eclampsia

Pharmacokinetics
Absorption IV administration results in complete bioavailability; well absorbed from IM sites.
Distribution Widely distributed. Crosses the placenta and is present in breast milk.
Metabolism and Excretion Excreted primarily by the kidneys
Half-life Unknown

Contraindications and Precautions
Contraindicated in Hypermagnesemia/hypocalcemia/anuria/heart block/active labor or within 2 hours of labor (unless used for preeclampsia or eclampsia)
Use Cautiously in Any degree of renal insufficiency

Adverse Reactions and Side Effects
Central Nervous System Drowsiness
Respiratory System Decreased respirations
Cardiovascular System Arrhythmias, hypotension, bradycardia
Gastrointestinal System Diarrhea
Dermatological System Flushing, sweating
Metabolic Hypothermia

Interactions Potentiates neuromuscular blocking agents

Route and Dosage
Eclampsia/Preeclampsia Piggyback a solution of 40 g of magnesium sulfate in 1000 mL of lactated Ringer's solution—use an infusion control device (pump) at the ordered rates; loading dose: initial bolus of 4–6 g over 15–30 min; maintenance dose: 1–3 g/hr.
IM: 4–5 g given in each buttock, can be repeated at 4-hour intervals; use Z-track technique

(Note: IM route rarely used because the absorption rate cannot be controlled and injections are painful and may result in tissue necrosis.)

Time/Action Profile for Anticonvulsant Effect IM: Onset is 60 minutes with peak unknown and duration is 3–4 hours. **IV:** Onset is immediate with peak unknown and duration is 30 minutes.

Nursing Implications
Remember that this is a very potent, high alert drug!
Explain the purpose and side effects of the medication to the patient and her companion.

Explain that she may feel very warm and become flushed and experience nausea and vomiting, visual blurring, and headaches.

Magnesium sulfate must never be abbreviated (i.e., $MgSO_4$ is not acceptable) and requires a written order by the physician for administration.

Always use an infusion pump for administration and run the medication piggyback, not as the main line.

Monitor pulse, blood pressure, respirations, and ECG frequently throughout parenteral administration. Respirations should be at least 16/min before each dose.

Monitor neurologic status before and throughout therapy.

Institute seizure precautions

Keep the room quiet and darkened to decrease the likelihood of triggering seizure activity

Patellar reflexes should be tested before each parenteral dose of magnesium sulfate. If absent, no additional dose should be administered until a positive response returns.

Monitor intake and output. Urine output should be maintained at a level of at least 100 mL/4 hr.

Serum magnesium levels and renal function should be monitored periodically throughout administration of parenteral magnesium sulfate.

Have 10% calcium gluconate available should toxicity occur. Administer 10 mL intravenously over 1–3 minutes until signs and symptoms are reversed.

After delivery, monitor the newborn, for hypotension, hyporeflexia, and respiratory depression.

Data from Deglin, J., & Vallerand, A. (2009). Davis's drug guide for nurses (11th ed.). Philadelphia: F. A. Davis.

Medications Used to Treat Chronic Severe Hypertension in Pregnancy

Agent (trade name)	Class	Dose	Contraindications and Adverse Effects	Breast feeding
Alpha-Methyldopa (Aldomet)	Central alpha-adrenergic inhibitor	Starting dose is 250 mg PO, tid or qid Maximum dosage of 2–4 g/24 hr	Methyldopa hypersensitivity, history of hepatitis, autonomic dysfunction, lethargy, or syncope. Can cause liver damage, fever, Coombs-positive hemolytic anemia.	Safe

(continued)

Medications Used to Treat Severe Hypertension in Pregnancy (Continued)

Agent (trade name)	Class	Dose	Contraindications and Adverse Effects	Breast feeding
Labetalol (Trandate, Normodyne)	Alpha/ beta-adrenergic blocker	100–400 mg PO bid–tid (maximum dose 2400 mg a day)	Labetalol hypersensitivity, bradycardia, asthma, heart block, heart failure. Can cause maternal and fetal bradycardia, hypotension, bronchospasm	Safe
Nifedipine (Adalat, Procardia)	Calcium channel blocker	10–30 mg PO tid. Slow release once a day. Maximum of 90 mg/day	Hypersensitivity to calcium channel blockers, persistent dermatologic reactions, congestive heart failure. Can potentiate cardiac depressive effect of magnesium sulfate.	Safe
Furosemide (Lasix)	Loop diuretic	20–80 mg PO, once or twice daily	Hypersensitivity to furosemide, anuria, or depleted blood count. Can cause profound diuresis with water and electrolyte depletions, sensitivity to sunlight exposure, hyperuricemia and gout, exacerbation of SLE, abdominal cramping, diarrhea, tinnitus, dizziness, pancreatitis, and cholestasis.	Safe
Hydrochloro-thiazide (HydroDIURIL)	Loop diuretic	25–50 mg PO daily	Anuria, renal disease, liver disease, SLE, hypersensitivity to hydrochlorothiazide or other sulfonamide derived drugs. Can cause weakness, hypotension, pancreatitis, cholestasis, anemia, allergic reactions, electrolyte disturbance, hyperglycemia, hyperuricemia, dizziness, renal dysfunction.	Risk is remote, but there are concerns about potential thromb-ocytope-nia in infants.

Source: Yankowitz, J. (2004). Pharmacologic treatment of hypertensive disorders during pregnancy. *The Journal of Perinatal & Neonatal Nursing, 18* (3), 230–240. Reproduced with permission.

Medications Used to Acutely Treat Severe Hypertension in Pregnancy

Agent (Trade Name)	Class	Dosage
Labetalol hydrochloride (Normodyne, Trandate)	Alpha/beta-adrenergic blocker	IV bolus 20 mg; if no response, double dose and repeat every 15 minutes, up to a cumulative maximum dose of 300 mg.
Hydralazine (Apresoline, Nepresol)	Peripheral/arterial vasodilator	IV bolus 5–10 mg every 15–20 minutes to a maximum dose of 30 mg
Nifedipine (Adalat, Procardia)	Calcium channel blocker	Nifedipine can be given PO in doses of 10 mg repeated every 15 minutes to a maximum of 30 mg.
Sodium Nitroprusside (Nipride, Nitropress)	Vasodilator	0.25 mcg/kg per minute (Increase by 0.25 mcg/kg per minute every 5 minutes to a maximum of 5 mcg/kg per minute.)

Source: Yankowitz, J. (2004). Pharmacologic treatment of hypertension during pregnancy. *The Journal of Perinatal & Neonatal Nursing, 18* (3), 230–240.

TEACHING THE FAMILY

Home Management of the Patient with Pregnancy-induced Hypertension

Before discharge, ascertain that the home environment is conducive to rest and the patient will be able to rest frequently throughout the day. Ensure that the patient can verbalize understanding of the importance of keeping all prenatal appointments and that she must immediately notify her physician or midwife at the first appearance of:

- Blood pressure values greater than those at the time of hospital discharge: MD or CNM should provide parameters.
- Visual changes
- Epigastric pain
- Nausea and vomiting
- Bleeding gums
- Headaches
- Increasing edema, especially of the hands and face
- Decreasing urinary output
- Decreased fetal movement
- "Just not feeling right"

ADDITIONAL INFORMATION FOR THE CLINICAL SETTING

Grading Reflexes and Checking for Clonus

During the assessment, grade maternal reflexes on a 0 to 4+ scale:

4+ Very brisk, hyperactive; often indicative of disease; often associated with clonus
3+ Brisker than average; possibly but not necessarily indicative of disease
2+ Average; normal
1+ Somewhat diminished
0 No response

Clonus is usually noted as "absent" or "present" but it may be rated as:

Mild (2 movements)
Moderate (3–5 movements)
Severe (6 or more movements)

SPASMS: A Memory Enhancer When Caring for a Patient with Preeclampsia

S: Significant blood pressure changes may occur without warning.
P: Proteinuria, a serious sign of renal involvement, is present.
A: Arterioles are affected by vasospasms that result in endothelial damage, leakage of intravascular fluid into the interstitial spaces, and edema.

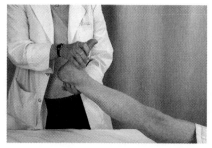

Figure 8-3 Assessing for clonus.

S: Significant laboratory changes (most notably, liver function tests and platelet count) signal worsening of the disease.

M: Multiple organ systems can be involved, including cardiovascular, hematological, hepatic, renal, and central nervous systems.

S: Symptoms appear after 20 weeks of gestation.

Endocrine Complications in Pregnancy
FOCUSED ASSESSMENT

Diabetes Mellitus		
Classification of Diabetes	Characteristics	Implications
Type 1	• Usually diagnosed in persons younger than 30 years of age • Polyuria, polydipsia, weight loss • An abrupt onset that requires emergency medical attention • Approximately 10% of those diagnosed with diabetes	• Requires insulin *Possible sequelae* (dependent on level of glycemic control; HbA$_{1c}$ level used to guide treatment): • 4 times more likely to develop preeclampsia or eclampsia • 5 times increase in perinatal death • 2–3 times increase in congenital malformations and poor fetal growth • Fetal demise
Type 2	• Usually diagnosed in adults older than age 30 • Slow onset with gradual progression of symptoms • Not ketosis prone	Does not always require insulin *Possible sequelae* (dependent on level of glycemic control; HbA$_{1c}$ level used to guide treatment): • 4 times more likely to develop preeclampsia or eclampsia • 5 times increase in perinatal death • 2 to 3 times increase in congenital malformations and poor fetal growth • Fetal demise

(continued)

Diabetes Mellitus (Continued)

Classification of Diabetes	Characteristics	Implications
Gestational	• Develops in the latter half of pregnancy • Symptoms are usually mild and not life threatening • May be treated with either diet or insulin *Risk factors:* • Women older than 25 years of age • Obesity • Insulin resistance • Polycystic ovary syndrome • History of a large-for-gestational age infant, hydramnios, stillbirth, miscarriage, infant with congenital anomalies • Family history of type 2 diabetes • Ethnicity	Increased risk for developing diabetes later in life *Possible sequelae:* (Dependent on level of glycemic control; HbA_{1c} level used to guide treatment): • Fetal demise • Growth abnormalities • Hydramnios • Macrosomia • Newborn hypoglycemia

Other Endocrine Disorders

Disorder	Signs/Symptoms	Tests and Treatment
Hyperthyroidism	Heat intolerance, diaphoresis, fatigue, anxiety, emotional lability, tachycardia, wide pulse pressure, weight loss, goiter, nausea, vomiting, diarrhea, cardiomyopathy	*Tests:* Decreased TSH with increased free T_4 *Treatment:* Antithyroid medications (thioamides, propylthiouracil, methimazole), subtotal thyroidectomy, radioactive iodine treatment *Potential effect on pregnancy:* Increased risk of preeclampsia, preterm labor, low birth weight, neonatal mortality
Hypothyroidism	Weight gain, decreased exercise tolerance, constipation, hoarseness, hair loss, brittle nails, dry skin	*Tests:* Increased TSH with normal to low T_3 and T_4 *Treatment:* Thyroid hormone supplement *Potential effect on pregnancy:* Increased risk of preeclampsia, placental abruption, stillbirth

Disorder	Signs/Symptoms	Tests and Treatment
Hyperemesis Gravidarum	Abnormal condition of pregnancy characterized by protracted, persistent vomiting, weight loss, and fluid and electrolyte imbalance	*Tests:* Electrolytes assessment *Treatment:* Rest; eat small frequent meals of dry, bland foods high in protein; avoid spicy foods; antiemetics; hospitalization if severe for parenteral or enteral feedings.

CLINICAL ALERT

Maternal Diabetes and Preterm Labor

Magnesium sulfate is the drug of choice for diabetic women who experience preterm labor. The use of terbutaline sulfate (Brethine) or antenatal corticosteroids to accelerate fetal lung maturation can cause significant maternal hyperglycemia and precipitate diabetic ketoacidosis (DKA). Follow patients closely in an acute care setting for at least 48 to 72 hours after corticosteroids have been given. An intravenous insulin infusion is usually required and is adjusted on the basis of frequent capillary glucose measurements (Landon, Catalano, & Gabbe, 2002).

DIAGNOSTIC TESTS

The Glucose Challenge Test (Glucola Screening)

- Administer a 50-g oral dose of glucose solution to the woman.
- Take a blood sample 1 hour after the glucose is consumed.
- Follow up with the formal 3-hour oral glucose tolerance test (OGTT) if the patient's 1-hour plasma glucose level is 140 mg/dL or higher.

Oral Glucose Tolerance Test (OGTT)

The 3-hour OGTT requires the fasting patient to ingest 100 g of glucose and have blood drawn at 1-hour intervals. For at least 12 hours before and during the test, the woman should avoid consuming caffeine (it may increase glucose levels) and refrain from smoking. The diagnosis of gestational diabetes mellitus is made when two or more of the threshold values are above the norm. According to the American Diabetes Association (ADA; 2006), normal plasma glucose values are:

Fasting blood sugar	<95 mg/dL
1-hour	<180 mg/dL
2-hour	<155 mg/dL
3-hour	<140 mg/dL

MEDICATIONS

Medications for Nausea and Vomiting of Pregnancy

- Pyridoxine (vitamin B$_6$, 25–75 mg (orally) per day, used alone or in combination with Doxylamine (Unisom), 25 mg (orally) per day
- Promethazine (Phenergan) 12.5–25 mg (intravenously, intramuscularly, orally, or rectally) every 4 hours
- Dimenhydrinate (Dramamine) 50–100 mg (orally or rectally) every 4–6 hours or 50 mg intravenously (in 50 mL of saline run over 20 minutes) every 4–6 hours
- Metoclopramide (Reglan) 5–10 mg (intravenously, intramuscularly, or orally) every 8 hours

(ACOG, 2004; Cunningham et al., 2005)

ETHNOCULTURAL CONSIDERATIONS

- Gestational diabetes occurs more often in Native Americans, African Americans, Hispanic Americans, Asian Americans, and Pacific Islanders (ADA, 2006).

TEACHING THE FAMILY

Complementary Care for Nausea and Vomiting of Pregnancy

- Ginger, a perennial native to many Asian countries, is effective in treating nausea and vomiting during pregnancy. The antiemetic effect of this root (taken in a dosage of 1 gram per day) is due to its ability to increase gastrointestinal motility. Ginger is available in tablet, capsule, and syrup form. Some concerns about taking ginger during pregnancy have been raised, but to date no significant side effects have been documented.

- Elasticized wristbands (i.e., Sea-Bands®) that use a firm object to place pressure on the Neiguan point (acupressure P6 point) are a nonpharmacological, noninvasive method that may lessen the frequency and severity of nausea and vomiting during pregnancy (Hunter, Sullivan, Young, & Weber, 2007).

ADDITIONAL INFORMATION FOR THE CLINICAL SETTING

Diet and Exercise for the Patient with Gestational Diabetes Mellitus (GDM)

Diet and exercise are important components of care for the woman with GDM. Typically, the patient is placed on a standard diabetic diet that is calculated to include 30 kcal/kg per day, based on a normal preconceptional weight. For the obese woman, the diet may be calculated to include up to 25 kcal/kg per day. On-going nutritional counseling is essential.

Physical activity such as walking and swimming is also important for the woman with GDM. Exercise helps to lower blood glucose levels and may decrease the need for insulin (ADA, 2006).

Planning Care for the Woman with GDM

Although diet and exercise are the mainstays of care for the woman with gestational diabetes mellitus, up to 20% require insulin during pregnancy to maintain euglycemia. If fasting blood glucose levels exceed 105 mg/dL, insulin therapy is initiated (ADA, 2006).

Anticipating Changes in Insulin Needs During Pregnancy

- During the first trimester, maternal blood glucose levels typically decrease and the insulin response to glucose increases. To avoid hypoglycemia, a woman with well-controlled diabetes may need a decreased insulin dosage when she becomes pregnant.

- Maternal insulin resistance begins at about 14 weeks of gestation and increases until it stabilizes during the final weeks of pregnancy.
- During the second and third trimesters, as insulin requirements steadily increase, the insulin dosage must be adjusted to prevent hyperglycemia.

Infections that May Adversely Affect Pregnancy

FOCUSED ASSESSMENT

Various Infections and Their Effects on the Pregnancy

Infection	Signs/Symptoms	Sequelae in Pregnancy	Treatment
Urinary Tract Infection (UTI), Cystitis	Urinary frequency, urgency, dysuria and suprapubic pain	Preterm labor, septic shock, adult respiratory distress syndrome	Anti-infectives for 7–10 days
Pyelonephritis	Flank tenderness, nausea, vomiting, fever and chills together with the symptoms of a lower UTI	If left untreated or inadequately treated, septic shock, adult respiratory distress syndrome and/or preterm labor may result.	Treated aggressively with hospitalization and intravenous antibiotics
Group B *Streptococcus* (GBS)	All women are now screened between 35 and 37 weeks of pregnancy and treated before childbirth.	May cause UTI, chorioamnionitis, or endometritis, preterm labor, neonatal infection	Penicillin-based anti-infective agent
Chlamydia	Vaginal discharge, dysuria, abnormal vaginal bleeding, or asymptomatic	Neonatal infection transmitted during birth (conjunctivitis and pneumonia)	Erythromycin or penicillin-based anti-infectives
Gonorrhea (GC)	Vaginal discharge, dysuria and abnormal vaginal bleeding	Ophthalmia neonatorum, amniotic infection syndrome	Oral or intramuscular cefixime (Suprax) or ceftriaxone (Rocephin)

Infection	Signs/Symptoms	Sequelae in Pregnancy	Treatment
Syphilis	Primary: Chancre Secondary: Palmar rash Tertiary: Neurosyphilis	Delayed treatment or untreated infection results in a range of fetal effects from minor anomalies to preterm birth or fetal death	Penicillin
Human Papillomavirus (HPV) Infection	Genital warts	May be transmitted to fetus transplacentally	Cryotherapy, trichloroacetic acid, dichloroacetic acid, surgical excision
Human Immunodeficiency Virus (HIV) and Acquired Immunodeficiency Syndrome (AIDS)		Vertical transmission to fetus (antepartally, intrapartally); transfer in breast milk (postpartally)	Without identification of HIV-infected women and the aggressive use of preventive therapy, 20%–30% of exposed children will become infected with HIV (CDC, 2006; Landry, 2004; Moran, 2004).
Tuberculosis (TB)	Inflammatory infiltrations in the respiratory tract, the gastrointestinal and genitourinary tracts, bones, joints, nervous system, lymph nodes and skin	The tubercle bacillus can spread to the fetus from the maternal blood by crossing the placenta, and entering the umbilical vein. Bacilli may settle in the fetal liver or the lungs.	Isoniazid (INH), ethambutol, and rifampin

TORCH Diseases

Infection/Agent	Mode of Transmission/ Detection	Maternal Effects	Neonatal Effects	Treatment	Incidence and Prevention	High Risk Potential
Toxoplasmosis Single-celled protozoan parasite *Toxoplasma gondii*	*Transmission:* Transplacental Eating raw meat, especially pork, lamb or venison Touching the hands or mouth after handling undercooked meat containing *T. gondii* Secreted in feces of infected cats Cyst is destroyed with heat. *Detection:* Serological antibody testing IgM specific antibody	Most infections in humans are asymptomatic. However, may include fatigue, muscle pains, and sometimes lymphadenopathy. In the immunocompetent person, toxoplasmosis can be a devastating infection.	Severity varies with gestational age. Congenital infection can occur if a woman develops acute toxoplasmosis during pregnancy (most likely in the third trimester). May have miscarriage if acquired early. Fetal infections are more virulent the earlier the infection is acquired but less frequent. Sequelae include low birth weight, hepatosplenomegaly, icterus, anemia, neurological disease, and chorioretinitis.	Pyrimethamine and sulfadiazine may reduce incidence of congenital toxoplasmosis. Treatment of the mother has been shown to reduce the risk of congenital infection. *Pyrimethamine is not recommended for use during the first trimester of pregnancy.*	ACOG does not recommend routine screening except for pregnant women with HIV infection. Incidence varies throughout the world (1–4 infants per 1000 live births). 30% of U.S. women have been exposed. Approximately 40%–50% of U.S. adults have an antibody to this organism. Frequency of seroconversion during pregnancy is ≤5% and approximately 3 in 1000 infants show evidence of congenital infection.	People who consume raw or poorly cooked meat High-risk gestational age is 10–24 weeks. Toxoplasmosis is more common in Western Europe, particularly France.

IgG seroconversion from negative to positive Most accurate confirmation of active infection is a rise in IgG titer in two appropriately spaced tests.	Clinically significant congenital toxoplasmosis occurs in approximately 1 in 8000 pregnancies.			Incidence of congenital toxoplasmosis infection in the United States is 1 in 1000–8000. More than 60 million people in the United States carry a parasite. Cook meat to a safe temperature. Peel or wash fruits and vegetables.
Other **HEPATITIS B** **HBV** Incubation usually 60–90 days *Transmission:* Direct contact with the blood or body fluids of an infected person Sexual Perinatal Percutaneous Transplacental Blood, stool, amniotic fluid, and saliva transmission	The course of the disease is not altered during the pregnancy. Symptoms are seen in only 30%–50% of patients; these include low-grade fever, nausea, anorexia, jaundice, hepatomegaly, malaise, preterm labor, and preterm birth.	Infants infected at birth have a 90% risk of becoming chronically infected with HBV (carrier) and 25% risk of developing significant liver disease—yet if they receive prophylaxis at birth, 95% can be prevented.	Mother: Rest Infant: Vaccine if mother is carrier, infant receives HBIg HBV vaccine is recommended (three doses).	Screen all pregnant women. The incidence of hepatitis B in the United States declined by >60% from 1985 to 1995. Estimated that 1–1.25 million people in the United States are chronically infected with HBV. High-risk categories: Pregnant women from China, Southeast Asia, Africa, Philippines, and Indonesia Eskimos Prostitutes Homosexuals IV drug users Hemophiliacs

(continued)

TORCH Diseases (Continued)

Infection/Agent	Mode of Transmission/ Detection	Maternal Effects	Neonatal Effects	Treatment	Incidence and Prevention	High Risk Potential
	Shared razors, toothbrushes, towels, and other personal items *Detection:* HBsAg identified 7–14 days after exposure Hepatitis B surface antibody present with HBsAg indicates noninfectious HBcAg, HBeAg, and anti-HBc evaluate stage and progression of the infection	No specific treatment, but may include bedrest and a high-protein, low-fat diet. Mother-to-child transmission of HBV occurs in 10%–20% of women who are seropositive for HBsAg and in 90% of women who are seropositive for both HBsAg and HBcAg. Transmission to the neonate appears to occur as a result of exposure to infected blood and genital secretions during delivery.	Increased risk of transmission to infant if mother is HBeAg-positive (indicating acute infection) Stillbirth Clinical illness is relatively infrequent. Most (90%–95%) of those infected are symptomatic and become chronic hepatitis B carriers. Infants born to women who have hepatitis B infection during pregnancy should be given HBIg within 12 hours of delivery.		Estimated that 300 million people worldwide are chronically infected with HBV. Approximately 8000 acute HBV infections were reported to the CDC. HBV vaccine has been available since 1982. Acute infection occurs in 1–2 per 10,000 pregnancies. Minimize exposure of close physical contact. Heptavax-B (Pregnancy does not contraindicate vaccination.)	Transfusion recipients People with other sexually transmitted diseases or multiple sex partners CDC recommends universal screening of all prenatal patients.

| Rubella (3-day German measles) Rubella virus incubation is 2–3 weeks. | *Transmission:* Nasopharyngeal secretions Transplacental *Detection:* Virus isolated from throat Rubella-specific IgM antibodies Hemagglutination-inhibition antibodies Complement-fixing antibodies Rubella antibody titer of 1:8 or more indicates immune status. | Erythematous maculopapular rash on face, neck, arms, and legs lasting 3 days Lymph node enlargement Slight fever, malaise, headache, and arthralgia History of exposure 3 weeks earlier | Overall risk of congenital rubella syndrome is approximately 20% for primary maternal infection in the first trimester. High incidence of congenital abnormalities in newborns whose mother contracted rubella within the first 4 months of pregnancy. Approximately 50% of infants exposed to the virus within 4 weeks of conception will manifest signs of congenital infection. When infection occurs in second 4 week period after conception, approximately 25% of | Women with rubella require no special therapy other than mild analgesics and rest. Infants born with congenital rubella may shed virus for many months and thus be a threat to other infants, as well as to susceptible adults. | Last epidemic in 1965; since introduction of vaccine in late 1960s, rubella has been rare. Absence of rubella antibody indicates susceptibility. Estimated that 6%–25% of women are susceptible. Occurs more commonly in the spring. Vaccinate immediately postpartum and use contraception for a minimum of 1 month after vaccination. |

(continued)

TORCH Diseases (Continued)

Infection/Agent	Mode of Transmission/ Detection	Maternal Effects	Neonatal Effects	Treatment	Incidence and Prevention	High Risk Potential
			fetuses will be infected; when infection develops in the third month, approximately 10% of fetuses will be infected. Spectrum anomalies: Deafness (60%–75%) Eye defects (10%–30%) CNS anomalies (10–25%) Cardiac malformation (10%–20%) Risks appear to be almost exclusively associated with women who previously have not been infected with CMV. Even in this case, two thirds of infants will not become infected and only 10%–15% of		Vaccination is contraindicated during pregnancy.	

Cytomegalovirus (CMV) DNA virus of the herpesvirus group	*Transmission:* Transmitted horizontally by droplet infection and contact with saliva and urine, and vertically from mother to fetus-infant, and as a sexually transmitted infection. Intimate contact with infected secretions (breast milk, cervical mucus, semen, saliva, tears and urine) Transplacental *Detection:* Isolation of virus from urine or endocervical secretions	Most infections are asymptomatic, but approximately 15% of adults have a mononucleosis-like syndrome characterized by fever, pharyngitis, lymphadenopathy, and polyarthritis. the remaining will have symptoms. Infection is most likely to occur with primary maternal infection. The timing of the infection during pregnancy is a major determinant of outcome (first and second trimester being more severely affected). CID includes low birthweight, IUGR, microcephaly, CNS abnormalities, mental and motor retardation, intracranial calcifications, sensorineural deafness, blindness with chorioretinitis, mental retardation, hepatosplenomegaly and jaundice	Mother: Treat symptoms. Infant: No satisfactory treatment is available. Isolate the infant. Approximately 50% of females in the United States have antibodies. It is estimated that approximately 2% of susceptible pregnant women in the United States acquire primary CMV infection during pregnancy.	Maternal immunity to CMV does not prevent recurrence. Found in 0.5%–2.0% of all neonates. Incidence of primary CMV infection in pregnant women in the United States varies from 1% to 3%. Maintain rigorous personal hygiene throughout the pregnancy.	Day care centers are a common source of infection. Prevalence depends on age, sex, SE class, sexual behavior, and occupational or institutional exposure. Serological screening is not recommended by ACOG. Vaccine is experimental.

(continued)

TORCH Diseases (Continued)

Infection/Agent	Mode of Transmission/ Detection	Maternal Effects	Neonatal Effects	Treatment	Incidence and Prevention	High Risk Potential
Herpes Simplex Virus (HSV) Herpes virus type 1 (more common with oral lesions) and type 2 (more common in genital lesions) Incubation is 2–10 days	*Transmission:* Ascending infection Intimate mucocutaneous exposure Transmission is more likely to occur from men to women. Passage through an infected birth canal Transplacental (although rare) if initial infection occurs during pregnancy	Painful genital vesicle lesions Vesicles on the cervix, vagina, or external genitalia area Primary infection is commonly associated with fever, malaise, and myalgia; numbness, tingling, burning, itching, and pain with lesions; lymphadenopathy; and urinary retention.	Rare transplacental transmission have resulted in miscarriage. Mortality of 50%–60% if neonatal exposure is with active primary infection.	Protect neonate from exposure at time of birth. Cultures are obtained when the mother has active lesions. Avoid routine use of scalp electrodes. If lesions are visible, delivery by cesarean section is the current standard of care. Acyclovir has been used near term to suppress viral outbreak.	An estimated 1 million Americans are newly infected with genital HSV annually. Seroprevalence of HSV is approximately 25%. Approximately 1%–2% of pregnancies. 1 in 3000–20,000 live births is at risk for the development of neonatal herpes. Up to 70% of women who give birth to infected infants have no history of genital herpes.	Risk factors include female sex, African-American, or Mexican-American ethnic background, older age, low educational level, poverty, cocaine use, a greater number of lifetime sexual partners, unprotected sex, and having a sexual partner with genital herpes.

Detection:	Neurological	Prophylactic
Tissue culture (swab specimen from vesicles) and immunofluorescent staining of the cell can differentiate HSV-1 from HSV-2. Presence of swelling, redness, and painful lesions	morbidity such as chorioretinitis, microcephaly, mental retardation, seizures, and apnea	treatment with oral acyclovir may be appropriate in women with frequent recurrent infections in pregnancy. If symptoms or lesions are present, cesarean delivery should be performed. Avoid genital contact when male partner has penile lesions. Use condoms.

ACOG = American College of Obstetricians and Gynecologists; Anti-HBc = antibody to hepatitis B core antigen; CDC = Centers for Disease Control and Prevention; CID = cytomegalic inclusion disease; CNS = central nervous system; DNA = deoxyribonucleic acid; HBV = hepatitis B virus; HbsAg = surface antigen to HBC; HbcAg = core antigen to HBV; HbeAg = hepatitis B early antigen; HBIg = hepatitis B immunoglobulin; IgG = immunoglobulin G; IgM = immunoglobulin M; IUGR = intrauterine growth restriction; IV = intravenous.

Source: Moran, B. (2004). Maternal infections. In Mattson, S. & Smith, J. (Eds), Maternal-child nursing core curriculum. 3rd ed. Philadelphia: W.B. Saunders. Reproduced with permission.

DIAGNOSTIC TESTS

Caring for the Patient with a UTI: Urine Specimens

- UTI is more likely during pregnancy, when urine becomes more alkaline and vaginal secretions have an increased glycogen level, both of which foster bacterial growth.
- Before collecting a midstream specimen, explain the importance of proper cleansing.
- Obtain a urinalysis and urine culture and sensitivity on all patients with signs of preterm labor.
- Remember that signs and symptoms of UTI commonly are similar to those of normal pregnancy (urgency, frequency).
- Urge the patient to take all prescribed antibiotic(s), even if she feels better before completing the prescription.
- When treatment is complete, expect to retest the patient's urine to confirm the UTI cure.

MEDICATIONS

Antibiotic Use During Pregnancy

- Sulfonamides should not be used near term because they interfere with protein binding of bilirubin.
- Tetracyclines should never be used during pregnancy because they cause retardation of fetal bone growth and staining of fetal teeth.
- Antibiotics that are safe to use during pregnancy include amoxicillin (Amoxil), ampicillin (Marcillin), and cephalosporins (cephalexin [Keflex]).

Immunizations During Pregnancy

- The ideal time for immunizations that prevent disease transmission from mother to fetus is before conception.
- After conception, maternal and fetal benefits of immunization still usually outweigh the theoretical risks of adverse effects.
- The risks of disease exposure and adverse effects on the mother and her fetus must be weighed against the risks, benefits, and efficacy of the vaccine.
- Nurses should educate women about the importance of immunizations and document each patient's immunization status on her permanent medical record.

Special Conditions and Circumstances that May Adversely Affect Pregnancy

Selected Conditions and Their Effects on Pregnancy

Condition	Definition	Implications
Preterm Labor (PTL)	Contractions and cervical dilation before the end of the 37th gestational week. Symptoms can be subtle: backache, pelvic aching, menstrual-like cramps, vaginal discharge, pelvic pressure, urinary frequency, intestinal cramping.	RhoGAM if indicated Preterm birth: >50% survive at 25 weeks, >90% survive at 28–29 weeks. Assess for infection and fetal fibronectins (fFN) (proteins produced by the fetal membranes).
Premature Rupture of Membranes (PROM)	Rupture of membranes before the onset of labor Diagnosed based on history of vaginal discharge and results of Nitrazine and fern tests	Implications depend on gestational age. Monitor for infection.
Multiple Gestation	More than one fetus	Considered a high-risk pregnancy; at risk for PTL, GDM, UTIs, PIH, placenta previa, IUGR, abnormal presentation, cord prolapse
Disseminated Intravascular Coagulopathy (DIC)	Pathological clotting disorder that consumes clotting factors and results in widespread bleeding.	Life-threatening, early detection is crucial. Observe for signs of bleeding, e.g., petechiae, oozing from injection sites, hematuria.
Venous Thromboembolic Diseases	Includes superficial and deep vein thrombophlebitis (DVT), pulmonary embolus (PE), septic pelvic thrombophlebitis, and thrombosis.	Account for 50% obstetric mortality.
Sickle Cell Disease	Recessive genetic disorder resulting in the production of S hemoglobin (HbS) Most commonly affects those of African or Mediterranean descent.	"Sickled" erythrocytes cannot change their shape and are unable to squeeze through the microcirculation, resulting in obstruction, progressive tissue, and organ damage.

(continued)

Selected Conditions and Their Effects on Pregnancy (Continued)

Condition	Definition	Implications
Thalassemia	Defective globin chains damage developing red blood cells	Predominately affects blacks and those of Italian, Greek, Middle-Eastern Indian, Asian, and West Indies descent.
Rho(D) Isoimmunization	Hemolytic disease of the fetus and newborn resulting from maternal production of antibodies against the $Rh_o(D)$ antigens present on the fetal red blood cells.	Fetal RBC deficiency, hyperbilirubinemia, erythroblastosis fetalis, neonatal kernicterus
ABO Isoimmunization	Hemolytic disease in response to ABO incompatibility between mother and fetus. Type O carries no antigens, type A carries A antigen and type B caries B antigen.	Milder reaction than $Rh_o(D)$ incompatibility
Psychiatric Complications	May represent an exacerbation of an ongoing disorder, a resurgence of previously remitted symptoms, or onset of a new illness.	Psychoactive medications cross the placenta; however, the effects of an untreated psychiatric disorder can also affect pregnancy outcome. The risk:benefit ratio must be carefully considered.
Substance Abuse	Frequent drug and/or alcohol use in pregnancy	See Chapter 4.

Other Special Circumstances

Circumstance	Potential Problems and Complications
Antenatal Bedrest	Muscle wasting, failure to gain weight, cardiovascular and psychological difficulties, difficulty regulating blood pressure, dizziness, fainting
Adolescence	Prenatal medical and behavioral risk factors can severely complicate adolescent pregnancy and result in poor birth outcomes, particularly when late or inadequate prenatal care occurs.

Circumstance	Potential Problems and Complications
Older Gravida	Pregnant women older than the age of 35 are more likely to experience obstetrical complications such as placenta previa, abruptio placentae, prolonged labor, cesarean birth, and mortality. The fetus is at a greater risk for low birth weight, macrosomia, chromosomal abnormalities, congenital malformations, and neonatal mortality.
Obese Patient	A pregnant woman is considered **overweight** if she is 20% above ideal weight or has a BMI over 26.1; she is considered **obese** if her weight exceeds 200 pounds, if she is 50% over ideal body weight for height, or if her BMI is above 29. Obesity is associated with a higher incidence of diabetes and hypertension, macrosomia, prolonged labor, shoulder dystocia, and higher cesarean rates. Cesarean delivery is often complicated by excessive operative blood loss, difficult intubations, postoperative wound complications, operative injury, the need for blood transfusions, thromboembolism, and hysterectomy.
Intimate Partner Violence (IPV)	Pregnancy is often a trigger for escalation of violence in a relationship.

FOCUSED ASSESSMENT

Recognizing Thromboembolism

Assess for the following signs and symptoms:

- Pain, tenderness, warmth in the extremity
- Asymmetrical swelling of lower extremities, with a difference of more than 2 cm between the normal and affected leg. (Thigh swelling is especially significant because the risk of pulmonary embolism is associated with femoral or iliac phlebitis.)
- Color change, especially in the left leg
- A palpable cord beneath the tender, painful area
- Positive Homans' sign
- Signs or symptoms of pulmonary embolism: Tachypnea, dyspnea, pleuritic chest pain, atelectatic rales, cough, fever, diaphoresis, tachycardia, hemoptysis, cyanosis, heart gallop or murmur, anxiety, apprehension (Cunningham et al., 2005; McPhedran, 2004)

Screening for Depression During Pregnancy

The U.S. and Canadian Task Forces on Preventive Health Care recommend using the following two "probe questions" to screen women for depression during pregnancy:

- "Over the past 2 weeks, have you felt down, depressed, or helpless?"
- "Over the past 2 weeks, have you felt little interest or pleasure in doing things?"

(Records & Rice, 2007)

CLINICAL ALERTS

Hemodynamic Changes in Pregnancy

A patient with a cardiac disorder is at greatest risk when hemodynamic changes reach their maximum, between the 28th and 32nd weeks of gestation.

Indicators of Decreased Cardiac Output During Labor and Birth

- Decreased or irregular pulse
- Increased respiratory rate
- Dyspnea
- Chest pain
- Abnormal breath sounds (crackles at lung bases)
- Decreased blood pressure
- Decreased urinary output (<30 mL/hr)
- Edema of hands, face, and feet
- Abnormal heart sounds (diastolic murmur at heart's apex)
- Signs or symptoms of air hunger (anxiety)
- Decreased oxygen saturation (<95%)
- Cool, clammy, cyanotic skin
- Increased capillary refill time (>3 seconds)
- EKG changes
- Mental changes (disorientation, fatigue, syncope)

DIAGNOSTIC TESTS

Kleihauer-Betke test: Estimates the number of fetal RBCs in the maternal circulation

Coombs test: Immunological test that is performed on newborn's blood at birth and that includes direct and indirect Coombs tests

Direct Coombs test: Identifies the presence of maternal Rh-positive antibodies in the neonate's blood and hemolysis or lysis of RBCs

Indirect Coombs test: Detects Rh-positive antibodies in maternal serum

Antepartum Fetal Assessment Tests

Name	Description	Nursing Implications
Chorionic Villus Sampling (CVS)	An invasive procedure in which a thin catheter is inserted vaginally into the intrauterine cavity and a sample of chorionic villus is aspirated from the placenta	Used to obtain a fetal karyotype. Performed between 10 and 12 weeks. The risk of complications with CVS is 1 in 200 and includes infection, fetal loss, rupture of membranes, Rh isoimmunization, and possible fetal limb reduction. After CVS, administer microdose Rh_o(D) immune globulin to the Rh_o(D) negative woman to prevent isoimmunization (Gilbert & Harmon, 2003).
Percutaneous Umbilical Blood Sampling (PUBS)	An invasive procedure in which a needle is inserted through the maternal abdomen and into the fetal umbilical cord	Used to obtain a sample of fetal blood for karyotyping and to test for anemia, isoimmunization, metabolic disorders, and infection. Complications include cord laceration, thromboembolism, preterm labor, premature rupture of the membranes, and infection (Jenkins & Wapner, 2004).
Amniocentesis	An invasive procedure in which amniotic fluid is removed via a needle inserted through the maternal abdomen and into the amniotic sac to obtain a sample of fetal cells	Performed after 12 weeks. May be used to analyze for chromosome abnormalities, fetal lung maturity, infection, the presence of bilirubin in Rh-sensitized pregnancies, amniotic fluid reduction for temporary alleviation of maternal symptoms associated with hydramnios. Complications include rupture of the membranes, preterm labor, infection, fetal injury, and fetal death. If the woman has Rh_o(D)-negative blood, Rh_o(D) immune globulin should be administered after amniocentesis to prevent isoimmunization.

(continued)

Antepartum Fetal Assessment Tests (Continued)

Name	Description	Nursing Implications
	L/S ratio (Lecithin to sphingomyelin) is determined from amniotic fluid, with a value of 2:1 or more indicating mature fetal lungs.	These proteins are components of surfactant formed by the alveoli beginning around the 22nd week of gestation.
	Phosphatidyl glycerol and desaturated phosphatidylcholine	These two substances are found only in the amniotic fluid once the fetal lungs are mature.
Ultrasonography	Use of high-frequency sound waves to detect differences in tissue density and visualize outlines of structures in the body	Noninvasive and painless. Often performed during the first trimester to confirm the viability and age of the pregnancy; determine the number, size, and location of the gestational sacs; identify uterine abnormalities (and rule out an ectopic pregnancy); and locate the presence of an intrauterine contraceptive device
Kick Counts	A count of the number of times the woman feels the fetus move in a specified time	Many variations have been developed but there are two major methods for performing kick counts: 1. While lying on her side, the woman counts and records 10 distinct movements in a period of up to 2 hours. Once 10 movements have been perceived, the count may be discontinued. 2. The patient counts and records fetal movements for 1 hour three times per week. The count is considered reassuring if it equals or exceeds the woman's previously established baseline.

Name	Description	Nursing Implications
Doppler Ultrasound Blood Flow Studies (umbilical velocimetry)	Used to study blood flow in the umbilical vessels of the fetus, placental circulation, fetal cardiac motion, and maternal uterine circulation by measuring the velocity of red blood cell movement through the uterine and fetal vessels	This noninvasive technology is useful in managing pregnancies at risk because of hypertension, diabetes mellitus, intrauterine growth restriction (IUGR), multiple fetuses, or preterm labor.
Fetal Biophysical Profile (BPP)	A noninvasive "fetal physical examination" that combines electronic fetal heart rate monitoring with ultrasonography to evaluate fetal well-being, producing a more accurate prediction than any single assessment	Comprises five components (Harmon, 2004): 1. Nonstress test 2. Fetal breathing movements (one or more episodes of rhythmic fetal breathing movements for 30 seconds) 3. Fetal movement (three or more discrete body or limb movements) 4. Fetal tone (one or more episodes of extension of a fetal extremity with return to flexion, or opening or closing of a hand) 5. Determination of the amniotic fluid volume (a single vertical pocket of amniotic fluid exceeding 2 cm - provides evidence of adequate amniotic fluid) Each of the five components is assigned a score of 2 (normal or present) or 0 (abnormal). A score of 8–10 is reassuring. *(continued)*

Antepartum Fetal Assessment Tests (Continued)

Name	Description	Nursing Implications
Non-stress Test (NST)	The use of electronic fetal monitoring (EFM) for 20 minutes based on the premise that a normal fetus moves at various intervals and that the central nervous system and myocardium respond to movement, with the response of a healthy fetus demonstrated by an acceleration of the fetal heart rate	Acceptable criteria: The presence of 2 fetal heart rate accelerations of 15 beats per minute that last for 15 seconds each during a 20-minute period (ACOG, 1999)
Acoustic Stimulation/ Vibroacoustic Stimulation	A hand-held instrument such as an artificial larynx (especially designed for this purpose) positioned on the maternal abdomen to produce a low-frequency vibration and a buzzing sound for 1 to 3 seconds	May be used as an adjunct to the NST to elicit an acceleration of the fetal heart rate.
Contraction Stress Test (CST)	Evaluates the fetal heart rate response to uterine contractions, with CSTs evaluated according to the presence or absence of late fetal heart rate decelerations.	A late deceleration, associated with fetal hypoxia, is one that begins at the peak of the contraction and persists after conclusion of the contraction. The test is considered negative (normal) if there is no evidence of late or significant variable decelerations; a positive CST (abnormal) is one in which there are late decelerations after 50% of contractions, even if the frequency is less than three in 10 minutes.
Electronic Fetal Heart Rate Monitoring (EFM)	Use of electronic techniques to give an ongoing assessment of fetal well-being, which can be accomplished by either external or internal means	EFM provides information related to the response of the fetal heart rate in the presence or absence of uterine contractions.

MEDICATIONS

Rho(D) Immune Globulin (arr aych oh **dee** im-**yoon glob**-yoo-lin) (RhoGAM, HypRho-D, BayRho-D, Gamulin Rh, Rhophylac)

Pregnancy Category C

Indications
Administered to Rh-negative women who have been exposed to Rh-positive blood by:

Delivering an $Rh_o(D)$-positive infant
Aborting an $Rh_o(D)$-positive fetus
Having chorionic villus sampling, amniocentesis, or intraabdominal trauma while carrying an $Rh_o(D)$-positive fetus
Having an accidental transfusion of $Rh_o(D)$-positive blood

Action Prevents production of anti-$Rh_o(D)$ antibodies in $Rh_o(D)$-negative patients who were exposed to $Rh_o(D)$-positive blood by suppressing the immune reaction of the $Rh_o(D)$-negative woman to the antigen in the $Rh_o(D)$-positive blood.

Therapeutic Effects Prevents antibody response and subsequently prevents hemolytic disease of the newborn (erythroblastosis fetalis) in future pregnancies of women who have conceived an $Rh_o(D)$-positive fetus. Prevents $Rh_o(D)$ sensitization after a transfusion accident.

Pharmacokinetics
Absorption Well absorbed from IM sites.

Contraindications and Precautions
Contraindicated in $Rh_o(D)$- or Du-positive patients and patients previously sensitized to $Rh_o(D)$ or Du.

Adverse Reactions and Side Effects Pain at IM site

Route and Dosage
One vial *standard* dose (300 mcg) administered intramuscularly:

- At 28 weeks of pregnancy and within 72 hours of delivery
- Within 72 hours after termination of a pregnancy of 13 weeks or more of gestation
- After an accidental transfusion, with dosage calculated based on the volume of blood that was erroneously administered

One vial *microdose* (50 mcg) within 72 hours after chorionic villus sampling (CVS) or termination of a pregnancy of >13 weeks' gestation

Notes:

- More than 300 mcg of RhoGAM may be indicated after a large transplacental hemorrhage or after a mismatched blood transfusion
- Rhophylac can be given IM or IV (prefilled syringes are available).

Nursing Implications

Do not give to infant, to Rh_o(D)-positive person, or to Rh_o(D)-negative person previously sensitized to the Rh_o(D) antigen. Note: There is no more risk than when given to a woman who is not sensitized – if in doubt, administer Rh_o(D) immune globulin.

Administer into the deltoid muscle.

Give within 3 hours if possible, but may be given up to 72 hours after delivery, miscarriage, abortion, or transfusion.

Explain the purpose of this medication to protect future Rh_o(D)-positive infants; before administering, obtain a signed consent form if required by your facility.

Data from Deglin, J., & Vallerand, A. (2009). Davis's drug guide for nurses (11th ed.). Philadelphia: F. A. Davis.

Administer and Document RhoGAM When Clinically Indicated

- Administering and properly documenting Rh_o(D) immune globulin (RhoGAM) is an important nursing action.
- If the mother is Rh-negative and nonsensitized and the baby is Rh-positive:
  - Always check to be sure the patient has received Rh_o(D) immune globulin (RhoGAM), if indicated, before discharge.
  - Make certain that she has received the appropriate dose.
- Patients who have miscarried also must be treated.
- In cases where it is not possible to determine the fetus' or baby's blood type, Rh_o(D) immune globulin (RhoGAM) is still given.
- Question if an order (for Rh_o(D) immune globulin) has not been written.

Safe Administration of Rh₀(D) Immune Globulin (RhoGAM)

- In a RhD-negative woman who is **non**-sensitized, RhoGAM should be given after delivery of an RhD-positive infant. In the United States, the standard dose is 300 mcg and it is given within 72 hours of delivery.
- Educate your patient as to the reason why she is receiving RhoGAM.
- Give your patient documentation that she has received RhoGAM.
- **Never** give RhoGAM to: (1) an Rh(D)-positive woman; (2) a sensitized Rh(D) negative woman; (3) an Rh(D)-negative woman who has given birth to an Rh(D)-negative infant; or (4) the infant or father of the infant.

Recognizing Cardiac Effects of Obstetric Medications

Obstetric medications such as tocolytics and uterine stimulants can have a major impact on circulatory function.

- Terbutaline, administered to suppress premature uterine contractions, may stimulate the heart. Adverse effects may include chest discomfort, dyspnea, irregular pulse, EKG changes, or pulmonary edema. Question the use of this medication in any patient with a cardiac history.
- Prostaglandin is a vasodilator and should not be used in patients with certain cardiac conditions. Oxytocin can cause hypertension and fluid retention and may lead to congestive heart failure.

Nursing Care of the Patient Receiving Tocolytic Therapy

- Explore the woman's understanding of what is taking place.
- Include the woman's partner in all discussions about medications and their effects.
- Provide anticipatory guidance regarding what is likely to happen during medication administration.
- Position the woman on her side for better placental perfusion.
- Explain the side effects and contraindications of the drug.
- Assess blood pressure, pulse, and respirations regularly according to hospital policies (every 15 minutes in many institutions).

- Notify the health care provider if systolic blood pressure is >140 mm Hg or <90 mm Hg.
- Notify the health care provider if diastolic blood pressure is >90 mm Hg or <50 mm Hg.
- Assess for signs of pulmonary edema (chest pain, shortness of breath).
- Assess for the presence of deep tendon reflexes (DTRs).
- Assess output every 1 hour.
- Notify the health care provider if the maternal output is <30 mL/hr.
- Limit intake to 2500 mL/day (90 mL/hr).
- Provide psychosocial support and opportunities for the patient to express anxiety.

(Source: *March of Dimes Nursing Module: Preterm Labor: Prevention and Nursing Management [2004]. Reproduced with permission.*)

Contraindications to the Use of Tocolytics in Preterm Labor

- Significant maternal hypertension (eclampsia, severe preeclampsia, chronic hypertension)
- Antepartum hemorrhage
- Cardiac disease
- Any medical or obstetrical condition that contraindicates the prolongation of pregnancy
- Hypersensitivity to a specific tocolytic agent
- Gestational age >37 weeks
- Advanced cervical dilation
- Fetal demise or lethal anomaly
- Chorioamnionitis
- In utero compromise: Acute—Non-reassuring fetal heart rate pattern; Chronic—Intrauterine growth restriction (IUGR) or substance abuse (Cunningham et al., 2005)

ETHNOCULTURAL CONSIDERATIONS

- RhoGAM is a blood product. Special considerations may be indicated for women who are members of Jehovah's Witness because this medication is made from human plasma.

ADDITIONAL INFORMATION FOR THE CLINICAL SETTING

Various Risk Factors Associated with Preterm Labor and Birth

- History of preterm birth
- Uterine or cervical anomalies
- Multiple gestation
- Hypertension
- Diabetes
- Obesity
- Clotting disorders
- Infection
- Fetal anomalies
- Premature rupture of membranes
- Vaginal bleeding
- Late or no prenatal care
- Illicit drug use
- Smoking
- Alcohol use
- Diethylstilbestrol (DES) exposure
- Intimate partner violence
- Non-Hispanic black race
- Age <17 years or >35 years
- Low socioeconomic status
- Stress
- Long working hours with long periods of standing
- Periodontal disease (ACOG, 2001; Freda and Patterson, 2004)

Considerations When Caring for the Obstetric Trauma Patient

- Maternal stabilization is the initial goal in resuscitation. Resuscitation during pregnancy proceeds as with any other trauma.
- Trauma in pregnancy involves at least two patients (more in the case of multiple gestation).
- The fetal heart rate is often the first vital sign to change. All pregnant trauma patients need continuous fetal monitoring.
- Risk factors predictive of fetal death include ejection during an automobile crash, motorcycle and pedestrian

collisions, abnormal fetal heart rate patterns, maternal tachycardia, and maternal death (Haney, 2004).

RESOURCES

The Association of Women's Health, Obstetric and Neonatal Nurses (AWHONN) (www.awhonn.org), the American College of Obstetricians and Gynecologists (ACOG) (www.ACOG.org), and the American Academy of Pediatrics (AAP) (www.aap.org) have partnered with the March of Dimes (MOD) (www.marchofdimes.com) in a multimillion-dollar research, education, and awareness campaign to address the problem of prematurity. Educating all women of childbearing age about preterm labor is a crucial component of prevention (MOD, 2005).

Sidelines is a national support group for women on bed rest (www.sidelines.org).

The Surgeon General's Call to Action to Prevent Deep Vein Thrombosis and Pulmonary Embolism: http://www.surgeongeneral.gov/topics/deepvein/calltoaction/call-to-action-on-dvt-2008.pdf.

REFERENCES

American College of Obstetricians and Gynecologists (ACOG). (1999). *Antepartum fetal surveillance* (Practice Bulletin No. 9). Washington, D.C.: Author.

American College of Obstetricians and Gynecologists (ACOG). (2001). *Assessment of risk factors for preterm birth* (Practice Bulletin No. 31). Washington, DC: Author.

American College of Obstetricians and Gynecologists (ACOG). (2002). *Diagnosis and management of preeclampsia and eclampsia* (Practice Bulletin No. 33).

American College of Obstetricians and Gynecologists (ACOG). (2004). *Nausea and vomiting of pregnancy.[miscellaneous]* (Practice Bulletin No. 52).

American Diabetes Association (ADA). (2006). Diagnosis and classification of diabetes mellitus. *Diabetes Care, 29*(Suppl), S543–S548.

Centers for Disease Control and Prevention, Workowski, K., & Berman, S. (2006). Sexually transmitted diseases treatment guidelines 2006. *MMWR Morbidity and Mortality Weekly Report, 51*(RR11), 1–23.

Cunningham, F., Leveno, K., Bloom, S., Hauth, J., Gilstrap, L., & Wenstrom, K. (2005). *Williams obstetrics* (22nd ed.). New York: McGraw-Hill.

Deglin, J., & Vallerand, A. (2009). *Davis's drug guide for nurses* (11th ed.). Philadelphia: F.A. Davis.

Freda, M., & Patterson, E. (2004). In Wieczorek R. (Ed.), *Preterm labor: Prevention and nursing management* (3rd ed.). White Plains, NY: March of Dimes.

Gilbert, E., & Harmon, J. (2003). *Manual of high risk pregnancy and delivery* (3rd ed.). St. Louis, MO: C.V. Mosby.

Haney, S. (2004). Trauma in pregnancy. In S. Mattson & J. Smith (Eds.), *Core curriculum for maternal-child nursing* (3rd ed., pp. 703–726). Philadelphia: W.B. Saunders.

Harmon, C. (2004). Assessment of fetal health. In R. Creasy, R. Resnik & J. Iams (Eds.), *Maternal-fetal medicine: Principles and practice* (5th ed., pp. 357–401). Philadelphia: W.B. Saunders.

Hunter, L.P., Sullivan, C.A., Young, R.E., & Weber, C.E. (2007). Nausea and vomiting of pregnancy: Clinical management. *The American Journal for Nurse Practitioners, 11*(8), 57–67.

Jenkins, T., & Wapner, R. (2004). Prenatal diagnosis of congenital disorders. In R. Creasy, R. Resnik & J. Iams (Eds.), *Maternal-fetal medicine: Principles and practice* (5th ed.). Philadelphia: W.B. Saunders.

Landon, M., Catalano, P., & Gabbe, S. (2002). Diabetes mellitus. In S. Gabbe, J. Niebyl & J. Simpson (Eds.), *Obstetrics: Normal and problem pregnancies* (4th ed., pp. 1081–1116). Philadelphia: Churchill Livingstone.

Landry, M. (2004). Viral infections. In G. Burrow, T. Duffy & J. Copel (Eds.), *Medical complications of pregnancy* (6th ed., pp. 347–374). Philadelphia: W.B. Saunders.

McPhedran, P. (2004). Venous thromboembolism during pregnancy. In G. Burrow, T. Duffy & J. Copel (Eds.), *Medical complications of pregnancy* (6th ed., pp. 87–101). Philadelphia: W.B. Saunders.

Moran, B. (2004). Maternal infections. In S. Mattson & J. Smith (Eds.), *Core curriculum for maternal-newborn nursing* (3rd ed., pp. 592–629). St. Louis, MO: W.B. Saunders

Poole, J. (2004). Hypertensive disorders in pregnancy. In S. Mattson & J. Smith (Eds.), *Core curriculum for maternal-newborn nursing* (3rd ed., pp. 554–591). St. Louis, MO: W.B. Saunders.

Records, K., & Rice, M. (2007). Psychosocial correlates of depression symptoms during the third trimester of pregnancy. *Journal of Obstetric, Gynecologic and Neonatal Nursing, 36*(3), 231–242.

Sibai, B.M., Dekker, G., & Kupfermine, M. (2005). Preeclampsia. *The Lancet. 365*(9461), 785–799.

Simpson, K., & Knox, G.E. (2004). Obstetrical accidents involving intravenous magnesium sulfate: Recommendations to promote patient safety. *The American Journal of Maternal/Child Nursing, 29*(3), 161–171

Yankowitz, J. (2004). Pharmacologic treatment of hypertensive disorders during pregnancy. *The Journal of Perinatal & Neonatal Nursing, 18*(3), 230–240.

The Process of Labor and Birth

KEY TERMS

acceleration – An increase in the fetal heart rate of 15 bpm above the baseline, lasting for at least 15 to 30 seconds.

acrocyanosis – Peripheral cyanosis; a bluish coloration of the hands and feet present in most infants at birth

active phase of labor – Phase in the first stage of labor from 4 to 7 cm of cervical dilation

amniotomy – Artificial rupture of the membranes (AROM)

Apgar score – Numeric expression of the condition of a newborn obtained by assessment at 1 and 5 minutes of age; evaluates five signs of cardiopulmonary adaptation and neuromuscular function

attitude (fetal) – Relationship of the fetal parts to each other in the uterus

baseline fetal heart rate – Average fetal heart rate (FHR) observed between contractions over a ten-minute period

bloody show – Expulsion of blood-tinged mucus plug

bradycardia – Baseline fetal heart rate (FHR) of less than 110 to 120 beats per minute

breech presentation – Presentation in which buttocks or feet are nearest the cervical opening and are born first

cephalic presentation – Fetal head is first into the birth canal

cervical ripening – Softening of the cervix

crowning – Stage of birth when the top of the fetal head is visible at the vaginal introitus as the widest part of the head distends the vulva

deceleration – Any decrease in fetal heart rate below the baseline FHR.

dilation – Stretching and enlargement of the cervix

effacement – Process of shortening and thinning of the cervix

electronic fetal heart rate monitoring (EFM) – Electronic surveillance of the fetal heart rate; may use external or internal methods

false labor – Uterine contractions that do not produce cervical change (dilation or effacement)

first stage of labor – Stage of labor from the onset of regular uterine contractions to full dilation of the cervix

fontanel – Unossified membrane or soft spot that lies between the cranial bones of the skull of a fetus or infant

involution – Reduction in uterine size following birth

latent phase of labor – Phase in the first stage of labor from 0 to 3 cm of cervical dilation

lochia rubra – Bright red vaginal flow that follows birth and lasts 2 to 4 days

long-term variability – Changes in fetal heart rate over a period of time (e.g., 1 minute)

malpresentation – Presentation other than cephalic (e.g., breech, shoulder)

molding – Overlapping or overriding of the fetal cranial bones to accommodate and conform to the bony and soft parts of the mother's birth canal during labor

position – Location of a fixed reference point on the fetal presenting part in relation to a specific quadrant of the maternal pelvis: front, back, or side

second stage of labor – Stage of labor from full dilation of the cervix to the birth of the infant

short-term variability – Beat-to-beat changes in fetal heart rate

station – Level of the presenting fetal part in relation to the maternal ischial spines

tachycardia – Baseline fetal heart rate greater than 160 beats per minute

tachysystole – Greater than 5 contractions in 10 minutes, averaged over a 30-minute window

third stage of labor – Stage of labor from the birth of the infant to the expulsion of the placenta

transition phase of labor – Phase in the first stage of labor from 8 to 10 cm of cervical dilation

uteroplacental insufficiency – Decline in placental function, leading to fetal hypoxia and acidosis

variability – Normal irregularity of fetal cardiac rhythm; fluctuations in the baseline fetal heart rate (FHR) observed on the fetal monitor; absence of variability is non-reassuring

Short-term: beat-to-beat changes in the FHR

Long-term: changes in FHR over a longer period of time (i.e., 1 minute)

FOCUSED ASSESSMENT

The 5 P's of Labor

- Powers: Primary (uterine contractions), secondary (use of maternal abdominal muscles for pushing)
- Passageway: Maternal pelvis and soft tissues
- Passenger: Fetus and fetal membranes (lie, attitude, presentation)
- Passageway/passenger relationship: Engagement, station, position
- Psychosocial influences: Factors other than the physical forces that have an effect on the labor and birth process

Powers

The coordinated efforts of the uterine contractions help to bring about effacement and dilation of the cervix (Fig. 9-1).

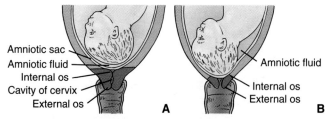

Amniotic sac
Amniotic fluid
Internal os
Cavity of cervix
External os
A

Amniotic fluid
Internal os
External os
B

Figure 9-1 Cervical effacement and dilation. The membranes are intact. *A.* Before labor. *B.* Early effacement.

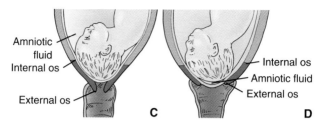

Figure 9-1 cont'd *C.* Complete (100%) effacement. The fetal head is well applied to the cervix. *D.* Complete dilation (10 cm).

Assess uterine contractions as follows:

- Frequency: Measured from beginning of one contraction to the beginning of the next contraction
- Duration: Measured from the start of one contraction to the end of the same contraction
- Intensity: Measured by uterine palpation, described as mild, moderate, or strong.

Passageway
The maternal bony pelvis is divided into the inlet, midpelvis, and outlet

Passenger (Figs. 9-2, 9-3, 9-4, 9-5, 9-6, and 9-7)

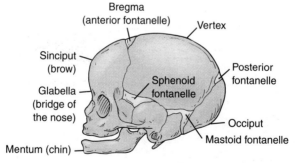

Figure 9-2 Bones, fontanelles, and sutures of the fetal head. An understanding of the placement and relationships of these structures is essential in making an accurate assessment during the labor process.

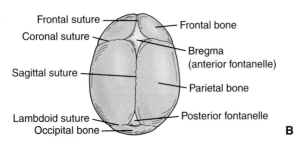

Figure 9-2 cont'd

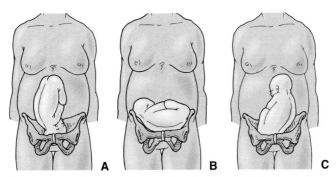

Figure 9-3 The fetal lie refers to the relationship of the long axis of the woman to the long axis of the fetus. *A.* Longitudinal lie. *B.* Transverse lie. *C.* Oblique lie.

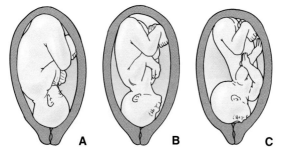

Figure 9-4 The fetal attitude describes the relationship of the fetal body parts to one another. *A.* Flexion (vertex). *B.* Moderate flexion (military). *C.* Extension.

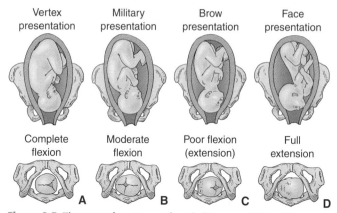

Vertex presentation	Military presentation	Brow presentation	Face presentation
Complete flexion	Moderate flexion	Poor flexion (extension)	Full extension
A	B	C	D

Figure 9-5 There are four types of cephalic presentation; the vertex presentation with complete flexion is optimal. Fetal presentation refers to the fetal body part that first enters the maternal pelvis.

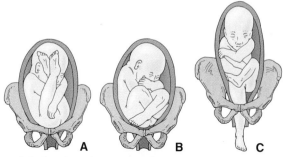

Figure 9-6 There are three types of a breech presentation. *A.* Frank. *B.* Complete or full. *C.* Footling breech (single or doubling). Frank breech is the most common variation.

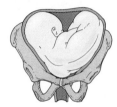

Figure 9-7 Shoulder presentation.

Passage/Passenger Relationship

The relationship between the passageway and the passenger is assessed when determining engagement, station, and the fetal position (Figs. 9-8 and 9-9).

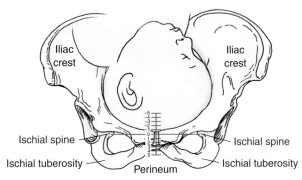

Figure 9-8 The maternal ischial spines represent the narrowest diameter through which the fetus must pass. When the presenting part lies above the ischial spines, it is at a minus station; when the presenting part lies below the ischial spines, it is at a positive station.

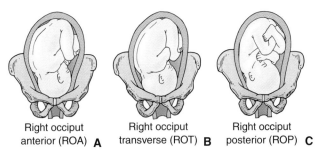

Right occiput anterior (ROA) **A**	Right occiput transverse (ROT) **B**	Right occiput posterior (ROP) **C**

Figure 9-9 Fetal presentations and positions. The presenting part can be right anterior, left anterior, right posterior, and left posterior. These four quadrants designate whether the presenting part is directed toward the front, back, right, or left of the passageway.

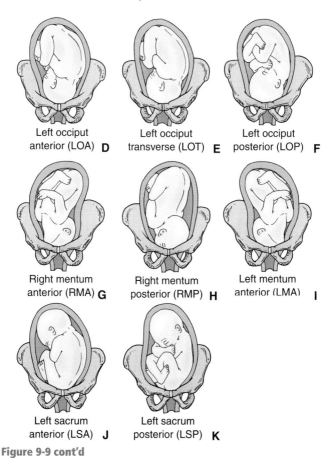

Left occiput anterior (LOA) **D**

Left occiput transverse (LOT) **E**

Left occiput posterior (LOP) **F**

Right mentum anterior (RMA) **G**

Right mentum posterior (RMP) **H**

Left mentum anterior (LMA) **I**

Left sacrum anterior (LSA) **J**

Left sacrum posterior (LSP) **K**

Figure 9-9 cont'd

Psychosocial Influences

Factors that influence the birth experience:

- Readiness for labor and birth
- Level of educational preparedness
- Emotional readiness
- Ethnicity and cultural influences
- Anxiety; fear; fatigue
- Previous experiences with childbirth

Assessment During Labor

Distinguishing True Labor from False Labor	
True Labor	**False Labor**
Contractions at regular intervals	Irregular contractions
Contractions increase in frequency, duration, and intensity.	Usually no increase in frequency, duration, or intensity of contractions.
Pains usually begin in the lower back, radiating to abdomen.	Pains usually occur in abdominal region.
Progressive dilation and effacement of the cervix	No change in the cervix
Activity such as walking usually increased labor pains.	Walking may lessen the pain.

Questions to Ask the Patient Who Calls the Birth Unit

Conduct the telephone assessment by asking the following questions:

"What is your due date?"
"Are your membranes ruptured?" or "Did your water break?" and "Are you having any bleeding or vaginal discharge?"
"Describe your contractions: When did they start? How frequent? How long? How strong?"
"Is the fetus active?"
"What helps to decrease the discomfort?"
"Who is with you?"

Hospital and Birth Center Admission Procedures

Assess the following factors:

- Is this true labor?
- Are the membranes ruptured?
- Is birth imminent?
- Are there any factors that increase risk to the mother and/or fetus?
- What is the gestational age and estimated date of delivery?
- What is the fetal status (FHR and response to contractions; fetal movement)?
- What is the mother's status (physical [vital signs]; psychosocial [coping, supports])?

- What is the contraction status (frequency, duration, intensity)?
- What are the findings from the vaginal exam (cervical dilation, effacement; fetal station, presentation, position)?

 Procedure 9-1 Auscultating the Fetal Heart Tones During Labor

Purpose

An auditory method of monitoring the fetal heart tones to assess the fetus. Performed intermittently during labor.

Equipment

- Fetoscope or hand held Doppler ultrasound with gel ("Doppler")
- Disposable wipes

Steps

1. Wash and dry hands and explain procedure and purpose of the examination to the patient

2. Help the patient assume a comfortable position that provides access to the abdomen.

3. Palpate the maternal abdomen using Leopold maneuvers to identify the fetal position to aid in obtaining the location of the fetal heart tones. Note that the fetal heart tones are heard most loudly over the fetal back.

4. Palpate the fundus of the uterus for the presence of uterine contractions. At the end of a uterine contraction place the fetoscope or Doppler over the location of the fetal back. Adjust the fetoscope or Doppler if necessary to obtain a clearly audible fetal heart rate (FHR). Depending on fetal position, the fetal heart sounds may be soft and muffled or loud and clear.

5. Listen for audible fetal heart sounds. Note that two distinctly different sounds can be heard: fetal heart tones that result from blood moving through the placenta and umbilical cord (funic soufflé) and the uterine soufflé, which is the same rate as the maternal pulse.

6. Palpate the maternal radial pulse to ensure that the auscultated fetal heart sounds are at a different rate than the maternal pulse.

(continued)

Procedure 9-1 (Continued)

7. Auscultate the fetal heart sounds for the rate and rhythm. The greatest accuracy for assessment of the fetal heart rate occurs when listening for 1 minute.

   Note: During active labor, 30-second intervals may be more feasible.

8. Count the FHR for 30 to 60 seconds between contractions to determine the baseline rate.

9. Interpret the fetal heart rate: Is the baseline normal between 110 and 160 bpm? Is there tachycardia (baseline >160 bpm) or bradycardia (baseline <110/bpm)? Is the rhythm regular or irregular? Can you note the presence of accelerations or decelerations?

10. Repeat the procedure as indicated according to agency policy.

11. Inform the patient of the findings.

12. Document fetal heart rate according to agency policy.

Procedure 9-2 Performing the Intrapartal Vaginal Examination

Purpose

Vaginal examination may be performed during the intrapartal period for many reasons including assessment of cervical dilation, effacement and station, position and presentation of the fetus, rupture of the membranes, and prolapse of the umbilical cord.

Equipment

- Sterile examination gloves (clean gloves may be used if the membranes are intact)
- Sterile lubricant
- Antiseptic solution and light source (if required)
- Disposable wipes

Steps

1. Wash and dry your hands. Explain the procedure and purpose of the examination to the patient.

2. Assess for latex allergies.

3. Ensure privacy.

4. Assemble necessary equipment including: clean gloves (if the membranes are intact) or sterile examination gloves (if the membranes are ruptured), sterile lubricant, antiseptic solution (if required).

5. Position the patient in a supine position with a small pillow or towel under her hip to prevent supine hypotension. Instruct the patient to relax and position herself with her thighs flexed and abducted. (Proper positioning facilitates the examination by providing access to the perineum.)

6. Don sterile gloves (clean gloves may be used if the membranes are intact).

7. Inspect the perineum for any redness, irritation or vesicles.

8. Using the nondominant hand, spread the labia majora and continue assessment of the genitalia. Check for discharge including blood or amniotic fluid and lesions. The presence of lesions may be indicative of an infection and possibly preclude a vaginal birth. The presence of amniotic fluid implies that the membranes have ruptured. Bleeding may be a sign of placenta previa.

   Note: Do not perform a vaginal examination if a placenta previa is suspected.

9. Gently insert the lubricated gloved index and third fingers into the vagina in the direction of the posterior wall until they touch the cervix. Stabilize the uterus by placing the nondominant hand on the woman's abdomen.

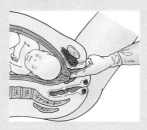

(continued)

Procedure 9-2 (Continued)

10. Assess the cervix for effacement and the amount of dilation.

11. Assess for intact membranes; if fluid is expressed, test for amniotic fluid.

12. Palpate the presenting part.

13. Assess fetal descent and station by identifying the position of the posterior fontanel.

14. Withdraw the fingers. Assist the patient in wiping her perineum from front to back to remove lubricant or secretions. Help her to resume a comfortable position.

15. Inform the patient of the findings from the examination.

16. Wash hands.

17. Document the procedure on the patient's chart and on the fetal monitor strip (if a fetal monitor is being used). Include the assessment findings and the patient's tolerance of the procedure.

Procedure 9-3 Assessing for Amniotic Fluid

Purpose

Assessing for the presence of amniotic fluid helps determine whether the membranes have ruptured. There are two tests commonly used to detect amniotic fluid: the Nitrazine tape test and the fern test.

Equipment

- Nitrazine test tape
- Sterile gloves
- Sterile speculum
- Sterile cotton swab and glass slide
- Microscope

Steps

1. Wash and dry hands and explain the procedure and purpose of the examination to the patient, noting what she will experience, and what the results will indicate.

Procedure 9-3 (Continued)

2. Assess for latex allergies.

3. Ask the patient if she has noticed any leakage of fluid from her vagina.

4. Assess for the presence of amniotic fluid before other tests that require the use of lubricant (such as vaginal examination).

5. Don sterile gloves.

6. With one hand, spread the labia to expose the vaginal opening. With the other hand, place a 2-inch (5 cm) piece of Nitrazine tape against the vaginal opening, ensuring contact with enough fluid to wet the tape. Alternately, a sterile cotton-tipped applicator may be used to obtain fluid from the vagina. Touch the applicator to the Nitrazine tape.

7. Remove the tape. Compare the color of the tape with the color guide on the Nitrazine tape container. If the tape turns blue-green, gray or deep blue, amniotic fluid is present. If the tape remains beige, no amniotic fluid has been detected.

   Caution: Blood, *Trichomonas vaginalis*, and other substances may also turn the Nitrazine test strip alkaline or blue.

8. When the Nitrazine test has *not* confirmed the presence of amniotic fluid, the nurse may insert a speculum and sterile cotton swab to collect a sample of fluid from the posterior vagina.

9. Smear the swab on a glass slide and allow it to dry. Then place the glass slide on the microscope. The presence of a ferning pattern confirms the presence of amniotic fluid. The fern test is often indicated if premature rupture of the membranes (PROM) is suspected.

10. Inform the patient of the findings.

11. Document the findings on the admission or labor record.

Characteristics of the First and Second Stages of Labor

	First Stage	Second Stage
Definition	Commences with the onset of regular contractions and ends with full dilation (10 cm) of the cervix	Begins with full dilation of the cervix (10 cm) and ends with the expulsion (birth) of the fetus
Contractions	Latent: 5–10 minutes, may be irregular in frequency, duration 30–40 seconds, mild to moderate strength Active: Regular pattern established (2–5 minutes apart), 40–60 seconds duration and moderate to strong by palpation Transition: 2–3 minutes apart lasting 60–90 seconds duration, strong by palpation.	Contractions continue at a similar rate as during the transition phase: 2–3 minutes apart lasting 60 seconds and strong by palpation.
Dilation	Latent: 0–3 cm Active: 4–7 cm Transition: 8–10 cm	Fully dilated
Physical Discomforts	Latent: Contractions often begin as painful menstrual-like cramps or low backache. Active: Increasing discomfort as contractions become stronger and more regular. May have backache. Transition: Increasing discomfort as contractions are very strong with little time for relaxation in between. As the fetal head descends there may be an increase in rectal pressure and the urge to push.	May have an urge to push that increases as the fetal head descends. Many women prefer to push so that they can use the contractions and work with them. When head is crowning may feel intense pain, burning.
Maternal Behaviors	Latent: Pain often well controlled; various behaviors may be present: excited, talkative, confident, anxious, withdrawn. This stage may be completed at home.	Often during this stage many women get a "second wind" as they see that they are making progress and are embarking on a new (labor) phase.

First Stage	Second Stage
Active: Needs to focus more on staying in control and managing the pain; often requires coaching at this stage; quieter and more inwardly focused Transition: Most intense phase. Often difficult to cope; may experience various emotions; irritable, agitated, hopeless (can't do it); tired (sleeps between contractions)	Intense concentration with pushing efforts

Friedman Curve

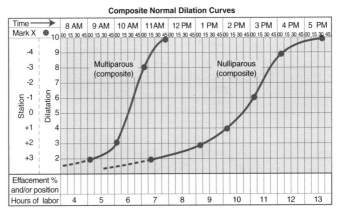

Figure 9-10 A labor curve assessment tool, often referred to as a "Friedman curve," helps to identify whether a patient's labor is progressing in a normal pattern.

Electronic Fetal Monitoring (EFM)

External Fetal Monitor

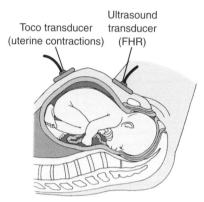

Figure 9-11 The external fetal monitor is composed of a Doppler ultrasound transducer and tocodynamometer that is applied to the maternal abdomen to monitor and display the FHR and contractions.

Internal Fetal Monitor

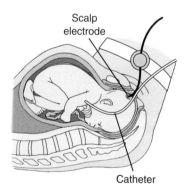

Figure 9-12 The internal fetal monitor is composed of a spiral electrode inserted into the fetal scalp or presenting part. Uterine activity is assessed by an intrauterine pressure catheter (IUPC).

Fetal Heart Rate Patterns

Normal Fetal Heart Rate

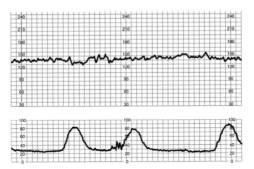

Figure 9-13 The normal baseline fetal heart rate at term is 110 to 160 bpm. *Top*: fetal heart rate. *Bottom*: Uterine contractions.

Fetal Heart Rate Accelerations

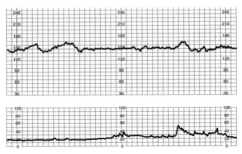

Figure 9-14 FHR accelerations: often associated with a normal FHR baseline and normal variability.

Early Decelerations

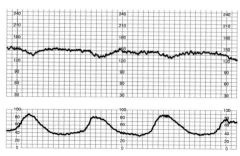

Figure 9-15 Early decelerations: Related to fetal head compression.

Variable Decelerations

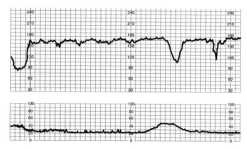

Figure 9-16 Variable decelerations: Related to umbilical cord compression.

Late Decelerations

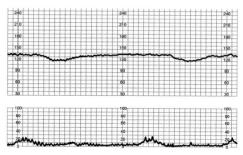

Figure 9-17 Late decelerations: related to uteroplacental insufficiency.

Interpreting Fetal Monitor Tracings

To aid in the interpretation of EFM tracings, the nurse should consider the following parameters:

Uterine Activity

What is the frequency, duration, and intensity of contractions?

Labor Progress

What is the stage of labor?

What is the dilation, effacement, station, presentation and position?

Baseline FHR

What is the baseline FHR?

Is tachycardia or bradycardia present?

Baseline Variability

What is the variability of the FHR (absent, minimal, moderate, marked, or other)?

Periodic Changes in FHR

Are there any FHR changes from the baseline?

Are accelerations present?

Are any decelerations present?

If decelerations are present, are they early, variable, late or prolonged?

Maternal History/Condition

Are there any preexisting conditions that increase the risk for this pregnancy?

Are there any intrapartum high-risk factors (e.g., meconium) that should be noted?

Characteristics of Reassuring and Non-reassuring FHR Patterns by EFM	
Reassuring Patterns	**Non-reassuring Patterns**
Normal baseline FHR (110–160 bpm)	Absence of variability (short-term and long-term)
Presence of short-term and long-term variability	Late decelerations
Presence of accelerations with fetal movement or contractions	Severe variable decelerations
Early decelerations may be noted in active labor.	Prolonged decelerations
	Severe bradycardia or tachycardia
Category I FHR tracing	Category III FHR tracing
Possible category II FHR tracing	Possible Category II FHR tracing

Sources: Macones et al. (2008); Tucker (2004).

Conditions Associated with Fetal Heart Rate Variations	
Tachycardia	**Bradycardia**
Fetal hypoxia	Late hypoxia
Maternal fever	Medications
Maternal medications	Maternal hypotension
Infection	Prolonged umbilical cord compression
Fetal anemia	Bradyarrhythmias
Maternal hyperthyroidism	

PROMOTING EFFECTIVE PUSHING

- Closed-glottis pushing: Encourage the patient to begin pushing at full cervical dilation, regardless of the urge to bear down, by taking a deep breath and holding it for at least 10 seconds while pushing as hard and as long as she is able throughout the contraction.
- Open-glottis pushing: Encourage the patient to hold her breath for only 5 to 6 seconds during pushing and to take several breaths between each bearing down effort. Instruct the woman to exhale throughout the bearing down attempts.

Characteristics of the Third and Fourth Stages of Labor		
	Third Stage	**Fourth Stage**
Description	Begins with the birth of the infant and ends with the delivery of the placenta. Usually 5–10 minutes, may take up to 30 minutes.	A time of physiological adaptation that begins after delivery of the placenta and lasts 1–2 hours.
Contractions	Uterus should be firmly contracted.	Uterus should be firmly contracted.
Assessment	Uterus becomes globelike. Uterus rises upward. Umbilical cord descends further. Gush of blood as placenta detaches.	Uterus remains firmly contracted. Lochia rubra, blood red flow with occasional small clots. Vital signs return to prelabor values.
Physical Discomforts	Discomfort or cramping as the placenta is expelled.	Some women experience perineal discomfort usually related to trauma from the episiotomy or tearing, or hemorrhoids.

	Third Stage	Fourth Stage
Maternal Behaviors	Focus on infant well-being	Excited, tired
	Crying common	Bonding and attachment with infant
	Expressions of relief	Initiation of breastfeeding
	Culturally influenced	Culturally influenced

CLINICAL ALERTS

Preventing Supine Hypotension

Much of the fetal assessment involves the maternal abdomen. To avoid supine hypotension, do not position the patient flat on her back. Slightly elevate the head of the bed or place a wedge under the patient's hip to prevent compression of the maternal vena cava caused by the gravid uterus.

Fourth Stage Risk Signs

The following risk signs that may occur during the fourth stage of labor are associated with hemorrhage and must be reported immediately: hypotension, tachycardia, excessive bleeding, or a boggy, non contracting uterus. If the uterus is boggy, the nurse must immediately initiate fundal massage and continue until the uterus becomes firm.

MEDICATIONS

Oxytocin (ox-i-**toe**-sin)

Pitocin, Syntocinon

Pregnancy Category B

Indications Induction of labor at term. Facilitation of uterine contractions at term. Control of postpartum bleeding after expulsion of placenta.

Actions Stimulates uterine smooth muscle producing uterine contractions similar to those in spontaneous labor (administered IV). Stimulates mammary gland smooth muscle facilitating lactation (administered intranasally). Has vasopressor and diuretic effects.

Therapeutic Effects Induces labor. Reduces postpartum bleeding. Induces breast milk letdown.

Pharmacokinetics

Absorption Well absorbed from the nasal mucosa when administered intranasally.

Distribution Through extracellular fluid. Small amounts reach the fetal circulation.

Metabolism Metabolized rapidly in kidneys and liver.

Excretion Small amounts excreted in urine, half-life 3–9 minutes

Contraindications and Precautions

Contraindicated in Cephalopelvic disproportion or deliveries that require conversion (e.g., transverse lie).

Use with caution in First and second stage of labor.

Adverse Reactions and Side Effects Maternal adverse reactions are associated with IV use only. Painful contractions and increased uterine motility most common. May contribute to maternal coma, seizures, hypotension. May contribute to fetal asphyxia or arrhythmias.

Route and Dosage May be added to IV for labor induction or given IV or IM to control postpartum bleeding (do not administer IM and IV routes simultaneously). Intranasal spray is administered 2 to 3 minutes before planned breastfeeding.

Nursing Implications Fetal maturity, presentation, and maternal pelvic adequacy should be assessed prior to administration to induce labor. Monitor contractions, resting uterine tone, and fetal heart rate frequently. Monitor the uterus for firmness and early detection of bogginess. Monitor lochia for signs of excessive bleeding.

Data from Deglin, J.H., & Vallerand, A.H. (2009). Davis's drug guide for nurses *(11th ed.). Philadelphia: F.A. Davis.*

The Apgar Scoring System

Physiological Parameter	Score		
	0	1	2
Heart Rate	Absent	Slow: Below 100	Above 100
Respiratory Effort	Absent	Slow: Irregular, weak cry	Good; strong cry
Muscle Tone	Flaccid	Some flexion of extremities	Well flexed
Reflex Irritability	No response	Grimace	Vigorous cry
Color	Blue, pale	Pink body, blue extremities	Completely pink

Range of Apgar Score: From 0 to 10

A score of 8–10 reflects a newborn in good condition who usually requires only nasopharyngeal suctioning. A score of <8 may warrant further resuscitation measures.

ETHNOCULTURAL CONSIDERATIONS

Assessing Cultural Influences on the Laboring Patient

To provide culturally sensitive care to the laboring patient, the nurse should consider:

- The patient's and family's level of comfort with the nurse's "language" and whether an interpreter is needed
- Who the designated birth support person is and the extent of this person's role
- The patient's level of comfort with touch
- If any special rituals or practices will be used during the childbirth experience

TEACHING THE FAMILY

Providing Patient Guidelines for Reporting to the Birthing Center	
Questions to Ask the Patient	Guidelines for Admission
Describe your contractions: frequency, duration, and intensity.	Primigravida: Contractions are regular, occur about every 5 minutes for at least 1 hour. Multipara: Contractions are regular, occur about every 10 minutes for at least 1 hour.
Have your membranes ruptured?	*Any* gush of fluid needs to be evaluated, even if there are no contractions.
Is there any vaginal bleeding?	The mucous plug or "bloody show" is usually pink or dark red. Any bright red bleeding requires immediate evaluation.
Has there been a decrease in the movement of the baby?	Any decrease in fetal movement signals the need to report to the birthing center.
Has there been any change in your health?	Any cause for worry or anxiety in the pregnant woman needs to be explored by the nurse and may lead to admission.

ADDITIONAL INFORMATION FOR THE CLINICAL SETTING

Determining and Documenting Fetal Position

During the assessment, the nurse determines that the fetal occiput is in the right anterior quadrant of the maternal pelvis. The position is correctly documented as ROA. If the fetus were presenting in the frank breech position with the buttocks positioned to the left maternal posterior quadrant, the position would be correctly documented as LSP (left sacral posterior).

RESOURCES

National Certification Corporation monograph (2006). *Applying NICHD terminology and other factors to electronic fetal monitor interpretation*. Retrieved on February 14, 2008 from http://www.nccnet.org/public/files/NICHDMonograph.pdf.

REFERENCES

Deglin, J.H. & Vallerand, A.H. (2009). *Davis's drug guide for nurses* (11th ed.). Philadelphia: F.A. Davis.

Macones, G.A., Hankins, G.D., Spong, C.Y., Hauth, J., & Moore, T. (2008). The 2008 National Institute of Child Health and Human Development Research Workshop Report on Electronic Fetal Heart Rate Monitoring. *Journal of Obstetric, Gynecologic, & Neonatal Nursing, 37*(5), 510–515.

Tucker, S.M. (2004). *Pocket guide to fetal monitoring and assessment* (5th ed.). St Louis, MO: C.V. Mosby.

chapter 10

Promoting Patient Comfort During Labor and Birth

KEY TERMS

acupressure – Massage technique applied to specific points along the body's energy pathways (meridians); also called "Chinese massage"

acupuncture – A form of treatment that involves the insertion of fine, stainless steel needles into specific points along the energy pathways to correct, enhance, and rebalance the flow of body energy

aromatherapy – The use of essential oils whose aroma is believed to have a therapeutic effect in treating illness and promoting health and well-being

autologous epidural blood patch – The administration of 10 to 20 mL of the patient's blood into the lumbar epidural space to form a clot in the hole in the dura mater around the spinal cord. The clot effectively seals the area from further cerebrospinal fluid (CSF) leakage.

analgesia – Relief, to some degree, from pain without loss of consciousness

anesthesia – the partial or complete loss of sensation with or without the loss of consciousness

biofeedback – Treatment method that uses monitors to provide patients with physiological information of which they are normally unaware. Practice during the prenatal period enhances the woman's body awareness and ability to recognize her responses to stimuli. She can then use various strategies (e.g., focal points, breathing techniques) during labor to control her response to uncomfortable stimuli.

cleansing breath – A slow, deep breath taken in through the nose and out through the mouth

effleurage – Gentle stroking technique performed in rhythm with uterine contractions

epidural anesthesia and analgesia block – Regional anesthesia produced by injection of a local anesthetic into the epidural space between L4 and L5

general anesthesia – Induced unconsciousness

hydrotherapy – Water therapy; the use of water to promote comfort and relaxation

hypnotherapy – Technique used to enable an individual to achieve a state of heightened awareness and focused concentration to alter the perception of pain

intrathecal analgesia – Injection of opioids into the subarachnoid space

postdural puncture headache – A complication following spinal anesthesia block; occurs from leakage of cerebrospinal fluid (CSF) from the puncture site in the dura mater

referred pain – During labor, pain that originates from the uterus and radiates to the abdominal wall, lumbosacral area, iliac crests, gluteus maximus, and down the thighs

regional anesthesia – Temporary and reversible loss of sensation

somatic pain – Perineal discomfort that results from stretching and distention of the perineal tissues

sympathetic blockade – Decreased cardiac output that results from vasodilation with pooling of blood in the lower extremities after the administration of an epidural anesthetic

transcutaneous electrical nerve stimulation (TENS) – Delivery of an electric current through electrodes applied to the skin over the painful region of a peripheral nerve

visceral pain – A slow, deep, diffuse pain, the predominant discomfort during the first stage of labor. Usually located over the lower abdomen, and radiates to the lumbar area and thighs. Related to cervical dilation and effacement, distention of the lower uterine segment, and uterine ischemia.

FOCUSED ASSESSMENT

Types of Pain During Labor and Birth

- Visceral pain
- Referred pain
- Somatic pain

Factors that Affect the Experience of Pain		
Physical	**Physiological**	**Psychological**
Labor intensity	History of dysmenorrhea	Anxiety
Cervical readiness	Maternal position	Fear
Fetal position	Maternal control	Previous experience
Pelvic dimensions	Fetal size	Support system
Fatigue		Childbirth preparation
Medical interventions		

Assessing Pain During Labor

- Using appropriate pain assessment tools, conduct an initial assessment and continuously evaluate the patient and address her needs for comfort measures.
- Develop an individualized plan of care that includes pain relief interventions acceptable to the patient.

Recognizing the Anxiety–Tissue Anoxia–Pain Connection

- Pain triggers the body's general stress response.
- The release of epinephrine causes peripheral and uterine vasoconstriction and results in tissue anoxia and increased pain.
- Decrease the patient's anxiety by assisting with relaxation techniques to reduce anxiety; administer antianxiety medications as needed to reduce vasoconstriction and pain.

Other Maternal–Fetal Assessments During the Intrapartal Period

- Assess for risk factors: Bleeding, infection, ruptured membranes, fetal presentation, prolapsed cord,

precipitous labor, meconinum-stained amniotic fluid, postmaturity, prematurity, or fetal heart rate irregularities.
- Assess maternal vital signs per facility protocol.
- Assess the patient's anxiety level, coping mechanisms, and labor support.
- Assess the progress of labor.
- Assess the fetal heart rate, lie, and presentation.
- Assess the maternal and fetal responses to each comfort measure.
- Carefully document all findings.

Nonpharmacological Pain Relief Measures for Labor

- Position of comfort (e.g., movement, slow dancing, squatting bar, hands/knees, birth ball, kneeling)
- Breathing techniques
- Music
- Relaxation techniques
- Guided imagery
- Massage, touch, effleurage
- Hydrotherapy
- Hypnotherapy
- Aromatherapy
- Heat/cold application
- Biofeedback
- Acupressure and acupuncture
- Transcutaneous electrical nerve stimulation

CLINICAL ALERTS

Flumazenil to Reverse the Effects of Benzodiazepine Sedatives

Flumazenil (Romazicon) is an intravenously administered medication that reverses the effects of benzodiazepine sedatives. Ensure that flumazenil is readily available in any childbirth setting where benzodiazepines are used.

Combining Butorphanol with Other CNS Depressants

Butorphanol (Stadol) is associated with respiratory depression in both the mother and fetus. When administering butorphanol with other central nervous system (CNS) depressants (e.g., hypnotic agents, phenothiazines, sedatives, other tranquilizers, and general anesthetics), closely monitor the patient's respiratory and cardiac status for signs of respiratory depression. Ongoing observation of the maternal level of consciousness, vital signs, and pulse oximetry, and continuous electronic fetal heart rate monitoring is recommended. Naloxone (Narcan), the specific antagonist for this medication, should be readily available to reverse the drug effects if needed.

Complications Associated with Spinal Anesthesia Block

- Maternal hypotension (before administration, assess fluid balance, administer intravenous fluids; after administration, assess and document pulse, blood pressure, respirations and fetal heart tones (FHTs) every 5 to 10 minutes).
- Decreased placental perfusion
- Ineffective breathing pattern
- Sympathetic blockade
- Postdural puncture headache

Severe Maternal Hypotension and Decreased Placental Perfusion

In the event of severe maternal hypotension, the nurse takes the following actions:

1. Place the patient in a lateral position or use a wedge under the hip to displace the uterus; elevate the legs.
2. Maintain or increase the IV infusion rate, according to institutional protocol.
3. Administer oxygen by face mask at 10 to 12 L/min, or according to institutional protocol.
4. Alert the primary care provider, anesthesiologist or nurse anesthetist.
5. Administer an IV vasopressor (e.g., ephedrine 5 to 10 mg) according to institutional protocol, if the above measures are ineffective.
6. Remain calm, offer reassurance, and continue to assess maternal blood pressure and fetal heart rate (FHR) every 5 minutes until stable or per order from the primary care provider.

Postdural Puncture Headache

- Develops within 48 hours after the puncture.
- Typically intensified when the patient assumes an upright position.
- Relieved when the patient assumes a supine position.
- Accompanying symptoms include auditory (tinnitus) and visual (blurred vision, photophobia) problems.
- Interventions include oral analgesics, bed rest in a darkened room, caffeine, hydration, and autologous epidural blood patch.

MEDICATIONS

General Guidelines

- Ensure that the woman understands the alternative methods of pain relief that are available in the birth facility. When indicated, ask the primary care provider for further details or clarification.
- Explain that nonpharmacological measures promote relaxation and potentiate the effects of analgesic agents.
- Obtain informed consent for interventions after fully explaining advantages and disadvantages. The patient must agree with the plan of care as it is described to her; the patient's consent must be given freely without coercion or manipulation from her health care provider (Lowe, 2004).
- Initiate pain control before the pain intensifies to the point that catecholamines are released and the labor is prolonged.

Types of Medications Used During Labor and Birth

- Sedatives and antiemetics: Used during early latent phase and to augment analgesics
- Barbiturates: Produce mild sedation; rarely used in labor because of undesirable effects (i.e., maternal and neonatal respiratory and vasomotor depression)
- Benzodiazepines: Used to treat anxiety
- H_1-Receptor antagonists: Used for sedation and antiemetic effects

- Systemic analgesia: Provides central analgesia to patient and fetus (opioid agonists, opioid agonist–antagonists)
- Nerve block analgesia and anesthesia (regional analgesia, regional anesthesia)

Pharmacological Interventions for Intrapartal Pain Control According to Stage of Labor

First Stage of Labor
Systemic Analgesia
- Opioid agonists, e.g., hydromorphone hydrochloride (Dilaudid), meperidine (Demerol), fentanyl citrate (Sublimaze), sufentanil citrate (Sufenta)
- Opioid agonist–antagonists, e.g., butorphanol (Stadol); nalbuphine (Nubain)

Nerve Block Analgesia
- Epidural
- Combined spinal–epidural

Second Stage of Labor
Nerve Block Analgesia and Anesthesia (Fig. 10-1)
- Local infiltration
- Pudendal block
- Spinal block
- Epidural block
- Combined spinal–epidural

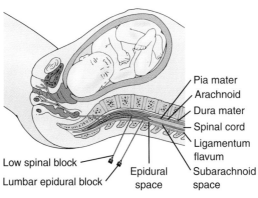

Pia mater
Arachnoid
Dura mater
Spinal cord
Ligamentum flavum
Subarachnoid space
Epidural space
Low spinal block
Lumbar epidural block

Figure 10-1 The spinal canal: Injection sites for regional anesthesia.

Opioid Agonist Analgesics		
Opioid-Agonist Analgesic	Route and Dosage	Nursing Considerations
Hydromorphone Hydrochloride (Dilaudid)	IV: 1 mg q–3hr prn IM: 1–2 mg q3–6hr prn	Monitor vital signs, FHR pattern, and uterine activity before and during administration; observe for maternal respiratory depression; encourage voiding q2hr, palpate for bladder distention; if birth occurs within 1–4 hours after administration, observe the neonate for respiratory depression.
Meperidine hydrochloride (Demerol)	IV: 25 mg q1–3hr prn IM: 50–100 mg q1–3hr prn	
Fentanyl Citrate (Sublimaze)	IV: 25–50 mg; 1–2 mg with 0.125% bupivacaine at rate of 8–10 mL/hr epidurally	
Sufentanil Citrate (Sufenta)	IV: 1 mg with 0.125% bupivacaine at a rate of 10 mL/hr	

Safety Measures for Women Who Receive Opioid Analgesics
- Administer cautiously to women with respiratory or cardiovascular disorders, as opioid analgesics may cause bradycardia/tachycardia, hypotension, and respiratory depression (Lehne, 2006).
- Assist with ambulation and observe for adverse effects because patients may experience sedation and dizziness after administration.

Pharmacological Interventions for Intrapartal Pain Control According to Birth Method
Vaginal Birth
- Local infiltration anesthesia
- Pudendal block
- Epidural block analgesia/anesthesia
- Spinal block anesthesia
- Combined spinal–epidural analgesia/anesthesia

Cesarean Birth
- Spinal block anesthesia
- Epidural block anesthesia
- General anesthesia

Commonly Used Regional Blocks for Labor and Birth

Type of Block; Areas Affected	When Used During Labor and Birth	Nursing Implications
Local Perineal Infiltration AFFECTED AREA: Perineum	Immediately before birth for episiotomy; after birth for repair of lacerations	Assess the patient's knowledge and understanding; provide information as needed. Observe the perineum for bruising or discoloration during the recovery period.
Pudendal Nerve Block AFFECTED AREAS: Perineum and lower vagina	Late in the second stage for episiotomy, forceps or vacuum extraction; during third stage for repair of episiotomy or lacerations	Assess the patient's level of knowledge and understanding; provide additional information as needed.
Spinal Anesthesia Block AFFECTED AREAS: Uterus, cervix, vagina, and perineum	First stage for both elective and emergent cesarean births; low spinal anesthesia block may be used for vaginal birth—not suitable for labor	Assess the patient's level of knowledge and understanding; provide additional information as needed. Monitor maternal vital signs and FHR status.
Lumbar Epidural Block AFFECTED AREAS: Uterus, cervix, vagina, and perineum	First and second stages	Assess the patient's level of knowledge and understanding; provide additional information as needed. Monitor maternal blood pressure—the major side effect is hypotension. Provide ongoing support.
Combined Spinal–Epidural AFFECTED AREAS: Uterus, cervix, vagina, and perineum	Spinal analgesia may be administered during the latent phase for pain relief. Epidural is given when active labor begins	Assess the patient's level of knowledge and understanding; provide additional information as needed. Monitor maternal vital signs and FHR status. Provide ongoing support.

Procedure 10-1 Assisting with the Administration of Spinal Anesthesia

Purpose

To facilitate safe, effective care during conduction of spinal anesthesia

Equipment

- Blood pressure cuff
- Stethoscope
- Fetal monitor

Steps

1. Wash and dry hands and explain procedure and purpose to the patient.
2. Assist the patient to a sitting position on the edge of the bed or operating table (as directed by the nurse anesthetist or anesthesiologist).
3. Provide support, promote comfort, and limit motion during the procedure.
4. Check the intravenous infusion for patency.
5. Assist the patient to lie down on her back after anesthesia administration (as directed by the nurse anesthetist or anesthesiologist).
6. Place a pillow under her head and a wedge under her right hip.
7. Monitor the pulse, blood pressure, and respirations every 1–2 minutes for the first 10 minutes, then every 5–10 minutes. Use electronic monitor to continuously monitor the FHR.
8. Document the procedure.

Nursing Consideration

The nurse informs the nurse anesthetist or anesthesiologist when a contraction is beginning so that the anesthetic will not be administered during a contraction.

Contraindications to Spinal/Epidural Block Anesthesia

- Maternal refusal
- Local or systemic infection
- Coagulation disorders

- Actual or anticipated maternal hemorrhage
- Allergy to specific anesthetic agents
- Lack of trained staff available (Cunningham et al., 2005)

Nursing Actions After Administration of Epidural and Intrathecal Opioids

- Monitor and record patient's respiratory rate every hour for 24 hours (or per institutional protocol) after administration of epidural or intrathecal opioids.
- Administer naloxone (Narcan) if the maternal respiratory rate decreases to <10 breaths per minute or if the maternal oxygen saturation rate decreases to <89%; administer oxygen by face mask and notify the anesthesiologist.

Epidural Block and Second Stage Labor

- The patient who has received an epidural block may need assistance with pushing owing to an inability to feel contractions or experience the urge to push. She may need someone to hold or control her legs in order to push.
- After the birth, ensure that full sensation has returned and the patient can control her legs before permitting ambulation (depending on drug and dose, it may take several hours).

Shiver Response After Epidural Block Administration

- If the patient exhibits a shiver response after administration of an epidural block, apply warm blankets and offer reassurance.

ETHNOCULTURAL CONSIDERATIONS

Realities of the Cultural Model

Cultural models of health care frequently stereotype women who share the same cultural heritage. In so doing, they may immobilize health providers who seek to change unfavorable health care situations in the name of protection of the cultural heritage (Meleis, 2003).

Recognizing Cultural Influences on the Experience of Pain

Culture strongly influences how one perceives and copes with pain. Women from certain cultures seek pain relief through prayer; others rely on herbal remedies, the application of cold or warmth, acupuncture, the "laying on of hands," and therapeutic massage. Assessment of cultural beliefs and practices, questions to identify specific needs, and encouragement and support to use safe interventions is key in providing culturally sensitive care that empowers the patient to maintain her sense of control over her labor and childbirth experience.

TEACHING THE FAMILY

Discharge Instructions After Autologous Epidural Blood Patch

- Maintain bedrest for 24 to 48 hours.
- Apply cold packs to the area as needed for pain relief.
- Increase oral fluids.
- Avoid the use of analgesics that affect platelet aggregation (e.g., nonsteroidal anti-inflammatory drugs) for 2 days.
- Observe for signs of infection at the site.
- Observe for signs of neurological complications (pain, numbness, tingling in the legs, difficulty with ambulation).

ADDITIONAL INFORMATION FOR THE CLINICAL SETTING

Environmental Strategies to Enhance Comfort During Labor

- Provide privacy, comfort, and a sense of security.
- Allow the patient to regulate the amount of noise, light, and temperature to foster relaxation and a sense of control.
- Keep medical equipment from the patient's view unless it needs to be used.

Precautions When Using Aromatherapy

Never apply essential oils to the skin in a full-strength form. Instead, dilute the oil(s) before application and caution patients that not all aromatherapy oils are safe to use during pregnancy.

Breathing Techniques for Labor and Childbirth
Slow-paced Breathing Pattern
- Use in early labor.
- Cleansing breath at the beginning of the contraction.
- Slowly breathe in through the mouth while the coach counts "one, two, three, four" and slowly breathe out as the coach counts "one, two, three, four."
- Rate = 6 to 8 breaths/min

Modified-paced Breathing Pattern
- Use as contractions increase in frequency and intensity.
- Shallower than slow-paced breathing pattern and faster rate.
- Rate = 32 to 40 breaths/min
- Cleansing breath at the beginning of the contraction.
- Inhale slowly; exhale at a faster pace.
- End with a cleansing breath.
- Requires more concentration.

Pattern-paced Breathing Pattern
- Use during the transition phase of labor.
- Cleansing breath at the beginning of the contraction.
- 3:1 pattern of breathing in and out 2 times, then breathe in and blow out; repeat throughout the contraction.
- End with a cleansing breath.

Assisting the Laboring Patient to Remain Focused During Contractions

Offer words of support and encouragement with statements such as:

- "You're doing a great job!"
- "You're almost there!"
- "I can see your baby's head - reach down and feel it!"
- "You can do it!"

Recognizing and Managing Hyperventilation

- Alert the patient and her support person to symptoms of respiratory alkalosis (light-headedness, dizziness, tingling of the fingers, or circumoral numbness)

- Instruct the patient to breathe into a paper bag held tightly around her mouth and nose. If a bag is not available, instruct her to breathe into her cupped hands.

Using Heat and Cold for Pain Relief During Labor

- Application of heat or cold over anesthetized body areas can cause tissue damage.
- Use hot and cold packs only after one to two layers of cloth have been placed between the pack and the patient's skin (Simkin & Bolding, 2004).

RESOURCES

American College of Obstetricians and Gynecologists: http://www.acog.org/index.cfm

Association of Women's Health, Obstetrical, and Neonatal Nursing (AWHONN): http://www.awhonn.org/awhonn/

Childbirth Connection: http://www.childbirthconnection.org/

Lamaze International: http://www.lamaze.org/

REFERENCES

Cunningham, F., Leveno, K., Bloom, S., Hauth, J., Gilstrap, L., & Wenstrom, K. (2005). *Williams' obstetrics* (22nd ed.). New York: McGraw-Hill.

Lehne, R. (2006). *Pharmacology for nursing care* (6th ed.). Philadelphia: W.B. Saunders.

Lowe, N. (2004). Context and process of informed consent for pharmacologic strategies in labor pain care. *Journal of Midwifery & Women's Health, 49*(3), 250–259.

Meleis, A. (2003). Theoretical considerations of health care for immigrant and minority women. In P. St. Hill, J.G. Lipson, & A.I. Meleis (Eds.), *Caring for women cross-culturally* (pp. 1–10). Philadelphia: F.A. Davis.

Simkin, P., & Bolding, A. (2004). Update on nonpharmacologic approaches to relieve labor pain and prevent suffering. *Journal of Midwifery & Women's Health, 49*(6), 489–504.

Caring for the Woman Experiencing Complications During Labor and Birth

KEY TERMS

amnioinfusion – The instillation of warmed normal saline or lactated Ringer's solution into the uterus via a sterile intrauterine catheter. Performed in an attempt to increase the fluid around the umbilical cord and prevent compression during contractions. Also used to dilute and help wash out thick meconium to avoid neonatal meconium aspiration syndrome.

amniotic fluid embolism (AFE) – Embolism that results from amniotic fluid entering the maternal circulation during labor and birth and after rupture of the membranes; may cause maternal death if it is a pulmonary embolism

artificial rupture of membranes (AROM) – Rupture of the membranes using a plastic device (Amnihook) or surgical clamp

augmentation of labor – The use of chemical modalities to stimulate uterine contractions after labor has begun spontaneously but is not progressing satisfactorily

Bishop score – A rating system to evaluate cervical inducibility; a higher score is associated with a greater likelihood for successful labor induction

cephalopelvic disproportion (CPD) – Condition in which the fetal head is of a shape, size, or position that prohibits it from

passing through the maternal pelvis; may also be caused by
maternal pelvic problems

cesarean birth – Birth of a fetus through an incision in the
maternal abdominal wall and uterus

dystocia – A long, difficult, or abnormal labor and birth

forceps – Instrument consisting of cephalic-curved blades
similar to the shape of the fetal head; used during birth to
protect the fetal head and to apply traction to assist the birth

hypertonic labor contractions – Uterine contractions that are
uncoordinated, frequent, and often painful but are
ineffective in producing cervical effacement and dilation

hypotonic labor contractions – Uterine contractions that are weak
and ineffective; this labor pattern usually occurs during the
active phase of labor

induction of labor – The use of chemical or mechanical
modalities to initiate uterine contractions before their
spontaneous onset to bring about childbirth.

intrauterine resuscitation – Interventions initiated when a
nonreassuring fetal heart rate pattern is noted; directed at
improving uterine and intervillous space blood flow and
cardiac output

macrosomia – Large body size; fetal birth weight above the 90th
percentile on an intrauterine growth chart for that
gestational age; often seen in neonates of diabetic or
prediabetic mothers

meconium – First stools of the infant; characteristically viscid,
dark greenish brown, sticky, sterile, and odorless

meconium stained amniotic fluid – In response to hypoxia, fetal
intestinal activity increases and the anal sphincter relaxes,
resulting in the passage of meconium into the amniotic
fluid. Normally seen in breech presentations

nuchal cord – Encircling of the fetal neck by one or more loops
of the umbilical cord

oligohydramnios – Less than 300 mL of amniotic fluid

pelvic dystocia – Occurs when contractures of the pelvic
diameters reduce the capacity of the bony pelvis: the
midpelvis; the outlet; or any combination of these planes

postdate pregnancy – A pregnancy that has gone past the
estimated date of birth

postterm pregnancy – A pregnancy that extends beyond 294 days or 42 weeks past the first day of the last normal menstrual period

precipitate (precipitous) labor – Rapid or sudden labor that lasts less than 3 hours from the beginning of contractions to birth

spontaneous rupture of membranes (SROM) – Rupture of the membranes by natural means

shoulder dystocia – Occurs when the fetal head is born but the anterior shoulder cannot pass under the maternal pubic arch

soft tissue dystocia – Occurs when the birth passage is obstructed by an anatomic abnormality other than that involving the maternal bony pelvis

trial of labor (TOL) – Observation period to determine if a woman in labor is likely to successfully progress to a vaginal birth

umbilical cord prolapse – Protrusion of the umbilical cord in advance of the presenting part

vacuum-assisted birth (also termed vacuum extraction) – Birth involving the attachment of a vacuum cup to the fetal head and using negative pressure to assist in the birth of the fetus

vaginal birth after cesarean (VBAC) – Giving birth vaginally after a previous cesarean birth

version – Act of turning the fetus in the uterus from one presentation to another

   external cephalic v. – Turning the fetus to a vertex position by externally exerting pressure on the fetus through the maternal abdomen

FOCUSED ASSESSMENT

Uterine Contraction Patterns (Fig. 11-1)

A – Normal uterine contraction pattern (brings about cervical effacement and dilation)

B – Hypertonic uterine contraction pattern (uncoordinated, frequent, painful)

C – Hypotonic uterine contraction pattern (weak, ineffective)

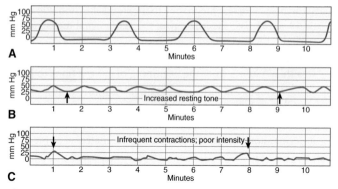

Figure 11-1 Uterine contraction patterns. *A.* Normal uterine contraction pattern. *B.* Hypertonic uterine contraction pattern. *C.* Hypotonic uterine contraction pattern.

Factors Associated with Increased Risk for Hypertonic Labor Contractions

- Increased maternal catecholamine release (e.g., epinephrine, norepinephrine)
- Maternal anxiety (primiparous labor, fear of loss of control, history of sexual abuse, lack of support, cultural differences)
- Fetal occiput–posterior malposition

Factors Associated with Increased Risk for Hypotonic Labor Contractions

- Fetal macrosomia
- Multiple gestation
- Hydramnios
- Maternal obesity unaccompanied by diabetes
- Pharmacological agents used for pain relief

Factors Associated with an Increased Risk for Uterine Dystocia

- Uterine abnormalities, such as congenital malformations and overdistention (e.g., hydramnios, macrosomia, multiple gestation)

- Fetal malpresentation or malposition
- Cephalopelvic disproportion (CPD)
- Maternal body build (>30 lbs. [13.6 kg] overweight, short stature)
- Uterine overstimulation with oxytocin
- Inappropriate timing of administration of analgesic/anesthetic agents
- Maternal fear, fatigue, dehydration, electrolyte imbalance (Gilbert, 2006)

How to Recognize Indicators of Dystocia

- Lack of progress in rate of cervical dilation, fetal descent, and expulsion
- Alteration in the pattern of normal uterine contractions

Assessment of the Patient Undergoing an Amniotomy

- Assess maternal understanding of the procedure.
- Assess vital signs, cervical effacement and dilation, station, fetal heart rate (FHR), and contractions.
- Ensure equipment is assembled (hip pad, padded bedpan, sterile gloves, lubricant, Amnihook, or Allis clamp; Fig. 11-2).
- Place the hip pad under the buttocks and position the padded bedpan to elevate hips.
- Assess the FHR immediately before and after artificial rupture of membranes (AROM).
  - Transient fetal tachycardia is common.
  - Bradycardia or variable decelerations may indicate cord compression or prolapse.
- Assess color, odor, consistency, clarity, and amount of amniotic fluid.
- Assess for signs of maternal infection.
  - Take temperature at least every 2 hours.
  - Assess for chills, uterine tenderness, foul-smelling vaginal discharge, fetal tachycardia.

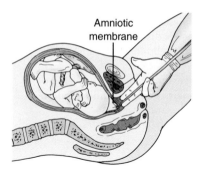

Figure 11-2 An Amnihook is used to rupture the membranes.

Assessing Cervical Inducibility with the Bishop Score				
Score	**0**	**1**	**2**	**3**
Dilation (cm)	0	1–2	3–4	≥5
Effacement (%)	0–30	40–50	60–70	≥80
Station (cm)	–3	–2	–1	+1, +2
Cervical Consistency	Firm	Medium	Soft	
Cervix Position	Posterior	Midposition	Anterior	

Source: Cunningham et al. (2005).

Assessment and Documentation During Oxytocin Administration

- Patient's vital signs (blood pressure, pulse, and respirations every 30 to 60 minutes and with every increment in medication dose)
- FHR (via electronic monitoring)
- Frequency, duration, and strength of contractions (note contraction pattern and uterine resting tone every 15 minutes and with every increment in medication dose during first stage; then monitor every 5 minutes during second stage).
- Cervical effacement and dilatation
- Fetal station and lie
- Rate of oxytocin infusion
- Intake and urine output (limit IV intake to 1000 mL/8 hr; output should be 120 mL or more every 4 hours)

- Any untoward effect of the medication administration (nausea, vomiting, headache, hypotension)
- Psychological response of the patient

(American College of Obstetricians [ACOG], 1999; Gilbert, 2006; Simpson, 2005)

CLINICAL ALERTS

Contraindications to the Use of Oxytocin to Stimulate Labor

- Vasa previa or complete placenta previa
- Transverse fetal lie
- Umbilical cord prolapse
- Previous transfundal uterine surgery

Conditions that Necessitate Special Precaution During Oxytocin Administration

- Breech presentation
- Multifetal pregnancy
- Presenting part above the pelvic inlet
- Severe hypertension
- Maternal heart disease
- Polyhydramnios
- One or more previous low-transverse cesarean deliveries (ACOG, 1999)

MEDICATIONS

Administering Oxytocin

1. Obtain written order for oxytocin for labor induction or augmentation from patient's primary health care provider.
2. Explain procedure and assess the patient's level of understanding.
3. Assist the patient to a side-lying or upright position.
4. Assess the patient and fetus and document the findings.
5. Prepare the primary IV solution and administer with a pump delivery system according to the prescribed orders.

6. Connect the piggyback solution with the medication to the intravenous infusion at the port nearest the point of venous insertion, and administer as ordered.
7. Perform ongoing maternal-fetal assessments according to institutional protocol.
8. Document:
   - Medication name and amount
   - Times of beginning infusion and any dose changes
   - Maternal–fetal reactions (FHR and pattern, maternal vital signs, pattern and progress of labor, and nursing interventions and maternal response)
   - Notification of primary health care provider of any change

Cervical Ripening Agents

Medication	Action	Adverse Effects	Dosage
Prostaglandin E₁ Misoprostol (Cytotec)	Induces labor contractions.	Diarrhea, abdominal pain, headaches, fever, tachysystole, uterine hyperstimulation	Intravaginally: 25 mcg; repeat every 4–6 hours until Bishop score equals 8 or greater
Prostaglandin E₂ Dinoprostone (Cervidil Insert, Prepidil Gel)	Promotes initiation of cervical ripening. May stimulate labor contractions.	Uterine hyperstimulation, fever, back pain, headache, nausea and vomiting, diarrhea, hypotension, tachysystole *Adverse effects are more common with intracervical administration.*	Cervidil insert: (10 mg dinoprostone gradually released over 12 hours). Remove after 12 hours or at labor onset. Keep insert frozen until ready to use. Prepidil Gel: (2.5-mL syringe containing 0.5 mg of dinoprostone). Repeat gel insertion in 6 hours as needed (maximum = 1.5 mg or 3 doses/24 hr). Allow the gel to reach room temperature before administration; do not heat. Continue administration until

Medication	Action	Adverse Effects	Dosage
			the maximum dose is reached, or uterine contractions are established (3/10 min) or the Bishop score equals 8 or greater or adverse reactions occur.

ETHNOCULTURAL CONSIDERATIONS

Communication Difficulties During Labor

Nurses need to be sensitive to cultural differences among women experiencing hypertonic labor, a pattern characterized by strong, painful contractions that do not produce cervical effacement and dilation. Maternal anxiety, related to factors such as fear of pain, loss of control, lack of support, and cultural differences, produces high levels of catecholamines, which can result in poor uterine contractility. Women who are unable to speak or understand the English language may have difficulty communicating their feelings. A therapeutic environment that fosters trust, comfort, relaxation, and rest, along with other measures such as hydration and sedation, help to reduce the irritability of the uterus and diminish the ineffective contractions.

Trends in Preterm Labor and Birth

Black women are at a higher risk for preterm birth than are Caucasian women. When preterm birth rates of married, educated women are compared with those of matched Caucasian women, a disparity continues to be noted among the Black women. The increase in cases of preterm labor results in a greater percentage of infant mortality in the Black population (Moore, 2003).

Minority Women and Level of Care Received

The Institute of Medicine (2003) reported that members of minorities do not receive the same level of quality care as do white Americans. A nurse working in the birth unit needs to be attentive to this problem. It is incumbent upon all nurses to advocate for patients any time there appears to be an ethnic bias in treatment. The nurse also must be aware of any personal prejudices that could affect care. In institutions that serve minority populations, it is essential that all hospital staff members undergo frequent in-service educational offerings that focus on heightening cultural sensitivity.

Cultural Aspects of Loss

Reactions to perinatal death vary among cultures. Tears and emotional outbursts are common to some cultures; others are quiet and introspective. The Hispanic culture that includes Mexicans, Puerto Ricans, and Cubans views children as their future. The loss of a child denies that future. Hispanic individuals tend to welcome touch from others and expect health care professionals to respect their need for extended family during this time frame (Gilbert, 2006).

TEACHING THE FAMILY

Preparing the Patient for an Amniotomy

- Ensure that the patient understands the procedure and the reason for it.
- Explain that the membrane rupture is painless for her and the fetus, but that she may feel some discomfort when the instrument is inserted.

Exploring Concerns of the Patient Experiencing Preterm Labor

- Use active listening; remain nearby; provide ongoing information.
- Encourage the patient to participate in decision making.
- Teach the patient and her partner about the process of labor and how they can support and help one another throughout the labor and birth experience.

Educating the Patient About Cervical Ripening Agents

- Assess knowledge of the medication.
- Explain the purpose of the medication and its side effects.

- Discuss comfort options to offset the side effects of the medication.
- Instruct the patient to void before insertion of the medication.
- Instruct the patient to maintain a supine position with a lateral tilt or side-lying position for 30 to 40 minutes after insertion of the medication.

(Deglin & Vallerand, 2009; Turkoski, Lance, & Bonfiglio, 2004)

ADDITIONAL INFORMATION FOR THE CLINICAL SETTING

Assisting with a Precipitous Birth

- Request a translator to interpret for patients unable to speak or understand English.
- Assist the laboring woman to breathe through each contraction to prevent pushing.
- Provide continuous emotional support.
- Provide perineal support with warm cloths.
- Frequently monitor the maternal and fetal vital signs and immediately report any abnormal findings to the physician or certified nurse midwife.
- After birth, carefully monitor the patient for signs of hemorrhage; assess for trauma to the perineum.
- Assess the neonate for evidence of trauma and report and document all findings.

Nursing Actions During a Trial of Labor (TOL)

Nursing responsibilities during a TOL include assessment of maternal vital signs and FHR and pattern. If complications arise, the nurse notifies the primary health care provider, and evaluates and documents the maternal–fetal responses to the interventions. Offering support and encouragement to the woman and her labor partner and ongoing information about labor progress are essential components of care.

Nursing Actions When a Non-reassuring FHR Pattern Is Detected

- Provide information to the patient; assist her to a lateral position.

- Encourage relaxation and mental imagery to reduce anxiety.
- Assess for and correct maternal hypotension by elevating the legs.
- Increase the rate of the maintenance IV fluids.
- Assess for hyperstimulation by palpating the uterus.
- Discontinue oxytocin if infusing.
- Administer oxygen at 8 to 10 L/min by mask.
- Consider internal monitoring to obtain more accurate fetal/uterine assessments.
- Apply fetal scalp or acoustic stimulation.
- Assist with fetal oxygen saturation monitoring if ordered.
- Assist with birth (cesarean or vaginal-assisted) if a non reassuring FHR pattern cannot be corrected.

Communicating Effectively When a Non-reassuring FHR Pattern Is Detected by Electronic Monitoring

When electronic monitoring reveals a non-reassuring FHR pattern, the nurse needs to maintain a calming presence and offer factual, simple explanations for all actions. For example, the nurse may say:

"We are concerned about your baby's heart rate pattern."
"I am going to change your position to your side to increase oxygen flow to your baby."
"I am also going to place this oxygen mask on your face to increase the oxygen flow to you and to your baby, and increase your IV rate."
"Do you have any questions?"
"I am here to help in any way and I will stay here with you. Please let me know what concerns you have."

Assisting with Intrauterine Resuscitation

Nursing priorities:

1. Open the maternal and fetal vascular systems.
2. Increase the blood volume.
3. Optimize oxygenation of the circulating blood volume.

These interventions are accomplished by:

- Changing the maternal position
- Increasing the rate of the primary IV
- Providing oxygen by face mask

Caring for a Patient Undergoing Amnioinfusion

1. Assess the patient's response to the fluid infusion.
2. Continually monitor the frequency and intensity of uterine contractions.
3. Stop the infusion if the following signs and symptoms are noted: Maternal shortness of breath, an over-distended uterus, hypotension, or tachycardia.

Recognizing and Responding to Problems During Labor Induction with Oxytocin

During induction of labor with oxytocin, be alert to signs indicative of complications: uterine hyperstimulation, nonreassuring fetal heart rate pattern, and suspected uterine rupture. Immediate emergency measures include discontinuing the oxytocin per institutional protocol; positioning the patient on her side; increasing the primary IV rate up to 200 mL/hr (unless there is evidence of water intoxication—in this situation, the rate is decreased to one that keeps the vein open); administering oxygen by face mask at 8 to 10 L/min or per physician order or institutional protocol.

Alternative Measures for the Induction of Labor

Herbal Remedies

Black haw, primrose oil, black and blue cohosh, chamomile, and red raspberry leaves are medicinal agents with some properties similar to those of oxytocin. Although used as labor inducers in some cultures, there is a lack of scientific research and validation of their effectiveness.

Nonherbal Methods

Nonherbal methods include acupuncture, the ingestion of a laxative (e.g., castor oil), and the stripping of membranes.

Assisting with External Cephalic Version (ECV): Nursing Responsibilities (Fig. 11-3)

1. Obtain consent.	The physician is responsible for explaining the procedure.
2. Assess for contraindications to a version.	Contraindications include previous cesarean birth, uterine anomalies, CPD, placenta previa, multifetal gestation, oligohydramnios
3. Provide teaching regarding the procedure.	Before the version, ultrasonography, non-stress testing, and/or electronic FHR monitoring is performed. The ECV may not be successful; complications include rupture of the membranes, fetal bradycardia, discomfort, and the potential for cesarean birth if maternal or fetal compromise occurs.
4. Administer medications if ordered.	Tocolytic agents (e.g., magnesium sulfate, terbutaline) may be ordered.
5. Maintain constant maternal and fetal surveillance.	Assess for fetal or maternal compromise.
6. Administer Rh immune globulin if the patient is Rh-negative	Manipulation may cause fetal–maternal bleeding.

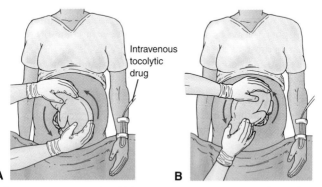

Intravenous tocolytic drug

A   B

Figure 11-3 External cephalic version is a maneuver performed through the maternal abdominal wall in an attempt to change the fetal position from a breech to a cephalic presentation.

Breech Presentation and the Presence of Meconium in the Amniotic Fluid

When the fetus is in a breech presentation, the presence of meconium in the amniotic fluid may not be indicative of fetal distress. Pressure exerted on the fetal abdomen during the birth process may cause the passage of meconium. It is important to assess the FHR and pattern to ensure there are changes indicative of fetal hypoxia. When the fetus is in a breech position, the FHR is best auscultated at or above the maternal umbilicus.

Intrapartal Neonatal Suctioning and Meconium-Stained Amniotic Fluid

The nasopharynx and oropharynx of the neonate born in the presence of meconium-stained amniotic fluid are often suctioned before the first breath to reduce the incidence and severity of meconium aspiration syndrome (MAS). However, because research does not support the efficacy of routine intrapartum suctioning to prevent MAS, this practice is no longer recommended (Vain et al., 2004).

Actions to Reduce the Risk of Umbilical Cord Prolapse

When SROM occurs, maintain the patient on bed rest until the fetal presenting part is engaged. AROM should not be attempted until engagement has occurred. To rule out umbilical cord prolapse, assess the fetal heart sounds immediately after spontaneous or artificial rupture of the membranes.

Nursing Actions After Prolapse of the Umbilical Cord (Fig. 11-4)

1. Call for assistance; notify the primary health care provider.
2. Using the gloved examining hand, insert two fingers into the vagina to the cervix. Place one finger on either side of the cord or both fingers to one side and quickly exert upward pressure against the presenting part to relieve compression of the cord.
3. Assist the woman into an extreme Trendelenburg, modified Sims, or knee–chest position.

4. If the cord is protruding from the vagina, wrap it loosely in a sterile towel saturated with a warmed, sterile normal saline solution.
5. Administer oxygen at 10 L/min by facemask.
6. Increase the IV fluids; administer a tocolytic agent as ordered.
7. Continuously monitor the FHR by internal fetal scalp electrode if possible.
8. Provide information and support to the patient and her birth partner.
9. Prepare for an immediate vaginal birth if the cervix is fully dilated or for cesarean birth if it is not.

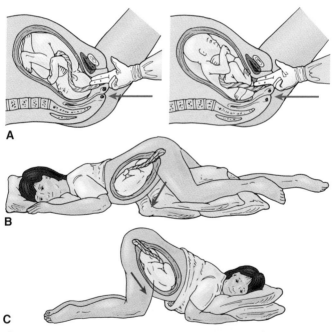

Figure 11-4 Interventions to relieve pressure on a prolapsed umbilical cord until birth can be effected. *A.* A gloved hand is placed in the vagina to lift the presenting part off the cord. *B.* The knee–chest position uses gravity to shift the fetus out of the maternal pelvis. *C.* The maternal hips are elevated with two pillows; this intervention is often combined with a Trendelenburg position.

Actions When Attending a Forceps-Assisted Birth

- Assess and record the FHR and pattern before the forceps application (there is a danger of compression of the cord between the fetal head and the forceps blade; cord compression causes a decrease in the FHR) (Fig. 11-5).
- Assess and record the FHR and pattern again *immediately* after the forceps application

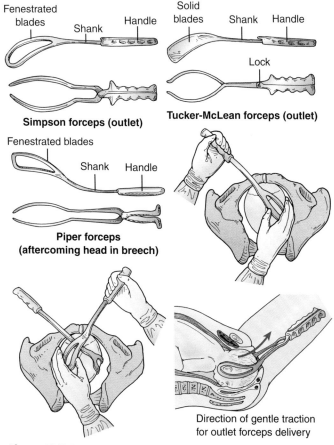

Fenestrated blades   Shank   Handle

Simpson forceps (outlet)

Solid blades   Shank   Handle

Lock

Tucker-McLean forceps (outlet)

Fenestrated blades

Shank   Handle

Piper forceps (aftercoming head in breech)

Direction of gentle traction for outlet forceps delivery

Figure 11-5 Forceps are instruments with curved blades that are used to facilitate birth of the fetal head.

Nursing Responsibilities Associated with a Vacuum-Assisted Birth (Fig. 11-6)

- Management of patient care.
- Control the vacuum gun and pressure while the physician applies the vacuum apparatus to the fetal head.
- Thoroughly document the sequence of events.
- Communicate progress or lack of progress to all members of the perinatal team.
- Assess maternal and fetal status and advocate for cesarean birth if maternal exhaustion and/or failure of descent indicates that the vacuum assistance is not effective.
- Be aware that after an assisted birth, the nurse who assesses the neonate is also liable with regard to the documentation of vital signs and the neonatal assessment (Mahlmeister, 2005).

Nursing Actions When Birth Is Complicated by Shoulder Dystocia

- Assist the patient in assuming the position ordered by the physician.
- Assist the physician with maneuvers (e.g., suprapubic pressure; McRoberts maneuver) to facilitate birth (Fig. 11-7).
- Document all procedures.
- Provide instruction to the patient to facilitate cooperation and understanding.

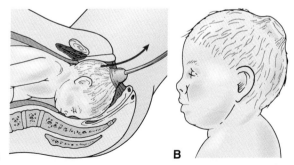

A   **B**

Figure 11-6 Vacuum extraction also facilitates the delivery of the fetal head and is associated with fewer lacerations of the maternal birth canal. *A.* Vacuum extractor is applied with a downward and outward traction. *B.* A caput succedaneum, or chignon, is formed from the suction cup.

- After birth, closely observe the mother for signs of hemorrhage and soft tissue trauma of the birth canal.
- Assess the neonate for birth asphyxia, fracture of the clavicle or humerus, and/or brachial plexus injuries

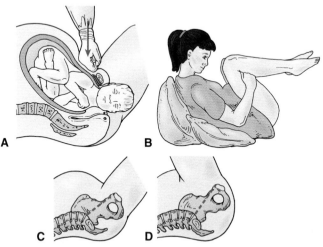

A **B**

C **D**

Figure 11-7 Methods to relieve shoulder dystocia. *A.* Pressure is applied immediately above the maternal symphysis pubis to push the fetal anterior shoulder downward. *B.* McRoberts maneuver. The woman's thighs are sharply flexed on her abdomen to straighten the pelvic curve. *C.* Angle of pelvis before maneuver. *D.* Angle of pelvis after maneuver.

Understanding Types of Uterine Rupture

Type	Description	Symptoms
Complete Rupture	Extends through the endometrium, myometrium, and peritoneum.	Sudden, severe, abdominal pain during a contraction followed by cessation of the pain and contractions with bleeding into the abdominal cavity and possibly into the vagina.
Incomplete Rupture	Extends into the peritoneum but not into the peritoneal cavity or broad ligament.	Bleeding is usually internal and the woman may be asymptomatic (a "silent" rupture) or complain of localized tenderness and aching pain over the lower uterine segment.

Umbilical Cord and Placental Variations

Variation	Description	Implications
Velamentous Insertion of Cord	The fetal vessels separate at the distal end of the cord and insert into the placenta at a distance away from the margin.	Vessels are not protected by Wharton's jelly and are subject to rupture and/or thrombosis. Most common with placenta previa and multiple pregnancies.
Vasa Previa	The umbilical cord is implanted into the fetal membranes rather than the placenta; the vessels cover the cervical os and precede the fetus.	Hemorrhage
Circumvallate Placenta	A ring composed of a double fold of amnion and chorion forms near the fetal surface.	Associated with antepartum hemorrhage, preterm birth, and fetal malformations.
Succenturiate Placenta	Placenta contains one or two separate lobes, each with its own circulation.	After childbirth, one of the separate lobes may be retained in the uterus and impede contractions, resulting in severe maternal hemorrhage. The remaining lobes must be manually removed from the uterus to prevent hemorrhage.
Battledore Placenta	The umbilical cord is implanted near the margin of the placenta.	Associated with fetal hemorrhage, especially after marginal separation of the placenta
Placenta Accreta	A slight penetration of the myometrium by the trophoblast.	Hemorrhage
Placenta Increta	A deep placental penetration of the myometrium.	Hemorrhage and possible hysterectomy
Placenta Percreta	Perforation of the uterus by the placenta.	Hemorrhage, hysterectomy

Disseminated Intravascular Coagulation (DIC)

Be alert for maternal clinical signs indicative of DIC:

- Bleeding from multiple sites: intravenous access site, venipuncture site, site of urinary catheter insertion

- Spontaneous bleeding from the gums and nose
- Widespread petechiae and bruising
- Gastrointestinal bleeding
- Tachycardia
- Diaphoresis

Care of the Patient Experiencing an Intrapartal Hemorrhage

Assessment	Plan	Intervention	Evaluation
Vital Signs	Establish maternal stability.	Take every 5 minutes if unstable, or every 15 minutes if stable. Use pulse oximetry. Auscultate respirations.	Vital signs are within normal range. Pulse is between 60 and 120 beats per minute. Respirations are between 14 and 26 breaths per minute. Temperature is <100.4°F (38°C); BP is >90/60 mm Hg.
Bleeding	Resolve hemorrhage. Prevent shock.	Start two large-bore IV sites. Infuse normal saline and lactated Ringer's solution. Estimate blood loss. 1 g = 1 mL for replacement Infuse blood products as necessary. Monitor circulatory volume using central venous pressure (CVP)/Swan-Ganz catheter as needed for extreme bleeding.	Bleeding is minimized. Homeostasis is established.

(continued)

Care of the Patient Experiencing an Intrapartal Hemorrhage (Continued)

Assessment	Plan	Intervention	Evaluation
		Send blood sample to lab for analysis of gases. Document blood loss.	
Intake/Output	Prevent volume depletion.	Insert in-dwelling urinary catheter. Measure and record output every hour. Measure and record input every hour.	Urine output will be >30 mL/hr.
Fetal Status	Prevent fetal injury.	Continuous electronic fetal monitoring	Fetal heart rate tracings remain between 120 and 160 bpm. There is no evidence of abnormal tracings.
Emotional Response	Assist the patient to cope with the condition.	Educate the patient regarding all procedures. Inform the patient of her status throughout the bleeding crisis. Provide relaxation and breathing techniques. Provide spiritual support as necessary.	The patient verbalizes an understanding of her condition. The patient's face displays no grimace. The muscles remain relaxed.
Pain	Reduce pain.	Provide relaxation and breathing techniques. Use guided imagery.	The patient reports pain on a rating scale of 1–10 as between 3 and 5.

Assessment	Plan	Intervention	Evaluation
		Offer massage. Monitor contractions. Offer limited pain medication as ordered.	

Sources: MacMullen, Dulski, & Meagher (2005); Curran (2003); Mandeville & Troiano (1999).

Nursing Actions When Amniotic Fluid Embolism (AFE) Develops

Immediately perform the following actions:

- Administer oxygen by facemask or cannula at a rate of 8 to 10 L/min; or resuscitation bag to deliver 100% oxygen.
- Prepare for intubation and mechanical ventilation.
- Initiate or assist with cardiopulmonary resuscitation (CPR). Position the pregnant patient in a 30-degree lateral tilt to displace the uterus.
- Administer intravenous fluids and blood (e.g., packed cells; fresh frozen plasma).
- Insert indwelling urinary catheter; measure hourly urine output.
- Continuously monitor maternal–fetal status.
- Prepare for emergency birth once the patient is stable.
- Provide ongoing information and emotional support to the patient and her family.

Risks Associated with Multiple Gestations

- Antepartal complications: Hypertension of pregnancy, anemia, gestational diabetes
- Intrapartal complications: Hemorrhage (related to atony from uterine overdistention); abruptio placentae, multiple or adherent placentas, abnormal fetal presentation(s), fetal distress (related to cord prolapse and the onset of placental separation after the birth of the first fetus)
- Fetal/newborn complications: primarily related to problems associated with low-birth-weight infants due to preterm birth and intrauterine growth restriction

Medical Indications for Elective Preterm Birth in Women with Diabetes

- Poor metabolic control
- Worsening hypertensive disorder
- Fetal macrosomia or fetal growth restriction (ACOG, 2001; Cunningham et al., 2005)

Postpartal Complications in Diabetic Women

Increased risk for:

- Preeclampsia/eclampsia
- Hemorrhage (more likely following uterine overdistention [e.g., hydramnios, macrosomia])
- Infection (e.g., endometritis)

Intrapartal Nursing Care for Patients with Preeclampsia

Blood Pressure
- Check every 4 hours (or more frequently according to physician orders or institutional protocol).
- Use the same arm at each assessment.
- Encourage a side-lying position to enhance uterine perfusion.
- Record all data.
- Notify the physician of an increase in blood pressure.

Medication Administration
- Administer as ordered and evaluate its effect.
- Adhere to hospital protocol for magnesium sulfate infusion.
- Monitor maternal vital signs, FHR, urine output, deep tendon reflexes (DTRs), IV flow rate, and serum magnesium levels.
- Assess for magnesium sulfate toxicity (e.g., depressed respirations, hyporeflexia, sudden onset of hypotension, oliguria, indicators of fetal compromise).
- Administer calcium gluconate (the antidote for magnesium sulfate toxicity) for respirations below 12/min and discontinue the magnesium sulfate infusion.

Renal Balance
- Assess edema on a scale of 1 to 4 (4 is generalized massive edema that includes the face, abdomen, and sacrum).

- Assess and record urinary output. An indwelling urinary catheter may be inserted to measure urinary output more accurately. A urine output <30 mL/hr is indicative of oliguria and the physician must be notified.
- Assess urine for protein every 4 hours. A dipstick reading >2+ is indicative of a worsening condition.

Neurological Status
- Assess DTRs every 4 hours (or more frequently) on a scale of 1 to 4. Reflexes >2+ are a sign of worsening status.
- If dorsiflexion of the foot produces clonus (convulsive spasm), the maternal condition is deteriorating.

Pulmonary
- Auscultate the lungs every 4 hours (or more frequently).
- Assess for dyspnea, crackles, and diminished breath sounds (may be indicative of pulmonary edema).
- Assess the respiratory rate every 4 hours (or more frequently).
- Patients who are receiving magnesium sulfate require more frequent respiratory assessments because a respiratory rate below 12 is an indicator of magnesium toxicity.
- Hemoglobin oxygen saturation can be assessed with a pulse oximeter.

Psychological Status
- Assess for indicators of anxiety and fear.
- Provide information to the patient and family about the treatment protocols and status of the maternal-fetal conditions.
- Assess the patient's and family's level of understanding and provide updates when indicated.

Advancing Symptoms
Headaches, blurred vision, severe right upper quadrant epigastric pain, and restlessness are all indicators of impending eclampsia. Prepare for immediate delivery.

Seizures
Protect the patient. Keep the airway patent: turn the head to one side and place a pillow or folded linen under one shoulder or back. Call for assistance. Ensure that the side rails have been raised. Observe and document all seizure activity. Notify the physician and prepare for delivery. Administer oxygen.

Fetal Status

Monitor the fetal heart rate every 4 hours or more frequently as indicated. Assess fetal movements. Notify the physician if indicators of fetal compromise are noted.

Factors that May Necessitate Immediate Intervention to Facilitate Birth in Patients with Hypertensive Disorders

- Uncontrolled severe hypertension
- Eclampsia
- Persistent oliguria (<500 mL/24 hr)
- Abruptio placentae
- Platelet count <100,000/mm^3
- Elevated liver enzyme levels with epigastric pain or right upper quadrant tenderness
- Pulmonary edema
- Persistent severe headache or visual changes
- Spontaneous labor
- Fetal death
- Rupture of the membranes
- Gestational age <34 weeks (an observational period may be initially attempted as a conservative management approach)
- Evidence of fetal compromise

Supporting the Mother Whose Newborn Has Died

When caring for the mother whose infant has died, the nurse conveys compassion by simply being available. Often, the mother finds comfort in talking about the birth experience, her infant, and how she will cope with her loss. The nurse can gain insights into the mother's support systems by asking the following questions:

"What are you most worried or fearful about?
"How supportive is the baby's father and your family or friends?
"What coping techniques have been helpful for you in the past?" (Gilbert, 2006)

REFERENCES

American College of Obstetricians and Gynecologists (ACOG). (1999). *Induction of labor.* ACOG Practice Bulletin No. 10. Washington, DC: Author.

American College of Obstetricians and Gynecologists (ACOG). (2001). *Gestational diabetes.* ACOG Practice Bulletin Number 30. Washington, DC: Author.

Cunningham, F., Leveno, K., Bloom, S., Hauth, J., Gilstrap, L., & Wenstrom, K. (2005). *Williams' obstetrics* (22nd ed.). New York: McGraw-Hill.

Curran, C. (2003). Intrapartum emergencies. *Journal of Obstetric, Gynecologic, and Neonatal Nursing, 32*(6), 802–813.

Deglin, J.H., & Vallerand, A.H. (2009). *Davis's drug guide for nurses* (11th ed.). Philadelphia: F.A. Davis.

Gilbert, E.S. (2006). *Manual of high risk pregnancy and delivery.* St. Louis, MO: C.V. Mosby.

Institute of Medicine. (2003). *The future of the public's health in the 21st century.* Washington, DC: National Academy Press.

MacMullen, N., Dulski, L., & Meagher, B. (2005). RED ALERT: Perinatal hemorrhage. *The American Journal of Maternal Child Health, 30*(1), 46–51.

Mahlmeister, L. (2005). Nursing responsibilities in preventing, preparing for and managing epidural emergencies. *Journal of Perinatal and Neonatal Nursing, 17*(1), 19–34.

Mandeville, L., & Troiano, N. (1999). *High-risk and critical care: Intrapartum nursing* (2nd ed.). Philadelphia: Lippincott.

Moore, M. (2003). Preterm labor and birth: What have we learned in the past two decades? *Journal of Obstetric Gynecological and Neonatal Nursing, 32,* 638–649.

Simpson, K. (2005). The context and clinical evidence for common nursing practices during labor. *MCN American Journal of Maternal/Child Nursing, 30*(6), 356–363.

Turkoski, B.B., Lance, B.R., & Bonfiglio, M.F. (2004). *Lexi comp's drug information for nursing: Including assessment, administration, monitoring guidelines, and patient education* (6th ed.). Hudson, OH: Lexi-Comp.

Vain, N., Szyld, E., Prudent, L., Wiswell, T., Aguilar, A., & Vivas, N. (2004). Oropharyngeal and nasopharyngeal suctioning of meconium-stained neonates before delivery of their shoulders: Multicentre, randomized, controlled trial. *Lancet, 364*(9434), 597–602.

*Caring for the Postpartal
Woman and Her Family*

KEY TERMS

afterpains (afterbirth pains) – Painful intermittent uterine
  contractions that occur for approximately 2 to 3 days,
  during the process of uterine involution.

couplet care – Situation when one nurse, who has been educated
  in both mother and infant care, serves as the primary nurse
  for the mother and the infant, even when the infant is kept
  in the nursery. Also known as "mother–baby care"

engorgement – Distention or vascular congestion

  breast e. Excessive swelling of the breast and areola brought
    about by an increase in blood and lymph supply to the
    breast, which precedes lactation. Typically occurs between
    the 3rd and 5th postpartum day and lasts about 24 hours.

involution – Reduction in uterine size after birth

lactogenesis – Process by which the breasts secrete milk

latch-on – Proper attachment of the infant to the breast for
  feeding

"let-down" reflex – Release of milk from the breast, caused by the
  contraction of the myoepithelial cells within the milk glands
  in response to oxytocin. Also termed "milk ejection reflex"

lochia – Vaginal discharge during the postpartal period; consists
  of blood, tissue, and mucus

  l. alba Thin, yellowish-white vaginal discharge that follows
    lochia serosa on approximately the tenth day after birth

  l. rubra Bright red vaginal flow that follows birth and lasts
    2 to 4 days

l. serosa Serous, pinkish-brown thin vaginal discharge that follows lochia rubra until about the 10th day after birth

maternal blues/baby blues/postpartum blues – Feelings that include sadness, forgetfulness, tearfulness and mood swings; usually begin 2 to 3 days after giving birth and disappear within 1 to 2 weeks

nipple confusion – Difficulty experienced by some infants when attempting proper latch-on to the breast; occurs after the breastfed infant is given supplemental feedings with a bottle

parturition – The act of giving birth

puerperium – Period that begins after the third stage of labor and lasts until uterine involution is complete, usually 3 to 6 weeks; also known as the "fourth trimester"

sitz bath – Application of moist heat to the perineum; may be accomplished by sitting in a tub or basin filled with warm water

subinvolution – Failure of a part (e.g., the uterus) to return to its normal size and condition after enlargement from a functional activity (e.g., pregnancy)

FOCUSED ASSESSMENT

Assessment of Vital Signs During the Early Puerperium		
Parameter	Frequency	Expected Findings
Temperature		May increase up to 100.4°F (38°C) during first 24 hours due to exertion and dehydration.
Heart Rate	All vital signs are assessed q15min × 4; q30min×2hr; qhr × 1; then q8hr	Bradycardia (50–70 bpm) is common for the first 6–10 days.
Blood Pressure		Compare with pre-pregnancy norms. Orthostatic hypotension is common.
Respirations		Should remain in a normal range.

BUBBLE-HE: Essential Components of a Postpartum Assessment

Letter	Assess	Assessment Includes
B	Breasts	Inspection of nipples: Everted, flat, inverted? Breast tissue: Soft, filling, firm? Temperature and color: Warm, pink, cool, red streaked?
U	Uterus	Location (midline or deviated to right or left side) and tone (firm, firm with massage, boggy)
B	Bladder	Last time the patient emptied her bladder (spontaneously or via catheter)? Palpable or nonpalpable? Color, odor, and amount of urine?
B	Bowels	Date/time of last bowel movement; presence of flatus and hunger (unless the colon was manipulated, do not need to auscultate for bowel sounds)
L	Lochia	Color, amount, presence of clots, any free flow?
(I) E	(Incision) Episiotomy	Type as well as other tissue trauma (lacerations, etc.) Assess using REEDA (redness, edema, ecchymosis, drainage/discharge, approximation of episiotomy, if present)
L/H	Legs (Homans' sign)	Pain, varicosities, warmth or discoloration in calves; presence of pedal pulses; sensation and movement (after cesarean birth)
E	Emotions	Affect, patient–family interaction, effects of exhaustion
(B)	Bonding	Interaction with infant—"taking in" phase: Presence of finger tipping, gazing, enfolding, calling infant by name, identifying unique characteristics

Performing the Uterine Assessment

- Assist the patient to a supine position.
- Observe the abdomen for contour to detect distention, striae, or diastasis (separation).
- Place one hand immediately above the symphysis pubis to stabilize the uterus.
- Place the other hand at the level of the umbilicus.
- Press inward and downward with the hand positioned on the umbilicus until the fundus is located.

- Note and document the findings: the fundus should feel like a firm, globular mass located at or slightly above the umbilicus (first hour after birth; Fig. 12-1).
- Uterus descends in the pelvis at a rate of about 1 cm/day (one fingerbreadth; Fig. 12-2).

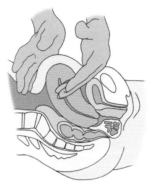

Figure 12-1 To palpate the uterus, the upper hand is cupped over the fundus; the lower hand stabilizes the uterus at the symphysis pubis.

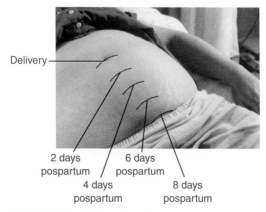

Delivery

2 days pospartum

4 days pospartum

6 days pospartum

8 days pospartum

Figure 12-2 Fundal heights postpartum.

Assessment and Documentation of Uterine Involution

Time	Location of Fundus	Documentation
Immediately after birth	Midline, midway between umbilicus and symphysis pubis	
1–2 hours	At the level of the umbilicus	at U (umbilicus)
12 hours	1 cm above umbilicus (1 fingerbreadth)	U+1
24 hours	1 cm below umbilicus	U–1
2 days	2 cm below umbilicus (2 fingerbreadths)	U–2
3 days	3 cm below umbilicus (3 fingerbreadths)	U–3
7 days	Palpable at the symphysis pubis	
10 days	Not palpable	

Assessment and Documentation of Lochia Flow

- Pattern of lochia flow progresses from lochia rubra to serosa to alba; should not reverse.
- Lochia should contain no large clots.
- Lochia odor is similar to that of menstrual blood.
- Document lochia in amounts described as scant, small, moderate, heavy (Fig. 12-3).
- Always include the time factor associated with the flow of lochia.

Scant: Blood only on tissue when wiped or 1- to 2-inch stain

Light: 4-inch or less stain

Moderate: Less than 6-inch stain

Heavy: Saturated pad

Figure 12-3 Assessment of lochia flow in 1 hour.

ASSESSMENT AND CARE OF THE PERINEUM

The REEDA Acronym to Guide the Perineal Assessment

Points	Redness	Edema	Ecchymosis	Discharge	Approximation
0	None	None	None	None	Closed
1	Within 0.25 cm of incision bilaterally	Less than 1 cm from incision	1–2 cm from incision	Serum	Skin separation 3 mm or less
2	Within 0.5 cm of incision bilaterally	1–2 cm from incision	0.25–1 cm bilaterally or 0.5–2 cm unilaterally	Serosanguineous	Skin and subcutaneous fat separated
3	Beyond 0.5 cm of incision bilaterally	Greater than 2 cm from incision	Greater that 1 cm bilaterally or 2 cm unilaterally	Bloody, purulent	Skin, subcutaneous fat, and fascial separation

Providing Early Episiotomy Care

1. Apply an ice bag or commercial cold pack, wrapped in a cover, to the perineum during the first 24 hours. Application of cold provides local anesthesia and promotes vasoconstriction while reducing edema and the incidence of peripheral bleeding.

2. After 24 hours, encourage the use of moist heat (sitz bath) between 100° and 105°F for 20 minutes three to four times/day. The sitz bath increases circulation to the perineum, enhances blood flow to the tissues, reduces edema, and promotes healing.

3. Dry heat, in the form of a commercial perineal "hot pack," may also be used. Women should be cautioned to apply a washcloth or gauze square between the hot pack and their skin to prevent a potential burn.

Assessment and Interventions for the Urinary System

Patient's Signs and Symptoms	Nursing Interventions
Location of fundus above the baseline level	Promote voiding: Provide privacy; turn on the lavatory faucet.
Fundus displaced from midline	Promote hydration.
Bulge of bladder above the symphysis pubis	Promote ambulation.
Frequent voiding of <150 mL of urine; urinary output disproportionate to fluid intake	Administer an analgesic before voiding, as prescribed.
Bladder discomfort	Place ice on the perineum to reduce swelling and pain. Encourage the use of a sitz bath.

Special Considerations for Assessment and Care After a Cesarean Birth

In addition to the BUBBLE-HE assessment:

- Facilitate bonding (recovery from anesthesia and incision pain may inhibit maternal–newborn bonding).
- Assess REEDA as well as warmth, redness, and tenderness around the incision.
- Monitor anesthesia recovery.
- Facilitate pulmonary exercises.
- Prevent deep venous thrombosis (DVT)—with leg exercises (flexion and extension of the knee) and application of compression boots as ordered by the physician.

PROMOTION OF INFANT NOURISHMENT

Assessing for Infant Feeding-Readiness

The infant demonstrates readiness for feeding when she:

- Begins to stir.
- Bobs the head against the mattress or mother's neck/shoulder.
- Makes hand-to-mouth or hand-to-hand movements.
- Exhibits sucking or licking.
- Exhibits rooting.
- Demonstrates increased activity; arms and legs flexed; hands positioned in a fist.

Assessing for Milk Let-down

Cues that indicate that the milk let-down reflex has occurred:

- The mother reports a tingling sensation in the nipples (not always present).
- The infant's quick, shallow sucking pattern transitions to a slower, more drawing pattern.
- The infant exhibits audible swallowing.
- The mother reports uterine cramping; increased lochia may be present.
- The mother states she feels extremely relaxed during the feeding.
- The opposite breast may leak milk.

Assessing Infant Weight Gain During the Early Days of Life

- Expected loss: Up to 5% of birth weight
- Greater than 7% weight loss indicates need for closer assessment/evaluation

Assessing Maternal–Infant Attachment

Assess for the following indicators:

Does the mother show eagerness to feed and care for her infant?

What is her response when the baby cries?

Does she make eye contact when holding and feeding her baby?

CLINICAL ALERTS

Proper Technique for Uterine Palpation

Never palpate the uterus without supporting the lower uterine segment. Failure to do so may result in uterine inversion and hemorrhage.

Assessing for a Hematoma After an Episiotomy

- Look for discoloration of the perineum.
- Listen for the patient's complaints or expression of severe perineal pain.
- Observe for edema of the area.
- Listen for the patient's expression of a need to defecate (the hematoma may cause rectal pressure).
- Don sterile gloves; gently palpate the area and observe for the patient's degree of sensitivity to the area by touch.
- Call the physician or nurse-midwife to report the findings immediately if hematoma is present. The bleeding that has produced the hematoma must be promptly identified and halted.

Teaching the Patient to Avoid the Knee–Chest Position

Teach the patient to avoid a knee–chest position until at least the third postpartal week. This position causes the vagina to open. Since the cervical os is still open to some extent, there is a danger that air can enter the vagina, pass into the cervix and enter the open blood sinuses inside the uterus. Entry of air into the circulatory system can cause an air embolus.

MEDICATIONS

Commonly Used Medications in the Postpartum Period			
Classification	Medication	Dose and Safety of Use in Breastfeeding Mothers	Indication for Use During the Postpartum Period
Stool Softener	Docusate sodium (Colace)	50–500 mg by mouth daily until bowel movements are normal Not contraindicated in breastfeeding mother	Used in the treatment of constipation

Classification	Medication	Dose and Safety of Use in Breastfeeding Mothers	Indication for Use During the Postpartum Period
Stool Softener	Bisacodyl (Dulcolax)	10–30 mg by mouth until bowel movements are normal Not contraindicated in breastfeeding mother	Used in the treatment of constipation
Topical Anesthetic	Lidocaine spray	Apply spray to the perineal area after sitz bath or perineum care. Not contraindicated in breastfeeding mother	Used on the skin to relieve pain and itching
Hemorrhoid Care	Witch hazel (Tucks)	Apply to the perineal area after sitz bath or perineum care. Not contraindicated in breastfeeding mother.	Used on the skin to relieve the itching, burning, and irritation associated with hemorrhoids
Nonsteroidal Anti-inflammatory Drugs (NSAIDs)	Ibuprofen (Motrin)	400 mg by mouth every 4–6 hours as needed for pain Not contraindicated in breastfeeding mother	Used for the treatment of mild to moderate pain
Opioid Analgesics	Propoxyphene napsylate and acetaminophen (Darvocet)	Take one tablet by mouth every 4 hours as needed for pain. Not contraindicated in breastfeeding mother	Used for the treatment of moderate to severe pain
Opioid Analgesics	Oxycodone and acetaminophen (Percocet)	Take one to two tablets every 4–6 hours as needed for pain. Not contraindicated in breastfeeding mother	Used for the treatment of moderate to severe pain

Breastfeeding and Afterpains

Analgesics such as ibuprofen (Advil, Motrin) or naproxen (Aleve, Anaprox) are frequently administered to lessen the discomforts of afterpains. Breastfeeding women should take pain medication approximately 30 minutes before nursing the baby to achieve maximum pain relief and to minimize the amount of medication that is transferred in the breast milk.

MEDICATIONS

Methylergonovine (meth-ill-er-goe-**noe**-veen); Methergine

Pregnancy Category C

Indications Prevention and treatment of postpartum and postabortion hemorrhage caused by uterine atony or subinvolution

Actions Directly stimulates uterine and vascular smooth muscle

Therapeutic Effects Uterine contraction

Pharmacokinetics
Absorption Well absorbed following oral or IM administration
Onset of Action Oral: 5 to 10 minutes; IM: 2 to 5 minutes; IV: Immediately
Distribution Oral: 3 hours; IM: 3 hours; IV: 45 minutes. Enters breast milk in small quantities
Metabolism and Excretion Probably metabolized by the liver
Half-life: 30–120 minutes

Contraindications and Precautions
Contraindicated in Hypersensitivity. Should not be used to induce labor.
Use cautiously in Hypertensive or eclamptic patients (more susceptible to hypertensive and arrhythmogenic side effects); severe hepatic or renal disease; sepsis
Exercise extreme caution in Third stage of labor

Adverse Reactions and Side Effects
CNS Dizziness, headache
Eye, ear, nose, throat Tinnitus
Respiratory Dyspnea
Cardiovascular Hypotension, arrhythmias, chest pain, hypertension, palpitations
Gastrointestinal Nausea, vomiting

Genitourinary Cramps
Dermatological Diaphoresis

Route and Dosage
PO: 200–400 mcg (0.4–0.6 mg) q6–12hr for 2–7 days
IM: IV: 200 mcg (0.2 mg) after delivery of fetal anterior shoulder, after delivery of the placenta, or during the puerperium; may be repeated as required at intervals of 2–4 hours up to 5 doses

Nursing Implications
1. Physical assessment: Monitor blood pressure, heart rate and uterine response frequently during medication administration. Notify the primary health care provider if uterine relaxation becomes prolonged or if character of vaginal bleeding changes.
2. Assess for signs of ergotism (cold, numb fingers and toes, chest pain, nausea, vomiting, headache, muscle pain, weakness)

Data from Deglin, J.H., & Vallerand, A.H. (2009). Davis's drug guide for nurses (11th ed.) Philadelphia: F.A. Davis.

Procedure 12-1 Preparing a Sitz Bath

Purpose
To facilitate healing through the application of moist heat.

Equipment
- Sitz bath tub/toilet insert with water receptacle
- Medications to be added to water or saline, as ordered
- Towels for drying the perineal area after the treatment
- Clean perineal pad to be applied after the treatment

Steps
1. Explain the procedure to the patient to ensure she understands that a sitz bath is a method for applying moist heat to the perineum to facilitate healing and comfort.
2. Wash your hands, identify the patient, and explain the procedure.

(continued)

Procedure 12-1 (Continued)

3. Assess the patient to confirm that she is able to ambulate to the bathroom.

4. Assemble equipment and ensure that all equipment is clean.

5. Raise the toilet seat in the patient's bathroom.

6. Insert the sitz bath apparatus into the toilet. The overflow opening should be directed toward the back of the toilet.

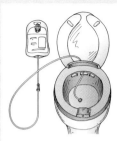

7. Fill the collecting bag with water or saline, as directed, at the appropriate temperature (105°F [41°C]).

8. Test the water temperature. It should feel comfortably warm on the wrist.

9. If prescribed, add medications to the solution.

10. Hang the bag overhead to allow a steady stream of water to flow from the bag, through the tubing, and into the reservoir.

11. Assist the ambulating patient to the bathroom. Help with removal of the perineal pad from front to back. Assist the patient to sit in the basin.

12. Instruct the patient to use the tubing clamp to regulate the flow of water. Ensure that the patient is adequately covered with a robe or blankets to prevent chilling.

13. Verify that the call bell is within reach and provide for privacy.

14. Encourage the patient to remain in the sitz bath for approximately 20 minutes.

15. Provide assistance with drying the perineal area and applying a clean perineal pad by grasping the pad by the ends or bottom side.

Procedure 12-1 (Continued)

16. Assist the patient back to the room.
17. Assess the patient's response to the procedure. Reinforce teaching about continued perineal care at home.
18. Document procedure and patient's response.

Clinical Alert The warm environment associated with a sitz bath may cause the patient to feel light-headed or dizzy. It is important to monitor the patient frequently throughout the intervention to ensure safety and tolerance.

Teach the Patient

1. The benefits of using the sitz bath, which include enhanced hygiene, comfort, and improved circulation
2. To use the sitz bath as often as recommended— usually three to four times per day or as needed for discomfort
3. To contact the nursing staff immediately if she becomes light-headed or dizzy
4. To check the temperature of the solution before use. Applying water or solution that is too warm may result in local trauma or burns to the area

Note

If the patient prefers to prepare a sitz bath in the tub at home, she should be instructed not to use the same water for bathing. Instead, fresh water should be drawn for washing to diminish the potential for infection.

Caution

The nurse must check the temperature of the water before administration of the sitz bath to ensure that it is not too warm.

ETHNOCULTURAL CONSIDERATIONS

Pregnancy-Related Skin Changes in the Puerperium

Although abdominal stretch marks (striae gravidarum) appear more pronounced immediately after childbirth, they tend to fade over the following 6 months. In Caucasian women, striae become pale and white in color; in African American women, they will appear as a slightly darker pigment.

Cultural Influences and Interventions for Breastfeeding Discomfort

Many non-Western cultures such as Asian, Latin, and African cultures embrace a hot and cold "humoral theory." Breastfeeding mothers from these cultures may choose not to use a cold modality for the relief of breast engorgement or discomfort. Although the nurse may explain the clinical rationale for applying ice packs to the breasts, the patient is culturally bound to adhere to her beliefs. Nurses must remain sensitive to culturally influenced customs and allow patients to use relief measures that do not conflict with their personal beliefs.

TEACHING THE FAMILY

Perineal Care

To enhance the patient's understanding about proper perineal care, provide the following instructions:

- Fill the squeeze/peri bottle with warm tap water (comfortable to your wrist).
- Sit on the toilet with the bottle positioned between your legs. Aim the bottle opening at your perineum and spray so that the water moves from front to back. Do not separate the labia and do not spray the water into your vagina. Empty the entire bottle over the perineum (takes about 2 minutes).
- Gently pat the area dry with toilet paper or cotton wipes. Move from front to back. Use each wipe once and drop into toilet.
- Grasp the bottom side or ends of a clean perineal pad and apply it from front to back.

Pain Relief Measures

- Suggest nonpharmacological methods for pain relief such as imagery, therapeutic touch, relaxation, distraction, and interaction with the infant.
- Provide pain relief by administering prescribed agents such as ibuprofen, propoxyphene napsylate/acetaminophen (Darvocet-N), or oxycodone/acetaminophen (Percocet).
- Suggest over-the-counter medications and alternative therapies such as tea tree oil for self-care after hospital discharge.

- Teach the patient that medications such as acetaminophen or ibuprofen may be equally as effective as narcotic analgesics.
- Reassure the patient that the pain and discomfort should not persist beyond 5 to 7 days, and that because the episiotomy sutures are made of an absorbable material, they will not need to be removed.
  - Instruct breastfeeding mothers to wash the nipples with warm water.
  - Avoid soaps because they have a drying effect and cause cracked nipples.
  - Avoid breast creams because they block the natural oil secreted by the Montgomery tubercles and may contain alcohol.
  - Avoid creams or oils that contain vitamin E because the infant may absorb toxic amounts of the fat-soluble vitamin.

Storage of Breast Milk

Freshly pumped breast milk can be safely stored:

- At room temperature for 4 hours
- Refrigerated at 34 to 39° F (0°C) for 5 to 7 days after collection
- Frozen at 0°F (−19°C) for 6 to 12 months (Lawrence & Lawrence, 2005)

Manual (Hand) and Electric Expression of Breast Milk

- Sometimes necessary due to medical complications or occupational reasons
- Frequent expression of breast milk during the early postpartum period helps to establish and increase the milk supply for later breastfeeding needs
- Once lactation is established, the mother may express milk either manually or with an electric breast pump, whichever method is most convenient

Preventing Infant Nipple Confusion

- The infant exhibits difficulty with latch-on.
- Teach parents to avoid bottles until breast feeding is well established (3 to 4 weeks).

Preparing Infant Formula

Provide the following safety instructions to parents who plan to formula feed their infant:

- Wash hands before beginning to prepare formula and after any interruptions.
- Always shake and wash tops of liquid formula cans before opening.
- Reconstitute the formula according to the manufacturer's recommendations.
- Store the ready-to-feed formula according to the manufacturer's recommendations.
- Shake the bottle well before feeding.
- Discard any formula that the infant does not drink.
- Wash thoroughly and sterilize all equipment used to prepare the infant formula and use a bottle and nipple brush to remove milk residue.
- Replace the nipples regularly.

Helping Older Siblings Adjust to the New Baby

- Talk with the child(ren) about their feelings regarding the new baby. Listen and validate their feelings.
- Teach the older sibling how to play with the new baby; encourage gentleness.
- Help develop the child's self-esteem by giving him/her special jobs (e.g., bringing the diaper when you are changing the baby). Praise each contribution.
- Praise age-appropriate behaviors and do not criticize regressive behaviors.
- Set aside time to be alone with the older sibling and remind him that he is loved very much.

Warning Signs Indicative of Poor Sibling Adjustment
Professional help may be needed if the child:

- Continually avoids or ignores the baby
- Shows the baby no affection
- Is consistently angry, taunting, or demonstrating aggressive behavior toward the baby or other family members
- Experiences nightmares and sleeping difficulties (International Childbirth Education Association [ICEA], 2003)

Maternal Mood Changes During the Postpartal Period

Teach the mother and her partner that:

- Emotional changes (e.g., sadness, weepiness) often appear on the second or third postpartal day
- "Mood swings" and periods of unexpected crying or anxiety occur in 70%–80% of postpartal women
- The health care provider should be contacted if the following symptoms persist for more than 2 weeks:
  - Crying excessively
  - Significant changes in appetite
  - Feeling helpless
  - Experiencing extreme worry, concern
  - Difficulty sleeping or wanting to sleep all of the time
  - Inability to care for self or for the baby
  - Experiencing panic attack(s)
  - Experiencing a fear of harming self or the baby

ADDITIONAL INFORMATION FOR THE CLINICAL SETTING

Actions to Protect the Infant from Abduction

- Educate personnel, parents, and significant others about various measures that have been implemented to protect the safety of the infant.
- During infant transport from the nursery to the mother's room, all staff must follow the hospital's protocol. In most facilities:
  - Infants may be transported only in a bassinet.
  - Parents are prohibited from carrying the infant in the halls.
  - When identification bracelets are used, they are matched before giving the infant to the mother.
- Instruct mothers to release the infant only to properly identified hospital personnel.
- Ensure that admission photographs and footprints, most likely taken after birth, are affixed to the permanent record
- Follow institutional protocol for infants that have a similar or same last name: frequently, the infants' cribs

and charts indicate the mother's first name, and bear a label that designates a "NAME ALERT."

- Follow institutional protocol for multiple births: the infants' cribs may be labeled with the infant's name followed by a letter of the alphabet (i.e., A, B, C, or D).
- Ensure that all hospital personnel follow institutional identification protocol: prominently displayed photo identification when working in the maternal–child unit; freedom to question any suspicious activity or individuals who are present on the maternal–child unit.
- Ensure that all visitors follow institutional identification protocol: prominently displayed identification badges while on the maternal–child unit.

Postpartum Discharge Teaching: Danger Signs to Report

Alert patients to signs and symptoms to report to the health care provider. Ensure that the patient is given written information and knows how to reach her care provider. She should immediately report any of the following:

- Temperature >100.4°F (38.0°C), chills, or flu-like symptoms
- Abdominal incision that is red, tender to touch, or painful, or if edges of the incision have separated.
- Difficulty initiating urination, urinary frequency, or painful urination
- Increased vaginal bleeding with or without clots, or foul-smelling vaginal discharge
- Persistent pain or marked swelling at the site of a perineal laceration or episiotomy
- Swelling or masses in the breasts; red streaks; shooting pain in the breasts; or cracked, bleeding nipples.
- Swelling, warmth, tenderness, or painful areas in the legs
- Blurred vision or persistent headache that is not relieved by pain medication
- Overwhelming feelings of sadness or an inability to care for self or the baby

RESOURCES

American Academy of Pediatrics (AAP):
http://www.aap.org/healthtopics/breastfeeding.cfm

American College of Obstetricians and Gynecologists (ACOG):
http://www.acog.org/navbar/current/publications.cfm

Association of Women's Health, Obstetric and Neonatal Nurses
(AWHONN): http://awhonn.org/awhonn/

International Childbirth Education Association (ICEA):
http://icea.org/

Lactation Education Resources: http://www.leron-line.com/

La Leche League International:
http://www.lalecheleague.org/philosophy.html

REFERENCES

Deglin, J.H., & Vallerand, A.H. (2009). *Davis's drug guide for nurses* (11th ed.). Philadelphia: F.A. Davis.

International Childbirth Education Association (ICEA). (2003). *Siblings and the new baby.* (Brochure). Minneapolis, MN: Author.

Lawrence, R., & Lawrence, R. (2005). *Breastfeeding: A guide for the medical profession* (6th ed.). Philadelphia: Elsevier Mosby.

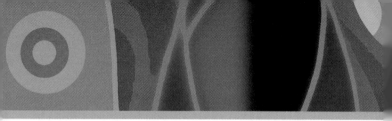

13

Caring for the Woman Experiencing Complications During the Postpartal Period

KEY TERMS

endometritis – Postpartum uterine infection

hematoma – Collection of blood in tissue; results from damage to a blood vessel

Homans' sign – Early sign of deep venous thrombosis in the leg – upon dorsiflexion, pain occurs from inflammation of the blood vessel. A negative Homans' sign does not rule out deep venous thrombosis.

magnetic resonance imaging (MRI) – Diagnostic test that uses electromagnetic energy to provide images of the heart, large blood vessels, brain, and soft tissues. In obstetrics, may be used to evaluate fetal structures, the placenta, and amniotic fluid volume.

mastitis – Infection in a breast; typically characterized by redness and tenderness in the affected breast along with influenza-like symptoms

postpartum – Occurring after birth (mother)

p. depression Symptoms including depressed mood or decreased interest in previously enjoyable activities, occurring within 6 months after giving birth and lasting longer than postpartum blues.

p. hemorrhage Excessive bleeding after childbirth; traditionally defined as a blood loss greater than 500 mL after a vaginal birth and 1000 mL or more after a cesarean birth.

p. psychosis Rare, severe form of mental illness; symptoms begin as postpartum blues or depression. However, distinguishing signs of psychosis, including hallucinations, delusions, agitation, confusion, and suicidal and homicidal thoughts can occur.

thrombophlebitis – Obstruction of a vein with secondary clot formation

thrombosis – Formation or presence of a blood clot within the vascular system

FOCUSED ASSESSMENT

Postpartum Hemorrhage (PPH)

Early hemorrhage: Occurs within first 24 hours after birth
Late hemorrhage: Occurs more than 24 hours after birth but <6 weeks postpartum

Early Postpartum Hemorrhage

Acronyms for Causes of Early Postpartum Hemorrhage	
"LARRY" (common causes of PPH)	**"4 T's" (factors associated with PPH)**
L: Lacerations	**T:** Tone (uterine)
A: Atony	**T:** Trauma (genital tract)
R: Retained placental tissue	**T:** Tissue (retained placenta)
R: Ruptured uterus	**T:** Thrombin (maternal coagulation disorders)
Y: "You pulled too hard on the cord!"	

Using a Standardized Assessment for Blood Loss After Childbirth

- Scant: Peripad blood stain <2 inches (<10 mL) within 1 hour
- Small: Peripad blood stain >2 inches, >4 inches (10–25 mL) within 1 hour
- Moderate: Peripad blood stain >4 inches but <6 inches (25–50 mL) within 1 hour
- Large: Peripad blood stain >6 inches to saturated peripad (50–80 mL) within 1 hour (Lugenbiehl et al., 1990)

Characteristics that Point to the Source of Postpartal Bleeding

Source	Color	Uterus
Uterine Atony	Dark red with clots	Soft/boggy
Retained Placenta	Dark red with clots	Soft/boggy
Lacerations of Cervix or Vagina	Bright red	Firm, contracted

Risk Factors for Uterine Atony

Uterine overdistention
  Large baby
  Multiple gestation
  Hydramnios
Bladder distention
Prolonged first and/or second stage labor
Precipitous labor

Labor induction/augmentation with Pitocin
Tocolytic therapy (especially with magnesium sulfate)
High parity
Retained placental fragments
Halogenated anesthetic agents
Prolonged/mismanaged third stage of labor

If hemorrhage results from uterine atony, perform continual fundal massage with lower uterine segment support.

Procedure 13-1 Performing Fundal Massage

Purpose

Fundal massage is used as an emergency measure to contract the uterus that is soft and boggy due to atony. It is performed to promote uterine tone and consistency and minimize the risk of hemorrhage. Uterine atony may result from prolonged labor, rapid or precipitous labor and birth, high parity, medications during labor (i.e., oxytocin, magnesium sulfate, inhalation anesthesia), intra-amniotic infection, operative delivery, and uterine overdistention from multiple gestation, hydramnios, or macrosomia.

Equipment

- Clean examination gloves
- Disposable cleansing wipes
- Two clean peripads

Procedure 13-1 (Continued)

Preexamination Preparation

1. Wash and dry hands; explain the procedure and its purpose to the patient. Ensure privacy.

2. Assemble necessary equipment, including clean examination gloves, disposable cleansing wipes, and clean peripads.

3. Ask the patient to void, unless fundal massage must be performed immediately due to excessive bleeding

4. Assist the woman to a supine position with the knees flexed and the feet placed together.

Steps

1. Don gloves, remove the peripad, and inspect the perineum. Observe the character and amount of drainage on the pad and the presence of clots. Apply a clean peripad.

2. Place one hand on the abdomen, just above the symphysis pubis.

3. Place the other hand around the top of the fundus.

4. With the lower hand maintained in a stable position, rotate the upper hand and massage the uterus until it is firm. Avoid overmassaging the uterus. Massaging a firm uterus may result in muscle fatigue and uterine relaxation. Overly aggressive fundal massage may result in uterine prolapse.

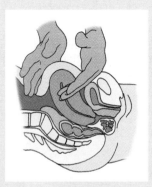

(continued)

Procedure 13-1 (Continued)

5. Once the uterus has become firm, *gently* press the fundus between the hands. Apply a slight downward pressure against the lower hand.

6. Observe the perineum for the passage of clots and the amount of bleeding.

7. Once the uterus remains firm, cleanse the perineum and apply a clean peripad. Dispose of the soiled gloves and pads according to institutional policy.

8. Document the findings. Continue to assess the fundus and vaginal drainage according to institutional protocol. Alert the physician or nurse midwife if the fundus does not remain contracted or if bleeding persists.

Risk Factors for Postpartum Hemorrhage from Tissue Trauma

- Rapid second stage labor
- Rapid/precipitous labor (<3 hours from onset to birth)
- Operative vaginal deliveries (forceps, vacuum extraction)
- Fetal manipulation (extrauterine or intrauterine version, corkscrew maneuver for shoulder dystocia [corkscrew maneuver: a progressive 180 degree manual rotation of the baby's posterior shoulder to release the impacted anterior shoulder])
- Large episiotomy, including extension
- Large infant
- Cesarean birth
- Uterine rupture (increased incidence with previous uterine surgery, tetanic contractions, labor stimulation, versions, placental attachment abnormalities)

Source: Cunningham et al. (2005).

CLINICAL ALERTS

Postpartal Blood Loss and Vital Signs

In the presence of a firm uterus, continuous vaginal bleeding in a slow but steady trickle, with or without clots, can result in significant blood loss. Normal physiological adaptations in pregnancy mean that a large loss of blood can occur before changes in vital signs (decreased blood pressure and increased pulse) are evident. The usual signs of shock (restlessness, anxiety, pallor, cool, clammy skin, increased pulse, tachypnea, shaking, decreased blood pressure) may not be evident until 30% to 40% of the patient's total circulating blood volume has been lost. A decrease in the mean arterial pressure (MAP) measurement may be the first indicator of hypovolemia. The lack of objective signs and symptoms may lead to a delay in treatment.

Postpartal Blood Loss and the Behavioral Assessment

Assess the patient for:

- Restlessness
- Level of consciousness
- Vague complaints
- Level of pain

Immediate Intervention for Uterine Atony

As soon as excessive blood loss is noted, begin fundal massage. Support the lower uterine segment by placing a hand in a slight "C" position just above the symphysis pubis. Do not express clots if the uterus does not become firm with massage. The clots may protect the patient from an even greater blood loss.

Lacerations of the Cervix or Vaginal Canal

Lacerations are usually internal and are not visible when the nurse examines the perineum. Identifying either a vaginal wall or cervical laceration usually requires that the physician or midwife examine the patient while she is in the lithotomy position. Often the physician locates and repairs a laceration before the patient's transfer to the postpartum unit.

Hematoma

- May cause excessive blood loss and severe discomfort and tenderness
- Occurs most frequently in the vulva; also occurs in the vagina and retroperitoneal area (Figs. 13-1 and 13-2).
- Risk factors
  - Genital tract lacerations

- Episiotomy
- Operative vaginal delivery
- Difficult or prolonged second stage of labor
- Nulliparity
- Examination may reveal discoloration, bulging of tissue at hematoma site
- Treatment: ice (first 24 hours); sitz baths (after 24 hours); analgesics; may require incision and drainage (if larger than 5 cm)

Late Postpartum Hemorrhage

- Causes
  - Retained placental fragments
  - Subinvolution
  - Uterine infection

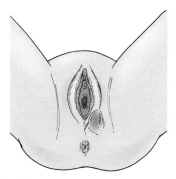

Figure 13-1 Vulvar hematoma.

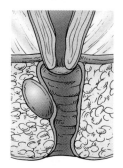

Figure 13-2 Vaginal wall hematoma.

- Treatment
  - Ergonovine medication (Ergotrate; methergine)
  - Antibiotics
  - Dilation and curettage

Postpartum Infection

May involve:

- Endometrium (endometritis)
- Operative wound (cesarean incision; episiotomy)
- Urinary tract
- Breasts (mastitis) (Fig. 13-3)
- Septic pelvic thrombophlebitis

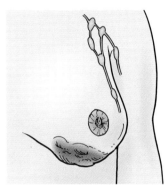

Figure 13-3 Mastitis.

Postpartum Infection: Endometritis

Type of Infection	Risk Factors	Onset	Signs and Symptoms	Causative Organisms	Diagnosis Based on	Collaborative Treatment	Prognosis and Complications
Endometritis (inflammation and infection of the inner lining of the uterus) Incidence: Vaginal birth: 1%–3% and cesarean birth 10%–20% (Kennedy, 2005)	Cesarean birth Prolonged rupture of the membranes, multiple vaginal examinations, internal electronic fetal heart rate (FHR) monitoring, low socio-economic status, poor nutrition, young age, diabetes, prior genital infection, lapse in aseptic technique, anemia, smoking, nulliparity, operative vaginal delivery, poor postpartum perineal care	2–4 days following childbirth	Prolonged fever ≥100.4°F (38°C), foul smelling lochia, uterine or abdominal tenderness, chills, poor appetite, malaise, increased pulse rate, cramping pain, increased WBC count (above 20–30,000)	Normal vaginal flora and enteric bacteria	Clinical signs and symptoms Vaginal and bimanual examination Laboratory test results: Culture of lochia; elevated WBC count (Must also rule out urinary tract infection.)	1. MD/CNM: Order antibiotics. 2. Treat symptoms: a. Rest b. Antipyretics c. Increase fluid intake. d. Encourage high-protein, high-vitamin C foods. e. Promote uterine drainage via ambulation and Fowler's position. f. Instruct in perineal care. 3. Explain treatments to patient/family.	90%–95% improvement within 48–72 hours after treatment. May be discharged on oral antibiotics. *Complication:* Extension of infections via lymphatic system to connective tissues (pelvic infection) Dehiscence of cesarean section incision or episiotomy Peritonitis

4. Home antibiotic therapy may need to be arranged with follow-up by a home care nurse.
5. Promote infant attachment.

Sources: The American Academy of Pediatrics (AAP) & The American College of Obstetricians and Gynecologists (ACOG), 2007; Cunningham et al. (2005); Gibbs, Sweet, & Duff (2004); Kennedy (2007).

Postpartum Infection: Wound Infections

Type of Infection	Risk Factors	Onset	Signs and Symptoms for ALL	Causative Organisms	Diagnosis Based on	Collaborative Treatment	Prognosis and Complications
Wound Infections *Perineal* Incidence: 0.35%–10% *Cesarean incision* Incidence: 3%–5%	Endometritis (infected lochia), poor hygiene, fecal contamination, hematoma ALL wound infections: obesity, diabetes, hypertension, immunosuppression, malnutrition, anemia, hemorrhage, prolonged labor, chorioamnionitis prolonged rupture of membranes, hematoma	Early: 48 hours Late: 6–8 days	Pain, foul-smelling discharge, edema, low-grade fever Sudden chills, high fever, abdominal tenderness, erythema, edema, warmth of incision, drainage from the incision	Polymicrobial, normal vaginal flora *Staphylococcus aureus*, aerobic streptococci, aerobic and anaerobic bacilli	Clinical signs and symptoms, subjective complaints Clinical signs and symptoms, along with a poor response to antibiotics given for endometritis. Laboratory test results: elevated white blood cell (WBC) count	1. Antibiotics per order 2. May require incision and drainage with placement of drain to facilitate healing by secondary intention.* If packing has been placed in the wound to keep it open and maintain drainage, alert the patient to exercise caution when changing her perineal pads to avoid dislodging the packing. 3. Perineal: Sitz baths; instruct in perineal care	Improvement usually within 24–48 hours; may require long-term antibiotic therapy **Complications** Necrotizing fasciitis, abscess, wound dehiscence

4. Cesarean: Wet to dry dressing changes 3+ times/day
5. Pain medication per order (usually nonsteroidal anti-inflammatory drugs [NSAIDs])
6. Instructions to patient and family about wound care
7. Possible referral for home health or community health nurse visits

*Secondary intention: Healing from the inside of the wound out to the skin.

Sources: Cunningham et al. (2005); Franzblau & Witt (2006); Gibbs, Sweet, & Duff (2004); Kennedy (2007).

Postpartum Infection: Urinary Tract Infections (UTI)

Type of Infection	Risk Factors	Onset	Signs and Symptoms	Causative Organisms	Diagnosis Based on	Collaborative Treatment	Prognosis and Complications
Urinary Tract Infections Incidence: 2%–4%	Catheterization, multiple vaginal exams, poor postpartum hygiene, genital tract trauma, epidural anesthesia, cesarean birth, premature rupture of the membranes, poor nutritional status, history of UTIs during pregnancy, diabetes, decreased bladder sensation after birth	Any time during pregnancy or after birth	May have none. Dysuria (painful urination), frequency, burning on urination, difficulty voiding and/or retention, costovertebral angle tenderness (CVAT), back or suprapubic pain, hematuria (blood in the urine); fever, fatigue, nausea, vomiting	Most common: *Escherichia coli* (60%–90% of all UTIs); *Proteus mirabilis; Klebsiella pneumoniae,* group B hemolytic streptococcus, *Staphylococcus saprophyticus*	Clinical signs and symptoms Laboratory test results: urine culture & sensitivity, presence of leukocytes and blood on urine dipstick	1. Antibiotics per order (usually sulfonamides, aminopenicillins, anti-infectives, nitrofurantoin, or cephalosporins × 3 to 10 days depending on symptoms). Teach importance of taking all medication. 2. Encourage increased fluid intake, including cranberry juice. 3. Encourage rest. 4. Instruct in perineal care.	Improvement within 48–72 hours after initiation of antibiotic therapy Can reoccur with bacteremia and scarring of the kidney followed by hypertension and kidney damage.

5. Instruct in monitoring temperature, bladder function, normal appearance of urine.
6. Instruct in/administer antipyretics, antispasmodics, analgesics, and antiemetics.
7. Educate the patient to avoid recurrence:
   - When intercourse resumes, void following
   - Clean from front to back

Data from Cunningham et al. (2005); Franzblau & Witt (2006); Kennedy (2007).

Postpartum Infection: Mastitis

Type of Infection	Risk Factors	Onset	Signs and Symptoms	Causative Organisms	Diagnosis Based on	Collaborative Treatment	Prognosis and Complications
Mastitis	Milk stasis, plugged milk duct, infrequent breastfeeding, fatigue, nipple trauma, primiparity	3–4 weeks postpartum	Warm, tender, hardened area on breast (usually only one), enlarged axillary lymph nodes, fever (up to 102°F [38.9°C]), chills, generalized aching, headache, malaise	Most common: *Staphylococcus aureus*; also: *Haemophilus parainfluenzae* (from infant's mouth and nose), *Candida albicans*, *Streptococcus viridans*	Clinical signs and symptoms Laboratory test results: culture of breast milk	1. Notify the MD/CNM. 2. Initiate antibiotics. 3. Continue breastfeeding or manual/electrical expression of milk to maintain lactation. May be instructed to discard the milk. 4. Promote rest. 5. Increase fluid intake. 6. Pump breast after infant feeding to ensure breast is empty. 7. Apply warm compress or ice to breast for comfort. 8. Administer antipyretics	Improvement within 24–48 hours after initiation of antibiotics *Complication:* Breast abscess If breast abscess occurs: Must discontinue breastfeeding on the affected side—may lead to decreased maternal–infant attachment, low self-esteem and feelings of disappointment and guilt.

9. Instruct in high-protein, high-vitamin C diet.
10. Educate regarding hygiene and prevention of future recurrence.
11. Assess the infant's mouth for signs of thrush (oral *Candida*), an overgrowth of fungal organisms related to the mother's antibiotic therapy.

Sources: Lawrence & Lawrence (2005); Mass (2004).

Postpartum Infection: Septic Pelvic Thrombophlebitis

Type of Infection	Risk Factors	Onset	Signs and Symptoms	Causative Organisms	Diagnosis Based on	Collaborative Treatment	Prognosis and Complications
Septic Pelvic Thrombophlebitis	Cesarean birth, genital tract lacerations, history of varicosities, immobility, operative vaginal delivery, prolonged labor, multiple vaginal exams	48 hours to 4–6 weeks post partum	Fever ≥ 102.2°F (39°C) with spikes after initiation of antibiotic therapy, abdominal and/or back pain, chills, increased pulse (resting tachycardia), few or absent bowel sounds	Normal vaginal flora and enteric bacteria—is usually an extension of endometritis	Clinical signs and symptoms. Pelvic CT or MRI to confirm the clinical picture. Laboratory test results: CBC; coagulation profile; blood chemistries	1. MD/CNM: prescribe antibiotics. 2. Add heparin therapy to increase APTT (activated partial thromboplastin time) to 1.5–2 times the normal value. 3. Rest in Fowler's position. 4. High-protein, high-vitamin C diet 5. Increased fluids 6. Comfort measures: Pain medications, antipyretics Complementary therapies: Heat, cold, relaxation, music, touch, etc. 8. Explain treatments. 9. Promote infant attachment.	Improvement usually within 48–72 hours of heparin initiation; may need to continue anticoagulant therapy for 6 months (7–10 days of heparin) followed by warfarin (Coumadin) *Complication:* Pulmonary embolism Possible decreased infant attachment; prolonged hospitalization

Sources: Cunningham et al. (2005); Franzblau & Witt (2006); Gibbs, Sweet, & Duff (2004).

Thrombophlebitis and Thrombosis

- Inflammation of the venous circulation and blood clot formation.
- Typically occurs in the lower extremities.
- Related to venous stasis and hypercoagulation associated with pregnancy.
- Early ambulation is key in prevention.
- Risk factors:
  - Smoking
  - Obesity
  - Age >35 years
  - Pregnancy-related complications (e.g., preeclampsia)
  - Immobility
  - Grand multiparity
  - Operative childbirth
  - Hemorrhage
  - Sepsis
  - Chronic health problems (e.g., inflammatory bowel disease, lupus erythematosus, varicose veins, factor V Leiden mutation)
  - History of DVT
- Symptoms may include tenderness, edema, redness, localized heat, decreased peripheral pulse, palpable cord, change in skin color, positive Homans' sign.
- Diagnosis with venous duplex ultrasonography (real-time imaging and Doppler flow studies); magnetic resonance imaging (MRI).
- Management:
  - Bedrest
  - Anticoagulation therapy (heparin; warfarin)
  - Analgesics
  - Elevation of affected extremity
  - Elastic support to affected leg
  - Increased fluid intake
  - Local application of moist, warm packs
- Nursing considerations:
  - Assess for bleeding.
  - Assess circulation to affected extremity.
  - Measure and document circumference to affected extremity.
  - Provide discharge teaching (e.g., medication side effects; avoidance of salicylic acid).

Recognizing Signs and Symptoms Indicative of DVT
Additional signs and symptoms that may be associated with DVT include elevated temperature, cough, tachycardia, hemoptysis, pleuritic chest pain and increasing apprehension. The presence of dyspnea and tachypnea may signal pulmonary embolism. Pulmonary embolism is a complication of DVT that occurs when part of a blood clot breaks away and travels to the pulmonary artery, where it occludes the vessel and obstructs blood flow to the lungs.

Clinical Alert
Avoid Extremity Massage When DVT Is Suspected
If DVT is present or suspected, it is essential to refrain from massaging the affected area. This action could loosen the clot and result in a pulmonary or cerebral embolism.

Postpartum Psychosocial Complications

May include:

- Postpartum blues (within first 2 weeks after childbirth; common; self-limiting)
- Postpartum depression (occurs in 8% to 15% of women; onset within the first year after childbirth; treated with psychotherapy, medications, and complementary therapies)
- Postpartum psychosis (rare, characterized by hallucinations, delusions, agitation, confusion, suicidal/homicidal thoughts, loss of touch with reality)

Signs and Symptoms of Postpartum Depression	
Decreased appetite	Excessive fears about the infant's health/safety
Insomnia or fragmented sleep	Hopelessness
Fatigue	Negativity
Inability to concentrate	Complaints about "loss of self" and a
Confusion	"sense of loneliness" (Clemmens
Withdrawal	et al., 2004)
Decreased self-esteem	Guilt
Suicidal thoughts	Decreased interest and functioning in
Infant neglect or abuse	both self and infant care

Data from Beck, Records, & Rice (2006); Clemmens, Driscoll, & Beck (2004); Franzblau (2006); Logsdon et al. (2005); Stoops & Mann (2004).

Recognizing Behavioral Cues that Signal Postpartum Psychosis
- Hyperactivity
- Agitation
- Confusion
- Suspiciousness
- Excessive complaints

DIAGNOSTIC TESTS

Tests to Help Identify a Postpartum Infection

- Complete blood count (CBC) with differential
- Blood cultures if sepsis is suspected
- Urinalysis with culture and sensitivity
- Cervical, uterine or wound culture as needed

Laboratory Findings with Disseminated Intravascular Coagulation (DIC)

- Low hemoglobin
- Low hematocrit
- Low platelets
- Elevated fibrin split/degradation products
- Low fibrinogen

MEDICATIONS

Medications and Nursing Considerations for Postpartum Hemorrhage

Name	Action	Dosage/Route	Contraindications	Nursing Considerations
Oxytocin (Pitocin)	Stimulates uterine smooth muscle and produces contractions similar to those that occur during spontaneous labor.	10 units IM if no IV access; 10–40 units in 1000 cc crystalloid IV fluid (lactated Ringer's or normal saline)	Hypersensitivity	Monitor uterine response. DO NOT administer a bolus of undiluted oxytocin, as it can cause hypotension and cardiac arrhythmias. Consider administration of pain medication for uterine cramping.
Methylergonovine (Methergine)	Causes uterine contractions by stimulating uterine and vascular smooth muscles.	0.1–0.2 mg IM followed by 0.2 mg PO q4–6hr × 24 hours	Hypersensitivity History of, or current elevation of blood pressure	Keep refrigerated. DO NOT add it to IV solutions or mix in a syringe with other medications.
Carboprost* (Hemabate)	Stimulates contractions of the myometrium.	250 mcg IM or directly into the uterus (by MD or CNM); may repeat dosage	Asthma or glaucoma	Do not administer if patient demonstrates shock, as it will not be well absorbed. Keep refrigerated. This medication is VERY expensive.

| **Misoprostol (Cytotec)** | Acts as a prostaglandin analogue; stimulates powerful contractions of the myometrium. | 400–1000 mcg rectally | Hypersensitivity to prostaglandins | Stable at room temperature Rectal absorption is likely slower than IV medication. Monitor uterine response. Note: Misoprostol is neither marketed by its manufacturer for obstetrical use nor approved by the FDA for obstetrical use although its effectiveness in abating postpartum hemorrhage is now generally accepted. |

*Eighty to ninety percent effective in stopping postpartum hemorrhage when unresponsive to Pitocin or Methergine (Smith & Brennen, 2006).

Sources: Adams, Josephson, & Holland (2005); Cunningham et al., (2005); Smith & Brennan (2006); Tucker (2004); Walters & Wing (2007).

MEDICATIONS

Herbal Medication: Echinacea Purpurea (Ek-i-**neigh**-sha)

Pregnancy Category Injectable form not recommended during pregnancy

Indications Treatment of wounds, injuries, enlarged lymph nodes; prevent and reduce symptoms and duration of common cold and bacterial infections of the upper respiratory tract; used by Native Americans to treat burns and insect and rattlesnake bites

Actions Boosts the immune system by increasing phagocytosis of the WBCs and by inhibiting the bacterial enzyme, hyaluronidase; also stimulates the production of interleukin and interferon; exerts an anti-inflammatory action

Therapeutic Effects Used by proponents to both prevent and treat infections; juice from leaves used as a supportive treatment for vaginal yeast infections; approved in Germany for treatment of the common cold and influenza

Contraindications and Precautions Herb–drug interactions with amiodarone, anabolic steroids, ketoconazole, methotrexate (possible increased hepatic toxicity)

  Possible exacerbation of autoimmune diseases (rheumatoid arthritis, lupus, multiple sclerosis, etc.) because of its immune system stimulation properties (no clinical evidence to support)

  Is a member of the daisy family: Possible cross-over allergic reaction

Adverse Reactions and Effects No toxicity noted with even extremely high doses of oral *Echinacea*; the most common side effects from oral form are gastrointestinal symptoms and increased urination. INJECTIONS: Side effects are short-term nausea, vomiting, shivering, headache, fever

Route and Dosage Tincture, oral, injection (dosage individualized)

Nursing Implications
  1. Be sure to ask every patient if she uses herbal remedies.
  2. Instruct the patient that daily dosages of *Echinacea* in an attempt to prevent infections may decrease the immunostimulating effects of this herb.
  3. Because the U.S. Food and Drug Administration (FDA) has not approved herbal treatments/remedies, encourage

the patient to be sure that she uses a reputable form of the herb to ensure its quality (Adams, Josephson, & Holland, 2005; Deglin & Vallerand, 2009; Lincoln & Kleiner, 2004).

Warfarin (**war**-fa-rin), Coumadin

Pregnancy Category X

Indications Prevention of thrombosis (clot) formation

Actions Inhibits the hepatic synthesis of coagulation factors II, VII, IX, and X; inhibits the action of vitamin K

Therapeutic Effects Used in patients who are at high risk for development of or who have a history of deep vein thrombosis or other thrombophilia (love of clot formation) conditions

Pharmacokinetics 99% binds to plasma proteins, thereby delaying the effects of warfarin

Route and Dosage Orally; dosage adjusted on the basis of international normalized ratio (INR) results (range is 2.5–15 mg daily)

Contraindications and Precautions
   Drug–drug interactions occur with NSAIDs, diuretics, antidepressants, steroids, some antibiotics, vaccines, and vitamin K. Concurrent use with NSAIDs may increase the risk of bleeding.
   Herbal supplements such as garlic, ginger, and feverfew may increase the risk of bleeding.
   Arnica may increase the anticoagulant effect of warfarin.
   Even after the drug is discontinued, its effects may continue for up to 10 days.
   Warfarin dosage must be individualized on the basis of prothrombin time results. The INR is now used for dosage adjustments. A normal INR is 2.0–3.5.

Adverse Reactions and Effects Overdosage leads to excessive blood loss that may appear via gastrointestinal bleeding, bleeding from the gums, nosebleeds, petechiae, excessive bruising, etc. The patient begins with heparin therapy for anticoagulation and transitions to warfarin. Because normal clotting factors circulate in the patient's blood stream routinely, several days of both heparin and warfarin therapy may be required for the anti-coagulant effect.

Nursing Implications

1. This drug is dangerous. The patient and family must receive detailed information regarding follow-up care and drug–drug, drug–herb, and food–drug interactions.
2. Instruct the patient to notify the doctor of excessive bruising, to take warfarin at the same time each day, and to avoid activities that could result in a bleeding injury.
3. Be sure the patient receives instructions on foods to minimize/avoid. (Involve the dietitian.)

Data from Deglin, J.H., & Vallerand, A.H. (2009). Davis's Drug Guide for Nurses (11th ed.). Philadelphia: F.A. Davis.

Medications Used to Treat Postpartum Depression		
Selective Serotonin Reuptake Inhibitors (SSRIs)	Serotonin–Norepinephrine Reuptake Inhibitors (SNRIs)	Tricyclics Pamelor (Nortriptyline)
Fluoxetine (Prozac) Paroxetine (Paxil) Sertraline (Zoloft)	Venlafaxine (Effexor) Duloxetine (Cymbalta)	Imipramine (Tofranil) Doxepin (Sinequan)

TEACHING THE FAMILY

Educating Patients About Risk Factors for Puerperal Infection

- Alert the patient about antepartum or intrapartum events that are risk factors for postpartum infection.
- Alert the family to the importance of promptly notifying the health care provider if symptoms (e.g., low abdominal tenderness; fever; red vaginal drainage beyond 1 week; foul smelling vaginal drainage) occur.
- Inform the family about arrangements for a community health nurse visit after hospital discharge.

Educating Patients About the Prevention of Infection

Teach the patient to:

- Thoroughly wash her hands before and after using the toilet, when changing peripads, changing the baby's diaper, etc. Hand washing with friction removes infection-causing microorganisms.

- Use a squeeze bottle with warm water to cleanse the perineum, then pat the perineum dry, and remove and replace peripads from front to back. Front to back patting and pad removal/application prevents bringing rectal organisms forward to the perineum and vagina.

- Drink extra fluids (eight 8-ounce glasses of water) to increase urine production. The increased blood flow and urine production will decrease the stagnation of microorganisms in the urinary tract.

- Gently wash incisions with soap and water. Be sure to dry the incision completely. If necessary, use a hair dryer set on low heat to ensure that the incision is dry. A dry incision is less likely than a wet one to promote bacterial growth.

- Feed the infant every 2–3 hours and alternate feeding positions if breastfeeding. Be sure that the baby gets as much of the nipple and areola in his mouth as possible. These actions reduce the likelihood of injury to the nipple.

- Properly care for the nipples. For a breast infection to occur, a cracked or blistered nipple is necessary. Use lanolin, vitamin E, cod liver oil, or express breast milk and rub any of these into the nipple to help reduce soreness and to protect the nipple from trauma.

- Consider alternative therapies to boost the immune system (e.g., *Echinacea*)

- Notify the health care provider if pain, redness, or swelling at the site of any incision develop.

- Notify the health care provider if a fever of 100.4°F (38°C) or greater develops. (If breastfeeding, a temperature elevation to 100.4°F [38°C] may occur when the milk production begins) (Lincoln & Kleiner, 2004).

Teaching Patients About Aspirin and Anticoagulants

- Caution patients to avoid medications that contain aspirin (salicylic acid) because it prevents blood clotting and increases the risk of bleeding.

ADDITIONAL INFORMATION FOR THE CLINICAL SETTING

Nursing Actions for the Patient Experiencing Hemorrhage

- Monitor and record intake and output (indwelling urinary catheter).
- Weigh pads, linens, and other bloody items on a gram scale.
- Administer oxygen at 10 to 12 L/min according to institutional protocol.
- Obtain appropriate lab studies (e.g., complete blood count; prothrombin time; partial thromboplastin time; fibrinogen degradation products).
- Type and cross-match for replacement blood.
- Assess for indicators of disseminated intravascular coagulation (DIC).

Alternative Therapies for Postpartum Depression

- Hypnosis: Enhances relaxation and an ability to focus on daily tasks.
- Exercise: Increases levels of neurotransmitters that communicate with brain cells to increase feelings of euphoria.
- St. John's wort (*Hypericum perforatum*): Believed to bind with neuroreceptors in the brain to prevent a response to the "depression" neurotransmitters (Lincoln & Kleiner, 2004). Do not use in combination with SSRI antidepressants.
- Biofeedback: Promotes relaxation and decreases anxiety.
- Meditation: Helps the woman to focus on "being rather than doing," thereby relieving stress and tension.
- Humor: Has been shown to decrease anxiety, fear, tension, anger, and frustration and to stimulate the immune system.
- Acupuncture, aromatherapy, and massage: Additional complementary therapies that may also be beneficial.

RESOURCES

Centers for Disease Control and Injury (CDC), National Center for Injury Prevention and Control: http://www.cdc.gov/ncipc/

Family Violence Prevention Fund: www.endabuse.org

LaLeche League International:
http://www.lalecheleague.org/philosophy.html

National Center for Complementary and Alternative Medicine (NCCAM): http://info@nccam.nih.gov/

The National Women's Health Information Center:
http://www.forwoman.gov/faq/depression-pregnancy.cfm

REFERENCES

Adams, M.P., Josephson, D.L., & Holland, L.N. (2005). *Pharmacology for nurses: A pathophysiologic approach.* Upper Saddle River, NJ: Pearson Education.

American Academy of Pediatrics (AAP) & The American College of Obstetricians and Gynecologists (ACOG). (6th ed.) (2007). *Guidelines for perinatal care.* Washington, DC: Author.

Beck, C.T., Records, K., & Rice, M. (2006). Further development of the Postpartum Depression Predictors Inventory-Revised. *Journal of Obstetric, Gynecologic, & Neonatal Nursing, 35*(6), 735–745.

Clemmens, D., Driscoll, J.W., & Beck, C.T. (2004). Postpartum depression as profiled through the postpartum depression screening scale. *The American Journal of Maternal/Child Nursing, 29*(3), 180–185.

Cunningham, F., Leveno, K., Bloom, S., Hauth, J., Gilstrap, L., & Wenstrom, K.D. (2005). *Williams obstetrics* (22nd ed.). New York: McGraw-Hill.

Deglin, J.H., & Vallerand, A.H. (2009). *Davis's Drug Guide for Nurses* (11th ed.). Philadelphia: F.A. Davis.

Franzblau, N., & Witt, K. (June 26, 2006). Normal and abnormal puerperium. Retrieved from http://www.emedicine.com/med/topic3240.htm (Accessed April 18, 2009).

Gibbs, R., Sweet, R., & Duff, P. (2004). Maternal and fetal infectious disorders. In R. Creasy, R. Reznik, & J. Iams (eds.), *Maternal-fetal medicine: Principles and practice* (5th ed., pp. 955–986). Philadelphia: W.B. Saunders.

Kennedy, E. (August 8, 2007). Pregnancy, postpartum infections. Retrieved from http://www.emedicine.com/emerg/topic482.htm (Accessed April 18, 2009).

Lawrence, R., & Lawrence, R. (2005). *Breastfeeding: A guide for the medical profession* (6th ed.). Philadelphia: C.V. Mosby.

Lincoln, V., & Kleiner, K. (2004). Holistic health: Complementary thera-peutic disciplines and remedies. In M. Condon (Ed). *Women's health: An integrated approach to wellness and illness* (pp. 195–225). Upper Saddle River, NJ: Pearson Education.

Logsdon, M.C., Birkimer, J.C., Simpson, T., & Looney, S. (2005). Postpar-tum depression and social support in adolescents. *Journal of Obstetric, Gynecologic & Neonatal Nursing, 34*(1), 46–54.

Luegenbiehl, D.L., Brophy, G., Artigue, G., Phillips, K., & Flack, R. (1990). Standardized assessment of blood loss. *MCN: American Journal of Maternal-Child Nursing,* 15(4), 241–244.

Mass, S. (2004). Breast pain: Engorgement, nipple pain, and mastitis. *Clini-cal Obstetrics and Gynecology, 47*(3), 676–682.

Smith, J.R. & Brennan, B. (June 13, 2006). Postpartum hemorrhage. Retrieved from http://emedicine.com (Accessed April 18, 2009).

Stoops, J., & Mann, N. (2004). Psychological/emotional wellness and illness. In M. Condon (Ed). *Women's health: An integrated approach to wellness and illness* (pp. 538–556). Upper Saddle River, NJ: Pearson Education.

Tucker, M.E. (2004). Treat before hypotension occurs: Avoiding hysterec-tomy for postpartum hemorrhage. *OB GYN News, 39(11),* 22–23.

Walters, K.C., & Wing, D.A. (2007). Misoprostol and postpartum hemor-rhage. *The Female Patient, 32*(7), 53–60.

Physiological Transition of the Newborn

KEY TERMS

acrocyanosis – Peripheral cyanosis; bluish coloration of the hands and feet present in most infants at birth

apnea – Temporary cessation of breathing that lasts more than 20 seconds, associated with generalized cyanosis

bilirubin – Yellow-orange pigment that is a breakdown product of hemoglobin

brown adipose tissue (BAT) – Unique neonatal heat source that is capable of greater thermogenic activity than ordinary fat. Deposits are located around the adrenal glands, kidneys, neck, between the scapulas and behind the sternum. Also termed "brown fat."

hyperbilirubinemia – Elevation of unconjugated serum bilirubin concentrations

icteric – Yellow discoloration of the body tissues (skin, sclera, oral mucous membranes) caused by the deposit of bile pigments (unconjugated bilirubin); jaundice

immunity – Protection from diseases, especially infectious diseases

  acquired i. Immunity that results either from exposure to an antigen (response to the infection) or from the passive injection of immunoglobulins

  active i. Immunity that develops in response to actual infection or vaccination

  natural i. Immunity that is genetically determined in a specific species; the first line of defense

  passive i. Immunity that is acquired by the introduction of preformed antibodies into an unprotected individual

(e.g., maternal antibodies that pass to the fetus through the placenta)

insensible water loss (IWL) – Evaporative water loss that occurs mainly through the skin and respiratory tract

jaundice – Yellow discoloration of the body tissues (skin, sclera, oral mucous membranes) caused by the deposit of bile pigments (unconjugated bilirubin); icterus

kangaroo care – Skin-to-skin infant care; provides warmth to the infant

kernicterus – Bilirubin encephalopathy that involves the deposit of unconjugated bilirubin in brain cells. Results in neurological damage or death.

neutral thermal environment (NTE) – Range of temperature in which the newborn's body temperature can be maintained (at least 36.5°C) with minimal metabolic demands and oxygen consumption

nonshivering thermogenesis – Infant's method of producing heat from brown adipose tissue by increasing the metabolic rate

periodic breathing – Sporadic episodes of cessation of respirations for periods of 5 to 15 seconds, not associated with cyanosis

polycythemia – Increased number of erythrocytes per volume of blood

respiratory distress syndrome (RDS) – Developmental disorder that results from decreased pulmonary gas exchange leading to carbon dioxide retention (increased arterial Pco_2). In the neonate, most commonly associated with prematurity, perinatal asphyxia, and maternal diabetes mellitus. Also known as hyaline membrane disease.

surfactant – Phosphoprotein necessary for normal respiratory function; prevents alveolar collapse and permits reexpansion after exhalation

thermogenesis – Production of heat

FOCUSED ASSESSMENT

Adaptation of the Respiratory System

Initiation of the neonate's first breath influenced by:

- Internal stimuli
  - Chemical factors (hypercarbia, acidosis, hypoxia)

- External stimuli
  - Sensory factors (tactile, visual, auditory)
  - Thermal factors (cool air)
  - Mechanical factors (chest compression – "thoracic squeeze") (Fig. 14-1)

Factors that interfere with initiation and maintenance of respirations include:

- Prematurity
- Birth asphyxia
- Trauma
- Maternal medications
- Mode of birth

Recognizing Normal Neonatal Lung Sounds During Early Auscultation

The neonate's lung sounds may sound moist during early auscultation, but should become clear within the following 24 hours as the lung fluid is gradually absorbed into the lymphatic and circulatory systems.

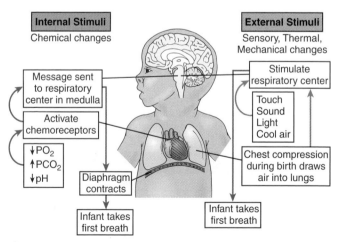

Figure 14-1 Internal and external factors involved in the initiation of respirations.

Cardiopulmonary Transitions

Conversion from fetal to newborn circulation: normal sequence of events (Fig. 14-2):

1. Air enters lungs, leading to increased P_{O_2} in the alveoli.
2. Relaxation of the pulmonary artery leads to decreased pulmonary vascular resistance.
3. Increased pulmonary blood flow leads to conversion to newborn circulation.

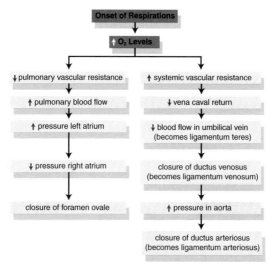

Figure 14-2 Major events that occur during the transition from fetal to neonatal circulation include closure of the foramen ovale, the ductus arteriosus, and the ductus venosus.

Structural Changes in Circulation After Birth		
Fetus	**Neonate**	**Mechanism**
Umbilical vein	Ligamentum teres	Constricts after placental separation.
Ductus venosus	Ligamentum venosum	Once the umbilical cord is clamped, cessation of umbilical venous blood return, along with mechanical pressure changes, lead to closure of the ductus venosus. Closure of the bypass route forces enhanced blood flow to the liver. Closure usually occurs by the end of the first week.

Fetus	Neonate	Mechanism
Foramen ovale	Closed atrial septum	Blood flow increases to the pulmonary veins, leading to increased left atrial pressure, which causes the foramen ovale flap to close. Fibrin and cells seal the shunt; it is physiologically closed by 1 month of age.
Ductus arteriosus	Ligamentum arteriosum	The pathway for most of the fetal blood due to the high pulmonary vascular resistance. Once the umbilical cord is clamped, placental blood flow ceases, and systemic blood pressure and vascular resistance increase. As the lungs oxygenate the blood, the increased Pao$_2$ stimulates the closure of the ductus arteriosus. Occurs within the first 72 hours of life.
Umbilical artery	Superior vesical (bladder) artery Lateral vesicoumbilical ligaments	Constricts after placental separation.

Thermogenic Adaptation

Mechanisms for Neonatal Heat Loss

Mechanism	Description	Nursing Actions
Evaporation	Heat loss when water is converted into a vapor.	Thoroughly dry the neonate immediately after birth, remove wet blankets, place hat on the head.
Conduction	Heat loss to a cooler surface by direct skin contact.	Place the infant on a pre-warmed radiant warmer, use warmed blankets, cover the scales with blankets before weighing, and avoid the use of cold instruments. The newborn can also be placed skin to skin with the mother to facilitate body warming and bonding (kangaroo care).
Convection	Heat loss from the warm body surface to the cooler air currents.	Prevent drafts in the birth area; place the newborn away from doors or windows; keep the neonate warmly clothed and possibly swaddled to prevent cooling from air currents.
Radiation	The transfer of heat between objects that are not in direct contact with one other (e.g., the walls of the nursery or the incubator)	Have a prewarmed radiant warmer present at the birth; avoid placing the crib or incubator by a cold window; and keep cold objects well away from the neonate.

Factors Related to Cold Stress

- Large body area in relation to body mass
- Limited subcutaneous fat
- Limited ability to shiver
- The skin is thin and the blood vessels are close to the body surface

Hematopoietic Adaptation

Changes in Hematopoietic Components	
Component	Change
Blood Volume	Approximately one half of the fetal blood volume is transferred from the placenta to the neonate by the end of the first minute of life.
Erythrocytes and Hemoglobin	Fetal RBCs have a shorter lifespan (90 days) than do adult RBCs, but carry 20%–50% more oxygen. The faster deterioration of fetal RBCs may cause physiological anemia of infancy and lead to higher bilirubin levels.
Platelets	Lack of vitamin K at birth places the neonate at risk for a blood clotting deficiency during the first few days of life.

Hepatic Adaptation

The liver is responsible for regulation of blood glucose, iron storage, bilirubin conjugation, and coagulation of the blood.

Risk Factors for Hypoglycemia in the Neonate

- Prematurity
- Postmaturity
- Intrauterine growth restriction (IUGR)
- Large or small for gestational age (LGA or SGA)
- Asphyxia
- Difficult transition at birth
- Cold stress
- Maternal diabetes
- Maternal intake of ritodrine (Yutopar) or terbutaline (Brethine)
- Infection

Conjugation of Bilirubin

1. Bilirubin is produced from hemolysis of erythrocytes (RBCs).

2. Reticuloendothelial system: Removes aging RBCs; converts hemoglobin to unconjugated bilirubin.
3. Bilirubin is transported via blood albumin to the liver.
4. In the liver, bilirubin is conjugated with glucuronic acid.
5. Resulting conjugated (direct) bilirubin is excreted into the common duct and duodenum.
6. Direct bilirubin is excreted in stools and urine (Fig. 14-3).

Factors that May Influence Bilirubin Levels in the Neonate

- Cultural background: Chinese, Japanese, Korean, and Native American neonates exhibit higher bilirubin levels than do European and American Caucasian neonates. The elevated levels of bilirubin persist for a longer period of time and cause no apparent adverse effects.
- Perinatal events (i.e., delayed cord cutting, breech presentation, the use of Pitocin)
- Prematurity
- Maternal diabetes

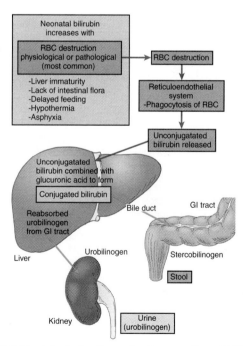

Figure 14-3 Physiological pathway for the excretion of bilirubin.

- Excess bilirubin production (e.g., hemolytic diseases such as Rh isoimmunization and ABO incompatibility; sepsis; metabolic disorders)
- Delayed feedings
- Liver immaturity (i.e., prematurity; glucose-6-phosphate dehydrogenase deficiency)
- Birth trauma
- Family history of jaundice or a previous child with jaundice
- Neonatal complications (i.e., asphyxia neonatorum, cold stress, hypoglycemia) (MacDonald, Mullett, & Seshia, 2005; Wong et al., 2006)

Types of Jaundice

Type	Definition	Comments
Physiological Jaundice (nonhemolytic)	Yellow tinge to skin and mucous membranes related to increased serum levels of unconjugated bilirubin	**Occurs in >60% term and >80% preterm newborns.** Typically occurs 24–48 hours after birth. Peaks between 5 and 7 days.
Pathological Jaundice (non-physiological jaundice)	Jaundice is usually noticeable within the first 24 hours of life. Caused by an abnormal condition such as Rh or ABO incompatibility. Results in bilirubin toxicity (i.e., kernicterus).	Total serum bilirubin (TSB) concentration increases by 5 mg/dL per day. Occurs within the first 24 hours of life. TSB >12.9 mg/dL in a term infant TSB >15 mg/dL in a preterm infant
Breastfeeding Jaundice (early onset)	Occurs between the 2nd and 4th days of life, peaks at 72 hours of life. Occurs when there is a decreased intake of breast milk and a decreased passage of meconium.	TSB peaks at 15–19 mg/dL by 72 hours of life. Believed to be associated with poor feeding practices, not related to the composition of the breast milk. Primary therapy centers on early and frequent feedings and avoidance of formula and glucose supplementation (Hertz, 2005).
Breast Milk Jaundice (late onset)	Typically occurs in the full term infant after the fifth day of life; peaks around day 10.	Infant thrives, stools appropriately, and gains weight. No evidence of hemolysis. Gradually declines over a few weeks.

Gastrointestinal Adaptation

- Bowel sounds are present within the first 15 to 30 minutes of life.
- First stool occurs within 8 to 24 hours of life (meconium).
- Stools may occur up to 10 times per day.
- Cardiac sphincter immature; regurgitation may occur after feedings.

Genitourinary Adaptation

Kidney Function

- The nephrons are fully functional by 34 to 36 weeks of gestation.
- The glomerular filtration rate is lower than that of the adult.
- There is a limited capacity for the reabsorption of HCO_3^- and H^+.
- Initially unable to dispose of fluid rapidly or to concentrate urine.
- Most newborns void immediately after birth; some may not void for up to 24 hours.

Immunological Adaptation

Recognizing and Preventing Newborn Infections	
Signs and Symptoms of Infection	**Nursing Interventions**
Subtle behavior changes Poor feeding patterns Respiratory distress Hypothermia	Maintain skin integrity. Assess for potential risk factors (e.g., maternal group B *Streptococcus* exposure). Assess all breaks in skin integrity (e.g., circumcision site, heel sticks, umbilical stump). Provide parents with thorough discharge instructions regarding infant hygiene, proper skin care, awareness of signs and symptoms of infection.

Psychosocial Adaptation

Early Stages of Activity	
Period	**Description**
First Period of Reactivity	First period of active, alert wakefulness displayed immediately after birth Rapid heart rate and respirations Increased muscle tone and activity Decreased body temperature Absent bowel sounds May last from 30 minutes to 2 hours Excellent time to initiate breastfeeding
Period of Inactivity and Sleep	Follows the first period of reactivity Decreased muscle activity Difficult to awaken Heart rate and respirations return to a normal range May last up to 4 hours
Second Period of Reactivity	Newborn becomes alert once again. Most infants show signs for feeding readiness. Infant becomes more responsive to stimulation. Lability in heart rate and respirations is common. Bowel sounds are usually present.

Newborn Behavioral States	
Sleep States	Sleep occurs in intervals of approximately 50 minutes.
Deep/Quiet	45% of sleep is "quiet" sleep.
Rapid Eye Movement (REM)	Approximately one half of the infant's total sleep is "active" (REM) sleep.
Alert States	
Drowsy/Semidozing	Open or closed eyes, fluttering eyelids; semidozing appearance; and slow, regular movement of the extremities. There is a delayed response to external stimuli.
Wide Awake	The infant is alert and follows and fixates on attractive objects, faces, or auditory stimuli. There is minimal motor activity and a delayed response to external stimuli.

Alert States	
Active Awake	The eyes are open; motor activity is intense, and the infant displays thrusting movements of the extremities. Environmental stimuli increase the motor activity.
Crying	Jerky movements accompany intense crying. Crying often serves as a distraction from unpleasant stimuli such as hunger and pain; it allows the infant to discharge energy and elicits a helpful response from the parents.

CLINICAL ALERT

Recognizing Hypoglycemia in the Neonate

When assessing the neonate during the transitional period, be alert to signs and symptoms of hypoglycemia: jitteriness; diaphoresis; poor muscle tone; poor sucking reflex; temperature instability (low temperature); respiratory distress; tachycardia; dyspnea; apnea; high-pitched cry; irritability; lethargy; and seizures or coma. Awareness of prenatal and perinatal risk factors that may predispose to postnatal hypoglycemia is essential as the infant may be asymptomatic.

DIAGNOSTIC TESTS

Laboratory Values for the Normal Term Neonate – Blood	
Blood Component	**Normal Range**
Albumin	3.6–5.4 g/dL
Amylase	0–1000 IU/hr
Bicarbonate	20–26 mmol/L
Bilirubin, direct	<0.5 mg/dL
Bilirubin, total	<2.8 mg/dL (cord blood)
0–1 days	2.6 mg/dL (peripheral blood)
1–2 days	6–7 mg/dL (peripheral blood)
3–5 days	4–6 mg/dL (peripheral blood)
Bleeding time	2 Minutes

(continued)

Laboratory Values for the Normal Term Neonate – Blood (Continued)

Blood Component	Normal Range
Arterial blood gases	
pH	7.35–7.45
$Paco_2$	35–45 mm Hg
Pao_2	50–90 mm Hg
Venous blood gases	
pH	7.35–7.45
$Paco_2$	41–51 mm Hg
Pao_2	20–49 mm Hg
Calcium, ionized	2.5–5 mg/dL
Calcium, total	7–12 mg/dL
Glucose	30–125 mg/dL
Hematocrit	48%–64%
	53% (cord blood)
Hemoglobin	17–18.4 g/dL
	16.8 g/dL (cord blood)
Platelets	150,000 – 300,000/mm³
Immunoglobulins, total	660–1439 mg/dL
Iron	100–250 mcg/dL
Red blood cell count	4,800,000–7,100,000/mm³
White blood cell count	9000–30,000/mm³

Sources: Nettina (2007); Pagana & Pagana (2006).

Laboratory Values for the Normal Term Neonate – Urine

Urine Component	Normal Range
Casts, WBC	Normal to be present for the first 2–4 days
Osmolality (maximum concentration ability)	800 mOsmol/L
(Maximum diluting ability)	25–30 mOsmol/L
pH	4.5–8.0
Phenylketonuria	No color changes
Specific gravity	1.002–1.010
Protein	May be present during first 2–4 days
Glucose	Negative
Blood	Negative
Leukocytes	Negative

Sources: Cloherty, Eichenwald, & Stark (2004); Nettina (2007).

MEDICATIONS

Betamethasone (bay-ta-**meth**-a-sone), **Dexamethasone** (dex-a-**meth**-a-sone)

Pregnancy Category C

Indications To prevent or reduce the severity of respiratory distress syndrome in preterm infants between 24 and 34 weeks of gestation (unlabeled use)

Action Stimulates fetal lung maturation by promoting the release of enzymes that induce the production or release of lung surfactant.

Classification(s)
Therapeutic Stimulates fetal lung maturation
Pharmacological Glucocorticoids (corticosteroids)

Pharmacokinetics
Absorption Preferred method of absorption is via injection
Distribution Crosses the placenta; enters the breast milk
Metabolism and Excretion Metabolized in the liver and excreted by the kidneys
Half-life 6.5 hours

Contraindications and Precautions Contraindicated in women in whom there is a medical indication for delivery (i.e., severe pregnancy induced hypertension [PIH], cord prolapse, chorioamnionitis, abruptio placentae) and in women with systemic fungal infection.

Adverse Reactions and Side Effects Seizures, headache, vertigo, hypertension, increased perspiration, petechiae, ecchymoses, and facial erythema, maternal infection, pulmonary edema (if administered with beta-adrenergic medications). May worsen certain maternal conditions such as diabetes and hypertension.

Route and Dosage 12 mg IM q24hr × 2 doses

Nursing Implications
1. Inform the woman of the benefit of medication and the need to administer to prevent respiratory distress syndrome in her preterm infant.
2. Teach the woman the signs and symptoms of pulmonary edema; assess lung sounds.
3. Shake the suspension well; prolonged exposure to heat and light must be avoided.

4. Administer the medication into a large muscle; avoid the deltoid to prevent local atrophy.
5. Vital signs must be monitored frequently and fetal monitoring should be performed according to institution policy.
6. Accurate intake and output must be monitored and recorded.
7. Monitor blood sugars if the woman is diabetic or at risk for diabetes.
8. Do not administer if the woman has an infection

NOTE: The FDA has not approved the medication for this use.

Data from Deglin & Vallerand (2009); Hayes, Kee, & McCuistion (2006).

ETHNOCULTURAL CONSIDERATIONS

Neonatal Jaundice and RBC Enzyme Defects

Jaundice occurs with greater frequency in infants of Chinese, Japanese, Korean, Native American, and Greek descent. In these populations there is an increased incidence of red blood cell enzyme defects, including glucose-6-phosphate dehydrogenase (G6PD) deficiency and pyruvate kinase deficiency. It occurs most frequently in Mediterranean, Middle-Eastern, Southeast Asian, and African infants. Pyruvate kinase deficiency is the next most common enzyme deficiency. Affected infants typically display symptoms of jaundice, anemia and reticulocytosis (MacDonald, Mullett, & Seshia, 2005).

ADDITIONAL INFORMATION FOR THE CLINICAL SETTING

Facilitating Newborn Transition in a Non-hospital Setting

When assisting with an unexpected birth in a non-hospital setting:

- Evaluate the mother before childbirth if possible.
- Manipulate the environment to facilitate immediate care for the neonate.
- Remain alert to signs of transitional difficulties.
- Ensure effective respirations.

- Facilitate a neutral thermal environment.
- Establish safe transport to the hospital for the mother and · newborn.
- Manage maternal–neonatal care until the transport team arrives.

Preventing Cold Stress in the Newborn

During nonshivering thermogenesis, the newborn metabolizes brown fat. This process increases the metabolic rate, oxygen consumption, and risk for metabolic acidosis. Decreased oxygen causes peripheral vasoconstriction and increases the likelihood of respiratory distress. Peripheral vasoconstriction can lead to increased pulmonary vascular resistance, and a return to fetal circulation as a compensatory mechanism.

Assessing Neonatal Blood Glucose

Capillary blood obtained from the neonate's heel is commonly used to assess blood glucose. When available, a heel warmer is used to increase blood flow to the sample site. Cleanse the area with a sterile alcohol pad. Gently puncture the heel, taking care to avoid the middle area, where there is a risk for nerve damage or puncture of the plantar artery. Place a large drop of blood on the test strip. Apply a sterile bandage to apply pressure on the sample site.

REFERENCES

Cloherty, J., Eichenwald, E., & Stark, A. (2004). *Manual of neonatal care* (5th ed.). Philadelphia: Lippincott Williams & Wilkins.

Deglin, J.H., & Vallerand, A.H. (2009). *Davis's drug guide for nurses* (11th ed.). Philadelphia: F.A. Davis.

Hayes, E., Kee, J., & McCuistion, L. (2006). *Pharmacology, a nursing process approach* (5th ed.). St. Louis, MO: W.B. Saunders/Elsevier.

Hertz, D. (2005). *Care of the newborn: A handbook for primary care.* Philadelphia: Lippincott.

MacDonald, M., Mullett, M., & Seshia, M. (2005). *Avery's neonatology, pathophysiology & management of the newborn* (6th ed.). Philadelphia: Lippincott Williams & Wilkins.

Nettina, S. (2007). *Lippincott manual of nursing practice.* Philadelphia: Lippincott Williams & Wilkins.

Pagana, K., & Pagana, T. (2006). *Mosby's manual of diagnostic and laboratory tests* (3rd ed.). St. Louis, MO: C.V. Mosby.

Wong, R., DeSandre, G., Sibley, E., & Stevenson, D. (2006). Neonatal jaundice and liver disease. In R. Martin, A. Fanaroff, & M. Walsh (Eds.), *Fanaroff and Martin's neonatal-perinatal medicine: Diseases of the fetus and infant* (8th ed., pp. 578–586). Philadelphia: C.V. Mosby.

15

Caring for the Normal Newborn

KEY TERMS

caput – Occiput of the fetal head appearing at the vaginal introitus preceding birth of the head

    c. succedaneum Swelling of the tissue over the presenting part of the fetal head; caused by pressure during labor

cephalhematoma – Extravasation of blood from ruptured vessels between a skull bone and its external covering (the periosteum). The hemorrhage does not cross the suture lines; swelling is limited by the margins of the cranial bone affected.

circumcision – Surgical procedure in which the prepuce (epithelial layer covering the penis; foreskin) is separated from the glans penis and excised

developmental dysplasia of the hip (DDH) – Abnormal development of the hip joint, resulting in instability of the hip causing one or both of the femoral heads to be displaced from the acetabulum

erythema toxicum – Transient pink papular rash in the neonate. Cause is unknown and it may persist up to 1 month of life. Also called "erythema neonatorum."

hypospadias – Anomalous positioning of the urinary meatus on the undersurface of the penis or close to or just inside the vagina

imperforate anus – Congenital absence of an opening in the anal ring

meningocele – Congenital hernia in which the meninges protrude through a defect in the skull or spinal column

microcephaly – Congenital anomaly characterized by abnormal smallness of the head in relation to the rest of the body; underdevelopment of the brain and mental retardation

molding – Overlapping or overriding of the fetal cranial bones to accommodate and conform to the bony and soft parts of the mother's birth canal during labor

myelomeningocele – Hernia of the spinal cord and meninges through the posterior vertebral column; results from failure of the neural tube to close during embryonic development

necrotizing enterocolitis (NEC) – Acute inflammatory bowel disorder that occurs primarily in preterm or low-birthweight infants. Occurs when bowel ischemia results in destruction of the intestinal mucosa; may lead to perforation and peritonitis.

nevus – Natural blemish or mark, a congenital deposit of pigmentation in the skin; mole

    n. flammeus "port wine stain"; a nonelevated capillary angioma located directly below the epidermis

    n. vasculosus (strawberry hemangioma) Elevated lesion of immature capillaries and endothelial cells – slowly regresses over a period of years

omphalitis – Inflammation of the umbilical stump, characterized by redness, edema, and purulent exudate in severe infections

ophthalmia neonatorum – Neonatal eye infection usually resulting from gonorrheal or other infection contracted during passage through the vagina at the time of birth

plethora – Deep purplish-red coloration of a newborn caused by an increased number of circulating red blood cells

simian crease – Single, straight crease that appears in the middle of the palm on one or both hands. May be present in a variety of developmental abnormalities including Down syndrome, Turner's syndrome and Klinefelter's syndrome

telangiectasia – Permanent dilation of groups of superficial capillaries and venules

telangiectatic nevus – "Stork bite"; "angel kiss." Small, red, localized area of capillary dilation frequently seen in neonates; may occur on the nape of the neck, eyebrows, eyelids, nose or upper lip

tetralogy of Fallot – Congenital heart defect that involves four distinct cardiac anomalies: transposition of the aorta and pulmonary artery; right ventricular hypertrophy; pulmonary stenosis; and ventricular septal defect

Wharton's jelly – Specialized white, gelatinous connective tissue that surrounds the umbilical vessels within the cord

FOCUSED ASSESSMENT

The Immediate Neonatal Assessment

- Follow universal precautions.
- Suction oral, pharyngeal, or endotracheal area according to policy (see Procedure 15-1).
- Place the infant on the mother's abdomen, if stable, or under a pre-warmed radiant warmer (unclothed).
- Dry the infant vigorously with warmed blankets (also stimulates respiratory effort).
- Place a cap on the infant's head.
- Observe the respiratory effort, color, and muscle tone.
- Assess the heart rate: May be done by palpating the base of the umbilical stump.
- Lightly flick the soles of the feet to prompt crying, if necessary.
- Document 1-minute and 5-minute Apgar scores.

 Procedure 15-1 Suctioning the Infant's Oral and Nasal Passages

Purpose
To clear secretions from the oral and nasal passages

Equipment
- One bulb syringe
- Tissue

Steps for Oral Suctioning
1. Assess the infant for oral secretions.
2. Position the infant's head to the side or downward if he is vomiting or gagging.
3. Compress the bulb syringe.
4. Insert the bulb syringe approximately 1 inch into one side of the infant's cheek.

   Avoid contact with the roof of the mouth and the back of the throat.

Procedure 15-1 (Continued)

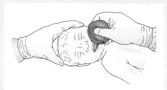

5. Gently release compression of the bulb syringe and allow it to fill with oral secretions.

6. Gently remove the bulb syringe; expel drainage into a tissue.

7. Repeat the process on the other side of the infant's cheek.

8. Repeat as needed.

9. Document procedure.

Steps for Nasal Suctioning

1. Assess the infant for nasal congestion.

2. Position the infant's head to the side or downward if he is vomiting or gagging.

3. Compress the bulb syringe.

4. Insert the bulb syringe into the tip of the infant's nostril. Avoid obstructing the nasal passageway.

5. Gently release the compression of bulb syringe to allow it to fill with mucus or nasal drainage.

6. Gently remove the bulb syringe; expel drainage into a tissue.

7. Repeat as needed.

8. Document the procedure.

Normal Neonatal Parameters at Birth

Parameter	Normal Finding
Respirations	Rate 30–60 breaths/min, irregular with no retractions or grunting
Apical pulse	Rate 120–160 beats/min
Temperature	97.8°F (36.5°C)
Skin color	Pink body, blue extremities
Umbilical cord	Contains two arteries and one vein
Gestational age	Full term: >37 completed weeks (should be 38–42 weeks to remain with parents for an extended time period)

The Later Neonatal Assessment

Vital Signs

Recognizing Normal Newborn Vital Signs			
Temperature	**Pulse**	**Respirations**	**Blood Pressure**
Normal 97.7°–99.4°F (36.5°–37.0°C) Axillary 97.5°–99°F (36.5°–37.2°C)	120–160 beats per minute (bpm) (count pulse rate for 1 full minute) During sleep the pulse rate can be as low as 80 bpm. During crying the pulse rate can be as high as 180 bpm.	30–60 respirations per minute (count respiratory rate for 1 full minute) Abdominal breathing is normal. Periodic breathing is considered normal; is classified as short pauses in the breathing of the newborn that last approximately 3 seconds. Apneic episodes are significant if they last more than 15–20 seconds; they may be accompanied by abrupt pallor, hypotonia, cyanosis, and bradycardia. Apnea must be differentiated from periodic breathing, which is normal in the newborn. *Caution:* Withhold the oral feeding if the respiratory rate is >60 respirations per minute.	Systolic: 60–80 mm Hg; diastolic: 40–50 mm Hg at birth Systolic: 95–100 mm Hg; diastolic: slight increase at 10 days of age

Importance of Temperature Assessment

If the newborn's temperature drops to 97.5°F (36.4°C) or below, immediately initiate temperature stabilization measures such as skin-to-skin contact by placing the infant directly on the mother's unclothed arms, chest, or abdomen or move him to a radiant warmer. Once the newborn's temperature reaches 98.6°F (37.0°C) or above, dress him in a T-shirt and hat and cover him with two or three blankets.

Assessment of the Neonate: A Systems Approach

Level of Reactivity Responsiveness, symmetrical movement, sleep pattern

Overall Size and Symmetry

Measurements Weight, length, head, chest, and abdominal circumference

- Average weight is 3400 grams; range is 2500 to 4300 grams.
  - Place a cover on the scale to prevent cross-infection (Fig. 15-1).
  - Protect the infant against heat loss.
  - Remain with the infant.
- Average length is 45 to 55 cm (18–22 in.) (See Procedure 15-2.)
- Average head circumference (frontal–occipital circumference) is 33 to 38 cm (13–15 in.).
  - Place the tape measure immediately above the eyebrows and pinna of the ears (Fig. 15-2).
  - Wrap the tape measure around to the occipital prominence at the back of the head.
  - Measure three times; record the largest finding.

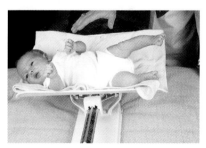

Figure 15-1 Weighing the infant.

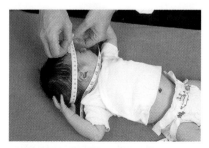

Figure 15-2 Measuring the head circumference.

- Average chest circumference is 30.5 to 33 cm (12–13 in.).
  - Place the tape measure on the nipple line (Fig. 15-3).
  - Wrap the tape measure around the entire thoracic area.
- The abdominal circumference should approximate the chest circumference.
  - Place the tape measure directly above the umbilicus (Fig. 15-4).
  - Wrap the tape measure around the infant's body.

Skin, Scalp, Body Hair, Nails Assess color, texture, distribution, disruptions, eruptions, birthmarks

Head Assess size, symmetry, suture lines, placement and condition of the eyes, nose, mouth, and ears, patency of both nares, integrity of the anterior and posterior fontanels, and the presence of a caput succedaneum or cephalhematoma

Respiratory System Assess symmetry in the movement of the chest, placement and size of the breast tissue, the respiratory rate and effort, and the presence of retractions or grunting

Cardiovascular System Palpate the point of maximum impulse (PMI), the heart rate, capillary refill, femoral pulses, brachial pulses; auscultate for murmurs or extra heart sounds

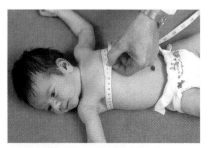

Figure 15-3 Measuring the chest circumference.

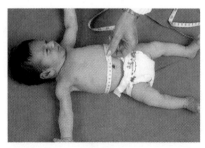

Figure 15-4 Measuring the abdominal circumference.

Gastrointestinal System Inspect the abdominal shape and the umbilical cord; auscultate bowel sounds, palpate and note structures; assess for the presence of a hernia

Genitourinary System: Assess patency of the anus, elicit the anal wink reflex, note passing of stool.

Males: Examine the scrotum and palpate for the presence of both testes; note location of urinary meatus; palpate the penis; note the presence of smegma.

Females: Examine the labia; note any discharge.

Musculoskeletal System Inspect extremities for differences in length or size, the number of digits, muscle tone and symmetry in movement; palpate the clavicles and hips for crepitus, perform passage range of motion on the remaining joints; assess rotation of the neck; assess for developmental dysplasia of the hip

Neurological System Assess reflexes, especially the gag reflex, Babinski, Moro, and Galant reflexes; assess integrity of the spine.

Procedure 15-2 Measuring the Newborn's Length

Purpose

To establish and document the newborn's length

Equipment

• Standard paper tape measure

Steps

1. Place the infant on a paper-covered flat surface.

2. Fully extend the infant's body by holding the head midline.

3. Gently grasp the knees and place them together.

4. Push down gently on the knees until they are fully extended and flat against the table surface.

5. Measure the crown-to-heel recumbent length by placing the paper tape measure beside the infant with the 0 end of the tape at the top of the head. Keep the infant's body in alignment and carefully extend one leg. Ensure that the tape measure remains straight.

(continued)

Procedure 15-2 (Continued)

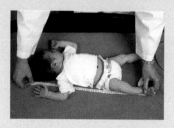

As an alternate measurement method, make a slash mark with a pen at the end points by the top of the infant's head and the heels of the foot. While providing continuous support, gently roll the infant to the side and measure between the two points with a paper tape measure that has increments designated in tenths.

6. Document the procedure and record the measurement.

Gestational Age Assessment (Fig. 15-5)

- Performed within the first 12 hours of life.
- Includes neuromuscular maturity and physical maturity components.
- Scores from each component are added together.
- Combined scores are mathematically extrapolated onto the maturity rating scale to determine the infant's gestational age by examination.
- Identifies the decreased levels of muscle and joint flexibility characteristic of the premature infant, and the mature term infant's ability to return to the original position after movement.
- The infant's maturity scoring does not directly translate to the gestational age in weeks (Ballard et al., 1991).

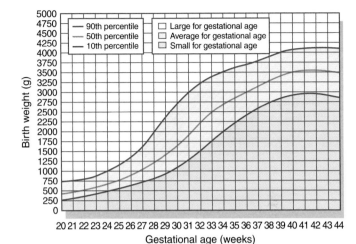

Figure 15-5 Gestational age assessment.

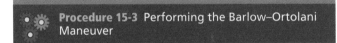

Procedure 15-3 Performing the Barlow–Ortolani Maneuver

Purpose

To assess for developmental dysplasia of the hips

Steps

1. Place the infant supine on a flat surface.

2. Place your thumbs on the infant's inner thighs and your fingers on the outside of the greater trochanters of the hips.

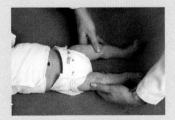

(continued)

Procedure 15-2 (Continued)

3. Flex the infant's knees and move the legs inward until your fingers touch.

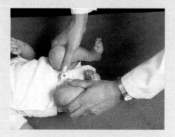

4. Using gentle but firm pressure, rotate the hips outward so that the knees touch the flat surface. No clicking or crepitus should be detected. The presence of clicking or crepitus indicates joint instability.

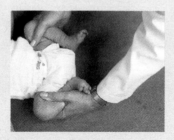

5. Document the procedure.

Newborn Reflexes

Reflex	Indicator/Method for Assessment
Palmar Grasp 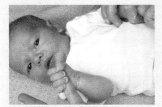	The infant curls his fingers around an object.
Toe or Plantar Grasp 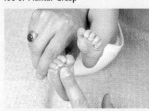	The infant curls his toes around an object that has been placed at the sole of the foot.
Rooting and Sucking Reflexes 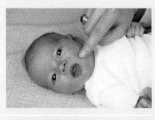 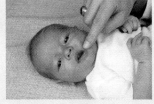	Stroke the infant's cheek and watch him turn toward the finger, open his mouth, and suck on an object placed in his mouth.
Extrusion Reflex 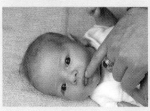	Touch the tip of the infant's tongue and the tongue will protrude outward.

(continued)

Newborn Reflexes (Continued)

Reflex	Indicator/Method for Assessment
Stepping Reflex 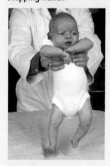	Hold the infant in an upright position with the legs flexed. The soles of the feet are lightly brushed against a flat surface. In response to the stimulation, the infant lifts his feet and then places them back down in a stepwise pattern that imitates walking.
Tonic Neck or Fencing Reflex 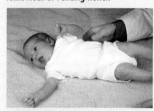	Observe the infant, in a supine position, extend his arm and leg on the side to which his head and jaw is turned while flexing his arm and leg on the opposite side.
Glabellar Reflex 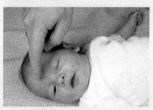	Tap on infant's forehead and observe him blink for the first few taps.
Babinski Reflex 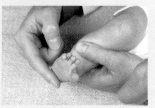	Lightly stroke the plantar surface of the foot from the heel toward the toes. The infant responds to this stimulation by first incurving the toes, then uncurling and stretching them out.

Reflex	Indicator/Method for Assessment
Moro Reflex 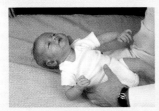	Observe the infant's head as it is lifted while the nurse mimics a release and watches for extension of both arms along with flexion of the legs.
Magnet Reflex 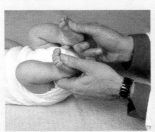 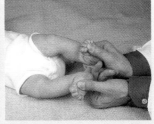	With the infant in a supine position, flex the leg and apply pressure to the soles of the feet. Observe the infant extend his legs against the pressure.
Galant Reflex or Trunk Incurvation Reflex 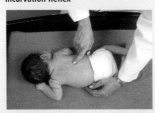	Hold or support the infant in a prone position. Stroke one side of the vertebral column. Observe the infant respond to this stimulus by moving his buttocks in a curving motion toward the side that is being stroked.
Crawling Reflex 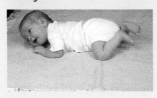	Place the infant on his abdomen; observe his attempts to crawl.

(continued)

Newborn Reflexes (Continued)

Reflex	Indicator/Method for Assessment
Crossed Extension	With the infant in a supine position, stimulate one foot; observe flexion, adduction, and then extension of the opposite leg.

Common Skin Findings in the Neonate

Finding/Condition	Description
Acrocyanosis	The bluish coloring of the hands and feet that results from vasomotor insufficiency and poor peripheral perfusion
Birthmarks	Distinct areas of color that may be red, tan, brown, white or red. Their appearance varies but generally these lesions are small and flat.
Blue Nevus	Appears as a distinct blue or blue-black birthmark often found on the buttocks, hands and feet, usually ≤1 cm in size.
Brown Nevi	Brown skin marks, or birth marks whose color can vary from brown to deep black
Café-au-lait	Flat, tan spots that are quite common and insignificant unless the infant exhibits six or more marks that are >1 cm in diameter
Coloboma	A disruption in the iris; appears as a keyhole in the circle of the iris and pupil and will affect vision in that eye.
Epstein's Pearls	Whitish hardened nodules found along the newborn's gum margins and at the junction of the soft and hard palates; disappear within a few weeks
Erythema Toxicum	Transient pink papular rash in the neonate. Cause is unknown and it may persist up to one month of life. Also called "erythema neonatorum."
Hypopigmentation	Diminished pigment in the tissue

Finding/Condition	Description
Jaundice	Yellow discoloration of the body tissues (skin, sclera, oral mucous membranes) caused by the deposit of bile pigments (unconjugated bilirubin); icterus
Milia	Small white papules or sebaceous cysts that may be present on the newborn's forehead, nose, cheeks and chin
Mongolian Spots	Gray, dark blue, or purple non-elevated pigmented area most often located on the back and buttocks in some neonates, especially those of nonwhite ethnicity
Nevus Flammeus	Often referred to as a "port wine stain," a capillary angioma located directly below the epidermis; a non-elevated, red to purple network of dense capillaries that varies in size, shape, and location, although it commonly appears on the face. It does not blanch on pressure, disappear, or grow in size.
Nevus Vasculosus	"Strawberry mark," a red, raised capillary hemangioma that can occur anywhere on the neonate's body. This birthmark usually has sharp borders and a rough surface that resembles a strawberry.
Periauricular Papillomas	Skin tags around the ear
Plethora	Deep purplish-red coloration of a newborn caused by an increased number of circulating red blood cells
Pustular Melanosis	A condition in which small pustules are formed before birth
Sturge–Weber Syndrome	A clinical condition involving the fifth cranial nerve; may be present when a nevus flammeus is accompanied by convulsions or other indicators of neurological problems.
Telangiectatic Nevus	"Stork bite"; "angel kiss": Small, red, localized area of capillary dilation frequently seen in neonates; may occur on the nape of the neck, eyebrows, eyelids, nose, or upper lip.
Torticollis	A deviation of the neck to one side caused by a spasmodic contraction of neck muscles. In the neonate, a torticollis is apparent when the head is positioned on one side while the chin points to the opposite side.

Obtaining an Accurate Assessment of the Infant's True Skin Color

- Use a variety of light sources (helps ascertain the "true" color).
- Examine the infant's entire skin surface.
- Carefully inspect the palms, soles of the feet, lips, and areas behind the ears.
- Gently palpate bony prominences (nose, sternum, sacrum, wrists, ankles):
  - Apply slight pressure for 1 second ("blanching").

- Observe for true skin color, reflective of the infant's ethnic heritage.
- Record true skin color; yellow is indicative of jaundice; white is indicative of pallor.

Understanding Classifications for Newborn Weight

Large for gestational age (LGA): Weight is above the 90th percentile at any week.

Appropriate for gestational age (AGA): Weight falls between the 10th and 90th percentiles for the infant's age.

Small for gestational age (SGA): Weight falls below the 10th percentile for the infant's age.

CLINICAL ALERTS

Safe Suctioning

Always suction the mouth before suctioning the nares because fluids and secretions that could obstruct the respiratory tract may be present in the mouth or the nares or both. Placing the syringe in the nares first may trigger an inspiratory gasp, causing the infant to pull mucus further into the respiratory tract.

Timely Recognition of Tachypnea

An increasing respiratory rate is often the first sign of respiratory comprise or obstruction. If this occurs, initiate and maintain effective ventilation.

Recognizing Immediate Neonatal Respiratory Distress

- During the neonatal assessment, the nurse is alert to the following signs and symptoms that are indicative of respiratory distress. If any of these symptoms are present, notify the physician immediately.
- Generalized cyanosis
- Tachycardia (heart rate >160 beats/min)
- Tachypnea (respiratory rate >70 breaths/min)
- Rib retractions
- Expiratory grunting
- Flaring nostrils

Safe Positions to Prevent Sudden Infant Death Syndrome (SIDS)

- Place all newborns on their backs to sleep.
- When using a side-lying position, place the infant's dependent arm forward to lessen the likelihood that the infant will roll into a prone position.

Recognizing an Ophthalmic Emergency in the Infant

Absence of the red reflex indicates an interference with the transmission of light to the retina. This is an ophthalmic emergency that requires immediate medical attention, as optic nerve suppression from obstructed light pathways may result in permanent blindness.

Recognizing Acute Abdomen in the Neonate

The following symptoms may indicate an acute abdomen:

- Rigid, board-like abdomen
- Inability to palpate abdominal organs
- Indicators of pain (continuous crying, facial changes, gross motor movements)

Scrotal Auscultation

If bowel sounds are present in the scrotum, immediately notify the physician. This is a medical emergency.

Protecting the Infant from the Sun

Advise parents to check with their health care provider about use of sunscreen products, as many do not recommend sunscreens until the infant is at least 6 months of age.

DIAGNOSTIC TESTS

Mandatory Newborn Metabolic Screening

- Mandatory in the United States to screen for inborn errors of metabolism (e.g., phenylketonuria (PKU), galactosemia, hemoglobinopathy, hypothyroidism)

- Serum sample obtained from a heel stick
- Performed 24 hours to 7 days after birth

MEDICATIONS

Eye Prophylaxis to Prevent Ophthalmia Neonatorum

- The Centers for Disease Control and Prevention (CDC) recommends that the medication (e.g., erythromycin, tetracycline, silver nitrate) be administered as soon as possible after birth.
- Some birth facilities delay neonatal eye prophylaxis up to an hour to allow eye contact to facilitate parent–infant bonding. If instillation is delayed, the facility should have a monitoring system in place to ensure that all infants receive the prophylaxis (CDC, Workowski & Berman, 2006).

Erythromycin (eh-rith-roe-**mye**-sin), Ilotycin

Pregnancy Category B
Indications
Infants Prophylaxis of ophthalmia neonatorum

Actions Suppresses protein synthesis at the level of the 50S ribosome

Therapeutic Effects Bacteriostatic action against susceptible bacteria spectrum: Streptococci, staphylococci, gram-positive bacilli

Pharmacokinetics
Absorption Minimal absorption may follow topical or ophthalmic use.

Contraindications and Precautions
Contraindicated in Hypersensitivity

Adverse Reactions and Side Effects Irritation

Route and Dosage Apply a thin strip to each eye as a single dose.

Nursing Implications
1. Inform the parents of medication administration.
2. Prepare to administer the eye ointment to the infant 1 hour after birth.

3. Apply a thin strip to each eye as a single dose.
4. Start at the inner canthus and move to the outer canthus.
5. Dab excess medication off gently, do not wash away the medicine.

Data from Deglin, J., & Vallerand, A. (2009). Davis's drug guide for nurses (11th ed.). Philadelphia: F.A. Davis.

AquaMEPHYTON Phytonadione (fye-toe-**na**-dye-one)
AquaMEPHYTON, Mephyton, Vitamin K

Classifications
Therapeutic Antidotes, vitamins
Pharmacological Fat-soluble vitamins

Pregnancy Category UK

Indications Prevention and treatment of hypoprothrombinemia, which may be associated with excessive doses of oral anticoagulants, salicylates, certain anti-infective agents, nutritional deficiencies, and prolonged total parenteral nutrition. Prevention of hemorrhagic disease of the newborn.

Action Required for hepatic synthesis of blood coagulation factors II (prothrombin), VII, IX, and X.
Therapeutic Effects Prevention of bleeding due to hypoprothrombinemia.

Pharmacokinetics
Absorption Well absorbed after oral, IM, or subcutaneous administration
Distribution Crosses the placenta; does not enter breast milk
Metabolism and Excretion Rapidly metabolized in the liver
Half-life Unknown

Contraindications and Precautions
Contraindicated in Hypersensitivity, hypersensitivity or intolerance to benzyl alcohol (injection only)
Use Cautiously in Impaired liver function.
Exercise Extreme Caution in Severe life-threatening reactions have occurred after IV administration; use other routes unless IV is justified.

Adverse Reactions and Side Effects
Gastrointestinal Gastric upset, unusual taste
Dermatological Flushing, rash, urticaria
Hematological Hemolytic anemia
Local Erythema, pain at injection site, swelling
Miscellaneous Allergic reactions, hyperbilirubinemia (large doses in very premature infants), kernicterus.

Route and Dosage IV use of phytonadione should be reserved for emergencies.

Prevention of hemorrhagic disease of the newborn:

IM (Neonates): 0.5–1 mg, given within 1 hour of birth. May be repeated in 2–3 weeks if the mother received previous anticonvulsant/anticoagulant/anti-infective/antitubercular therapy. 1–5 mg may be given IM to the mother 12–24 hours before delivery.

Nursing Implications
- Inform the parents of medication administration.
- Prepare to administer the injection to the infant 1 hour after birth.
- Administer IM injection into the anterolateral muscle of the newborn's thigh.
- Report any symptoms of unusual bleeding or bruising (bleeding gums, nose bleed, black, tarry stools, hematuria, bleeding from the base of the umbilical cord or other open wounds)
- A decrease in hemoglobin and hematocrit levels or any bleeding may indicate that the desired effects of the medicine have not been achieved and that more vitamin K may be necessary. Call the physician for further instruction.

Data from Deglin, J., & Vallerand, A. (2009). Davis's drug guide for nurses (11th ed.). Philadelphia: F.A. Davis.

Hepatitis B Vaccine (Recombivax HB, Enerix-B)
- Series of three doses, beginning at birth
- Recommended for all infants
- Parental consent required
- Administered into the vastus lateralis muscle
- Repeat doses at 1 and 6 months of age

ETHNOCULTURAL CONSIDERATIONS

Accepting Customs and Traditions

Valued health beliefs from various ethnic backgrounds frequently extend to the area of infant care. For example, some Asians, Hispanics, Eastern Europeans and Native Americans delay the initiation of breastfeeding because of the belief that colostrum is "bad" (D'Avanzo & Geissler, 2003; Dillon, 2007). Be respectful and accepting of cultural beliefs such as these.

TEACHING THE FAMILY

Proper Bulb Suctioning

- Ensure that parents understand the proper technique for use and care of the bulb syringe; ask for a return demonstration.
- Compress the bulb syringe first, then insert it into the infant's nostril or mouth; if the bulb syringe is inserted and then compressed, secretions may be forced further back into the nose or throat and cause obstruction.
- Position the infant's head to the side or downward if he is vomiting or gagging.
- Always wash the bulb syringe in warm, soapy water each day and after each use.
- Store the bulb syringe at the infant's bedside.

How to Recognize Breathing Difficulties

Teach parents the signs of breathing difficulties in their infant:

- Above normal respirations
- Prolonged (>15 seconds) periods of breath holding
- Sucking-in and see-saw movements around the rib cage
- Nasal flaring
- Grunting

Umbilical Cord Care

- Teach parents about the cord's normal appearance and when to expect complete cord detachment.

- Show parents how to fold and position the diaper below the cord stump; emphasize the need to keep the area free from urine and wetness during bathing.
- Alert parents to potential danger signs such as bleeding or a foul odor.

Basics of Newborn Care	
Topic	**Essential Instructions**
Bathing	Use a warm area that is free from drafts. Use only warm water for the first few days of life. Sponge bathe until the umbilical stump falls off (approximately 2 weeks). Use unscented products. There is no need to bathe every day.
Clothing	At home, dress as other family members, appropriate for temperature and season. Protect from wind or drafts and sun.
Diapering	Wash cloth diapers separately from other clothing. Infants may develop rash from perfumes in disposable diapers; if so, try another brand. Contact a health care professional if the rash persists.
Circumcision	Use petroleum gauze dressing for 1-2 days to prevent the diaper from adhering to the surgical site (unless a Plastibell is used). Cleanse with water only until healed.

How to Care for the Infant/Child Who Has Not Been Circumcised

Teach the parents:

- Keep the uncircumcised penis clean by gently washing the genital area while bathing. No special cleansing (e.g., with cotton swabs or antiseptics) is necessary.
- The foreskin usually does not fully retract for several years and should not be forced.
- When the foreskin fully retracts (4–5 years of age), teach your son to clean his foreskin by gently pulling it back away from the head of the penis and then rinsing the head of the penis and inside fold of the foreskin with soap and warm water every day. After washing, the foreskin should be pulled back over the head of the penis.

Safe Car Seat Use

- Ensure that the car seat meets federal guidelines; look for a label on the seat tag or packaging box that confirms this; guidelines are also available at the American Academy of Pediatrics Web site (www.AAP.org).
- Follow car seat instructions when installing the car seat.
- Car seats for initial hospital dismissal may be obtained through various community resources (e.g., hospital or birthing center, American Red Cross, local health and safety council, State Department of Health).
- Dress the infant in clothing that facilitates ease of positioning and strap placement.
- Provide infant head support: Use a commercially made product or place a rolled-up receiving blanket around the head and neck area.
- To prevent burns and overheating in warm weather, check the temperature of the car seat by touching the surface.
- Trained professionals may be available to perform safety checks to help parents with proper car seat use. New cars are required to be equipped with tethers and lower anchors to ensure safe car seat installation and use.

How to Plan for and Assess Child Care Arrangements

Encourage the family to:

- Communicate their needs and express their concerns about child care.
- Interview the facility director along with other individuals who may be involved in the child's care.
- Evaluate the educational programs related to qualification of teachers and structure of the learning environment (structured or unstructured).
- Investigate the provision of meals, nutrition, and related sanitation.
- Visit the child care facility on a few occasions, announced and unannounced.
- Identify practical aspects of child care such as location, hours of operation, fee requirements and payment schedule, child to worker ratio, environmental safety, indoor and outdoor space, sick day policies, and availability of care during a holiday or inclement weather.

- Evaluate the infection control and injury prevention measures.
- Gain broader information about the facility related to breast feeding, discipline, nurturing, diapering/toileting, stimulating growth and development, play, nap/rest time, and field trips.
- Discover state regulations and read the care facility's policies and related public records.
- Become familiar with early childhood programs that offer voluntary accreditation such as the National Academy of Early Childhood Programs.

ADDITIONAL INFORMATION FOR THE CLINICAL SETTING

Documenting Appropriate Birth Information

- Exact time of birth
- Status of infant's respirations (spontaneous or assisted)
- 1- and 5-minute Apgar scores
- Birth weight in pounds and kilograms
- Axillary temperature
- Number of vessels in the umbilical cord
- Type and amount of medication instilled for eye prophylaxis
- Injection sites for vitamin K and hepatitis B vaccine administration
- Findings from the general physical assessment
- Observations of voiding or stooling
- All laboratory testing obtained, such as blood glucose or cultures
- Legally register the neonate with the State Bureau of Vital Statistics (mother's name, father's name [if the mother gives permission], date, time, place of birth)

Fostering Family Attachment

- Provide time in the first few hours after birth for privacy and time for the new family to get to know one another.
- After birth, delay any procedures that are not immediately necessary such as measurements and other admission procedures, to allow the family adequate time alone.

- Encourage early breast-feeding by providing proper education and support.
- Teach parents about infant behavioral cues for feeding (rooting, sucking on their fingers or fist, increasing motor activity or crying) and how to respond to them.
- Help parents understand that crying is the infant's way of communicating, and all newborns have distinguishable cries for hunger, pain, tiredness, fussiness, or getting attention.
- Teach parents that newborns have a built-in capacity to console themselves and do so by sucking, motion, and distraction.
- Help parents to recognize the joys and frustrations that go along with ongoing parenting. Assure them that it takes time to feel comfortable in meeting their newborn's unique needs.
- Introduce the concept of anticipatory guidance to help prepare parents for important developmental milestones that will occur.
- Encourage the parents to invite siblings and other family members to visit for short periods of time to share the joy and to provide support.
- Provide consistent nurses throughout the hospital or birthing center stay.

RESOURCES

Centers for Disease Control and Prevention (CDC). National Center for Health Statistics. (2007). *National Health and Nutrition Examination Survey.* Available at:
http://www.cdc.gov/nchs/about/major/nhanes/growthcharts/charts.htm

National Newborn Screening and Genetic and Resource Center: *National newborn screening status report.* Available at:
http://genes-r-us.uthscsa.edu/nbsdisorders.pdf

Recommended Childhood and Adolescent Immunizations Schedule - United States (2007). Approved by the Advisory Committee on Immunization Practices (www.cdc.gov/nip/acip), the American Academy of Pediatrics (www.aap.org), and the American Academy of Family Physicians (www.aafp.org). Available at: http://www.cdc.gov/vaccines/recs/acip/default.htm

U.S. Preventive Services Task Force (USPSTF) (2001). *Screening for newborn hearing. Recommendation statement*. Available at: www.ahrq.gov/clinic/uspstf/uspsnbhr.htm

REFERENCES

Ballard, J.L., Khoury, J.C., Wedig, K., Wang, L., Eilers-Waisman, B.L., & Lipp, R. (1991). New Ballard score, expanded to include extremely premature infants. *Journal of Pediatrics, 119*, 417–423.

Centers for Disease Control and Prevention (CDC), Workowski K., & Bergman, S. (2006). Sexually transmitted disease treatment guidelines, 2006. *MMWR Morbidity and Mortality Weekly Report, 55*(RR-11), 1–94.

D'Avanzo, C., & Geissler, E. (2003). *Pocket guide to cultural assessment* (3rd ed.). St. Louis, MO: C.V. Mosby.

Deglin, J., & Vallerand, A. (2009). *Davis's drug guide for nurses* (11th ed.). Philadelphia: F.A. Davis.

Dillon, P.M. (2007). *Nursing health assessment: A critical thinking, case studies approach* (2nd ed.). Philadelphia: F.A. Davis.

Caring for the Newborn at Risk

KEY TERMS

preterm – An infant born before 37 completed weeks of gestation

term newborn – Live infant born between weeks 38 and 42 of completed gestation

postterm – An infant born after week 42 of completed gestation

FOCUSED ASSESSMENT

- Lung maturity: Fetal lung maturity develops in utero progressively until term. Fetal lung is determined via the lecithin/sphingomyelin (L/S) ratio and phosphatidyl glycerol (PG) values, which are essential in promoting oxygenation of the lung alveoli.
- Circulatory maturity: Fetal circulation functions in utero to oxygenate the organs needed for intrauterine growth.
- Neurological maturity: The neurological system, including the central and peripheral nervous systems and the parasympathetic and sympathetic nervous systems, is underdeveloped at birth. The preterm newborn is at an increased risk resulting in the inability to cope with the extrauterine stimuli at birth.

Viability Related to Newborns Classified According to Gestational Age (GA)

- Viable: Newborns whom all neonatal clinicians agree should be treated (gestational age [GA] greater than or equal to 25 weeks)

- Nonviable: Newborns whom nearly all neonatal clinicians agree should not be treated (GA less than or equal to 22 weeks)
- Viability uncertain: Newborns for whom the need for resuscitation or treatment (GA 23–24 weeks) is debated and discussed by clinicians, often with disagreement (Taeusch, Ballard, & Gleason, 2005).

Newborn Classification by Birth Weight and Gestational Age

Birth weight is compared to gestational age for a more accurate assessment of risk factors and specific growth patterns

- Small for gestational age (SGA): Weight below the 10th percentile for gestational age
- Average for gestational age (AGA): Weight between the 10th and 90th percentile for gestation age
- Large for gestational age (LGA): Weight above the 90th percentile for gestational age

Signs of Cold Stress

- Poor feeding
- Lethargy
- Central cyanosis or pallor
- Respiratory distress
- Bradycardia (Klaus & Fanaroff, 2005)

Temperature

- Normal skin temperature: 97–98°F (36.2–36.8°C)
- Normal axillary temperature: 97.7–99.5°F (36.5–37.5°C)
- Normal rectal temperature: 97.9–100.4°F (36.6–38°C)

Pain

High-risk newborns undergo numerous life-saving interventions, many of which produce pain. Pain should be assessed during both procedural and routine care. The Premature Infant Pain Profile is commonly used for pain assessment in the NICU (Fig. 16-1).

	0	1	2	3
GA	>/= 36 Wks	32–36 6/7 Wks	28–31 6/7 Wks	</= 28 Wks
Behavioral state	Active/awake	Quiet/awake	Active/sleep	Quiet/sleep
HR	0–4 beats/ minute Inc	5–14 beats/ minute Inc	15–24 beats/ minute Inc	25 beats or > Inc
O2 Sats	0–2.4% Decrease	2.5–4.9% Decrease	5–7.4% Decrease	7.5% or Decrease
Brow bulge	None	Minimum	Moderate	Maximum
Eye squeeze	None	Minimum	Moderate	Maximum
Nasolabial furrow	None	Minimum	Moderate	Maximum

Figure 16-1 Premature infant profile.

Relationship Between pH and Concentration of Arterial Blood Gases

	pH	pco_2	pao_2	$pHCO_3$
	Measures blood acidity	Partial pressure of carbon dioxide in blood	Partial pressure of oxygen in blood	Partial pressure of bicarbonate (alkaline or base) in blood
Normal Neonatal Values	pH = 7.25–7.45	pco_2 = 35–40 mm Hg	pao_2 = 50–80 mm Hg	$pHCO_3^-$ = 20–22 mEq/L
Respiratory Acidosis (due to poor ventilation)	↓pH	↑pco_2	WNL	WNL
Metabolic Acidosis (anaerobic metabolism from hypoxia, diarrhea, or kidney disease)	↓pH	WNL	WNL	↑$pHCO_3^-$
Respiratory Alkalosis (hyperventilation)	↑pH	↓pco_2	↑pao_2	WNL
Metabolic Acidosis (vomiting, diarrhea, hypocalcemia)	↑pH	WNL	WNL	↑$pHCO_3^-$

WNL = within normal limits.
Adapted from Noerr, B. (2000). Neonatal respiratory disease and management strategies, May 18, Hershey, PA. A continuing education service of Penn State's College of Medicine at the Milton S. Hershey Medical Center.

Assessment of the Preterm Infant

Skin	Head	Chest	Cardiac	Abdomen	Musculoskeletal	Genitalia	Neurological/Sensory
Skin tags	Irregular shaped head, molding after delivery, caput succedaneum cephalhematoma	Funnel or pigeon chest	Apical heart rate is assessed for a full minute.	Cord does not have two arteries and one vein.	No flexion of extremities resulting in increased susceptibility to heat loss and skin breakdown	Male scrotum has no rugae and the testes are often undescended.	Marked head lag in all positions
Translucent	Large anterior and posterior fontanels present. Fused sutures. Bulging or depressed fontanels	Supernumerary nipples or nipples are flat on the chest wall	The heart rate may normally be above 160 bpm but it should not be above 180 bpm.	Palpate for masses.	Assess for fractures or developmental hip dysplasia or fractured clavicle.	Female clitoris is often prominent and not covered by the labia minora. The labia majora is also small.	Consistent caregivers read the cues and notice subtle changes.
Lanugo covering the shoulders, back, thighs, forehead and ears	Ear pinnas are flat and readily fold upon themselves	Ribs are visible.	Heart auscultation is done in the second and fourth right and left intercostal spaces as well as the apex and axillae area	Auscultate bowel sounds.		Inguinal hernias are common.	Sucking and gagging reflexes are often absent until 32–34 weeks of gestation.

Little subcutaneous fat	Eyes are fused before 24 weeks of gestation.	Grunting, nasal flaring, or retractions (subcostal, sternal or suprasternal) are signs of respiratory distress.	Auscultation of heart sounds should be done routinely to detect murmurs that may or may not be innocent	Abdominal circumference is measured to assess for distention that may indicate necrotizing enterocolitis (NEC).	Female absence of vaginal or male urethral opening covered by prepuce	Moro reflex may be absent to weak.
Fragile and easily injured	Nose flattened or bruised Nasal patency Low placement of ears	Auscultate anterior, posterior, and at the sides of the chest	Blood pressure readings are taken on all four extremities to determine any wide variations that may be indicative of a ductal defect.		Meconium found in the vaginal opening	Any signs or symptoms of increased intracranial may be related to cerebral insults.
Mottled related to poor peripheral perfusion	Facial anomalies	Auscultate respiratory rate for a full minute.	Persistent central cyanosis	Enlarged liver or spleen	Ambiguous genitalia	Hypotonia or hypertonia
Prominent veins	Respiratory rate is between 60 and 80 respirations per minute.	Displacement of apex			Bladder exstrophy	Twitches, jittery, myoclonic jerks

(continued)

Assessment of the Preterm Infant (Continued)

Skin	Head	Chest	Cardiac	Abdomen	Musculoskeletal	Genitalia	Neurological/Sensory
Covered in vernix		Respiratory rates above 80 breaths per minute are not within normal limits.	Cardiomegaly				Eye lids edematous, drainage present, minimal reactivity to light, congenital cataracts, absence of red reflex, inability to follow object or bright light
Pale (pallor) related to anemia from blood loss		Asymmetrical chest movement may suggest respiratory conditions such as pneumothorax or diaphragmatic hernia.					Eyes have nystagmus, or strabismus, or ruptured capillaries.
Congenital strawberry hemangiomas		Excessive secretions will affect the oxygen intake.					

Diaper rash is common and related to the increase in irritation of the stool when the newborn is on antibiotics and the fragility of the skin

Soles of the feet are smooth.

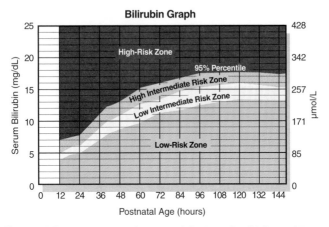

Figure 16-2 Laboratory evaluation of the jaundiced infant of 35 or more weeks' gestation.

Jaundice

Jaundice is diagnosed in term infants with a serum bilirubin level greater than 12.9 mg/dL and in preterm infants with a serum bilirubin >15 mg/dL. If jaundice appears, a bilirubin level to determine the bilirubin factor is plotted on the bilirubin graph in relation to hours of age (American Academy of Pediatrics [AAP], 2004) (Fig. 16-2).

Neonatal Abstinence Syndrome (NAS)

The following are signs and symptoms of withdrawal or neonatal abstinence syndrome (NAS) to determine if a newborn is an infant of a drug-abusing mother (IDAM):

- Irritability
- Tremors
- Wakefulness
- Uncoordinated feeding pattern
- Loose stools
- Yawning or hiccups
- Poor weight gain

- Hypertonia
- Seizures
- Exaggerated rooting reflex
- Regurgitation and vomiting
- Tachypnea or apnea
- Sneezing and stuffy nose
- Lacrimation

CLINICAL ALERTS

Fractured Clavicle

- The T-shirt is sometimes pinned so that the arm is in a flexed position to produce a loose splint.
- The affected arm is pinned to the opposite shoulder by the hand cuff of the newborn T-shirt.
- Pain management may be needed if the newborn appears uncomfortable.
- Keep the newborn off the injured side to decrease pain and promote alignment.

Microcephaly

- It is critical to maintain accurate and consistent head measurements by plotting them on the growth chart and monitoring the newborn for neurological symptoms.

Taking the Newborn's Blood Pressure

Attempt to take the blood pressure while the newborn is sleeping or use a pacifier to quiet the newborn for the procedure.

Aspiration

Never feed newborns with greater than 60 respirations/minute orally because they have an increased risk of aspiration pneumonia.

Calculating Standard Newborn Formulas

To maintain adequate growth, newborns need a caloric intake of 100 to 120 kcal/kg per day and a fluid intake of 150 to 180 mL/kg per day (Gomella, 1999).

$$\text{kcal/kg per day} = \frac{\text{kcal/mL} \times \text{total mL of formula}}{\text{weight}}$$

DIAGNOSTIC TESTS

Hypoglycemia and Hyperglycemia

- Hypoglycemia is diagnosed when glucose levels fall below 60 mg/dL. The newborn may also start building up ketones.

- Hyperglycemia is rarer than hypoglycemia but is still significant. A blood glucose level above 150 mg/dL is considered hyperglycemia and can cause dehydration and weight loss. Severe hyperglycemia may also cause cerebral hemorrhage (Treusch et al., 2005).

Hemoglobin and Hematocrit Levels

- Closely monitor hemoglobin, hematocrit, and bilirubin levels.
- Exchange transfusions may be ordered for hematocrits greater than 65% in the first 24 hours of life to prevent neurological deficits.
- Exact hematocrit values at which complications will occur are difficult to determine because different newborns become symptomatic at different levels.
- Monitor questionable hematocrit levels by venous blood because capillary hematocrits are less exact.
- Assess the newborn for neurological symptoms such as high pitched cry, feeding problems, irritability, and apnea.
- Test urine for blood and macroscopic analysis (Klaus & Fanaroff, 2005).

Normal Newborn Blood Counts

Value	28 Weeks' Gestation	34 Weeks' Gestation	Term
Hemoglobin (g/dL)	14.5	15	16.8
Hematocrit (%)	45	47	53
Red blood cells (mm³)	4	4.4	5.25
MCV (μm³)	120	118	107
MCH (pg)	40	38	34
MCHC (%)	31	32	31.7
Reticulocytes (%)	5–10	3–10	3–7
Platelets (1000/mm³)			290

Source: Klaus & Faranoff (2005).

Radiology

The radiographs of respiratory distress syndrome (RDS) show a reticulogranular pattern that looks like "ground glass," possible atelectasis that looks like white correction fluid, and obscure heart borders (Noerr, 2000).

Differential White Blood Cell Count

The formula for a total neutrophil ratio (I/T ratio) is bands divided by segs + bands:

$$\frac{\text{bands}}{\text{segs} + \text{bands}}$$

For example:

$$\frac{7 \text{ bands}}{54 + 7} = 0.11 \text{ shift}$$

This is a less than 0.3 shift and is not indicative of an infection.

White Blood Cell Count for a 1-Week-Old Newborn		
	<1500 g	1500–2500 g
Total WBC count	16.8 ($\times 10^3$/mm³)	13.0 ($\times 10^3$/mm³)
Segmented	54	55
Unsegmented	7	8
Eosinophils	2	2
Basophils	1	1
Monocytes	6	5
Lymphocytes	30	29

Source: Klaus & Faranoff (2005).

MEDICATIONS

In high-risk infants, after an airway has been established, the administration of synthetic surfactant within 15 to 30 minutes of the birth is required. Newborns larger than 1000 g benefit from surfactant therapy at any time during the first 2 to 6 hours of life.

Beractant (Survanta)

Classifications Sterile nonpyrogenic pulmonary surfactant.

Indications Lowers minimum surface tension and increases pulmonary compliance and oxygenation in preterm newborns. Prevents and treats respiratory distress syndrome.

Action Lowers surface tension at the alveolar level.

Storage Refrigerate and protect from light.

Pharmacokinetics
Absorption Absorbed only in lungs.
Distribution Is not absorbed systemically.

Contraindications and Precautions Monitor heart rate and respiration.

Adverse Reactions and Side Effects Transient bradycardia, oxygen desaturation, possible increased nosocomial infections.

Route and Dosage Intratracheal 4 mL/kg q6hr × 4 (maximum of 4 doses in first 48 hours)

Nursing Implications
1. Give within 15 minutes of birth to premature newborns.
2. Perform naso-oral suction before administration.
3. Warm the vial 20 minutes to room temperature or 8 minutes by hand.
4. Do not suction for 1 hour after administration.
5. Discard vial after use; do not re-refrigerate once it is warmed.

Data from RxList (2008).

Drugs that Can Cause Withdrawal Symptoms in Newborns

Opiates	Barbiturates	Others
Codeine	Butabarbital	Alcohol
Heroin	Phenobarbital	Amphetamine
Meperidine	Secobarbital	Chlordiazepoxide
Methadone		Clomipramine
Morphine		Cocaine
Pentazocine		Desmethylimipramine
Propoxyphene		Diazepam
		Diphenhydramine
		Ethchlorvynol
		Fluphenazine
		Glutethimide
		Hydroxyzine
		Imipramine
		Meprobamate
		Phencyclidine

Source: Gomella (1999).

Medications Used to Treat Infant of a Drug-abusing Mother (IDAM)

- Paregoric (camphorated tincture of opium)
- Phenobarbital (Luminal)

- Clonidine (Catapres)
- Chlorpromazine (Thorazine)
- Diazepam (Valium)

Naloxone (Narcan) in a Newborn with Neonatal Abstinence Syndrome

Do not use Naloxone (Narcan) if the mother is a suspected drug abuser. It may increase the severity of drug withdrawal.

ETHNOCULTURAL CONSIDERATIONS

Racial Disparities in Preterm Deliveries

- White and Asian women: 10.7%
- Hispanic women: 11.4%
- African American women: 17.6% (Cuevas et al., 2005)

Recording Weights

Record the newborn's weight in units corresponding to the parents' culture:

- North American: pounds
- European and Asian: kilograms

TEACHING THE FAMILY

Communicating to Parents About Cleft Lip and Palate Repair

- Provide parents emotional support related to their newborn's cleft lip and palate repair.
- Refer parents to Web sites that contain valuable information (see Resources at end of chapter).

Orienting Family Members to the Neonatal Unit

Orient parents to the neonatal intensive care units' (NICU) environment and policies and procedures and Health Insurance Portability and Accountability Act of 1996 [HIPAA] regulations.

- Assign one primary care nurse as the main contact for the parents.

- Explain the rationale for policies and procedures.
- Listen to the parent's expectations of their role in the NICU.
- Explain the integration of caretaking roles between parents and staff.
- Use a white board at the newborn's bed to relay messages back and forth.
- Encourage parents to call the NICU and inquire about their newborn 24/7.
- Encourage parents to bring in the newborn's personal clothes when the newborn can be dressed.
- Encourage parents to verbalize if there is dissatisfaction with newborn's care. Try to incorporate parent's suggestions into care when possible.

ADDITIONAL INFORMATION FOR THE CLINICAL SETTING

Weaning the Newborn from the Incubator

- When the newborn is being "weaned" from the servo (skin) mode of the incubator the temperature is decreased gradually every few hours while the body temperature is checked.
- When the newborn can maintain his temperature above 97.7°F (36.5°C) axillary, switch to air mode and dress the newborn.
- Closely observe the newborn's temperature, weight gain, and behavioral status during the weaning process.

Hypoglycemia in the Newborn

The nurse must understand the dynamics of hypoglycemia and remember that not all newborns are symptomatic:

- Monitor glucose levels carefully in SGA newborns. Glucose testing is often performed via heelstick (capillary blood sampling). A heelstick is done by pricking the heel and scooping the dripping heel blood into the appropriate neonatal laboratory tubes. Approximately 1 mL of blood is required for testing.
- Optimal glucose levels are 70 to 100 mg/dL, as they are in adults. The lowest clinically acceptable level is 60 mg/dL.

At a level of 40 mg/dL the newborn may become symptomatic.

- Many NICUs have protocols requiring blood glucose levels at specific intervals for SGA newborns (e.g., at birth, 1, 2, 4, and 8 hours of age; Klaus & Faranoff, 2005). Some NICUs repeat glucose levels at 12 and 24 hours of age.
- For newborns on IV therapy, since a basic component of the parenteral fluid is glucose, nurseries maintain routine blood glucose checks. IV therapy consists of providing glucose at a rate of 4 to 8 mg/kg per minute.
- If a stable newborn is found to be hypoglycemic on routine blood glucose check, start enteral feedings immediately. Recheck the glucose level 30 minutes after feeding.

Transient Tachypnea of the Newborn

The nurse must perform an accurate assessment of the respiratory system because immediately after birth or into the transitional period (within 1–2 hours) the neonate's respiratory rate should be **below 60** breaths/min with **no** retractions, nasal flaring, or grunting and a peripheral pulse oximeter reading of **>92%**. If any of these parameters are not met immediately after birth or in the transition period, immediate attention and supplemental oxygen are warranted.

Caring for the Infant with Jaundice

- Shield the newborn's eyes with an opaque mask during phototherapy. Remove the mask during feedings so the infant can receive visual stimulation.
- Assess the newborn's eyes every 4 hours for discharge or corneal irritation.
- Cover the infant's genital area.
- Keep the newborn warm during phototherapy. The infant is susceptible to hypothermia due to skin exposure and his temperature needs to be monitored closely.
- Provide proper nutrition to ensure the clearance of the bilirubin. Encourage the mother to feed the child as often as every 2 hours.
- Explain treatment measures to parents to help decrease their anxiety.

- Instruct parents to report any changes in the infant's condition such as an increase in jaundice, poor feeding, lethargy, or vomiting.

Retinopathy of Prematurity

Because retinopathy of prematurity (ROP) may be a complication of oxygen therapy, the nurse must maintain the lowest level of oxygen possible to maintain the pulse oximeter reading above 92%.

Extracorporeal Membrane Oxygenation

- Extracorporeal membrane oxygenation (ECMO) is used for newborns who are not responding to conventional or high-frequency ventilation.
- ECMO has only an 80% success rate and it is used as a last resort for respiratory support.
- Delivering ECMO is complicated, and it is a heart and lung bypass procedure used mainly for newborns with meconium aspiration pneumonia, neonatal pneumonia, and congenital diaphragmatic hernias.
- Newborns less than 34 weeks' gestation or 2000 g are not candidates owing to the need for heparinization of the blood, which can cause a cerebral hemorrhage in small or preterm newborns.
- ECMO is accomplished by inserting a catheter into the right internal jugular vein that extends into the right atrium and another catheter inserted into the right carotid artery into the aorta arch. The system drains venous blood and replaces arterial blood with oxygenated packed red blood cells, platelets, and fresh frozen plasma.
- The procedure is expensive, work intensive, and carries a multitude of complications.
- ECMO is available only at select Level III neonatal centers (Taeusch et al., 2005).

Necrotizing Enterocolitis

- Measure and record frequent abdominal circumferences.
- Auscultate bowel sounds before every feeding, and observe the abdomen for distention (observable loops or shiny skin indicating distention).

- Before a feeding, check for aspirates at each feed for undigested formula or breast milk. If excessive (20%) undigested breast milk or formula is found, follow the hospital's protocol, which may suggest that the next feeding be held and the primary care practitioner notified.
- Record all bowel movements (amount, consistency, and frequency).
- Hematest of stools may be needed to detect occult (nonvisible) fecal blood.

Most Common Causes of Neonatal Sepsis According to Onset of Symptoms

Neonatal sepsis is a systemic infection and can be due to any number of causes.

Early Onset and Late Onset	Nosocomial Onset
Group B *Streptococcus* (GBS)	*Staphylococcus epidermidis*
Listeria monocytogenes	*Pseudomonas*
Staphylococcus	*Klebsiella*
Streptococcus	*Serratia*
Haemophilus influenzae	*Proteus*

Procedure 16-1 Taking a Newborn's Blood Pressure

Purpose
Blood pressure is the pressure of blood as it is forced against the arterial walls during a cardiac contraction and is an indicator of a newborn's state of health.

Equipment
- Appropriate size cuff
- Blood pressure (B/P) machine
- Method to record results

Steps
1. Choose the appropriate size cuff by measuring the midpoint of the limb.
2. Do not use an extremity that has an IV.
3. Do not apply to broken skin areas.
4. Do not extend the cuff over a joint.

(continued)

Procedure 16-1 (Continued)

5. Inspect the cuff for intactness and decompress it to ensure it is not leaking.
6. If the cuff has an arterial mark, palpate the artery and line up the mark.
7. Wrap cuff snugly.
8. Connect the cuff to the air hose.
9. Start the blood pressure device.
10. Remove the cuff and inspect the skin (Stebor, 2005).
11. Document the procedure.

Clinical Alert Attempt to take blood pressures while the newborn is sleeping or use a pacifier to quiet the newborn for the procedure.

Note

The blood pressure is usually slightly higher in the legs.

Caution: A wide pulse pressure may indicate: Arteriovenous malformation, truncus arteriosus, or patent ductus arteriosus (PDA). A narrowed pulse pressure may indicate: peripheral vasoconstriction and cardiac failure. A systolic pressure in the arms that is 20 mm Hg or higher may indicate aortic coarctation.

Teach Parents

The nurse can teach the parents that the blood pressure is an indicator of the newborn's state of health.

Developmental Care

Providing an environment for optimal growth is the primary philosophy of developmental care. Developmental care assists in modulating the preterm newborn's behavioral states. Some of the environmental issues that can be controlled by the nurse in order to promote developmental growth include:

- Decrease noise level.
- Keep lighting subdued, and use light–dark cycles.
- Promote non-nutritive sucking.
- Provide cluster care (1–3 hours of undisturbed time between vital signs, feedings, and treatments).
- Include parents in discharge planning.

- Encourage nesting (a concept in which the linen is used to safely contain the newborn in a flexed position).

Acquainting Parents with the NICU

Explain to parents that HIPAA [Health Insurance Portability and Accountability Act of 1996 from the U.S. Department of Health and Human Services (HHS)] is taken seriously within the unit:

- Parents may be asked to step out of the unit during medical rounds, nursing report times, and possibly in emergencies to protect the privacy of all newborns.
- Phone inquiries can be done by the parents only after they identify themselves by the infant's medical record or bracelet number and they have signed a consent permitting nursing and medical personnel to discuss information on the phone with them.
- Nurses and physicians will not answer questions regarding the condition of other newborns in the unit.
- Pictures of their own newborn are allowed but they cannot photograph other newborns in the unit.

The Transport Team

The S.T.A.B.L.E. Program is designed to assist health care professionals in the postresuscitation/pretransport phase of neonatal care. It is an acronym for aspects critical to stabilization of the high-risk newborn.

S Sugar
T Temperature
A Airway
B Blood pressure
L Lab work
E Emotional support (S.T.A.B.L.E., 2006).

Endotracheal Tube (ET Tube) Size According to the Newborn's Weight and Gestational Age		
500–1000 g	<28 weeks' gestation	2.5 mm internal diameter
1000–2000 g	28–34 weeks' gestation	3.0 mm internal diameter
2000–3000 g	34–38 weeks' gestation	3.5 mm internal diameter
>3000 g	>38 weeks' gestation	3.5–4.0 mm internal diameter

Source: American Academy of Pediatrics (2000).

Types of Mechanical Ventilation Used for the Newborn

Conventional Ventilation	Conventional ventilators are set at rate of 20–60 (usually 30) breaths/min. The inspiratory time is 3-5 seconds and the peak inspiration pressure is set at 12–20 cm H_2O based on tidal volume. The flow rate is set at 6–8 L/min and they can be set to work on a timed cycle or volume cycled. Ventilators can also be patient triggered, whereby the newborn can take a spontaneous breath in between timed ventilations.
High-frequency Ventilation (HFV)	This machine uses small tidal volumes at rapid frequency (60–150 breaths/min) to decrease dead space. This is used when lower volumes would be less stressful for the neonate's respiratory system.
High-frequency Jet Ventilation (HFJV)	This method is used to limit air leaks that are problematic with atelectasis. It delivers very minute volumes at high frequency (60–600 breaths/min).
High-frequency Oscillatory Ventilation (HFOV)	This method also increases frequency to decrease volume and minimize pressure to the newborn lung. These machines are set at 300–3000 breaths/min.
Liquid Ventilation	Uses fluorocarbons, which absorb respiratory gases even better than blood. It has a low surface tension and is easily eliminated by vaporization. To date there have been no clinical trials using liquid ventilation in the newborn population (Taeusch et al., 2005).
Nitric Oxide	Used to reduce pulmonary hypertension.

RESOURCES

Parent information on discharge topics:
http://www.advanceinneonatalcare.org

Cleft Lip and Palate Association: http://www.clapa.com/

American Society of Plastic Surgeons:
http://www.plasticsurgery.org/public_education/procedures/CleftLipPalate.cfm

March of Dimes: http://www.marchofdimes.com/pnhec/4439.asp

S.T.A.B.L.E. Program: http://www.stableprogram.org/addinfo.html

National Association of Neonatal Nurses: http://www.nann.org

Cleft lip and palate information: http://www.rxlist.com/

Wide Smiles: http://www.widesmiles.org/

REFERENCES

American Academy of Pediatrics (AAP), Clinical Practice Guidelines. (2004). Management of Hyperbilirubinemia in the Newborn Infant 35 or More Weeks of Gestation, Subcommittee on Hyperbilirubinemia. *Pediatrics*, *114*(1), 297–316.

Cuevas, K., Silver, D., Brooten, D., Younglut, J., & Bobo, C. (2005). The cost of prematurity: hospital charges at birth and frequency of rehospitalizations and acute care visits over the first year of life. *AJN 105*(7), 56–64.

Gomella, T. (1999). *Neonatology*. Stamford, CT: Appleton & Lange.

Klaus, M., & Fanaroff, A. (2005). *Care of the high-risk neonate* (5th ed.). Philadelphia: W.B. Saunders.

Noerr, B. (2000). Neonatal respiratory disease and management strategies, May 18. Hershey, PA. A continuing education service of Penn State's College of Medicine at the Milton S. Hershey Medical Center.

S.T.A.B.L.E. Program (2006). Retrieved from http://www.stableprogram.org/addinfo.html (Accessed April 3, 2009).

Stebor, A.D. (2005). Basic principles of noninvasive blood pressure measurement in infants. *Advances in Neonatal Care: Official Journal of the National Association of Neonatal Nurses, 5*(5), 252–261.

Taeusch, H., Ballard, R., & Gleason, C. (2005). *Avery's diseases of the newborn*. (8th ed.) Philadelphia: Elsevier Saunders.

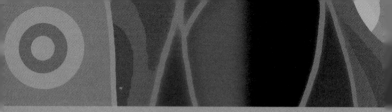

chapter

17

Caring for the Developing Child

KEY TERMS

age groups

Newborn: birth to 1 month

Infant: 1 month to 1 year

Toddler: 1 to 3 years

Early childhood/preschool: 3 to 6 years

School-age: 6 to 12 years

Adolescence: 12 to 19 years

FOCUSED ASSESSMENT

Principles of Childhood Growth and Development

- It is important for the pediatric nurse to have a working knowledge of growth and development in order to tailor care to the specific needs of the child and help the family understand the normal limits of behavior and development.
- *Nature* describes the traits inherent in the infant: biologically imposed idiosyncratic factors that create what and how each person "is."
- *Nurture* refers to the influence of external events such as parenting received, culture, or the "times" in which a child lives. Both are intrinsically influential.
- Each child moves at her own pace and in her own way. One child may move quickly through physical tasks, only to be slower with words.

- Growth refers to the continuous adjustment in the size of the child, internally and externally.
- Development refers to the ongoing process of adapting throughout the lifespan.
- Growth and development is a continuous process from conception to death.
- Development advances in an orderly sequence and each child progresses through the predictable stages within a predictable timeframe.
- Development proceeds in a cephalocaudal direction from head to tail (top to bottom).
- Development proceeds proximodistally, meaning from near to far and midline to periphery.
- Development proceeds from gross motor skills (e.g., walking, jumping, riding a bike) to fine motor skills (using utensils, coloring, cutting with scissors).
- Growth and development can be discussed in terms of theoretical approaches as well as developmental domains. A theoretical approach explains, describes, and predicts the various aspects of growth and development. A developmental domain refers to a way of understanding the total child in relation to the mind, body, and spirit. Understanding both the theoretical and developmental aspects is important because each contributes to a broader understanding about the child.

CLINICAL ALERTS

Reflexes

It is imperative to note important infant reflexes:

- Rooting: The infant's head turns and she begins to suck when her cheek or lower lip is stroked
- Sucking: Motion of lips, mouth, and tongue allowing the infant to take in sustenance
- Moro: Startle response when the infant is surprised
- Grasping: When palm of hands or soles of feet are stroked
- Babinski: Turning in of foot and spreading out of toes when sole of foot is stroked

Privacy

Guard the privacy of a school-age and adolescent child. Be aware of self-conscious behavior related to physical changes in the body that are occurring. Pay attention to other issues affecting the child and family such as menstruation, development of secondary sexual characteristics, hormonal imbalances, mood swings, family dynamics, social needs and other specific areas identified by the child and family.

ETHNOCULTURAL CONSIDERATIONS

Attachment

Infants from various cultures bond with parents and caregivers in the manner appropriate to their culture. Some cultures are more comfortable with physical touch and others with verbal exchange. Infants respond based on the cultural norms.

Puberty

African American girls tend to develop secondary sexual characteristics and begin menses somewhat earlier than Caucasian girls do.

TEACHING THE FAMILY

Introducing Solid Foods

- The infant is ready for the introduction of solid foods at approximately 6 months of age. To help determine if the infant is ready for solid foods, look for developmental cues such as the ability to sit well with support and the decrease or disappearance of extrusion reflex. The infant may also watch very intently as you eat, and may seem hungry between bottles or breastfeeding.
- Iron-fortified rice cereal is recommended as the infant's first solid food because it is the least allergenic of the grains, and the iron helps the infant replenish the iron stores received in utero. Mix the rice with formula, breast milk, or boiled and cooled water until it is soupy. As the infant adjusts to solids, you can increase the consistency of the cereal.

- When the infant is eating about 4 tablespoons of cereal twice per day, you can begin introducing vegetables and fruits. Starting with vegetables may help to increase acceptance by an infant not yet exposed to the sweet taste of fruits.
- Introduce one food at a time, waiting 3 to 5 days between new foods so you will be able to identify any reactions to particular foods.
- Introduce food before formula or breastfeeding when the infant is hungry, and then follow each solid food meal with a bottle or breast.
- If the infant is not growing or gaining weight, cannot suck or swallow, or shows any sign of allergic reaction it is important to seek help from the primary health care provider, nearby clinic, or emergency room if the problem is urgent.
- Keep salt, sugar, and additives to a minimum or avoid them altogether. If you make your own baby food, do not add salt or sugar.
- To prevent aspiration, **never** put solid food in bottles or mix with formula.
- Pay close attention while feeding and keep bites small to prevent choking

When Parents Inquire About the Development of Their Child

- Each child does not always reach the appropriate developmental stage based on chronological age alone.
- Certain events or variables, such as illness, may stunt the child's attempts to advance developmentally.
- Certain events or variables may move the child toward maturity.
- The child must successfully complete one stage before advancing to the next.

Anticipatory Guidance

Provide caregivers with information of what to expect with the child's next developmental phase (e.g., discipline, nutrition, safety, schooling, elimination, immunizations, and play).

Discipline

- Discipline teaches the child socialization and safety.
- Discipline corrects, molds, or enhances mental capacities and moral character.
- Early forms of discipline take place when the caregiver molds and structures the infant's daily routines and responds to the infant's needs.
- Parents often learn how to discipline from their own experiences as children.
- Teach parents what to expect at each of the developmental stages and how to recognize appropriate strategies for teaching and limit-setting.

Discipline Strategies

Distraction: Providing a toy or activity to divert the child's attention.

Time-out: Moving the child to a "cooling-off" place where the child can calm down or redirect. This can be a predetermined chair, step, or space that is associated with calming down.

Removal of privileges: Withholding a favorite toy or refusing to show a favorite video until the child's behavior is appropriate.

Verbal reprimands: Spoken warnings or disapprovals without berating the child or judging the child as "bad."

Corporal punishment (not recommended): e.g., spanking, swatting, grabbing.

ADDITIONAL INFORMATION FOR THE CLINICAL SETTING

Newborn and Infant

- The newborn or neonatal period of development refers to the first 4 weeks of life.
- The infant period of development encompasses the development from 1 to 12 months of life. This period of development continues to be a time of intense change in all aspects of development.
- Sensory development (the infant uses the five senses to explore and to learn about the world).
- Touch is extremely important and is the first sense to develop. The ability to feel objects, textures, and other people opens up the newborn's world of learning.

- The infant responds to smells within the first few days and has an innate preference for sweet tastes.
- Hearing is well developed at birth. A newborn can immediately recognize the difference between male and female voices and will generally turn toward the female voice.
- Vision is the least developed of the senses at birth. Newborns are fascinated with faces and with designs or objects that resemble faces. They may also demonstrate the beginnings of eye–hand coordination.
- Gross motor skills (the ability to use large muscles for movement) are the first to develop in the newborn and infant.
- Fine motor skills (the use of muscles to accomplish minute tasks such as pinching or picking up food) build on the gross motor skills.
- The infant must achieve three major tasks during this phase of development (separation, object permanence, mental representation)
- Infants initially communicate through cries (a universal language) that indicate physical discomfort or loneliness.

Infant Temperament

- Temperament refers to the characteristics present at birth that govern the way in which an infant responds to her surroundings. Understanding an infant's temperament is essential in her care to help both the parent and infant adapt to these experiences.
- Based on the work by Thomas, Chess, and Brich (1956), the following descriptors can be used to help recognize the infant's unique personality:
  - Regularity: Regularity refers to the need for reliability in sleeping, eating, and bowel habits. A child who is "easy" is one who can adapt to relatively flexible schedules. A child who is "difficult" has trouble when the schedule has been disrupted.
  - Reaction to new people and situations: The easy child responds easily to new people in her environment. Another child may stand back or withdraw when something or someone new is present.
  - Adaptability to change: This trait refers to a child's willingness to change routine. An easy child makes transitions with little or no discomfort. A slow-to-adapt child will become distressed with even the smallest changes, for instance, taking a different route home from school.

- Sensory sensitivity: An easy child with lower sensitivity appears much less meticulous or disturbed by her senses. A difficult child with high sensitivity may react strongly when exposed to sensory stimuli. The child may chafe against certain textures, tastes, smells, or sounds.
- Emotional intensity: An easy child may show little or no response to a situation. An intense child reacts dramatically and profoundly, whether that reaction is loud or withdrawn.
- Level of persistence: This trait refers to the child's willingness to stay engaged regardless of setbacks. A persistent child has difficulty giving up until the goal is reached. A less persistent child may be more flexible and give up easier.
- Activity level: An easy child is less frenetic with activity. A difficult child has difficulty with inactivity, preferring to always be on the move.
- Distractibility: The distractible child has difficulty concentrating on tasks in which he is not immersed. This is not the same as attention deficit disorder (ADD). A less distractible child is able to stay with a task longer.
- Mood: An easy child tends to see the world in a more positive way. A difficult child reacts more negatively.

Toddler (1 to 3 years)

- As the physical growth rate slows, the toddler develops skills (physical, cognitive, and emotional) that help her become more independent.
- As the toddler develops mobility, he is in a wonderful position to start exploring how things work and his senses become more refined.
- The toddler uses newly acquired gross motor skills.
- Tantrums are the toddler's way of working things out internally and are normal for the toddler. It may be possible to anticipate when tantrums are most apt to occur. For instance, when the toddler is tired, hungry, or overwhelmed by new situations, reserves are low; therefore, he may be more likely to explode or "melt down."
- If tantrums can be anticipated, they may be avoided or minimized.

- Finding a way for a tired toddler to rest or feeding a hungry child will do wonders in decreasing her frustration level.
- When the child is wailing and thrashing, but not doing any harm, the toddler should be ignored. Often this is not possible, and it may be necessary for a parent to intervene quickly and decisively to remove the child to a quieter or safer place.
- Some children respond to soothing touch, others can be distracted, and still others may need to continue the tantrum under the watchful eye of a parent.
- The goal is for the child to feel (and be) safe without being reinforced (positively or negatively) for having a tantrum.

Early Childhood (Preschooler; 3 to 6 years)

- The preschooler is much more agile; he can climb stairs using alternating feet and is able to ride his tricycle.
- As the brain becomes more developed the preschooler is better able to pick things up with the fingers.
- The preschooler engages in magical thinking.
- The preschooler has increased ability to verbalize; vocabulary has increased, from 1500 to 2000 words between the ages 3 and 5.
- Tantrums generally begin to subside.
- The preschooler is still egocentric (focused only on his own sense of things) and therefore is limited socially.
- It is a time of exploration of new skills and figuring out how to get and do things for oneself.

School-Age Child (6 to 12 years)

- There are many variations in size and shape of children in this period. These variations are influenced not only by familial and cultural genetics, but also by environmental factors such as diet and exercise.
- Sexual development begins.
- The school-age child is more able than the younger child to think logically.
- The school-age child builds on experience and begins to recognize consequences of actions.
- The school-age child is more able to determine what is important to remember and what is not.

- Language improves considerably; the child uses words more accurately and is able to elaborate on concepts that she wants to get across.
- The school-age child has a more definite sense of self-esteem or competence based on the ability or lack of ability to perform.
- Best friends tend to be of the same gender, although mixed-gender groups of school-age children become common as they reach the preteen and early teen years.

Adolescence (12 to 19 years)

- Adolescence technically begins with the onset of puberty when the pituitary gland relays messages to the sex glands to manufacture hormones necessary for reproduction.
- It is a period of great growth.
- The adolescent thinks abstractly and uses logic to solve problems and to test out hypotheses.
- Three major tasks must be confronted: choose an occupation or course of study, subscribe to a set of values, and develop a satisfactory sexual identity.

The Adolescent and the Informed Consent Process

- An informed consent is a way to elicit permission that is given freely that protects a person's right to autonomy and self-determination. Informed consent is given when the person understands the usual procedures and their rationales and associated risks.
- A legal parent or guardian customarily gives informed consent on behalf of the child.
- As children gain critical thinking skills they can become more active in the consent process.
- Depending on state law, people 18 to 21 years of age can give legal informed consent in the following situations: when they are minor parents of a child patient, when they are between 16 and 18 years of age seeking birth control, counseling or help for substance abuse, or when they are self-supporting (emancipated).
- In many states, a pregnant teen is considered emancipated.
- The physician is ultimately responsible for explaining the procedure and related risks while the nurse's role is to

serve as a witness to the parents' signature for the child or an emancipated adolescent's signature

- The nurse has a responsibility to notify the physician if the parent (or legal guardian) does not understand the procedure or related risks.
- This is a time of great questioning and consternation as the adolescent learns that it is possible for several views of morality to exist.

Helping the Teen Make Healthy Decisions

- Listen: Pay close attention not only to what the adolescent is saying, but also to his nonverbal cues. Try to understand his view of the world and the situation. Stay open minded when listening to the teen's views.
- Discuss without judging: The nurse can share his understanding of the issues and his perspectives while respecting those of the teenager.
- Encourage critical thought: Allow the teenager to explore and further develop his options.

RESOURCES

American Academy of Pediatrics. Topics on children and adolescents. http://www.aap.org

REFERENCE

Thomas, A., Chess, S., & Birch, H.G. (1968). *Temperament and behavior disorders in children*. New York: New York University Press.

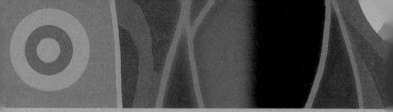

18

Caring for the Child in the Hospital and in the Community

KEY TERMS

acute pain – Pain that occurs 24 to 48 hours after trauma and surgery; severe pain that gradually subsides over time

chronic pain – Pain that lasts more than 3 months

informed consent – Involves providing the patient with the necessary knowledge to make a decision regarding health; implies that the person understands the benefits and risks of treatment or the refusal of treatment

FOCUSED ASSESSMENT

Gathering the Child's Health History

Use the mnemonics Old Cat and SODA to gather a child's health history (Bickley & Szilagyi, 2007, p. 31).

Old Cat

Onset: "When did the child become ill?"

Location: "Where is the pain?"

Duration: "How long does the pain last?"

Character: "Can you tell me on a scale of 1 to 10 how bad it is?" Or, for a younger child, ask the parents, "How much pain do you think the child is experiencing?"

Aggravating/Alleviating: "What has made the pain better or worse?"

Timing: "When does the pain start/stop?"

SODA

Sleep: "How has your child been sleeping?"

Output: "How many times per day do you _____?" (Use the expression the family has adopted to convey urine/stool output.) Or, for the younger child ask, "How many wet diapers has he had today?"

Diet: "How much fluid has your child taken in today?" "Has the illness affected the child's appetite or diet?"

Activity: "Has the child's activity level changed since he has been ill?"

Comprehensive Health History

Family Medical and Social History

- Ages and cause of death of any deceased parents, grandparents, and siblings
- Chronic illnesses experienced by family members
- Inherited diseases
- Parents' professions, religious affiliations or spiritual beliefs, and family activities
- For the older child, interviewed without the presence of the parent, the social history must also include information regarding grade level, friendships, drug or alcohol use, smoking, sexual activity, and safe sex practices

Past Medical History

- History of the pregnancy
- Labor and delivery
- Health of the baby at birth (birth weight and APGAR scores, difficulties with feeding, breathing, jaundice, or other medical problems in the early neonatal period)
- Acute illness(es)
- Chronic illness(es)
- Medication(s)
- Herbal product(s) and home remedy(ies)
- Review all encounter form(s) and determine the reason for the visit(s), resultant medical diagnose(es), and outcome(s) of previous treatment(s)
- Immunizations
- Patterns of daily activities: sleep, nutrition, play (activities and schoolwork)

Developmental Milestones

Age	Gross Motor	Fine Motor	Sensory/Language/Play
Newborn Birth–1 Month	Reflexes present Absence of head control, but can momentarily hold the head in midline Hand lag when the newborn is pulled from a lying to a sitting position Assumes flexed position When supine assumes tonic neck flex position Kicks legs and waves arms Rounded back when sitting Rolls over accidentally	Hands predominately closed Strong grasp reflex	Touch: First sense to develop Smell: Recognizes mother and has a taste preference for sweets Hearing well developed; Becomes quiet when hears a familiar voice Limited visual acuity 20/100, fascinated with faces, follows moving objects, contrasting colors (black and white) Language: Cries and smiles during sleep Play: Interaction with parents and caregivers
Infant 1–2 Months	Less head lag when pulled to sitting position When prone can slightly lift head off of floor Improved head control, turns and lifts head from side to side when prone	Hold hands open Grasp reflex absent Call pull at clothes and blanket, bats at objects	When supine follows dangling toys Visually searches for sounds Turns head to sound Language: Coos, has social smile Play: Interaction with parents and caregivers, through gross and fine motor skills and senses

Infant 3–6 Months

- Can hold head more erect when sitting, still some babbling, by 6 months sturdy head control
- Only slight head lag, by 6 months no head lag
- Raises head to 45 degrees to 90 degrees off of floor
- In sitting position (tripod) back is straight and balances head well, sits alone by 8 months
- When held in a standing position can bear some weight, by 8 months readily bears weight
- Rolls from back to side and then abdomen to back
- When supine puts feet to mouth
- Begins to creep on hands and knees

- Plays with toes
- Clutches own hands, inspects and plays with hands
- Pulls blanket over face
- Rakes objects
- Grasps objects with both hands (palmer grasp)
- Shakes rattle and holds bottle
- Eventually able to put objects in container and bang them together
- Carries objects to mouth
- Transfers objects from hand to hand
- Reaches and bangs toys on table
- Likes mirror images

- Follows object 180 degrees
- Good vision
- Locates sound by turning head
- Beginning eye–hand coordination
- Pursues dropped object visually
- Sees small objects
- Responds to name
- Language: Coos and babbles
- Play: Interaction with parents and caregivers, through gross and fine motor skills and senses

Infant 9–12 Months

- Creeps on hands and knees
- Pulls self to standing position
- Stands while holding onto furniture and begins to cruise
- Stands alone
- Changes from prone to sitting position
- Can reach backwards while sitting
- Can sit down from standing position alone
- Begins to walk holding hand and then independently, takes first step

- Uses pincer grasp
- Hand dominance evident
- Releases and rescues an object
- When sitting, purposely reaches around back to retrieve object
- Can randomly turn pages in a book
- Can make a simple mark on paper
- Waves bye-bye and plays pat-a-cake
- Begins to feed self finger foods

- Increasing depth perception
- Moves toward sound
- Thoroughly explores and experiences objects
- Points to simple objects
- Language: Says "mama" and "dada"
- Play: Plays alone, continues interaction with parents and caregivers, through gross and fine motor skills and senses

(continued)

Age	Gross Motor	Fine Motor	Sensory/Language/Play
Toddler 1–3 Years	Stands without support Walks independently Creeps upstairs Pulls toys while walking Runs with wide stance Jumps in place with both feet Climbs Begins to stand on one foot momentarily Can walk up and down stairs with alternate feet	Holds a pencil or a large crayon Makes artwork that is more representative of the object Copies a circle Knows colors Feeds self with a spoon and drinks from a cup Constantly throws objects on floor Builds tower of 3–4 cubes eventually building tower of 7–8 cubes Screws/unscrews Turns pages in a book one page at a time Turns knobs Removes shoes and socks, learns to undress self	Well developed vision Can identify geometric objects Intense interest in book's pictures Distinguishes food preferences based on senses Language: Single words and simple phrases, "I do," "Want drink." By 15 months knows 15 words Play: Play along side another child
Early Childhood (preschooler) 3–6 Years	Dress self Throws and catches ball Pedals tricycle Kicks ball forward Stands on one foot for 5–10 seconds Skips and hops on one foot Walks down steps with alternate feet Jumps from bottom step Balances on alternate feet with eyes closed	Moves around in more balanced fashion Builds a tower or 9–10 cubes Draws stick figure with 6 parts Uses scissors to cut outline of picture Copies and traces geometric patterns Ties shoe laces Uses fork, spoon, and knife with supervision Colors, prints letters Mostly independent toilet training	Well developed senses Preferences based on the use of senses Language: Vocabulary has increased from 1500 to 2000 words, eventually speaks in complete sentences Play: Plays with peers, make believe, dramatic play

School-age 6–12 Years	Gradual increase in dexterity and becomes limber Improves coordination and balance, rhythm Climbs, bikes, skips, jumps rope, swings Learns to swim, dance, do somersaults and skate	Good eye–hand coordination Balance improves Can sew, draw, makes arts and crafts, build models, play video games Prints and writes Likes activities that promote dexterity such as playing a musical instrument	20/20 Visual acuity Color discrimination fully developed Mature sense of smell Hearing deficits may be discovered as language develops Language: Accelerated, vocabulary expands to 8000–15,000 words Play: Play with peers, solitary activities and active play (e.g., dance, karate)
Adolescence 12–19 Years	Begin to develop endurance Speed and coordination Focuses skills on interest area	Manipulates complicated objects High skill level playing video games and computer Good finger dexterity for writing and other intricate tasks Precise eye–hand coordination	Increased concentration so can follow complicated instructions Senses tied into body image Develops adult preferences based on senses Language: Continues to develop and refine with increased vocabulary up to 50,000 words; improved communication skills Play: Peer groups, team sports, solitary time, school or community activities, dating

Review of Systems

- General: Usual weight, change in weight, weakness, fatigue, fever, or allergies
- Skin: Rashes, pruritus, turgor, changes in color, indications of injury, acne, changes in nails or hair
- Head, eyes, ears, nose, throat (HEENT): Injury to head, headaches, dizziness; eye infections, itching or watering eyes, behaviors indicating change in visual acuity, use of glasses, date of last eye exam; ear infections, behaviors indicating change in hearing; nose bleeds, colds, hay fever, sinus infections; sore throats, tonsils, dentition, caries
- Neck: Neck pain, enlarged lymph glands, neck range of motion
- Chest: Respiratory infections, asthma, chronic cough, wheezing, shortness of breath, breast changes
- Cardiovascular: Heart murmur, anemia, palpitations, date of last blood work
- Gastrointestinal: Regurgitation, vomiting, changes in bowel habits, constipation, diarrhea, food intolerance, abdominal pain, changes in appetite or eating pattern
- Genitourinary: *General*—dysuria, urgency, odor to urine, date of last urinalysis; signs of puberty, urethral or vaginal discharge, presence of lesions, sexual habits, contraceptive use, and symptoms or history of sexually transmitted infections; *males*—changes in groin/scrotum/glans, presence of circumcision; *females*—menarche, date of last menstrual period, dysmenorrhea, and date of last Pap smear (if appropriate)
- Musculoskeletal: Injuries, fractures, weakness, clumsiness, gait, muscle pains
- Neurological: Seizures, tics, psychiatric diseases, anxiety, depression
- Endocrine: History or symptoms of thyroid disease or diabetes or diseases that affect normal growth

Health Assessment

Anthropometric Measurements
- Length
- Weight
- Body mass index (BMI)
  - Calculate by measuring the weight in kilograms and the height in meters squared

- Help the family calculate their child's BMI by accessing the Centers for Disease Control and Prevention (CDC) Web site. This Web site has a BMI Percentile Calculator for the Child and the Teen: http://apps.nccd.cdc.gov/dnpabmi/Calculator.aspx
- Access growth charts from the National Center for Health Statistics (NCHS) are available at http://www.cdc.gov/nchs/about/major/nhanes/growthcharts/charts.htm
- Head circumference (Fig. 18-1)
- Skinfold thickness

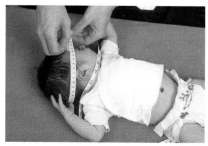

Figure 18-1 Measuring head circumference.

Vital Signs

Expected Temperatures in Children		
Age	Degrees Fahrenheit (°F)	Degrees Centigrade (°C)
2 months	99.4	37.5
4 months	99.5	37.5
1 year	99.7	37.7
2 years	99.0	37.2
4 years	98.6	37.0
6 years	98.3	36.8
8 years	98.1	36.7
10 years	98.0	36.7
12 years	97.8	36.6

Centigrade to Fahrenheit Temperature Conversions

°F = (°C × 9/5) + 32, or (°C × 1.8) + 32
°C = (°F − 32) × 5/9, or (°F − 32) × 0.55

°C	°F
35.0	95.0
35.2	95.4
35.4	95.7
35.6	96.1
35.8	96.4
36.0	96.8
36.2	97.2
36.4	97.5
36.6	97.9
36.8	98.2
37.0	**98.6**
37.2	99.0
37.4	99.3
37.6	99.7
37.8	100.0
38.0	100.4
38.2	100.8
38.4	101.1
38.6	101.5
38.8	101.8
39.0	102.2
39.2	102.6
39.4	102.9
39.6	103.3
39.8	103.6
40.0	104.0
40.2	104.4
40.4	104.7
40.6	105.1
40.8	105.4

Average Range for Pediatric Vital Signs

Age Group	Heart Rate (beats/min)	Respiration Rate (breaths/min)	Blood Pressure Systolic	Blood Pressure Diastolic
Infant	80–150	25–55	65–100	45–65
Toddler	70–110	20–30	90–105	55–70
Preschooler	65–110	20–25	95–110	60–75
School-age Child	60–95	14–22	100–120	60–75
Adolescent	55–85	12–18	110–125	65–85

Physical Assessment

General Impression

As the nurse meets the child and the parents and engages in conversation with them, an impression begins to take form. This subjective feeling about the child encompasses many areas of assessment.

- How does the child react to questions?
- What is the child's speech like?
- Is the child quiet, pleasant, talkative, uninterested, or angry?
- For the younger child: Does the child listen to parents, interact in a meaningful way, or engage in age-appropriate behavior?
- Is the child clean and appropriately dressed for the season?
- Observe body size, skin color, eyes, and the condition of the hair for evidence of a good overall nutritional state.

Skin

- Assess the skin for color, turgor, and lesions.
- Skin color reflects ethnicity, diet, disease, and injury.
- Assess for evidence of dehydration by grasping a small area of skin and pulling up. Once released, the skin should quickly return to its normal position.
- Inspect the texture of the hair and the condition of the scalp, palms, and nails. Normal nails are pink and convex, with white edges extending over the end of the fingers.
- Examine the palms for the normal flexion creases.

Head

- Observe the head for symmetry and shape.
- Palpate the skull to evaluate fontanels, sutures, contusions, or other swellings.
- The posterior fontanel closes within 1 to 3 months after birth, while the diamond-shaped anterior fontanel remains open until 12 to 18 months of age. The anterior fontanel is the most significant fontanel for evaluation (Fig. 18-2).
- Examine the face for general appearance and compare features with those of the parents.

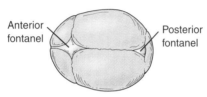

Anterior fontanel

Posterior fontanel

Figure 18-2 Anterior and posterior fontanels.

Neck

- Palpate the lymph nodes of the head and neck systematically, starting at the preauricular area, proceeding to the postauricular area, and then to the occipital nodes (Fig. 18-3).
- Palpate the trachea for midline placement and masses. A lateral deviation of the trachea may be due to a mass or a collapsed lung.
- Examine the thyroid gland for enlargement, nodules, and goiters.

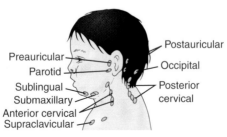

Postauricular

Preauricular

Parotid

Occipital

Sublingual

Submaxillary

Posterior cervical

Anterior cervical

Supraclavicular

Figure 18-3 Lymph nodes of the head and neck.

Eyes

- Observe the eyes to assess symmetry, shape, and placement in relation to the nose.
- Assess for symmetry and size of the pupils and their response to light.
- Observe the conjunctiva and lids for conjunctivitis, styes, or chalazia.
- Inspect the color of the sclera.
- Note erythema, swelling, or discharge from the eyes.

Ears

- Examine the external ears for size, shape, placement, pain, and presence of drainage from the ear canal.
- Examine the tympanic membrane for the presence of normal anatomic landmarks (Fig. 18-4).
- The pinna of the ear should be above the imaginary horizontal line drawn from the medial and lateral canthi toward the occiput.
- Low-set ears may indicate a congenital anomaly such as Down syndrome.
- To assess for pain, move the pinna of the ear up and down.
- Check for purulent drainage. This may indicate a foreign body in the external ear canal or a ruptured tympanic membrane.
- Immediately report any clear drainage from the ear, particularly after head trauma or with cranial infections. This fluid may indicate a cerebrospinal fluid leak.

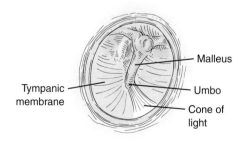

Figure 18-4 Tympanic membrane landmarks.

Nose/Sinuses

- Inspect the nasal mucosa for color and inflammation. Pale, boggy mucosa is a typical finding in a child with allergic rhinitis.
- Purulent discharge from the nose may indicate a viral or bacterial condition.
- Purulent discharge occurring in one nostril is suggestive of a foreign object in the other nostril.
- Inspect the septum for the midline position.
- Palpate maxillary sinuses for tenderness, using the thumbs of both hands and holding the child's head.

Throat/Mouth

- Eliciting the sound *eeehh* flattens the tongue better than the sound *aaahh* and visualization of the posterior pharynx is possible without the use of the tongue blade.
- Assess the palate, uvula, tonsils, and mucous membranes for color, exudate, and odor.
- Observe the lips for shape, symmetry, color, dryness, fissures at the corners of the mouth indicative of vitamin B_2 (riboflavin) deficiency, and clefts.
- Inspect teeth for number present, condition, color, alignment, and caries.
- Inspect the color and condition of gingival tissue. The gingival tissue should be the same color as the surrounding mucous membranes and should not be hypertrophied or show evidence of bleeding.

Chest

- Inspect the chest for size, shape, symmetry, respiratory effort, and breast development in infants. The anteroposterior diameter is fairly equal to the lateral diameter. By 2 years of age, the lateral diameter is greater than the anteroposterior diameter. Equal anteroposterior and lateral diameter after the age of 2 years may indicate chronic lung disease.
- A chest that is larger on the left than on the right may indicate an enlarged heart or a collapsed right lung.
- Pectus carinatum is a protrusion of the sternum.
- Pectus excavatum is a depression of the lower portion of the sternum.
- Retractions may also be seen in the suprasternal, substernal, subcostal, and suprasternal notch regions.

- Lung sounds are best auscultated with the child in a sitting position.
- Using a stethoscope with an appropriately sized pediatric diaphragm, auscultate the five lobes of the lungs, anteriorly and posteriorly, beginning with the apices and then moving side to side to compare bilateral lung sounds.
- Direct observation of breathing can also indicate inadequate oxygenation.
- The child's posture can be indicative of adequate or inadequate oxygenation. The child in respiratory distress sits in a tripod position sitting upright, leaning forward on outstretched arms with the jaw thrust forward. This particular position helps maximize opening up the airway and use of accessory muscles of respiration.
- Normal breath sounds are classified as bronchial (crackles), bronchovesicular (wheezes), or vesicular (rhonchi). Bronchial breath sounds are loud, high-pitched, and heard only over the trachea. The inspiratory and expiratory sounds are equal in length. Bronchovesicular breath sounds are of intermediate intensity and pitch, with equal inspiratory and expiratory phases.

Cardiac

- The chest is inspected for symmetry and pulsations and all peripheral pulses are palpated
- The nurse begins palpation with the carotid pulse, noting any distended neck veins, and continues with the brachial and radial pulses.
- Capillary refill is assessed as well as changes in the fingernails, e.g., clubbing of the fingers is noted.
- Peripheral edema and cyanosis are assessed during palpation of the femoral, popliteal, posterior tibial, and dorsalis pedis pulses.

Cardiac Assessment Techniques

Assessment Technique	What to Look for	Normal Findings	Abnormal Findings	Rationale
Inspection	Skin color, shape, and symmetry of chest, clubbing	Pink, symmetrical chest	Pallor, cyanosis, asymmetry of chest shape and movement, hyperdynamic precordium	Poor cardiac output. Deoxygenated circulating blood, ventricular failure or hypertrophy, tachycardia
Palpation	Skin and body temperature, moisture, chest movement, point of maximal impulse (PMI)	Warm, dry, symmetrical movement. PMI at 4th or 5th intercostal space at midclavicular line	Cold extremities, dry flaky skin, diaphoresis. Thrills or heaves	Poor circulation, heart failure, ventricular hypertrophy
Percussion	Heart shape and size	Normal size and shape for age and weight	Enlarged heart, axis deviation	Heart failure and hypertrophy
Auscultation	Murmurs, other sounds	No murmurs, innocent murmurs. Quiet precordium	Murmurs, clicks, rub, snaps.	Structural defects, increased workload of heart and volume overload

© Judith M. Marshall (2006).

- The point of maximal impulse (PMI), or area of most intense pulsation, and the point of apical impulse, or the impulse corresponding to the apex of the heart, are usually located in the same area of the chest.
- To assess for the first heart sound (S_1— the *lub* sound), begin at the fourth or fifth *left* intercostal space at the midclavicular line. The first heart sound reflects the closure of the mitral and tricuspid valves and signifies the beginning of ventricular contraction or systole.
- The second heart sound (S_2—the *dub* sound) reflects the closure of the pulmonary and aortic valves and signifies the beginning of atrial contraction or diastole. You hear *lub dub*.
- Murmurs are attributed to turbulent blood flow within the vessels. Assess for intensity, location, radiation, timing, and quality.

Abdominal

- Inspect the abdomen and its contour, which may be flat, round, protuberant, or scaphoid (shaped like a boat).
- Visible peristalsis may be noted in a thin child, and should be documented and reported.
- Inspect the umbilicus and inguinal areas for bulging. Note any scars, rashes, and lesions or piercings.
- The abdomen is divided into four quadrants: right upper quadrant (RUQ), left upper quadrant (LUQ), right lower quadrant (RLQ), and left lower quadrant (LLQ) (Fig. 18-5).
- Listen for up to 1 minute before determining the absence of bowel sounds in any one quadrant.
- After inspection, auscultate the abdomen in all four quadrants to assess for bowel motility. These high-pitched sounds occur every 5 to 10 seconds. Allow enough time to adequately assess frequency and character of the bowel sounds.
- Palpate the abdomen last so as not to disrupt bowel sounds. Palpation is divided into light palpation and deep palpation. Light palpation assists in identifying abdominal tenderness; these areas should be palpated last. Deep palpation is useful when assessing for masses in the liver, kidneys, spleen, inguinal and lymph nodes.
- Throughout the abdominal assessment, observe for changes in facial expression, guarding, and tensing of the abdominal muscles.

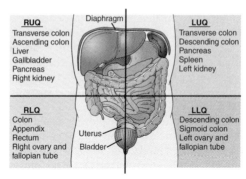

Figure 18-5 Abdomen divided into quadrants and organs in each quadrant.

Genitourinary and Perineal

- Assess boys and girls for Tanner staging of hair growth, evidence of normal development for the age of the child, signs of sexual abuse, and precocious puberty.

Tanner Staging of Development of Secondary Sex Characteristics

Sex Characteristics	Scoring				
	1	2	3	4	5
Breast Development in Females	Slight to no elevation of papilla	Breast buds appear; areolar widening with slight elevation	Entire breast enlarged with no protrusion of the papilla or nipple	Enlargement of the entire breast with formation of secondary mound of areola and papilla	Mature breast with protrusion of nipple only. No protrusion of the papilla
Pubic Hair Development in Females	None	Sparse, lightly pigmented, straight along border of labia	Darker and increasing amount on labia and pubis. Distribution in typical female inverted triangle	Coarse, thicker, curly. Increasing amount, less than adult.	Adult female triangle with extension of hair onto medial thighs
Pubic Hair and Genital Development in Males	No pubic hair. Preadolescent genitalia	Scant, long, slightly pigmented pubic hair. Slight enlargement of scrotum and testes; scrotum reddens and becomes more textured	Pubic hair darker, starting to curl and extends across pubis. Scrotum and testes continue to enlarge. Penis becomes longer and slightly wider.	Pubic hair is coarse, curly, less quantity than adult. Scrotum is darker; penis increases in length and breadth. Glans is broader.	Adult distribution of pubic hair with extension to medial thighs; genitalia adult in size and shape

Adapted from Tanner, J.M. (1962). *Growth at adolescence* (2nd ed.). Oxford: Blackwell.

- The anus is not routinely examined in children unless indicated due to abdominal, bowel, rectal, or stool abnormalities.

Musculoskeletal

- Perform the musculoskeletal exam while observing the child for range of motion, symmetry of movement, general alignment, and any deformities.
- Palpate each joint for range of motion and the presence of erythema or swelling.
- Assess the muscles for strength of movement.
- To test upper extremity strength, ask the child to hold both arms out to the sides and then out to the front. Ask the child to hold these positions as you apply downward pressure to both arms.
- Assess the symmetry of strength in both hands by having the child squeeze your index fingers.
- Test the strength of the legs by asking the child to lie supine and raise his legs while you apply downward pressure on the legs.
- Screen for scoliosis by age 14. A scoliometer can be used to assess for the condition as well as noting if the back appears straight and the hips are even.

Neurological

- Assess mental status by observing the infant's interaction with the parents, or by asking the older child to answer questions and listening for clear speech in the responses.
- Assess motor functioning during the skeletal examination. Ask the child to hop, skip, or jump to assess symmetry of movement.
- Sensory testing is done if there is a question regarding sensory functioning.
- Check cerebellar function by observing the child's posture and gait or by using the finger-to-nose test.
- Use the Romberg test to assess cerebellar functioning; the child stands with eyes closed and arms outstretched and is assessed for the ability to stand without swaying.
- Assess for persistence of primitive reflexes, which normally disappear during infancy (e.g., Babinski, Moro), palmar, plantar, and tonic neck reflexes are a few that are seen in the neonate but that disappear over time. Persistence of these reflexes may indicate cerebral dysfunction.

- Check deep-tendon reflexes (DTRs) with the reflex hammer. DTRs are difficult to elicit in some children and a distraction may be needed while testing reflexes.
- Cranial nerve assessment is an integral part of the physical examination and may be completed throughout the exam or as a separate part of the exam.

Cranial Nerve Testing

Cranial Nerve (CN)	How to Test
I. Olfactory	Ask the child to close both eyes and have the child identify smells. Rarely done during a routine examination.
II. Optic	Perform vision screen for test of visual acuity and color vision, test for peripheral vision, and examine the optic disc with the ophthalmoscope.
III. Oculomotor	Ask the child to follow an object through the six cardinal positions of gaze. Assess for papillary response and drooping of upper lids.
IV. Trochlear	CN III, IV, and VI are tested together.
V. Trigeminal	Observe the child chewing on a cracker. With eyes closed, gently stroke different areas of the face with a cotton ball to assess sensory function.
VI. Abducens	CN III, IV, and VI are tested together.
VII. Facial	Observe the child's facial expressions during the interview and exam. May need to ask child to frown and then smile.
VIII. Acoustic	Cause a loud sound and assess if child turns toward the sound.
IX. Glossopharyngeal	Stimulate gag reflex.
X. Vagus	Assess the uvula in midline. Assess the ability to swallow by asking child to do so.
XI. Accessory	While providing resistance, ask the child to shrug his shoulders and turn his head side to side.
XII. Hypoglossal	Observe infant sucking on a bottle. Ask the child to stick out the tongue. Listen for clarity of speech.

Feeding

- Basic knowledge of nutritional requirements is essential when working with children.
- Formula-fed infants require no more than 24 to 32 ounces of iron-fortified formula daily.
- Assess the older child, by taking a diet history and asking about routines at mealtimes.
- Children are often prescribed an "as tolerated" diet and they are able to select foods that appeal to them.
- Encourage the intake of wholesome and nutritious foods and snacks.
- Foods ingested are also important for their fluid content (e.g., gelatin and ice pops).
- Encourage parents to bring in favorite foods from home.
- Cultural preferences may make a difference in whether or not a child eats while hospitalized.
- Evaluate if foods and caloric intake are appropriate for age and developmental level.

Average Daily Caloric Requirements for Children	
Age	Daily caloric requirements
0–1 month	100–110 kcal/kg per day
2–4 months	90–100 kcal/kg per day
5–60 months	70–90 kcal/kg per day
>5 years	1500 kcal for first 20 kg + 25 kcal for each additional kg/day

Source: Hay W.W. Jr. et al. (2005). *Current pediatric diagnosis & treatment* (19th ed.). New York: Lange Medical Books/McGraw-Hill.

Measuring Intake and Output
Calculation of Daily Maintenance Fluid Requirements

- The surface area method is the most common and used for children weighing more than 22 lbs. (10 kg): 1500 to 2000 mL/m² per day.

- Daily maintenance fluid requirements:

Calculation of Daily Maintenance Fluid Requirements

Child's Weight	Daily Maintenance Fluid Requirement
0–10 kg (0–22 lbs.)	100 mL/kg of body weight
11–20 kg (24.2–44 lbs.)	1000 mL + 50 mL/kg for each kg >10
>20 kg (>44 lbs.)	1500 mL + 20 mL/kg for each kg >20

Example:
A child weighs 48 kg. For the first 20 kg the child needs 1500 mL. For the next 28 kg the child needs 20 mL/kg. So,
500 mL + (28 kg × 20 mL) = 1500 mL + 560 mL = 2060 mL/day.

- Normal urinary output is 1 to 2 mL/kg per hour.

Pain

- Remember that *"pain is whatever the child says it is."*
- Mild pain is a slight discomfort and is managed with minor analgesics along with comfort measures or distraction.
- Moderate pain may be relieved by using distraction and in conjunction with regularly timed analgesic administration, including milder opioids such as codeine in varying combinations of acetaminophen (Children's Tylenol).
- Severe pain causes pallor, sweating, piloerection (elevation of the hair above the skin), dilated pupils, increased respiration and blood pressure, and muscle tension. Management of severe pain, often associated with surgical interventions, is usually managed with strong analgesics such as morphine (Astramorph).
- Pain may be either acute or chronic. Acute pain occurs 24 to 48 hours after trauma or surgery. It is initially experienced as severe pain, and gradually subsides over time. Chronic pain in children is any pain lasting more than 3 months. It can result in fear of reinjury, anorexia, weight loss, changes in sleep patterns, guarded movements, a rigid facial expression, and diminishment of the child's joy of living.

Characteristics of Acute and Chronic Pain

Acute Pain	Chronic Pain	Chronic Cancer Pain
Identifiable cause	Cause difficult to determine	Usually identifiable cause
Short duration	Lasts longer than 3 months	Duration varies
Sudden onset		Onset varies
Well defined	Begins gradually and persists	May or may not be well defined
Limited	May or may not be well defined	
Decreases with healing		Unlimited
Reversible	Unlimited	May persist beyond healing
Objective signs and symptoms	Persists beyond healing time	Exhausting and useless
Anxiety	Exhausting and useless	Objective signs absent
	Objective signs absent	Depression, fatigue, and anxiety
	Depression and fatigue	

Source: Otto, S. E. Oncology nursing. St. Louis: C.V. Mosby, 1991. Reprinted in Mosby's medical, nursing and allied dictionary (4th ed.), p. 1144.

Several statistically reliable pain scales are available for use with children of different ages and stages of cognitive development. The most commonly used pain scales are the numeric scale, the Wong Faces Scale, and the FLACC pain scale (Fig. 18-6).

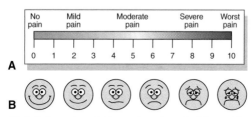

Figure 18-6 Pain scales. *A.* Numeric pain scale (about 12 years or older). *B.* Wong-Baker Faces pain scale (preschool through school-age).

FLACC Pain Scale

Categories	Scoring		
	0	1	2
Face	No particular expression or smile; disinterested	Occasional grimace or frown; withdrawn	Frequent to constant frown, clenched jaw, quivering chin
Legs	Normal position or relaxed	Uneasy, restless, tense	Kicking, or legs drawn up
Activity	Lying quietly, normal position, moves easily	Squirming, shifting back and forth, tense	Arched, rigid, or jerking
Cry	No cry (awake or asleep)	Moans or whimpers, occasional complaint	Crying steadily, screams or sobs, frequent complaints
Consolability	Content, relaxed	Reassured by occasional touching, hugging, or talking to. Distractible.	Difficult to console or comfort.

Each of the five categories—(F) Face; (L) Legs; (A) Activity; (C) Cry; (C) Consolability—is scored from 0 to 2, which results in a total score between 0 and 10

CLINICAL ALERTS

Important Respiratory Signals

Normal breath sounds are equal bilaterally in intensity, rhythm, and pitch. The following respiratory signals may indicate the presence of a respiratory condition in a child:

- Noisy breathing or snoring (air passing through a narrowed upper airway) may indicate nasal polyps, foreign body obstruction, choanal obstruction, hypertrophied adenoid tissue, or obesity.
- Grunting is caused by the glottis closing at the end of expiration and may suggest respiratory distress or pneumonia.
- Nasal flaring (intermittent outward movement of the nostrils) occurs on inspiration and is a form of accessory muscle use found in a variety of conditions such as respiratory distress syndrome (RDS) (Venes, 2005).

- Coughing (a forceful expiratory effort) is a normal process that clears the throat, but can indicate an infection, asthma, lung disease, or sinusitis.
- Stridor (a high-pitched, harsh sound occurring during inspiration) results from air moving through a narrowed trachea and larynx and can indicate croup (Venes, 2005).
- Wheezing (a musical noise) results from air moving through mucus or fluids in a narrowed lower airway that is associated with asthma.
- Hoarseness is a rough quality in the child's voice and can mean that the airway is inflamed.
- Crackles is a fine, high-pitched sound lung heard on inspiration or expiration produced by air passing over retained airway secretions or the sudden opening of collapsed airways found in several respiratory conditions (Venes, 2005).
- Rhonchi is a low-pitched wheezing, snoring, or squeaking sound indicating a partial airway obstruction. Mucus or other secretions in the airway, bronchial hyperreactivity, or tumors that occlude respiratory passages can cause the airway obstruction (Venes, 2005).
- Color changes in the skin (pallor, mottling and cyanosis) are significant respiratory signals and usually indicate cardiac involvement.
- Chest pain is caused by alteration in chest structures, nonpulmonary involvement, or a variety of respiratory conditions
- Clubbing (excessive growth of the soft tissues at the ends of the fingers or toes) is usually associated with chronic hypoxia and pulmonary disease.

Safety Measures

Keeping Children Safe in the Home or Hospital

- Parents must imagine how a child thinks. Suggest that parents get down on the floor in their home to see what their child sees (e.g., electrical plugs and outlets, tablecloths ready to be pulled, hot coffee mugs or tea saucers perched on the edge of the coffee table).
- In the hospital, store toxic and nontoxic materials in a locked utility room, on the top shelf of a cabinet, or in another location where children do not have ready access. Keep utility rooms, kitchens, medication carts, treatment rooms, and supply rooms locked. Lock play areas unless the child is accompanied by an adult.

Handwashing

- Wearing gloves does not replace the need for handwashing. Gloves may have small defects that allow the hands to become contaminated during removal of the gloves. Handwashing is essential if the caregiver touches any item in the child's room, as objects may have been touched by the child and are considered contaminated.

Risk of Infection

- With any procedure where the skin barrier is compromised, adhere to sterile techniques for dressing changes over IV sites and to monitor for signs and symptoms of infection (change in temperature, erythema, edema, pain at IV site, tenderness on palpation).

Gastrostomy Tubes

- A gastrostomy tube may move into the duodenum and cause an obstruction as it occludes the pyloric sphincter. Mark the tube with indelible ink to make it easy to observe for migration. Report any vomiting, abdominal distention, or evidence of bile drainage as aspirate.

Naloxone (Narcan)

- When giving morphine sulfate, be sure to have the opioid antagonist naloxone (Narcan) available. Narcan completely blocks the respiratory depression caused by the opioids, including central nervous system (CNS) effects. The dose for children is 5-10 mcg/kg (0.01 mg/kg) (Deglin & Vallerand, 2009).

DIAGNOSTIC TESTS

Body Mass Index (BMI)

- A BMI-for-age plotted below the 5th percentile indicates that a child is underweight; a BMI-for-age between the 5th and 85th percentile is considered a healthy weight; a child with a BMI-for-age between the 85th and 95th percentile are considered at risk for obesity; and those with a BMI-for-age greater than 95% are considered obese.

Eye Assessment Tools

- Visual screening for children can begin at the age of 2 $^1/_2$ years. Various charts are available to assist in the assessment of visual acuity.

- Visual acuity for each eye is assessed by occluding the contralateral eye with a plastic paddle.

- With all charts the objects, letters and numbers decrease in size. The Allen chart requires the child to identify common objects; the "tumbling E" requires the child to identify in which direction each E is facing; and the Snellen charts require the child to identify letters or numbers (Fig. 18-7).

- A common method for assessing ocular alignment is the Hirschberg corneal light reflex test, in which a light is shone directly into the child's eyes and note is taken of the position of the corneal light reflection in both eyes. The reflection should fall in the same location on the cornea of each eye.

- The second screening test is the cover–uncover test, in which the child is asked to focus on a distant object across the room. Cover the first eye while watching the second eye for any movement. Remove the cover and observe for any movement. If no movement is detected, ocular alignment is intact. Repeat the examination on the opposite eye.

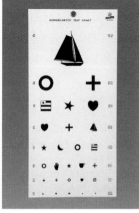 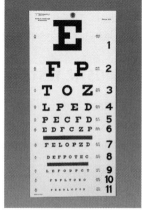

A   B

Figure 18-7 Eye charts used to assess vision.

- Test the red reflex by viewing the pupil through an ophthalmoscope from a distance of ten inches. If the pupil appears red, the finding is normal. A white retinal reflex may indicate cataracts, retinoblastoma, or chorioretinitis.
- Children should be screened at least once during the school-age years for the ability to discriminate between red, yellow, and green. A common method for detecting color blindness is the use of the Ishihara pseudochromatic charts. The inability to identify the numbers indicates color blindness.

Hearing Screening Techniques

- Hearing screening should be done before any injections, vaccines, or laboratory work. Assess for frequency (pitch) and the decibel level (loudness). Frequency is defined as the number of vibrations a sound creates per second. As the frequency increases, the pitch of the sound also increases. The frequency range is 250 to 6000. For a normal finding, the child should hear at all frequencies at the 20-decibel range.
- Conditioned play audiometry (CPA) is a common test for children older than 3 years. Engage the child in a play-oriented activity (e.g., placing a colorful block in a box each time a sound is heard). The child is subjected to sounds of different frequencies that a child with normal hearing could hear.
- A conventional audiogram assesses hearing acuity by asking the child to raise his hand or press a button each time a sound is heard. The child must be able to understand the language spoken, be able to follow directions, pay attention, and wait to listen to the sounds.
- Use tympanometry to assess the status of the middle ear. Places a probe into the ear canal. The amount of sound that is reflected by the tympanic membrane is measured along with the pressure in the canal. The tympanogram delineates the movement of the eardrum as stiffness, floppiness, or normal eardrum movement.
- The Weber test involves striking the tines of the tuning fork and immediately placing the handle of the tuning fork midline on top of the child's head. Ask the child in which ear he hears the sound best. If hearing is normal, sound is heard equally in both ears. Sound heard in one ear better than the other indicates a conductive hearing loss.

- Use the Rinne test to assess air and bone conduction of sound. Bone conduction is tested by placing the handle of the vibrating tuning fork on the mastoid process behind the ear. The child informs the nurse when he no longer can hear the sound of the vibrating tuning fork and the nurse immediately moves the tines forward to within 1 to 2 inches of the auditory meatus. The child should hear the air-conducted sound of the vibrating tines twice as long as he heard the bone-conducted sound.

Analysis of Cerebrospinal Fluid (CSF)

- With the lumbar puncture, a needle is inserted into the subarachnoid space at the level of L4 or L5 to withdraw CSF for analysis. CSF samples are sent for culture, glucose, red blood cell (RBC) and white blood cell (WBC) count, and protein.
- Normal values for total WBC and differential in adult males and females are:
  - Total WBC: 4500 to 10,000
  - Bands or stabs: 3% to 5%
  - Granulocytes (or polymorphonuclears)
    - Neutrophils (or segs): 50% to 70% relative value (2500–7000 absolute value)
    - Eosinophils: 1% to 3% relative value (100–300 absolute value)
    - Basophils: 0.4% to 1% relative value (40–100 absolute value)
  - Agranulocytes (or mononuclears)
    - Lymphocytes: 25% to 35% relative value (1700–3500 absolute value)
    - Monocytes: 4% to 6% relative value (200–600 absolute value)

Analysis of Cerebrospinal Fluid

	Pressure (mm Hg)	Protein (mg/dL)	RBCs	Glucose (mg/dL)	WBCs (%)
Infant	<200	20–170	None	34–119	0–30
Child	<200	5–40	None	60–80	0–20

MEDICATIONS

Pain Management with Acetaminophen

Acetaminophen is an over-the-counter medication that is used for mild to moderate pain and fever control in children. Acetaminophen comes as a liquid in drop or elixir form; as a tablet in the form of chewable tablets, swallowable caplets, and capsules; and as a suppository. Acetaminophen is the generic name for Tylenol, Panadol, Tempra, Liquiprin, in drop form; Paracetamol, St. Joseph Aspirin-Free Chewable, and Chewable Anacin 3 in tablet form; and Fever-all in suppository form.

How to Determine the Recommended Dose of Medication Based on the Child's Age and Weight

	3 mo	4–11 mo	12–23 mo	2–3 yr	4–5 yr	6–8 yr	9–10 yr	11 yr	12 yr
Weight (lbs.)	6–11	12–17	18–23	24–35	36–47	48–59	60–71	72–95	>96
Dose (mg)	40	80	120	160	240	320	400	480	650
Liquids									
Drops (1 dropper = 80 mg/0.8 mL)	$1/2$	1	$1–1\,1/2$	2	—	—	—	—	—
Elixir/suspension 160 mg/5 mL (1 tsp)	—	$1/2$ tsp	$3/4$ tsp	1 tsp	$1\,1/2$ tsp	2 tsp	$2\,1/2$ tsp	3 tsp	—
Tablets									
Chewable 80 mg/tab	—	—	—	2	3	4	—	—	—
Swallowable 160 mg/tab	—	—	—	1	$1\,1/2$	2	$2\,1/2$	3	4
Capsules 80 mg	—	—	—	2	3	4	—	—	—
Capsules 160 mg	—	—	—	1	—	2	—	3	4

Suppository									
Infant strength 80 mg	½	1	—	—	—	—	—	—	—
Child strength 120 mg	—	½	1	1	2	—	—	—	—
Junior strength 325 mg	—	—	—	—	—	1	1	1½	2

- Age-appropriate doses can be repeated every 4 to 6 hours according to instructions on the label and the recommendation of your health care provider.
- Do not exceed five doses in 24 hours.
- There are few side effects associated with acetaminophen when the appropriate dose for age and weight are followed.
- Gastrointestinal (stomach) upset can occur in some people. If this occurs, food or milk may be given to reduce the stomach upset.
- Signs of an allergic reaction may include fever and rash and should be reported to your health care provider if suspected.
- Signs of toxicity (overdose of the medication) that require immediate reporting to your health care provider include paleness, bluish discoloration of the skin or nails, weakness, irregular or rapid heart beat, shortness of breath, unexplained bleeding or bruising, sore throat, fatigue, headache or dizziness, and nausea or vomiting.
- Signs of chronic poisoning or overdose include abdominal pain, yellow skin and eyes, dark urine, itchy skin, and clay-colored bowel movements.

Essential Information

Acetaminophen is also found in other medications, such as cold and flu preparations. To prevent accidental overdose, check with your pharmacist or health care provider to ensure that your child is not receiving too much medication if you are using a combination of over-the-counter preparations that contain acetaminophen.

Commonly Used Herbal Preparations

Herb	Use	Concerns
Aloe Vera	Minor skin wounds and irritations.	No known side effects for topical applications.
Bilberry	The tea form is used for the treatment of diarrhea.	Can affect clotting time by decreasing platelet aggregation.
Cayenne Pepper	Relief of pain associated with tonsillitis (capsule form) and sore muscles (ointment).	Ointment may cause burning sensation when used topically.
Chamomile	Pain associated with colic, teething and stomach aches.	Hypersensitivity reaction. Contraindicated in those allergic to daisies, marigolds or ragweed.
Echinacea	Symptoms of the common cold and mild infections.	Do not use for autoimmune disorders, diabetes, AIDS, HIV. Use for short-term illnesses only.
Fennel	Colic, stomach spasms and cough associated with respiratory infections.	May have a laxative effect.
Feverfew	Migraines	Not safe for children younger than 2 years of age. Administration of nonsteroidal anti-inflammatory drugs (NSAIDs) inhibits the effect of feverfew.
Licorice	The oral form treats cough; the topical form is used in the treatment of eczema.	Safe for children if taken for short-term illness. Contraindicated in diabetes, hypertension, and liver and kidney disease.
Nettle	Asthma and allergy symptoms	May increase blood sugar.
St John's Wort	Mild depression	May cause photosensitivity; many herb–drug interactions
Tea Tree Oil	The topical form is used as an antibacterial	Use restricted to topical application.
Valerian	Mild to moderate insomnia	May potentiate sedative effects of barbiturates, anesthetics, and CNS depressants. May cause GI upset

Source: Bascom (2002).

Ibuprofen (Children's Advil)

- A common nonsteroidal anti-inflammatory drug (NSAID) given to children as a fever-reducing measure
- Given every 6 hours and may be an advantage when rest is crucial or when administering medications to the child is a challenging task.
- Dyspepsia and nausea are common side effects.
- Can be given (chewable tablet, caplet, or liquid) with food or after meals if gastrointestinal (GI) upset occurs.
- Monitor the child for GI bleeding.
- Dosing for ibuprofen is dependent on the temperature of the child. A fever below 102.6°F (39.2°C) warrants a dose of 5 mg/kg of body weight.
- Increase the dose to 10 mg/kg of body weight, if a child's temperature is over 102.6°F (39.2°C).
- Assess the efficacy of antipyretic medication by retaking the child's temperature one hour after administration.

Morphine Sulfate (Astramorph)

- Morphine sulfate (Astramorph) is an opioid analgesic that is frequently used for children with chronic pain.
- Administer PO, IV, IM, epidurally, or via a patient-controlled analgesia (PCA) pump. For children weighing less than 50 kg the dose is:

0.3 mg/kg PO every 3 to 4 hours, or 0.1 mg/kg IV or IM every 3 to 4 hours (Deglin & Vallerand, 2009).

ETHNOCULTURAL CONSIDERATIONS

Stereotyping

Avoid stereotyping an individual or family based on a specific racial or cultural background, or assuming that all members of a particular culture subscribe to the traditions, beliefs, and customs associated with that culture. Length of time in the country, level of education, level of acculturation, and economic status affect the degree to which the culture shapes the parent's approach to health care (Salimbene, 2005).

Skin Assessment

The sclera is white in light-skinned individuals. It is normal for the sclera to be slightly yellow with small black marks in darker-skinned individuals.

Lead Exposure in Folk Medicines

Folk medicines used by Indian, Middle Eastern, West Asian, and Hispanic cultures may contain high levels of lead. Inquire as to the use of greta, azarcon (coral, *luiga*, *maria luisa*, or *rueda*), ghasard, or ba-baw-san.

TEACHING THE FAMILY

Caring for the Child with a Disability

- Maintain a respectful attitude toward the parents and the child.
- Listen carefully to the parents' concerns. They know their child best.
- Evaluate how social and health care agencies can assist the parents and the child to manage the disability (financial, medical, community services).
- Assess the child's skills for coping with pain or fatigue
- Evaluate the need for respite care and reliable community resource providers.

Using Cotton Swabs

Instruct parents to use cotton swabs to clean only the external ear (not the ear canal) to avoid pushing cerumen into the canal, where it cannot be removed by the mechanical action of the tiny ear hairs. Cerumen dries, hardens, and becomes difficult to remove over time. Impacted cerumen in the ear canal may lead to hearing deficits.

Decreasing Exposure to Lead

- Encourage parents to contact the water authority to determine the lead content in the water. The EPA states that 15 parts per billion is acceptable.

- If mixing formula from powder or concentrate, advise parents to flush water from the system by running the tap for 1 to 2 minutes before using the water. Most of the lead comes from the corrosion of older pipes that leak into the water supply after sitting in the pipes for several hours.

Preparing Children for Procedures

Infant

- Describe the procedure to the parents; explain what will happen and how long it will take.
- Encourage the parents to stop you at any point if they have a question.
- Remind parents that infants often cry for reasons other than discomfort, but be honest about any discomfort the infant may experience with the procedure.
- Identify what restraints may be used and provide an explanation as to why they are needed. Allow parents to decide whether they would like to be present for the procedure. Parents may prefer to leave the room and return immediately after the procedure to comfort their child.

Toddler

- Describe the procedure to the parents, explaining what will happen and how long it will take.
- Use play to demonstrate the procedure to the toddler. Encourage him to demonstrate/practice with a doll or teddy bear.
- Use simple, concrete language to describe the procedure and how it might feel to the toddler.
- Limit preparation to 5 to 10 minutes due to the shorter attention span of the toddler.
- Identify the restraints that may be used and give an explanation as to why they are needed. Allow parents to decide whether they would like to be present for the procedure. Parents may prefer to leave the room and return immediately after the procedure to comfort their child.

Preschooler

- Explain the procedure in terminology the child can understand.

- Begin preparation immediately before the procedure so the child does not worry for hours or days.
- Use play to demonstrate the procedure to the child; encourage her to demonstrate/practice with a doll or teddy bear.
- Set limits for the child so she is aware of expectations (e.g., tell her she can yell and scream as much as she wants, but must hold very still).
- Give legitimate choices to the child whenever possible.
- Allow parents to decide whether they would like to be present for the procedure. Parents may prefer to leave the room and return immediately following the procedure to comfort their child.
- Use distraction techniques such as deep breathing, singing, or squeezing a parent's or nurse's hand.

School-age Child

- Explain the procedure in terminology that the child can understand. Children in this stage of development have a good concept of time, so preparation can begin in advance of the procedure.
- For the younger school-age child, use play to demonstrate the procedure and if possible have the child demonstrate on and practice positioning with a doll or teddy bear. Allow the child to touch and explore equipment to be used in the procedure, and involve the child in simple tasks during the procedure when possible. Set limits for the child so she is aware of expectations (e.g., tell her she can yell and scream as much as she wants, but must hold very still). Give legitimate choices to the child whenever possible.
- Allow parents and the child to decide together whether parents will be present for the procedure. Some school-age children may be modest about exposing body parts in front of family members.
- Teach the child techniques such as deep breathing, counting, reciting a silly rhyme, or anything else that might help distract and relax the child during the procedure.

Adolescent

- Describe the procedure, explaining exactly what will happen and how long it will take.
- Encourage the adolescent to stop you at any point if she has a question.

- Be honest. Describe potential risks and pain associated with the procedure, but do not dwell on it.
- Allow the adolescent to take as active a role as possible in the procedure. Practicing positioning or demonstrating the equipment prior to the procedure helps give the adolescent a sense of control.
- Provide a peer video of the procedure if possible.
- Allow the adolescent to make decisions such as when the procedure should take place, if possible.
- Offer tips for distraction such as deep breathing, relaxation, counting, or squeezing an object or parent's hand.

Insurance for Children

- Teach the family how to obtain health insurance for their child.
- Encourage the family to call 1-877 KIDS NOW (1-877-543-7669) or go to your state's program: http://www.insurekidsnow.gov/states.asp
- Children who are eligible for Medicaid cannot enroll in the state program because Medicaid provides comprehensive health benefits.

Promoting Resiliency

- Express love and gratitude.
- Foster competency and positive attitudes.
- Nurture positive emotions.
- Encourage helping others.
- Teach peace-building skills.
- Reinforce positive behaviors.
- Reduce stress.

ADDITIONAL INFORMATION FOR THE CLINICAL SETTING

Use of Herbal Products

- The use of herbal products and home remedies is common (Lanski et al., 2003), but often parents do not divulge herbal product use for their children in encounters with health care providers.

- Ask about the use of herbal products to avoid inadvertent drug interactions.

Key Actions in Caring for the Child Confined to Bed

- Keep skin clean and dry.
- Assess nutritional status for adequate protein.
- Use the draw sheet for position changes.
- Assess skin for irritated areas.
- Assess for pressure ulcers by looking for the "red flush" (the first sign of tissue compromise and ischemia).

Encouraging Adequate Intake

- Offer small portions at frequent intervals.
- Host a "tea party" using medicine cups filled with the child's favorite drink.
- Make food into fun shapes (trace a smile face with mayonnaise on a sandwich, use a cookie cutter to make different shapes for sandwiches).
- Offer incentives of more time doing a favored activity.
- To provide autonomy, offer two choices (e.g., a straw or a colored cup).

Spiritual Care

Comfort may be found in dialogue with a priest, monk, chaplain, deacon, rabbi, imam, or other trusted person with a religious affiliation. At times when parents ask "why is this happening to my child?" it may be beneficial for the nurse to arrange a meeting to discuss the parents concerns and issues.

Before, During, and After a Procedure

Before

- Think through the procedure in advance and anticipate problems.
- Gather all equipment and check to make sure it functions properly.
- Establish trust. Get to know the child first.
- Through the use of play, allow the child to "perform" the procedure on her doll, teddy bear, or other appropriate surrogate.

- Offer a coping strategy such as guided imagery or relaxation breathing.
- Give the child realistic choices.
- Be sure informed consent is signed.
- Wash hands.
- Let the child know that it is "OK" to cry.

During

- Whenever possible, schedule all treatments away from the child's bed or "safe area."
- Expect the child to do well.
- Talk to the child and ask how he is doing.
- Keep the child informed as to the progress of the procedure.
- Use distraction techniques such as pop-up picture books, bubbles, "shutting off the pain switch," or other techniques that have been practiced before the procedure.
- When appropriate, give the child some control by allowing him to make some of the decisions.
- Encourage the parent to provide comfort to the child, if the parent is able. Sometimes a parent's presence at the procedure may not be beneficial for the child.

After

- Praise the child for completing the procedure.
- Provide an opportunity for the child to verbalize feelings.
- If the parents were not involved in the procedure, comment on a positive aspect involving the child during the procedure (e.g., "Jill was able to help out and keep still when she was asked to do so! She did a great job!").
- Give a reward (stickers, small toy, previously agreed-upon reward negotiated with parents).
- Document the child's response to procedure and outcomes.

Using Developmentally Appropriate Words

- For children with beginning language skills, use simple terms that are familiar to the child, such as "go potty," "owie," and "boo boo."
- For the concrete thinker who takes what is said literally, do not use words that may frighten the child: "*dye* in your vein," "*shot* in the arm," "*cut* out the tonsils," and "*take* your temperature."

- Instead use "*special medicine* in your vein," "*special medicine* in your arm," "*make* your tonsils *better*," "*check* to see if your temperature *is working.*"
- Be honest and patients will learn to trust you.

Obtain Written Consent Before a Procedure

- Obtain informed consent before a procedure is performed.
- It is the physician's responsibility to explain the procedure and the risks and benefits of treatment.
- Alternatives to the prescribed treatment should be discussed.
- When signed by the emancipated minor or parent, an informed consent is a legal document denoting that the emancipated minor or parent understands the nature of the procedure, risks, and benefits.
- The nurse is a witness to the signature.

 Procedure 18-1 Guidelines for Inserting an Oro- or Nasogastric Tube

Purpose

To maintain the child's nutrition using a feeding tube that is passed through the mouth or nares and into the stomach

Equipment

- Oro- or nasogastric tube
- Tap water or a water soluble lubricant
- Syringe
- pH indicator paper

Steps

1. Wash hands and don gloves.
2. Determine tube length required by measuring from the nose to the earlobe and to the midway point between the end of the xiphoid process and the umbilicus.
3. Note the measurement by finding the manufacturer's black mark on the appropriately sized feeding tube.

(continued)

Procedure 18-1 (Continued)

4. Lubricate the tube with tap water or a water-soluble lubricant. Follow the manufacturer's guidelines. Using the dominate hand gently direct the tube toward the back of the throat. If using the nose, direct toward the occiput.

5. Aspirate stomach contents.

6. Check for proper placement using the method following the institution's policy:

   • Use pH indicator paper for assessment of gastric aspirate.

   • Inject a small amount of air into the tube while auscultating over the stomach; the nurse should hear a "swoosh" as the air enters the stomach.

   • Obtain an X-ray film to verify placement. This method is not practical for every feeding, but is often used after initial placement of the oro- or nasogastric feeding tube when used for continuous feeding.

7. Document the procedure.

Clinical Alert There are some risks with an oro- or nasogastric tube. The liquid from the feeding or medication may enter the lungs and possibility cause pneumonia. In addition, the feeding tubes may cause the child discomfort. The tube can also become plugged, causing pain, nausea, or vomiting.

Teach Parents

It is important to teach parents about artificial nutrition and hydration as well as the function of the oro- or nasogastric tube. Parents can be encouraged to report displacement of the tube, noted distress in the child and tube placement if necessary.

Psychosocial Needs of the Infant Receiving Gavage Feedings

• Place the infant comfortably in the mother's arms with the head elevated.

• Provide the infant with a pacifier to help simulate an actual feeding.

- Nonnutritive sucking has been shown to increase weight gain and decrease crying, and allow for the normal muscular development of the mouth and tongue.

Care of the Child in Restraints

- Remove restraints every 2 hours to assess skin and provide range of motion (ROM) exercises to the affected extremity.
- Provide supervised time with restraints off, if appropriate, to allow the child to engage in activities of daily living (toileting, feeding, reading a book, watching TV, etc.).
- Encourage games and activities that promote growth and development.
- Reapply restraints.
- Document condition of skin, nursing care given with restraints off, removal, and reapplication of restraints.
- Teach parents how to remove and reapply restraints.

Myths About Pain Management

- Children don't feel pain with the same intensity as adults.
- Neonates do not feel pain because their nervous systems are not mature.
- Children cannot tell where they hurt.
- Children will tell you if they are really having pain.
- Children become accustomed to pain.
- Narcotic analgesics are dangerous for children because they will become addicted or go into respiratory distress.
- If children can be distracted, they are not in pain.
- If children say they are in pain, but don't look in pain, they don't need to be medicated.
- Being in pain for only a little while isn't that bad.
- After children have undergone surgery, they should not be given analgesia until they can vocalize pain, because they received enough anesthetic to "cover" their pain.
- The best way to give analgesics is intramuscularly.
- Children with neurological impairments do not feel pain as much as other children.
- Children, especially boys, should learn to tolerate pain; they will make better, stronger adults.

Pain Management Strategies

Age (Guideline only)	Reactions	Concerns/ Distraction	Environment	Involvement	Parental Preparation	Positions	Post Procedure Comforting
Infant/Toddler (0–3 years)	Separation anxiety Protest Despair Denial	Pacifier Swaddling Rocking Eye contact Music Picture books	Controlled lighting and noise Use treatment room	Encourage parental presence, provide guidance, comfort/cuddle baby during procedure.	Prepare parent: offer explanations of what they will see and hear. Develop a plan "who will do what"	Swaddle Cuddle	Soothe Swaddle Hold and rock Soft music Soothing voice
Preschool (3–6 years)	Separation anxiety Concerns with body image Develops fantasies with illness and treatment Battle for control	Distraction kit Deep breathing Bubble blowing Counting Singing	Use treatment room Music Controlled lighting and noise	Encourage parental presence and provide guidance in encouraging participation during strategies.	Medical play with relevant medical equipment and participation Pre-procedural teaching Reassurance of what child is to expect (focus on senses)	Lap Parent or staff may support patient or have other close physical contact.	Praise and reward stickers Medical play Play Stories
School-age (6–11 years)	Has questions regarding body and illness	Deep breathing Hand squeezing Riddles/trivia Pretend games	Use treatment room Music Controlled lighting and noise	Encourage parental presence and provide guidance	Simple medical terms to describe what will happen	Lap	Praise, reward stickers Play, medical play

Concerns of helplessness, passivity, and dependency Tend to be phobic and develop fears Anger	Talking Distraction kit		Encourage parents to be part of the team.	Allow appropriate play with medical equipment. Explain reasons for various components of tests and allow appropriate participation by patient.	Parent may support patient or have other close physical contact. Present patient with choices.	Stories Evaluate procedures and discuss suggestions for next time.
Teens (12 years and older) Illness interferes with struggle for independence Illness is a major threat to developing self-image Very threatened by helplessness and loss of privacy Denial, withdrawal, anger, hostility, disappointment	Imagery Walkman Deep breathing Hand squeezing Talking Jokes Distraction kit	Use treatment room Music Controlled lighting and noise	Ask permission of patient for parental involvement Encourage parents to be part of the team.	Clarify misconception and initiate discussions about the past experiences with procedures. Allow appropriate participation by patient. Pre-procedural teaching utilizing medical play	Present patient with choices. Plan positioning with teen	Praise, reward stickers Play, medical play Stories Evaluate procedures and discuss suggestions for next time.

Distraction
A distraction kit is a set of materials that help divert the child's attention to a more pleasant experience than the painful experience.

- Appropriate for any age
- Use before, during, and after procedure
- Other suggestions: Hold someone's hand really tight, say 'ouch' really loud, count to 10 or count backwards, sing a song, pretend to be somewhere else.

Environment
- Use designated treatment rooms when possible.
- The child's inpatient room should be kept as a "safe area" whenever possible.
- Ensure lighting is sufficiently bright and focused on safety, without glare.

Preparations
- Relieve parental anxiety so they can help prepare and reassure the child/youth. Provide an explanation of what they will see and hear.
- Relieve patient anxiety. Use simple explanations that are developmentally appropriate to explain how, why, where, and when

(Stollery Children's Hospital, Edmonton, Alberta, Canada).

RESOURCES

U.S. Department of Health and Human Services. Insure Kids Now! http://www.insurekidsnow.gov/questions.asp#why1

Child immunization schedules: http://www.cdc.gov/vaccines

Denver II Developmental Screening Test:
http://www.denverii.com/DenverII.html

Food Guide Pyramid for Young Children:
http://www.mypyradmid.gov/kids/index.html

Lead Poisoning:
http://www.cdc.gov/nceh/lead/publications/books/plpyc/chapter3.htm#top

Insurance for children: http://www.insurekidsnow.gov/states.asp

REFERENCES

Bascom, A. (2002). *Incorporating herbal medicine into clinical practice.* Philadelphia: F.A. Davis.

Bickley, L.S., & Szilagyi, P.G. (2007). *Bates' guide to physical examination and history taking* (9th ed). Philadelphia: Lippincott Williams & Wilkins.

Deglin, J.H.L., & Vallerand, A.P. (2009). *Davis's drug guide for nurses* (11th ed). Philadelphia: F.A. Davis.

Karch, A. (2009). *Lippincott's nursing drug guide.* Philadelphia: Lippincott Williams & Wilkins.

Lanski, S.L., Greenwald, M., Perkins, A., & Simon, H.K. (2003). Herbal therapy use in a pediatric emergency department population: Expect the unexpected. *Pediatrics, 111*(5), 981–986.

Otto, S.E. (1991). *Oncology nursing.* St. Louis: C.V. Mosby. Reprinted in *Mosby's medical, nursing, and allied dictionary* (4th ed.), p. 1144.

Salimbene, S. (2005). *What language does your patient hurt in?* St. Paul, MN: EMCParadigm.

Stollery Children's Hospital, 8440-112 Street, Edmonton, Alberta, Canada

Venes, D. (Ed.). (2005). *Taber's cyclopedic medical dictionary* (20th ed.). Philadelphia: F.A. Davis.

19

Caring for the Family Across Care Settings

KEY TERMS

despair – Phase of separation experienced by a hospitalized child in which he seems to withdraw from the environment and becomes very apathetic

detachment – Final phase of separation experienced by a hospitalized child when he has begun to internalize the stressor and seems outwardly happy, although the stressor is still present

health screening – To test or examine children for the presence of a disease, illness, chronic condition, developmental delay, or mental health issue

health surveillance – Continuous observation related to tracking health conditions and risk behaviors

protest – Phase of separation experienced by a hospitalized child that begins when he realizes his parents are leaving or that he is separated, even if for a brief period, from his parents

therapeutic play – The use of play as therapy to help children who have had or will have a stressful experience decrease their fear and anxiety of the experience

FOCUSED ASSESSMENT

Developing a Plan of Care

Ask parents the following questions:

- What are your child's daily routines related to eating, elimination, sleeping, bathing, and play?

- Who are the important people in your child's life?
- Does your child have a favorite toy or attachment object?
- What has your child been told about hospitalization?
- Does your child have any fears that the staff should know about?
- Have there been any recent changes or problems in your child's life?
- How does your child usually react to pain or when frightened?

Include the Parents in the Plan of Care When Their Child Is Admitted to the Hospital

- Request information about the child's personal routine and schedule at home.
- Inquire about previous hospitalizations.
- Ask about the child's anxieties and fears.
- Encourage the parent's presence, involvement, and participation in caring for the child.
- Recognize the parent's concerns, including possible guilt, fear, or other anxieties about the child's hospitalization.
- Provide positive reinforcement for the family to alleviate as much stress as possible.

The Nurse's Role in Health Screening and Surveillance

- Pay attention to voiced parental concerns.
- Ask questions about the child's growth and development.
- Observe the child's mental, physical, and spiritual state (not just a diagnosed condition).
- Note any risk factors that may be present.
- Document specific observations and findings.
- Provide community resources and make appropriate referrals.
- Track disease incidence and demographics of illnesses.
- Implement policies that may prevent further spread of diseases.
- Initiate follow-up care for any concerns and conditions.

CLINICAL ALERT

Common Problems of Critical Illness

Common problems of critical illness are shock, acute respiratory failure, chronic respiratory failure, infection, sepsis, renal failure, neurological conditions, bleeding and clotting disorders, and multiorgan dysfunction.

TEACHING THE FAMILY

Teaching Tips for Families

Ask the family to bring a list of questions or concerns to discuss when visiting the primary care physician's office:

- Bring a list of any allergies that the child has, as well as medications the child is currently taking.
- Be ready to share information as to how the child is growing and changing. Keep track of the child's developmental progress.
- Inquire about resources including community organizations that may provide assistance.
- Request to meet the health care team members who will be working the child (a nurse, a referral coordinator, and a medical assistant).

Caring for the Child at Home After Minor Surgery

Teach parents how to care for their child at home after minor surgery. Explain:

- How to take the child's axillary temperature.
- How to assess the child's level of consciousness.
- When to begin giving the child liquids based on type of surgery, prescribed diet, and age.
- When to offer solid food based on type of surgery, prescribed diet, and age.
- What type of activity is expected or should be encouraged.
- The actions and side effects of medications.
- The signs and symptoms of infection.
- The signs of poor airway exchange.

- How to use assistive devices and medical equipment and perform home treatments.
- How to contact a nurse, pharmacist, health care professorial, or community agency.
- When to call the doctor.

Follow-up Care

- Inform the family of the following: Rehabilitation services are generally provided in a hospital or community center where the child can begin to recuperate and receive physical, occupational, audiology, or speech assessment and therapy.
- Other health care professionals will assist the child in working toward the achievement of optimal function and the relief of pain.
- The ultimate goal is to assist the child's physical recovery and reentry into the community, home, and school.
- A social worker may also be involved in the child's care to assess the capacities of the family's ability to cope with the impact of the condition and situation.
- A social worker can also offer a broad range of community services and may serve as emotional support to referrals for community resources.

ADDITIONAL INFORMATION FOR THE CLINICAL SETTING

Outcomes of a Medical Home and Coordinated Care

Children with special needs receive coordinated ongoing comprehensive care within a medical home (provides comprehensive primary care services on an ongoing basis, in a manner encouraging a positive relationship with the child, family, and the health care team) based on these outcomes:

- Families of children with special health care needs have adequate private and/or public insurance to pay for the services needed.
- Children are screened early and continuously for special health care needs and will have increased wellness.
- Services for children with special health care needs are organized in a manner that fosters trust, considers the

family's cultural and religious beliefs, and builds support for the child and family.

- Families of children with special needs will partner in decision making at all levels, and will be satisfied with the services they receive.
- All youth with special needs receive the services necessary to make appropriate transitions to adult health care, work, and independence.
- Families will have increased satisfaction with their health care.

Benefits of a Medical Home

- A child regularly sees the same primary care physician and staff.
- There is coordination of care for the child.
- There is an open exchange of information in an honest and respectful manner.
- There is support for finding resources and information related to all stages of growth and development and medical conditions.
- The family is connected to information and family support organizations.
- The medical home partnership promotes health and quality of life as the child grows and develops.

Primary Health Care Provider or Clinic Setting

- A private medical office or clinic
- Provision of health information
- Discussions about how to take care of the child at home
- Comprehensive and safe nursing care
- Education about child's condition
- Recommendations for additional community resources
- Reasonable cost of care and continuity of care (child remains in the care of the family)

The Hospitalized Child

- Hospitalization is required when the child becomes ill.
- It may be a new experience wherein both the child and family are exposed to an unfamiliar medical environment.

- Children are more vulnerable to the stress of hospitalization because they do not have a full range of coping mechanisms.
- The child and family are also introduced to an entirely new group of people
  - Children's hospital: Specialty pediatric hospital that is specially designed and managed specifically for children
  - Day hospital: Specialized hospital that serves children who require medical treatments
  - Ambulatory surgery center: Surgical center is where children receive minimal surgical treatment, recover from the procedure, and are discharged soon after the surgery

Stages of Separation with a Hospitalized Child

- Protest phase: The child realizes parents are leaving and could cry, cling, and act aggressively.
- Despair phase: The child seems to withdraw and becomes apathetic.
- Detachment phase: The child represses pain at the sense of loss and shows disinterest on parent's return.

Ways to Decrease the Stress of Hospitalization

- Rooming-in is when parents stay in the room both during the day and through the night
- Encourage child to do the following:
  - Bring something from home.
  - Draw a picture that can be hung up.
  - Watch a movie or select a game.

Therapeutic play is the use of play as therapy to help children who have had or will have a stressful experience. Therapeutic play may decrease the child's fear and anxiety. It also may help to correct misconceptions the child may have about being in the hospital. There are two types of play techniques:

- Directed therapeutic play is guided by an adult who facilitates the play, including determination of the goals.
- In nondirected therapeutic play, the child is in control of the activity, although an adult may select the materials.

Guided imagery is a relaxation technique that aims to ease stress and to promote a sense of peace and harmony during a difficult time.

- Guided imagery can be used by persons of all ages.
- Guided imagery encompasses the power of the mind, to help heal the body, while maintaining a relaxed state including all of the body's senses (touch, smell, sound, sight and visual) (Tusek, 2008).

Role modeling refers to a process by which the child learns certain behaviors by observing the behavior of others. Role models can also come from videotapes, movies, or even their peers. Role models who are similar in age, sex, race, and attitudes are more likely to be imitated as well as models who have a caring demeanor (Watson, 1996). For example, a child might view a video about another child and his or her experience preparing for hospitalization and surgery. Viewing how the child in the video prepares for surgery may help the child who is facing surgery to find ways to cope with the anxiety and stress of the procedure.

Assist Parents in Adapting to the Child's Hospitalization

- Involve the parents.
- Assess home routines, preferences, and developmental and special needs.
- Allow parents to tell their story.
- Promote trust.
- Give prompt attention to the child's needs.
- Allow the parents to participate in care.
- Give positive reinforcement.
- Conduct ongoing evaluation.

Nursing Interventions to Help Parents Cope with a Child's Hospitalization

- Encourage parents to visit the hospital to see where the child will be staying.
- Encourage constant and open communication with the health care team.
- Encourage visitation of parents, friends, and family members.

- Perform ongoing assessment to ensure that the nurse fully understands any changes in the child's plan of care.
- Observe for the need for crisis intervention, should the child's condition deteriorate or change.
- Encourage the parents to participate in the child's care, while being supportive of the child and family.

Twenty-Four-Hour Observation Unit

- Short-stay hospitalization experience.
- Sudden illness; most likely will recover quickly.
- Nurse provides acute nursing care.
- Quickly begins to prepare the child and family for discharge.

Ambulatory Surgery Center

- Surgical treatment is minimal.
- The child recovers from the procedure and then is discharged home soon after the surgery.
- Minimizes separation between the child and family (emotionally less stressful).
- Teaches the family about the surgery and ways to care for the child at home.

Critical Care Unit

- The child is admitted to the critical care unit through the emergency department or operating room, or transferred from a medical-surgical floor.
- After delivery, a newborn who requires intensive care is transferred to a neonatal intensive care unit.
- Other types of critical care units include cardiac, surgical, or psychiatric critical care units.
- The child is extremely ill and receives specialized care, medication, intravenous fluid, respiratory, or ventilator support.

Emergency Department

- Used for quick treatment for children who have become suddenly ill or experienced a severe injury
- Open 24 hours/day, 7 days/week
- Rapid screening or triage assessment

- Several areas of treatment
- Patient may be admitted to the hospital from emergency department

Community Settings

- The majority of a child's health care is provided in a community setting today.
- Community settings are on the front line of prevention and early detection.
- These settings may be located in neighborhood clinics, schools, shopping malls, or health care centers.

RESOURCES

Maternal and Child Health Bureau:
http://www.mchb.hrsa.gov/programs/

The National Center for medical home initiatives for children with special needs: http://www.mchb.hrsa.gov/programs/

The National Center for medical home initiatives for children with special needs: http://www.medicalhomeinfo.org/

Guided imagery: http://www.guidedimageryinc.com/guided.html

National Association of School Nurses: http://www.nasn.org/

Web MD, 2008: http://www.webmd.com

REFERENCES

Tusek, D. (2008). What is guided imagery? Retrieved from http://www.guidedimageryinc.com/guided.html (Accessed April 4, 2009).

Watson, J. (1996). Watson's theory of transpersonal caring. In P.H. Walker & B. Neuman (Eds.). *Blueprint for use of nursing models: Education, research, practice, and administration* (pp. 141–184). New York: National League for Nursing Press.

Caring for the Child with a Psychosocial or Cognitive Condition

KEY TERMS

developmental psychopathology – A discipline that evolved from the contribution of multiple fields of study with the goal to provide understanding between psychopathology and normal adaptation

encopresis – Repeated passage of feces into inappropriate places (e.g., clothing or floor)

enuresis – Occurrence of wetting clothing or the bed at least two times per week for at least 3 months, or that causes significant embarrassment or restriction of activities for the child

obesogenic – Role that environment plays in the development of obesity

FOCUSED ASSESSMENT

Assessing the Child for Posttraumatic Stress Disorder (PTSD)

After a trauma, a child with posttraumatic stress disorder (PTSD) exhibits symptoms within each of the following sets of reactions:

- Reexperiencing the trauma, perhaps in the form of a flashback (intense "remembering" of the event while feeling as if it were happening at the present moment), or nightmares, or sensations

- Avoidance of anything that could trigger the memories, through dissociation (a sense of being detached emotionally, mentally, and perhaps even physically) or avoiding places or events reminiscent of the trauma
- Physiological symptoms of anxious arousal (insomnia, startle response, sense of panic) (Commission on Adolescent Anxiety Disorders, 2005).

Assessing the Child for Bipolar Disorder (BPD)

As bipolar disorder (BPD) is a combination of major depression and mania, the nurse must be aware of symptoms of depression.

Manic and Depressive Symptoms	
Mania	**Depression**
Severe changes in mood—either extremely irritable or overly silly and elated	Persistent sad or irritable mood
Overly inflated self-esteem; grandiosity	Loss of interest in activities once enjoyed
Increased energy	Significant change in appetite or body weight
Decreased need for sleep—able to go with very little or no sleep for days without tiring	Difficulty sleeping or oversleeping
	Physical agitation or slowing
	Loss of energy
Increased talking—talks too much, too fast; changes topics too quickly; cannot be interrupted	Feelings of worthlessness or inappropriate guilt
Distractibility—attention moves constantly from one thing to the next	Difficulty concentrating
	Recurrent thoughts of death or suicide
Hypersexuality—increased sexual thoughts, feelings, or behaviors; use of explicit sexual language	
Increased goal-directed activity or physical agitation	
Disregard of risk – excessive involvement in risky behaviors or activities	

Source: National Institute of Mental Health (2000). Child & adolescent bipolar disorder: An update from the National Institute of Mental Health. NIH Publication No. 00-4778.

Assessing the Child for Suicide

The nurse should suspect suicide potential when faced with any of the following:

- Symptoms of depression or other mental illness
- Alienation or withdrawal from friendships or relationships
- Personality changes
- Decline in schoolwork
- Giving away personal possessions that were once prized

- Preoccupation with death in writing or drawings
- References to dying or to no longer being around
- Access to a method of suicide (e.g., medications, weapons)

Continued Assessment for Suicide

The nurse must ask the child about suicidal thoughts or behaviors. Examples of questions that the nurse might ask include:

"Have you thought about doing something to hurt yourself or take your life?"

"Do you ever wish you were not alive?"

"What would you do if you were to hurt yourself?"

Assessing the Child for Failure to Thrive

During a nursing assessment, the nurse can discern:

- How does the caretaker interact with the child?
- Are there signs of abuse or neglect?
- Does the caretaker understand appropriate feeding amounts and routines?
- Does the caretaker mistakenly believe that a healthy adult diet (i.e., lower fat) is also healthy for an infant?

Assessing the Child for Attention-Deficit/ Hyperactivity Disorder (ADHD)

Developmentally inappropriate or maladaptive symptoms consist of either inattentive symptoms, hyperactive or impulsive symptoms, or a combination

Symptoms of ADHD	
Inattention	**Hyperactivity or Impulsivity**
Distractibility	Excessive energy and activity
Inability to complete projects	Restlessness
Easily bored	Overactivity
Disorganized	Inability to sit still or stay in one place for long
Inattentiveness	Excessive talking
Avoidance of detailed tasks	Poor boundaries—interrupts or intrudes
Forgetfulness	Difficulty delaying

Assessing the Child for Maltreatment of Children

Type of Abuse	Tactics of Abuse	Possible Signs and Symptoms in the Child
Physical: Bodily injury caused by intentional or unintentional physical aggression.	Beating, hitting, slapping, poisoning, kicking, pinching, biting, choking, pulling hair, burning Excessive corporal punishment Shaken baby syndrome Munchausen by proxy	Suspicious bruises, welts, or burns Unexplained fractures or dislocations New and healing or healed lacerations or abrasions Wariness of adults or caregivers Fearful of going home Acting out with aggression Retinal hemorrhages CNS injury Prolonged or recurrent illnesses or injuries that cannot be explained
Sexual: Sexual acts between an adult and a child.	Penetration, incest, rape, Violations of bodily privacy Exposing children to adult sexuality Commercial exploitation Sexual exploitation (prostitution or pornography)	Inappropriate or precocious interest in or knowledge of sexuality Poor peer relationships Sudden changes in behavior Running away from home Substance abuse Declining school performance Suicide attempts
Emotional: Attitude, behavior, or failure to act that interferes with a child's mental health or social development	Intimidation, belittling, shaming, lack of affection and warmth, habitual blaming, ignoring or rejection, extreme punishment, exposure to violence, child exploitation, child abduction	Apathy, depression Hostility Difficulty concentrating
Neglect: Pattern of failing to meet basic needs	Physical, educational, emotional	Clothing unsuited to the weather Poor hygiene Hunger Lack of supervision

Evaluating the Child for Substance Abuse

Two common ways of evaluating for substance abuse are CRAFFT and CAGE.

CRAFFT	CAGE
Have you ever ridden in a **C**ar driven by someone (including yourself) who was high or had been using alcohol or drugs?	Have you ever felt like **C**utting down on your drinking?
Do you ever use alcohol or drugs to **R**elax, feel better about yourself, or fit in?	Have people made you **A**ngry by talking about your drinking?
Do you ever use alcohol or drugs while you are by yourself **A**lone?	Have you ever felt **G**uilty about your drinking?
Do you ever **F**orget things you did while using alcohol or drugs?	Do you ever need a drink first thing in the morning to have enough **E**nergy or to feel ready for the day?
Do your **F**amily or **F**riends ever tell you that you should cut down on your drinking or drug use?	Scoring: 2 or more positive answers = an alcohol problem.
Have you ever gotten into **T**rouble while you were using alcohol or drugs?	*Note: This tool is used with individuals 16 and older.*
Scoring: 2 or more positive items indicate the need for further assessment.	

Source: Reprinted from Center for Adolescent Substance Abuse Research at Children's Hospital, Boston.

Source: Ewing, J.A. (1984). Detecting alcoholism: The CAGE questionnaire. Public domain.

Assessing the Child for Sleep Disorders

Sleep disorders can be diagnosed based on a positive answer by the caregiver to one or more of these questions:

- Is it hard for your child to fall asleep?
- Is it hard for your child to stay asleep though the night?
- Does your child wake up feeling tired?
- Is your child sleepy during the day?

CLINICAL ALERTS

Suicidal Behavior Related to Antidepressant Therapy

The Food and Drug Administration (FDA) requested that pharmaceutical companies manufacturing selective serotonin reuptake inhibitors (SSRIs) add a "black box" warning to the packaging because of an apparent rise in suicide in children and adolescents recently prescribed an SSRI for depression. Several factors have been proposed to explain the occurrence of suicide ideation in children treated with these medications:

- The prescription may be an inadequate dose and therefore the depression is not treated.
- An energizing phenomenon, which describes a situation in which the depressive symptoms related to energy decrease before the mood symptoms, may occur, thus making it more possible for the depressed individual to have the energy to attempt suicide.
- The emergence of an activation syndrome may be related to a toxic reaction to the medication.
- Motor restlessness related to akathisia (motor restlessness that may appear as a side effect of antipsychotic medication)
- The shift from depression to mania in a not-yet-diagnosed bipolar child may occur
- Idiosyncratic reactions (perhaps related to gene-drug reactions) may occur

(Goodman, Murphy, & Storch, 2007).

Attachment Therapies to Avoid

Because there have been child deaths related to the following treatments, they should be avoided:

- Holding therapy
- Rage reduction
- Rebirth

(Barth et al., 2005; Stafford & Zeanah, 2006).

Anorexia Nervosa

Anorexia nervosa can become a life-threatening problem or cause death because the severe weight loss can result in electrolyte imbalance and hemodynamic instability.

MEDICATIONS

Somatic Therapies for Depression

Serotonin Selective Reuptake Inhibitors (SSRIs)

- Open-label studies suggest that fluoxetine (Prozac) is an effective medication in the treatment of pediatric major depression and dysthymia in patients with and without co-occurring mental health disorders (Findling et al., 2004).
- This type of medication has been used in children as young as 8 years of age (National Institute of Mental Health [NIMH], 2001).
- Other SSRIs are used off-label (i.e., use other than specifically approved for by the Food & Drug Administration [FDA]) such as sertraline (Zoloft), paroxetine (Paxil), citalopram (Celexa), escitalopram (Lexipro), or fluvoxamine (Luvox) have also been prescribed by some clinicians (NIMH, 2001).
- Recent evidence that SSRIs can contribute to suicidal ideation in adolescents and children have left many parents and physicians wary of using medication to treat depression in young people.

Valproate (Depakote)

- The nurse needs to be aware that most medications used for the treatment of bipolar disorder have not been studied specifically with children.
- Lithium carbonate (Eskalith, Lithobid) has been the most common treatment. It is a mood stabilizer that calms the manic symptoms.

Pharmacological Treatments for Psychological Difficulties		
Category	**Medications**	**Uses**
Antianxiety	Beta blockers Propanolol (Inderal) Alpha blockers Clonidine (Catapres)	Anxiety
Antidepressants	**SSRIs** Fluoxetine (Prozac) Sertraline (Zoloft) Paroxetine (Paxil) Citalopram (Celexa) Escitalopram (Lexapro) Fluvoxamine (Luvox)	Depression Anxiety Obsessive–compulsive disorder (OCD) Selective mutism

Category	Medications	Uses
	Tricyclics Imipramine (Tofranil) Clomipramine (Anafranil) **Other** Bupropion (Wellbutrin) Venlafaxine	Enuresis Autism
Mood Stabilizer	Lithium carbonate (Lithobid, Lithane, or Eskalith)	Bipolar disorder (BPD) Mania Oppositional defiant disorder (ODD) Attention-deficit/hyperactivity disorder (ADHD)
Anticonvulsants	Valproate (Depakote)	Bipolar disorder (BPD) Mania
Antipsychotics	Traditional: Haloperidol (Haldol) Atypical: Risperidone (Risperdal) Olanzapine (Zyprexa) Quetiapine (Seroquel) Ziprasidone (Geodon) Aripiprazole (Abilify)	Autism Psychosis Tourette's syndrome Behavioral problems related to other psychiatric disorders (oppositional conduct disorder), Attention-deficit/hyperactivity disorder (ADHD), and developmental disabilities
Stimulants	Methylphenidate (Ritalin and Concerta) Dextroamphetamine (Dexedrine and Adderall)	Attention-deficit/hyperactivity disorder (ADHD)
Nonstimulants	Atomoxetine (Strattera)	Attention-deficit/hyperactivity disorder (ADHD)

Enuresis
- Early pharmacological treatments included the use of the tricyclic antidepressant imipramine (Tofranil).
- It is important to note that other tricyclics do not stop bedwetting.
- DDAVP (desmopressin), a vasopressin analogue, has been shown to work to decrease nighttime enuresis. It is administered either nasally or orally.

ETHNOCULTURAL CONSIDERATIONS

Promoting Understanding of Culture in Diverse Families

- Nurses working with children and families of various diverse and socioeconomic backgrounds must take an approach of listening, providing as much positive feedback as possible for what families are doing well, and keep resilience-promoting strategies in mind.
- Using anticipatory guidance, nurses working with children and their families might be most effective suggesting alternative ways of handling a specific cognitive or psychosocial-related concern.

Differences in Incidence of Childhood Obesity

Despite the fact that African American and Latino children and adolescents have higher prevalence rates of obesity compared to white children and adolescents, researchers have found that:

- African American and Latino children receive much less attention related to obesity. African American and Latino are also more likely to develop obesity related problems, such as type 2 diabetes (Caprio, 2006).
- Children of low-income families also experience higher levels of obesity. Access to high-quality, low-fat foods is limited, as is often the education of the parents in providing such foods. Lower-income families often have less access to educational programs on weight management that more privileged families may have (Kumanyika & Grier, 2006).
- Nurses, especially nurses of African American and Latino backgrounds, can help eliminate these disparities by becoming involved or taking leadership roles in programs that identify and involve these youngsters and their families in interventions.

TEACHING THE FAMILY

Therapeutic Parenting Techniques

The nurse can teach the family and the child, as well as model the following therapeutic parenting techniques (Child and Adolescent Bipolar Foundation [CABF, 2008]).

- Practice and teach the child relaxation techniques.
- Use firm restraint to help the child contain rages.
- Prioritize battles and let go of less important matters.
- Reduce stress in the home.
- Use good listening and communication skills.
- Use music, sound, lighting, water, and massage to assist the child with waking, falling asleep, and relaxation.
- Become an advocate for stress reduction and other accommodations at school.
- Help the child anticipate and avoid, or prepare for stressful situations by developing coping strategies beforehand.
- Engage the child's creativity through activities that express and channel gifts and strengths.
- Provide routines, structure, and freedom within limits.
- Remove objects from the home (or lock them in a safe place) that could be used to harm self or others during a rage, especially guns.
- Keep medications in a locked cabinet or box.

Maltreatment

- Educate parents about what to expect from parenthood and from child rearing.
- Help parents develop resources for support such as babysitters, family members, community sites, and health care resources that may help them find ways to cope with parenting.
- Provide parents with information regarding "normal" stages of growth.
- Discuss with parents ways to discipline the child that does not involve physical or verbal aggression.
- Educate children and adolescents about the body and personal boundaries.

Sleep Hygiene

- Provide a quiet, dark, and comfortable environment or bedroom.
- Set a strict bedtime and awake routine that remains consistent on a daily basis.
- Avoid long daytime naps.
- Allow a long space of time between daytime nap and bedtime.

- Provide a healthy snack before bedtime so the child is not hungry.
- Avoid substances such as caffeine, chocolate, medication containing alcohol, and other foods/beverages that are stimulating to children.
- Cut down on fluids before bedtime so that a full bladder or wetness does not interrupt sleep.
- Avoid a high level of activity and television viewing before bedtime and replace it with quiet activities (e.g., reading books).
- Encourage children to fall asleep without a caregiver in the room (Sheldon, 2005).

Toilet Training

Indications to begin toilet training (American Academy of Family Physicians, 2006; Child Welfare Information Gateway, 2007):

- When the child indicates his diaper is soiled or wet or when he indicates he wants to use the toilet (generally 18 to 24 months, but could be 2 1/2 to 3 years)
- When parents can devote about 3 months of time to offer lessons and encouragement
- When the child shows interest in other people using the bathroom or interest in wearing underwear

ADDITIONAL INFORMATION FOR THE CLINICAL SETTING

Mindful Breathing

The pediatric nurse can teach deep breathing to avoid or help with an anxious episode:

- Consciously direct your attention to your breathing.
- Breathe in slowly, paying attention as the air enters your nose or mouth and fills your lungs.
- Breathe out slowly, paying attention as the air leaves your body.
- Allow your mind to follow your breath in and out.
- Imagine yourself in a rubber raft riding the gentle waves of your breath.

Understanding Autism Spectrum Disorder

Developmental disorders have subtle signs and may be easily missed.

The "First Signs" program uses the acronym Autism A.L.A.R.M. to highlight important clinical guidelines (Wiseman, 2006):

Listen to parents:

- Early signs of autism are often present before 18 months.
- Parents usually do have concerns that something is wrong.
- Parents generally do give accurate and quality information.
- When parents do not spontaneously raise concerns, ask if they have any.

Act early:

- Make screening and surveillance an important part of your practice.
- Know the subtle differences between typical and atypical development.
- Learn to recognize red flags.
- Improve the quality of life for children and their families through early and appropriate intervention.

Refer:

- To early intervention or a local school program (do not wait for a diagnosis).
- To an autism specialist, or team of specialists, immediately for a definitive diagnosis.
- To audiology department to rule out a hearing impairment.
- To local community resources for help and family support.

Monitor:

- Schedule a follow-up appointment to discuss concerns more thoroughly.
- Look for other features known to be associated with autism.
- Educate parents and provide them with up-to-date information.
- Advocate for families with local early intervention programs, schools, respite care agencies, and insurance companies.

- Continue surveillance and watch for additional or late signs of autism and/or other developmental disorders.

Youth Violence: Fact Sheet

The Youth Violence: Fact Sheet (http://www.cdc.gov/ncipc/factsheets/yvfacts.htm) offers a comprehensive resource about the problem of violence (compiled and referenced from research and refereed articles). The nurse can access this information to be used as an educational tool when talking to youth and families about violence. Examples of fact sheet topics are the following:

- Occurrence
- Consequences
- Groups at Risk
- Risk Factors
- Individual Risk Factors
- Family Risk Factors
- Peer/School Risk Factors
- Community Risk Factors
- Protective Factors
- Individual Protective Factors
- Family Protective Factors
- Peer/School Protective Factors

Child Abuse

- All states in the United States have mandatory reporting guidelines for cases of child abuse; the national hotline in the United States is 1-800-4-A-Child.
- All allegations must first be investigated before confirmed.
- After documented confirmation, the child is placed in an environment safe and free of abuse.

Prevention of Childhood Obesity in Schools

- Ensure that the school provide healthy meals and replace soda machines with water.
- Encourage improved physical activity.
- Provide education about nutrition, physical activity, and acceptable weight.
- Provide health education to promote healthy eating, physical activity, and well-being.
- Research and advocate for changes in school policy.

RESOURCES

de Benedictis T, Jaffe-Gill E, & Segal J. (2007). Child abuse: Types, signs, symptoms, causes and help.
http://www.helpguide.org/mental/child

Child & Adolescent Bipolar Foundation: http://www.bpkids.org

Could it be autism? http://www.firstsigns.org

Office of Science Policy National Institute of Health:
http://www.science.education.nih.gov

The Youth Violence: Fact Sheet:
http://www.cdc.gov/ncipc/factsheets/yvfacts.htm

REFERENCES

American Academy of Family Physicians (AAFP). (updated 2006). Toilet training your child. Retrieved from http://familydoctor.org/online/famdocen/home/children/parents/toilet/179 (Accessed April 4, 2009).

Barth, R.P., Crea, T.M., John, K., Thoburn, J., & Quinton, D. (2005). Beyond attachment theory and therapy: Towards sensitive and evidence-based interventions with foster and adoptive families in distress. *Child and Family Social Work, 10*(4), 257–268.

Caprio, S. (2006). Treating child obesity and associated medical conditions. *The Future of Children, 16*(1), 209–224. Retrieved from www.futureofchildren.org (Accessed April 4, 2009).

Child and Adolescent Bipolar Foundation. Retrieved from http://www.bpkids.org/site/PageServer (Accessed April 4, 2009).

Child Welfare Information Gateway (2007). Surviving toilet training. Retrieved from http://www.childwelfare.gov/preventing/supporting/resources/toilettraining.cfm (Accessed April 4, 2009).

Commission on Adolescent Anxiety Disorders. (2005). Anxiety disorders. In D.L. Evans, E.B. Foa, R.E. Gur, H. Hendin, C.P. O'Brien, M.E.P. Seligman, & B.T. Walsh (Eds.). *Treating and preventing adolescent mental health disorders: What we know and don't know: A research agenda for improving the mental health of our youth* (pp. 162–253). New York: Oxford University Press.

Ewing, J.A. (1984). Detecting alcoholism: the CAGE questionnaire. *JAMA, 252*(14), 1905–1907.

Findling, R.L., Feeny, N.C., Stansbrey, R.J., Delporto-Bedoya, D., & Demeter, C. (2004). Special articles: Treatment of mood disorders in children and adolescents: Somatic treatment for depressive illnesses in children and adolescents. *Psychiatric Clinics of North America, 27*(1), 113–137.

Goodman, W.K., Murphy, T.K., & Storch, E.A. (2007). Risk of adverse behavioral effects with pediatric use of antidepressants [Electronic version]. *Psychopharmacology, 191*(87), 87–96.

Kumanyika, S., & Grier, S. (2006). Targeting interventions for ethnic minority and low-income populations. *The Future of Children, 16*(1), 187–207.

National Institute of Mental Health (NIMH). (2000). Child & adolescent bipolar disorder: An update from the National Institute of Mental Health. (NIH Publication No. 00–4778). Retrieved from http://www.nimh.nih.gov/publicat/index.cfm (Accessed April 4, 2009)

National Institute of Mental Health (NIMH). (2001). Blueprint for change: Research on child and adolescent mental health: Report of the National Advisory Mental Health Council's Workgroup on Child and Adolescent Mental Health Development and Deployment. Washington, DC: Office of Communications and Public Liaison (ERIC Document Reproduction Service No. ED462650).

Sheldon, S.H. (2005). Introduction to pediatric sleep medicine. In S.H. Sheldon, R. Ferber, & M.H. Kryger (Eds.). *Principles and practice of pediatric sleep medicine* (pp. 1–16). Philadelphia: Elsevier Saunders.

Stafford, B.S., & Zeanah, C.H. (2006). Attachment disorders. In J.L. Luby (Ed.). *Handbook of preschool mental health: Development, disorders, and treatment* (pp. 231–251). New York: Guilford Press.

Vieth, V., Bottoms, B.L., & Perona, A. (2006). *Ending child abuse: New efforts in prevention, investigation, and training.* Binghamton, NY: The Haworth Maltreatment & Trauma Press.

Wiseman, N.D. (2006). *Could it be autism? A parent's guide to the first signs and next steps.* New York: Broadway Books.

Caring for the Child with a Respiratory Condition

KEY TERMS

retractions – Drawing back of the chest wall with inspiration; seen when the accessory muscles are used for breathing. Common sites for retractions include suprasternal, supraclavicular, intercostal, subcostal, and substernal (Ball & Binder, 2006).

status asthmaticus – Persistent and intractable asthma where the child does not respond to therapy and a medical emergency ensues

FOCUSED ASSESSMENT

Nursing Assessment

The nurse must use a complete nursing assessment to assess the child's respiratory condition:

- Watch for subtle changes in the child's color, respiration, behavior, heart rate, and general health.
- Subtle changes can occur before they can be recognized by technological methods.
- Use innate instincts when caring for the child; if the nurse senses impending crisis it is important to pay attention to this instinct and act accordingly (getting emergency equipment ready).
- Remember that children have an uncanny ability to compensate. When a child is no longer able to compensate, he or she "crashes" and may then have a poor probability of recovery.

Pediatric Respiratory Emergencies

Assessment	Critical	Unstable	Potentially Unstable	Stable
Airway	Completely or severely obstructed	Partially obstructed, excessive secretions or blood	Open with secretions	Open
Breathing Rate	May be slow, absent, or very fast with periods of slowing	Increased	Occasionally increased	Normal
Breathing Effort	Absent or greatly increased with periods of weakness	Increased	Normal	Normal
Breath Sounds	Grunting, faint, or absent	Wheezing or stridor, decreased breath sounds	Normal or slight wheezing	Normal
Skin Color	Pale, mottled, or blue	Pink or pale	Pink	Pink
Inspection	Normal, decreased, or absent chest movement	Normal or decreased chest movement	Runny nose, red eyes, fever	Runny nose
Actions	Immediately open airway, suction, give high concentration oxygen with assisted ventilation, and transport	Move at moderate pace; give high concentration oxygen; prepare for transport; reassess frequently	Move at moderate pace; help into position of comfort; give high concentration oxygen; prepare for transport	Begin focused history and physical exam

Based on CUPS Assessment table in Sanddal, N., et al. (1997). *Critical trauma care by the basic EMT* (4th ed.). Bozeman, MT: Critical Illness and Trauma Foundation.

Classification of Asthma Severity

Severity	Day Symptoms	Night Awakenings	SABA Use*	Limit to Activity
Criteria for Classification of Asthma Severity in Children 0–4 Years of Age				
Intermittent	**≤2 days/week**	None	≤2 times/week	None
Mild Persistent	**3–6 days/week**	**1–2X/month**	**>2 days/week**	**Minor**
Moderate, Persistent	Daily	3–4X/month	Daily	Some
Severe, Persistent	Several X/day	>1X/week	Several X/day	Extreme

*Short-acting beta 2 agonists (SABA) such as albuterol use does not include prevention of exercise induced bronchospasm (EIB).

The U.S. Department of Health and Human Services 2007, the National Asthma Education and Prevention Program. Expert panel report 3: Guidelines for the diagnosis and management of asthma.

CLINICAL ALERTS

Respiratory Rate Exceeding 60 Breaths/Minute

A respiratory rate that exceeds 60 breaths/min is dangerous! At this high rate, sufficient oxygen does not reach the alveoli for adequate gas exchange. **Never** feed an infant or child orally if the respiratory rate exceeds 60 breaths/min because of potential aspiration.

Retractions

- Retractions are a drawing back of the chest wall with inspiration and are seen when the accessory muscles are used for breathing.
- Common sites for retractions include suprasternal, supraclavicular, intercostal, subcostal, and substernal.

The Mother's Obstetrical History

- If the nurse caring for a newborn observes the infant to be drooling excessively and/or having persistent choking spells and color change with feedings, it is important for the nurse to check the mother's obstetrical history.

- These symptoms are highly suspicious of esophageal atresia and tracheoesophageal fistula.
- If there is history of polyhydramnios, the nurse must immediately report the observed symptoms to the baby's pediatrician.

Suctioning

- Preoperatively, nasogastric, or orogastric tube placement for suctioning must be done extremely carefully and gently, and progression stopped immediately if any resistance is met to avoid perforating the esophageal tissue of an infant with an anomaly.
- Postoperative oral or nasal suctioning of the infant with esophageal atresia (EA), tracheoesophageal fistula (TEF), or congenital diaphragmatic hernia (CDH) must be done extremely carefully to avoid disruption of the repairs. Ensure that the tube is not inserted any further than the distance from the nares to the ear lobe.

Assisted Mechanical Ventilation

Neonates with severe respiratory distress syndrome (RDS) and those with complications require assisted mechanical ventilation.

Signs of Bleeding After Tonsillectomy

Continuous swallowing is indicative of bleeding. Additional signs to be observed are restlessness, increased pulse rate, and pallor (late symptom).

Rupture of the Tympanic Membrane

Rupture of the tympanic membrane brings immediate pain relief, a gradual decrease in temperature, and the presence of a purulent discharge in the external auditory canal. However, rupture of the tympanic membrane may lead to scarring and hearing loss.

DIAGNOSTIC TESTS

Common Diagnostic Tests

Test	Indications	Preparation	Post-test Care
Bronchoscopy Insertion of a rigid or flexible fiberoptic bronchoscope to evaluate lungs, larynx, vocal cords, trachea, bronchi	Recurrent and persistent pneumonia or atelectasis, unexplained and persistent wheezes, presence of a foreign body, hemoptysis, congenital anomalies, and unexplained interstitial conditions	Explain procedure: IV inserted to infuse anesthetics and analgesics, general anesthetic in most cases, NPO 6 hours. Written and informed consent required.	Monitor vital signs. Explain that the patient may have sore throat or hoarseness. Observe for hemoptysis, difficulty breathing, cough, pain, absent breath sounds over affected area. Evaluate for symptoms of pneumothorax: dyspnea, tachypnea, anxiety, decreased breath sounds, restlessness.
Chest X-ray Radiologic study to identify and detect abnormalities in size, structure, and shape of bony structures and tissues.	Pneumonia, bronchitis, pleural effusion, atelectasis, tuberculosis, pneumothorax, tumors, presence of foreign body	Explain procedure. Record date of last menstrual period and determine the possibility of pregnancy.	
Computed Tomography (CT) Noninvasive cross-sectional and three dimensional study of internal structure of thorax	Mediastinal and pleural effusions, suspected bronchiectasis.	Explain the procedure: IV may be inserted for infusion of contrast medium or sedatives. The patient may experience a feeling of warmth and a salty or metallic taste if contrast medium is given. Fluids may be restricted before the test. Remove jewelry and metallic objects. Written and informed consent is required.	If contrast is used, observe for delayed allergic reactions such as rash, urticaria, tachycardia, nausea, or vomiting.
Lung Biopsy (surgical) Removal of living tissue from lungs for diagnostic purposes	Inflammatory diseases, infections	Explain the procedure: IV line will be inserted, NPO 6 hours. Record date of last menstrual period and determine possibility of pregnancy. Written and informed consent is required.	Monitor vital signs according to agency protocol. Observe the biopsy site for bleeding. Observe patient for hemoptysis, difficulty breathing, cough, pain, or absent

Test	Indications	Preparation	Post-test Care
			breath sounds over the affected area. Monitor chest tube patency and drainage after a thoracotomy.
Pulmonary Function Studies Tests measuring the volume, pattern, and rates of airflow of lungs	Differentiate between restrictive and obstructive conditions. Determine progression of disease. Determine responsiveness to respiratory therapies.	Explain the procedure. Obtain height and weight data. No smoking for 4 hours before procedure.	
Sweat Chloride Noninvasive study to assist in diagnosis of cystic fibrosis	Screen for suspected cystic fibrosis.	Explain that sweat is collected on filter paper disks by introducing a small electrical current to the skin which may result in a stinging sensation.	Observe site for unusual color, sensation, or discomfort.

Adapted from Van Leeuwen, A.M., Kranpitz, T.R., & Smith, L. (2006). *Davis's comprehensive handbook of laboratory and diagnostic tests with nursing implications.* Philadelphia: F.A. Davis.

Pulmonary Function Tests

Category	Test	Definition
Slow Vital Capacity Tests	Tidal volume (TV)	The amount of air inhaled and exhaled during normal respiration
	Inspiratory capacity (IC)	The maximum amount of air inhaled after the end of tidal volume expiration during normal respiration
	Expiratory reserve volume (ERV)	The maximum amount of air exhaled after the end of tidal volume expiration during normal respiration
	Inspiratory reserve volume (IRV)	The maximum amount of air inhaled after the end of tidal volume inspiration during normal respiration

(continued)

Pulmonary Function Tests (Continued)

Category	Test	Definition
	Vital capacity (VC)	The maximum amount of air exhaled following a maximal inhalation (VC = ERV + IC)
Lung Volume Studies	Residual volume (RV)	The amount of air that remains in the lungs after maximal exhalation
	Functional residual capacity (FRC)	The amount of air left in the lungs after normal exhalation (FRC = ERV + RV)
	Total lung capacity (TLC)	The total amount of air in the lungs at maximal inhalation (TLC = V + RV or TLC = FRC + IC)
Lung Volumes and Capacity	Forced vital capacity (FVC)	The maximum amount of air that can be exhaled as hard, fast, and long as possible after a maximum inhalation
	Forced inspiratory volume (FIV)	The maximum amount of air that can be inhaled after a maximum exhalation

Normal Values for Arterial Blood Gases

Component	Definition	Normal Values	Interpretation
pH	Acid–base status of the body	Preterms: 7.3–7.4 Full term: 7.3–7.4 Children 7.35–7.45	Acidosis <7.35 Alkalosis >7.45
$Paco_2$	Pressure exerted by CO_2 in blood	Newborn: 30–40 mm Hg Infant: 30–41 mm Hg Children: 35–45 mm Hg	Acidosis >45 mm Hg Alkalosis <35 mm Hg
HCO_3^-	Buffering effect of acid in blood	Children >7 yr 20–22 mEq/L	Acidosis: 22 mEq/L Alkalosis: 26 mEq/L
Base Excess	Status of bases in blood	Newborn: −10 to −2 mEq/L Infant: −7 to −1 mEq/L Children: −4 to +2 mEq/L Thereafter: −3 to +3 mEq/L A positive or negative number indicate increasing or decreasing range of bicarbonate ion concentration	Acidosis more + Alkalosis more −

Component	Definition	Normal Values	Interpretation
Pao$_2$	Pressure exerted by dissolved O$_2$ in blood	Newborn: 60–90 mm Hg Infant: 80–100 mm Hg Children: 80–100 mm Hg	Acidosis: <80 mm Hg Alkalosis: >100 mm Hg

Sputum Culture and Sensitivity

To be able to establish the causative organism and most effective antibiotic a culture and sensitivity test of the sputum is done.

- A specimen may be obtained by a direct throat swab immediately after coughing.
- In some cases, a sterile catheter may be inserted directly into the trachea through the endotracheal tube or during direct laryngoscopy.
- An early morning fasting specimen obtained by gastric aspiration may also be obtained.

Tuberculin Skin Test (TST)

The tuberculin skin test (TST) is an exact indicator of whether a child has been infected with the tubercle bacillus.

- Inject a measured amount of the intermediate strength of 5 tuberculin units of tuberculin purified protein derivative (PPD) intradermally to form a small wheal in the forearm.
- In 48 to 72 hours, a positive reaction is marked by an area of red induration (an area of hardened tissue).
- Reactions greater than 10 mm in size are considered positive in non-immunocompromised patients.

MEDICATIONS

Erythromycin (eh-rith-roe-**mye**-sin)

Indications IV, PO: Infections caused by susceptible organisms including upper and lower respiratory tract infections and otitis media.

Action Suppresses protein synthesis at the level of the 50S ribosome.

Therapeutic Effects Bacteriostatic action against susceptible bacterial spectrum: streptococci, staphylococci, gram-positive bacilli.

Pharmacokinetics
Absorption Variable absorption from the duodenum after oral administration.

Contraindications and Precautions
Contraindicated in Hypersensitivity

Adverse Reactions and Side Effects Irritation

Route and Dosage Children **PO:** 30–50 mg/kg divided doses q6–8hr Neonates **PO:** 20–50 mg/kg per day divided q6–12hr.

Nursing Implications Inform parents of medication administration.

Prepare to administer around the clock. Use a calibrated measuring device for liquid preparations. Do not crush or chew delayed–release capsules or tablets; swallow whole.

> *Data from Deglin, J., & Vallerand, A. (2009).* Davis's drug guide for nurses *(11th ed.), pp. 498–501. Philadelphia: F.A. Davis.*

Oseltamivir (o-sel-**tam**-i-vir) (Tamiflu)

Pregnancy Category C

Indications Uncomplicated acute illness due to influenza infection in adults and children older than 1 year of age who have symptoms for ≤2 days. Prevention of influenza in patients ≥13 years of age.

Actions Inhibits the enzyme neuraminidase, which may alter virus particle aggregation and release.

Therapeutic Effects Reduced duration of flu related symptoms

Pharmacokinetics
Absorption Rapidly absorbed from the GI tract and converted by the liver to the active form, oseltamivir carboxylate; 75% reaches the systemic circulation as the active drug.

Contraindications and Precautions
Contraindicated in Hypersensitivity and children <1 year old

Adverse Reactions and Side Effects
CNS Insomnia, vertigo
Respiratory Bronchitis

Gastrointestinal Nausea, vomiting

Route and Dosage PO: Children >40 kg: 75 mg twice daily for 5 days. Children 23–40 kg: 60 mg twice daily. Children 15–23 kg: 45 mg twice daily. Children ≤15 kg and 1 year or older: 30 mg twice daily.

Nursing Implications Monitor influenza symptoms. Additional supportive treatment may be indicated to treat symptoms. Treatment should be started as soon as possible at the first sign of flu symptoms. Administer with food or milk to minimize GI irritation. Drug should be used within 10 days of the infection. Caution patients/parents that Tamiflu should not be shared with anyone even if they have the same symptoms.

According to immunization guidelines, Tamiflu is not a substitute for flu shots. Advise patient to consult a health care professional before taking any medications concurrently with Tamiflu.

Data from Deglin, J., & Vallerand, A. (2009). Davis's drug guide for nurses (11th ed.), pp. 916–917. Philadelphia: F.A. Davis.

Albuterol (al-**byoo**-ter-ole) (Ventolin, Salbutamol)

Indications Control and prevent reversible airway obstruction caused by asthma or COPD Inhalant: Used as a quick relief agent for acute bronchospasm. **PO:** Used as a long-term control agent in patients with chronic/persistent bronchospasm.

Actions Binds to beta adrenergic receptors in airway smooth muscle.

Therapeutic Effects Bronchodilatation

Pharmacokinetics
Absorption Well absorbed after oral administration but rapidly undergoes extensive metabolism.

Contraindications and Precautions
Contraindicated in Hypersensitivity to adrenergic amines and to fluorocarbons (some inhalers).

Adverse Reactions and Side Effects Nervousness, restlessness, tremors, chest pains, palpitations.

Route and Dosage PO: Children 2–6 years: 0.1 mg/kg 3 times daily, not to exceed 2 mg 3 times daily initially; children 6–12 years: 2 mg 3–4 times daily or 0.3–0.6 mg/kg/day not to exceed 8 mg/day; children older than 12 years: 2–4 mg 3–4 times daily not to exceed 32 mg/day. **Inhalant:** Children older than 4 years – via metered-dose inhaler 2 inhalations every 4–6 hours. For acute asthma exacerbations: 4–8 puffs every 20 min for 3 doses, then every 1–4 hours; children older than 12 years: via nebulization or intermittent positive pressure breathing (IPPB): 2.5–5 mg every 20 minutes for 3 doses then 2.5–10 mg every 1–4 hours. PRN; children 2–12 years: via nebulization or IPPB: 0.15 mg/kg per dose (minimum dose 2.5 mg) every 20 minutes for three doses, then 0.15–0.3 mg/kg (not to exceed 10 mg) every 1–4 hours PRN or 1.25 mg 3–4 times daily for children 10–15 kg or 2.5 mg 3–4 times daily for children weighing more than 15 kg; children older than 4 years via Rota inhaler inhalation device: 200 mcg (as Ventolin Rotacaps) every 4–6 hours (up to 400 mcg every 4–6 hours).

Nursing Implications Assess lung sounds and vital signs before administration and during peak of medication. Note the amount, color, and characteristics of the sputum produced. Monitor pulmonary function test (PFT) periodically. If wheezing occurs, withhold medications and notify the physician immediately.

Data from Deglin, J., & Vallerand, A. (2009). Davis's drug guide for nurses (11th ed.), pp. 120–122. Philadelphia: F.A. Davis

ETHNOCULTURAL CONSIDERATIONS

Asthma

- In the United States, the poor, especially of black or Hispanic background, experience disproportionally high rates of both asthma and morbidity (Castro et al., 2001; Mannino et al., 2002).
- There is great worldwide variability in prevalence with industrialized areas having consistently high rates.

TEACHING THE FAMILY

Esophageal Atresia with or without Tracheoesophageal Fistula

- Teach parents proper sterile technique of suctioning and how to handle the equipment appropriately.
- Ensure that all emergency calling numbers are written down so emergency care can be provided in a serious situation.
- Ensure that parents know how to identify respiratory distress.
- Ensure that parents know feeding techniques for a gastrostomy tube and how to handle tube plugging and dislodging.
- Instruct parents in performing CPR before the child goes home.
- Encourage parents to use different toys and games to promote stimulation during regular care.
- Mobilization can be as simple as holding or rocking while action play can be games, toy figures, or crafts.
- Involve other siblings in adapting the young child with EA or TEF.
- Ensure the family knows how to operate equipment and knows proper maintenance of the equipment used at home.

Caring for the Child with Cystic Fibrosis at Home

- Teach the family about the nature of the disease and prepare them to manage day-to-day minor complaints.
- Assist in arranging for the portable suction machine and about the proper suctioning technique at home.
- Instruct the parents to perform respiratory therapy before meals because chest physiotherapy may induce vomiting of the thick tenacious mucus.
- Teach the parents different techniques for chest physiotherapy and postural drainage and about coughing exercises based on their child's age. The child needs to be suctioned followed by chest physiotherapy and inhalation to liquefy the thick secretions.
- Teach the family about the preferred meal plans, high-calorie diet, and mixing pancreatic enzymes with meals.

- Instruct the family to monitor the child's weight to ensure proper growth patterns.
- Teach the family how to administer medications properly.
- Inform the family how to access community resources and how to contact their home health nurse.

Avoiding Sinusitis

- Use an oral decongestant or a nasal spray decongestant when initial signs and symptoms appear.
- Have the child gently blow his nose, blocking one nostril while blowing through the other.
- Ensure the child drinks plenty of fluids to keep nasal discharge thin.
- Apply warm compresses or heating pad on low heat over the inflamed area.
- Use a cool mist humidifier.
- Avoid air travel. If it cannot be avoided, use a nasal spray decongestant before "take off" to help prevent blockage of the sinuses, allowing mucus secretions to drain.
- Avoid contact with main allergens.
- Use air conditioning to ensure even room temperature.
- Use electrostatic filters attached to heating and air conditioning systems to help remove allergens (American Academy of Otolaryngology, Head and Neck Surgery, 2008).

Home Discharge Instructions After a Tonsillectomy

- Keep the child away from highly seasoned food and "sharp" foods (nacho chips) for a period of 2 weeks. The postsurgical scab is most likely to be dislodged at the 8–12-day period.
- Ensure the child avoids gargling and vigorous tooth brushing.
- Instruct the child to avoid coughing or clearing the throat.
- Limit activities that may result in bleeding.

Preventing External Otitis Media

- Advise children to limit their stay in the water to less than an hour. Ears should be completely dry before entering the water again.

- Shaking the head and judicious use of the corner of a towel or small tuft of cotton can remove most excess water.
- To keep the ear dry, the parent can pull the auricle up and out to straighten the canal, then use a conventional hair dryer set on low or no heat held at a distance of 18 to 24 inches for 30 seconds, three times a day.
- Earplugs may be recommended.
- Advise against swimming in dirty water and in public swimming pools that do not maintain good control of the chlorine and pH pool testing and treatment.

Salicylates (Aspirin)

- Avoid giving salicylates (aspirin) because of the possibility of Reye syndrome.
- Watch for symptoms (nausea, vomiting, lethargy, and indifference). In severe cases there may be irrational behavior, delirium, and rapid breathing.

The Heimlich Maneuver

Conscious Child Older Than 1 Year of Age

1. Give five blows to the child's back with the heel of your hand with the child sitting, kneeling, lying.
2. If the obstruction persists, go behind the child and pass your arms around the child's body; form a fist with one hand immediately below the child's sternum. Place the other hand over the fist and pull upwards into the abdomen. Repeat five times.

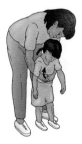

3. Check the child's mouth for any obvious obstruction that can be removed.
4. If necessary, repeat the sequence and ask for help to call 911 or rush to the nearest hospital.

Heimlich Maneuver on an Infant

1. Lay the infant on your arm or thigh with the infant's head down.
2. Give five blows to the infant's back using the heel of your hand.

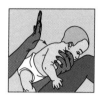

3. If the airway obstruction continues, turn the infant over with the head down and give five chest thrusts using two fingers at a distance of 1 fingerbreadth below the nipple level in midline.

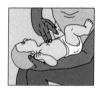

4. Check the infant's mouth for any obvious obstructions that can be removed.
5. If necessary, repeat the sequence and ask for help to call 911 or rush to the nearest hospital (The AHA Subcommittee on Pediatric Resuscitation, 2006. http://pediatrics. appublications.org/cgi/content/full/117/5/e989).

Peak Flow Meter

  Procedure 21-1 Using a Peak Flow Meter

Purpose

The purpose of a peak flow meter is to keep track of the results and help the parents and child learn about asthma. Keeping a daily record may also help determine if the child's asthma is getting worse.

Equipment

- Peak flow meter
- Peak flow record

Procedure 21-1 (Continued)

Steps

1. Before each use, make sure the sliding marker or arrow on the peak flow meter is at the bottom of the numbered scale (zero or the lowest number on the scale).

2. Instruct the child to stand up straight and to remove gum or any food from the mouth.

3. Instruct the child to take a deep breath and to put the mouthpiece of the peak flow meter into the mouth. Close the lips tightly around the mouthpiece. Be sure to keep the tongue away from the mouthpiece.

4. Instruct the child to take in one breath and to then blow out as hard and as quickly as possible. Blow a "fast and hard blast" rather than "slowly blowing" until all of the air is emptied from the lungs.

5. Teach the parents that the force of the air coming out of the lungs causes the marker to move along the numbered scale. Record the number where the marker landed on a peak flow record.

6. Repeat the entire routine three times (if the routine is done correctly the numbers from all three tries are very close together).

7. Record the highest reading. Do not calculate an average.

8. Measure the peak flow rate at the same time each day. A good time to measure the peak flow rate is between 7 and 9 A.M. and between 6 and 8 P.M. Note: It may be a good idea to measure the peak flow rate before or after using asthma medicine.

9. Keep a chart of the peak flow rates on a peak flow record.

Clinical Alert A peak flow meter package usually contains a peak flow record when the peak flow readings are recorded regularly.

Teach Parents

Teach parents about the child's personal best. The "personal best" peak flow is determined when the child is symptom free. It is important for the child, parents,

(continued)

Procedure 21-1 (Continued)

and the physician to discuss what is considered "normal." Remind parents of the need to discuss the readings with the physician.

● **Spacers**

The nurse understands that for children less than 5 years of age, a spacer or a valved holding chamber (VHC) is recommended which is attached to the MDI. A spacer may deliver the medication to the child's lungs better than an inhaler alone and may be easier for the child to use than an MDI alone. In addition, for ease of delivery, child sized masks are available that fit the VHC. With this device there is more medication deposited in the lungs and less systemic side effects. After VHC use the nurse can have the child follow with mouth washing and spitting to decrease swallowing medication and side effect including, in the case of inhaled corticosteroids (ICS), prevention of oral *Candidiasis* (U.S. Department of Health and Human Services, 2007).

Asthma Action Plan

The Asthma Action Plan is an educational tool used for communication between the health care provider and the patient, with their family and caregivers, to properly manage asthma and respond to asthma episodes. Found at http://www.lungusa.org

- Ensure it is completed by the child's primary care provider.
- It includes the symptoms and management for each color zone including peak flow measurements appropriate for each color zone.
- Provide adequate instructions on how to use, interpret, and complete the form.

ADDITIONAL INFORMATION FOR THE CLINICAL SETTING

Assessing Respiratory Status

- Assess the infant's respiratory status including increasing respiratory rate and decreasing oxygenation. The child who has a severe case of bronchopulmonary dysplasia (BPD) may need recurrent hospitalization; therefore, the nurse must be able to provide emotional support to parents during these crucial moments.

Preventing Respiratory Illnesses in Patients with BPD

- Instruct all visitors to wash their hands before touching the neonate. The nurse should politely ask visitors with current respiratory infections to leave the room, explaining that the infant is at an increased risk for infection.

Promoting Respiratory Function

- To ensure respiratory function, a multidisciplinary approach should be taken. A physician, nurse, respiratory therapist, social worker, dietitian, and psychologist are the important professionals in the management of a child with cystic fibrosis (CF).

Nutrition

- The best outcome for a child with CF is a well-balanced, high-protein, high-caloric diet. Pancreatic insufficiency results in malabsorption of fat-soluble vitamins (vitamins A, D, E, K). Daily vitamin supplementation is recommended. The nurse can also work closely with the family to prevent infection as well as optimize nutrition and growth of a child.

Acute Epiglottitis or Supraglottitis; a Medical Emergency

Acute epiglottitis or supraglottitis is a sudden, potentially lethal condition characterized by high fever, sore throat, dyspnea, and rapidly progressing respiratory obstruction. It is considered a serious obstructive inflammatory condition and a medical emergency that requires immediate attention.

- The child goes to bed asymptomatic and awakens with complaints of sore throat and pain on swelling accompanied by a febrile state.

- The child typically assumes the tripod position: leaning forward and sitting upright with chin thrust, mouth open while bracing on the arms, and tongue protruding with drooling of saliva.
- The child is irritable and restless with a thick and muffled voice and there is a froglike croaking sound on inspiration.
- Suprasternal and substernal retractions may be visible.
- The child breathes slowly, the throat is red and inflamed, and there is a distinctive large, cherry red edematous epiglottis.
- The nurse must never assess the child's throat with a tongue blade unless a respiratory therapist or medical doctor is present.

Preventing RSV

- RSV immunoglobulin (RSV-IGIV), an intravenous preparation of immunoglobulin G that provides neutralizing antibodies against RSV, may be given just before the start of the RSV season to prevent RSV.

What to Do in Cases of an Acute Asthma Attack

An asthma attack may occur anytime and anywhere. It may happen in the home, at a school, in a mall, or in a park. To guide parents, teachers, and people who work in places where children go, the nurse can provide the following tips:

Teachers and school administrators should be familiar with the health history of the child. It is important to coordinate care and share information with the school health nurse. The nurse should also know the school district's rules and regulations regarding carrying asthma medications to school, including where the medications are to be kept and how to use the medications. In coordination with the child's physician and parents the nurse can fill out an emergency asthma action plan, including the child's triggers. The nurse needs to post emergency phone numbers in case of an attack. In addition, the nurse must know the child's peak flow readings, the child's personal best, and when the child runs into trouble. The nurse can also educate the teachers and other personnel who come in contact with the child.

Parents should be sure to carry the child's quick relief medications. It is helpful if the school-age child carry it too, along with the instructions about how the medication is used.

Nurses can give information on environmental control and creating an allergen-free environment. In addition, through community health education, the nurse can emphasize that when child exhibiting difficulty breathing, wheezing, and coughing, it is important to be calm and reassure the child. It is important to find out if the child's medicine is available; if not, call 911.

Personnel in parks, mall, and play areas should be briefed about possible pediatric emergencies including management in an emergency situation.

RESOURCES

American Academy of Family Physicians. (2005). Asthma action plan. http://www.familydoctor.org/online/famdocen/home.html

American Lung Association: http://www.lungusa.org

Cystic Fibrosis Foundation: http://www.cff.org

REFERENCES

American Academy of Otolaryngology, head and neck surgery (2008). Retrieved from: http://entmd.org/healthinfo/sinus/sinusitis.cfm (Accessed June 20, 2008).

Castro, M., Schechtman, K., Halstead, J., & Bloomberg, G. (2001). Risk factors for asthma morbidity and mortality in a large metropolitan city. *Journal of Asthma, 38*(8), 625–635.

Deglin, J. & Vallerand, A. (2009). *Davis's drug guide for nurses* (11th ed.). Philadelphia: F.A. Davis.

Mannino, D.M., Homa, D.M., Akinbami, L.J., Moorman, J.E., Gwynn, C., & Redd, S.C. (2002). Surveillance for asthma—United States, 1980–1999. *MMWR. Surveillance Summaries: Morbidity and Mortality Weekly Report. Surveillance Summaries / CDC. 51*(1), 1–13.

U.S. Department of Health and Human Services. (2007). National asthma education and prevention program. Expert panel report 3: Guidelines for the diagnosis and management of asthma. Full report 2007. NIH Publication No. 07-4051. Bethesda, MD: NHLBI Health Information Center. Retrieved from http://www.nhlbi.nih.gov/guidelines/asthma/asthgdln.htm (Accessed July 8, 2008).

Venes, D. (Ed.). (2005). *Taber's cyclopedic medical dictionary* (20th ed.). Philadelphia: F.A. Davis.

Caring for the Child with a Gastrointestinal Condition

KEY TERMS

biliary atresia – Extrahepatic biliary atresia (EHBA), an idiopathic, progressive, inflammatory process that causes both intrahepatic and extrahepatic bile duct fibrosis and obstruction

constipation – Difficult or infrequent passage of hard stool, which is often associated with straining, abdominal pain, or withholding behaviors

encopresis – Stool incontinence beyond the age when children should normally be able to control their bowels, which is usually after the age of 4 years

intussusception – Condition that occurs when a proximal section of the intestine and the mesentery (the peritoneal fold that encircles the small intestine and connects it to the posterior abdominal wall) "telescopes" into a distal section of the intestine

irritable bowel syndrome (IBS) – A functional disorder that is commonly cause of recurrent abdominal pain in children

lactose intolerance – Inability to digest milk and some dairy products, which leads to symptoms of bloating, cramping, and diarrhea

nissen fundoplication – Wrapping the gastric cardia with adjacent portions of the gastric fundus

omphalitis – Infection of the umbilical stump; occurs once the umbilicus is colonized with streptococci, staphylococci, or gram-negative organisms, which may cause a local infection

probiotics – Food preparations containing microorganism, such as *Lactobacillus*; can improve lactose intolerance when live cultures are fermented in dairy products

FOCUSED ASSESSMENT

Classic Symptomatic Triad for Intussusception

- Paroxysmal, episodic abdominal pain with vomiting every 5–30 minutes.
- Screaming with drawing up of the legs with periods of calm, sleeping, or lethargy between episodes.
- Stool, possible diarrhea in nature, with blood (currant jelly) (Petersen-Smith, 2004, p. 862).

Appendicitis Physical Examination

- The child diagnosed with appendicitis experiences a progression of symptoms, with no single test providing overall confirmation of the diagnosis.
- Laboratory findings may demonstrate an elevated white blood cell (WBC) count.
  - An elevated WBC count does not distinguish simple appendicitis from perforated appendicitis.
  - Children with appendicitis may also have a normal WBC count (Burd & Whalen, 2001).
- An abdominal radiograph may reveal fecal matter, or some other obstruction, although this rarely confirms the diagnosis.
- If there is uncertainty in young children, ultrasound and computed tomography (CT) scan may help differentiate abdominal pain from other causes, although the usefulness is variable (Mow, 2005).

Appendicitis	
Signs and Symptoms	**Reaction**
Rebound Tenderness	Presence of involuntary guarding, rebound tenderness with pain over McBurney's point, which is located 1.5–2 inches in from the right anterior superior iliac crest on a line toward the umbilicus and is best elicited on palpation
Heel-drop Jarring Test	Stand on toes for 15 seconds, then drops on heels; inability to stand straight or climb stairs; winces when getting off examination table.

(continued)

Appendicitis (Continued)	
Signs and Symptoms	Reaction
Psoas Sign	Abdominal pain with right hip flexion against resistance
Obturator Sign	Pain on passive internal rotation of the flexed right thigh
Rovsing Sign	Deep pressure in lower left quadrant elicits pain with a sudden release (Petersen-Smith, 2004).

Comparison of Hepatitis A (HAV), Hepatitis B (HBV), and Hepatitis C (HCV)			
Clinical Features	HAV	HBV	HCV
Onset	Usually rapid, acute	More insidious	Usually insidious
Fever	Common and early	Less frequent	Less frequent
Anorexia	Common	Mild to moderate	Mild to moderate
Nausea and Vomiting	Common	Sometimes	Mild to moderate
Rash	Rare	Common	Sometimes
Arthralgia	Rare	Common	Rare
Pruritus	Rare	Sometimes	Sometimes
Jaundice	Present	Present	Present

Sources: Diagneau (2007) and Sokol & Narkewicz (2007).

CLINICAL ALERTS

Abdominal Pain in Children

- In children, abdominal pain can be referred from an extra-abdominal source (e.g., pneumonia, urinary tract infection, or testicular torsion) or it can be associated with a systematic disease.
- Abdominal pain is a common complaint in ill children and can be found in conditions such as streptococcal pharyngitis, lower lobe pneumonia, sickle cell disease, cystic fibrosis, or in other conditions (Duderstadt, 2006).
- A child's abdominal pain experience is usually limited and the child may be unable to accurately describe or pinpoint the location or sensation.

Vomiting

- Projectile vomiting is the classic and most common symptom of hypertrophic pyloric stenosis.

Signs of Perforation and Peritonitis

- The nurse is responsible for monitoring the infant for signs of perforation (a hole), peritonitis (inflammation of the abdominal cavity), or shock in addition to evidence of increased pain. The nurse also monitors and records the child's stools. The nurse understands that the spontaneous passing of a stool may indicate a resolution of the obstruction.
- Perforation: Acute pain, beginning over the perforated area and spreading over the abdomen; abdomen may become rigid; nausea; vomiting; tachycardia; fevers; chills; sweats; confusion; decreased urinary output (Venes, 2005).
- Peritonitis: Moderate or mild abdominal pain that worsens with movement; fever; change in bowel habits; malaise; nausea; loss of appetite; fever; hypothermia; distended abdomen with decreased bowel sounds (Venes, 2005).

Shock

- Signs of shock include tachycardia, tachypnea, hypotension, and cool, clammy, or cyanotic skin (Venes, 2005).

Irritable Bowel Syndrome (IBS)

- Symptoms of IBS include fever, severe abdominal pain and/or vomiting blood require immediate attention; surgical evaluation and/or intervention may be necessary.

Appendicitis

- Children with suspected appendicitis who respond with a "yes" to being hungry most likely do not have appendicitis because in most cases the child does not feel like eating (Potts, 2002).

Constipation

- Most children who are constipated usually have some abdominal pain due to cramping.
- If the onset of constipation and severe abdominal pain is acute and/or accompanied by fever, vomiting, or other symptoms, the child must be evaluated for a bowel obstruction.

Probiotics

- Concern regarding the potential for decreased bone mineral density and osteoporosis in children and adolescents with lactose intolerance reinforces the recommendations for the ingestion of small amounts of dairy products with meals.
- Probiotics (food preparations containing microorganism) such as *Lactobacillus* can improve lactose intolerance when live cultures are fermented in dairy products.
- *Lactobacillus* is a non-pathogenic bacterium that produces lactic acid from carbohydrates. The active culture in yogurt provides a source of calcium for persons with lactose intolerance in addition to producing some of the lactose enzyme required for proper digestions.

Complications of a Central Venous Line

Observe infusion site at least every 4 hours for the following complications (Venes, 2005):

- Infiltration
- Thrombophlebitis
- Fluid or electrolyte overload
- Air embolism

DIAGNOSTIC TESTS

- Diagnosis of hypertrophic pyloric stenosis can be made by palpating the pyloric mass. The mass is olive-shaped, movable, firm, and best palpated from the left side and located above and to the right of the umbilicus in the mid-epigastrium (the superior central portion of the abdomen) beneath the liver edge (Bishop, 2006).

- An abdominal x-ray film may show an enlarged stomach with diminished or absent gas in the intestine (Bishop, 2006).
- Examination of the pylorus on ultrasound shows elongation and thickening of the pylorus, which may be confirmed by a barium upper GI series.
- Confirmation by an upper GI series demonstrates a "string sign," which is caused by the barium passing through narrowed pylorus (Bishop, 2006).

Ultrasound

A diagnosis is often made after the history and physical examination. The diagnosis can be established 60% to 80% of the time by an experienced examiner. For example, if the diagnosis of hypertrophic pyloric stenosis is inconclusive, an ultrasound can be used to demonstrate an elongated muscular mass surrounding a long pyloric canal. Ultrasound confirms the diagnosis of hypertrophic pyloric stenosis.

Intussusception

- A flat-plate x-ray film in the child can appear normal early in the course of the disorder. However, an abdominal "ultrasound establishes the diagnosis in 90% of the cases" (Petersen-Smith, 2004, p. 862).

Laboratory Findings for Ulcerative Colitis

Laboratory findings for ulcerative colitis may include elevated sedimentation rate, microcytic anemia, and elevated white blood cell count with left shift, antineutrophil cytoplasmic antibodies (ANA) present in 80% (Petersen-Smith, 2004).

Conditions, Laboratory Tests, and Their Implications

Condition	Laboratory Tests	Implication
Cyclic Vomiting Syndrome	Complete blood count (CBC) with differential, electrolytes, glucose, liver function tests, metabolic screening, urinalysis, urine culture, urine organic acids	Rule out other conditions

(continued)

Conditions, Laboratory Tests, and Their Implications (Continued)

Condition	Laboratory Tests	Implication
Crohn's Disease	CBC with differential, serum iron, total iron-binding capacity, serum albumin, sedimentation rate, C-reactive protein	Inflammation, malnutrition
Ulcerative Colitis	CBC with differential, sedimentation rate	Inflammation, malnutrition
Short Bowel Syndrome	Electrolytes	Diarrhea, malnutrition, dehydration
Biliary Atresia	CBC, electrolytes, bilirubin, liver enzymes, TORCH titer, urine cytomegalovirus, sweat test	For diagnosis and to rule out other conditions

Tests, Purpose, and Condition

Test	Purpose	Condition
Anorectal Manometry	Measures pressure of the internal and anal sphincters	Hirschsprung disease
Barium Enema	Allows visualization of bowel; may reduce intussusception	Intussusception, Hirschsprung disease
Barium Swallow	Allows visualization of upper gastrointestinal tract	Post swallowing reflux
Intraesophageal pH Monitoring Study	Records presence of acid reflux	Gastroesophageal disease
Intravenous Pyelogram	Provides information about structure and function of the kidney, ureters, and bladder	Anorectal malformations
Liver Biopsy	Establishes degree of disease	Hepatitis
Radionuclide or Meckel Scan	Creates images of body parts through injection and detection of radioactive isotopes	Meckel diverticulum
Ultrasound	Outlines shape of tissues and organs	Anorectal malformations; hypertrophic pyloric stenosis; intussusception; appendicitis
Voiding Cystogram	Allows visualization of bladder and urethra	Urinary tract defects associated with anorectal malformations

Chronic Diarrhea

- Chronic diarrhea is defined as "one or more liquid to semiliquid stools passed per day for 14 days or longer" (Petersen-Smith, 2004, p. 878).
- Diagnostic assessment may include stool for culture and sensitivity, ova and parasites.

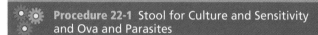

Procedure 22-1 Stool for Culture and Sensitivity and Ova and Parasites

Purpose

Collecting stool for culture and sensitivity and ova and parasites is used to detect the presence of bacterial overgrowth; to confirm bacterial gastroenteritis; and to assess sensitivity of specific antimicrobials.

Equipment

- Gloves
- Patient identification label
- Sterile culture tube and cotton swab to collect specimen
- Biohazard container

Steps

1. Don gloves.
2. Using the sterile cotton swab collect (scrape) a fresh, warm specimen of stool from the diaper or stool receptacle and place it into the sterile culture tube.
3. Label both the sterile culture tube and the biohazard bag with the patient's identification information.
4. Place the sterile culture tube into the biohazard bag.
5. Deliver the fresh specimen of stool to the laboratory promptly after collection.
6. Document the procedure.

Clinical Alert

- Avoid external contamination of stool and deliver to laboratory promptly.
- Provide samples from several areas of the stool to assure that organisms are isolated. Failure to do so may yield a false-negative result.
- Inform the lab of antimicrobial or antiamebic therapy within 10 days as it may yield false-negative results.

(continued)

Procedure 22-1 (Continued)

- Medications such as antacids, antibiotics, antidiarrheals, iron, and castor oil may interfere with analysis.

Teach Parents

Teach the parents that a stool for culture and sensitivity is used to detect the presence of bacterial overgrowth; confirm bacterial gastroenteritis; and to assess sensitivity of specific antimicrobials.

Teach parents that a stool for ova and parasites (O & P is used to aid in diagnosis of parasites or their eggs).

Source: Schnell, Van Leeuwen, & Kranpitz (2003).

MEDICATIONS

Medications for Gastrointestinal Conditions		
Category	Examples	Treatment of
Antiemetics	Promethazine Ondansetron Trimethobenzamide	Cyclic vomiting syndrome
Antispasmodics	Atropine Hyoscyamine Scopolamine	Irritable bowel syndrome
Laxatives	Milk of magnesia Polyethylene glycol	Constipation
Prokinetics	Metoclopramide	Cyclic vomiting syndrome Gastroesophageal reflux
Proton Pump Inhibitors	Lansoprazole Omeprazole	Gastroesophageal reflux

Steroid Side Effects

In gastrointestinal disorders steroids can help with inflammation. However there are side effects the nurse needs to be aware of:

- Cardiovascular: Edema, hypertension, congestive heart failure
- Central nervous system: Vertigo, seizures, psychoses, headache

- Dermatologic: Acne, skin atrophy, impaired wound healing, petechiae, bruising
- Endocrine and metabolic: Cushing's syndrome, growth suppression, glucose intolerance, sodium and water retention
- Gastrointestinal: Peptic ulcer, nausea, vomiting
- Genitourinary: Menstrual irregularities
- Neuromuscular and skeletal: Muscle weakness, osteoporosis, fractures
- Ocular: Cataracts, elevated intraocular pressure, glaucoma (Deglin & Vallerand, 2009).

Medications Used for Vomiting

- A combination of medications is used for sedation and the relief of pain and nausea and vomiting, which may include a combination of diphenhydramine (Benadryl), lorazepam (Ativan), promethazine (Phenergan), and meperidine (Demerol).
- Metoclopramide (Reglan) is a prokinetic agent that accelerates gastric emptying.
- Migraine relief includes sumatriptan (Imitrex) for acute episodes; amitriptyline (Elavil), cyproheptadine (Periactin), phenobarbital (Luminal), propranolol (Inderal) for prophylaxis; and ethinyl estradiol (Loestrin) for menstrual pain relief.
- Erythromycin (E-Mycin, E.E.S., EryPed) as a prokinetic is not used much in children secondary to the gastric effects and questionable efficacy.

ETHNOCULTURAL CONSIDERATIONS

Occurrence of Hypertrophic Pyloric Stenosis

- Hypertrophic pyloric stenosis occurs in approximately 6–8 of 1000 live births in the United States (Bishop, 2006).
- The incidence of pyloric stenosis is more common in the Caucasian population compared to 1.8 per 1000 live births in the Hispanic population and 0.7 in the African American population (Letton, 2001).

- Males, especially firstborns, are affected two to four times more often than females are, and there may be a positive family history (Letton, 2001).

Colic

- Chamomile, vervain, licorice, fennel, and balm mint have antispasmodic properties that are found in herbal teas and are used as a remedy for colic in Israel.

Occurrence of Lactose Intolerance

- Asians, southern Europeans, Arabs, Israelis, and African-Americans experience a high incidence of primary lactase deficiency.

Occurrence of Celiac Disease

- Celiac disease primarily affects people of northern European descent. The average incidence of celiac disease in Europe is 1 per 1000 live births with a ratio of 1 per 250 in Sweden to 1 per 4000 in Denmark (Potts, 2002).

TEACHING THE FAMILY

Inguinal Hernia

- If the child has an inguinal hernia, tell the parents that the surgery will repair the defect caused by the hernia.
- Recovery for an inguinal hernia is usually rapid and the child will return home the same day as the surgery.
- After surgery, the nurse can inform the parents that the child's vital signs are monitored frequently and that the child's position will be changed often to avoid undue stress on the surgical area.
- Postoperative care includes keeping the wound clean and dry and managing the child's pain.
- For a child who is not toilet trained, changing diapers as soon as possible is important to prevent wound irritation and infection.

- Discharge instructions include informing the parents on wound care and the importance of keeping the surgical site clean and dry.
- The nurse can also tell the parents that the child can resume normal activity within 4–6 weeks and that they may be given a prescription for stool softeners for the child to prevent straining during defecation (Venes, 2005).

Irritable Bowel Syndrome (IBS)

- Explain to the family that stress can trigger the symptoms of IBS (school, family circumstances).
- Instruct parents and children to keep a food diary to determine the triggers that cause flares of IBS.
- Family counseling may be recommended.

Dealing with Food Jags with Young Children

- Reassure the parents that food jags are normal and that these tendencies will pass. Stress that a little patience will keep both parents and child from further gastrointestinal upsets.
- Suggest that the parents not force the child to eat foods he is not interested in but to provide a variety of nutritious foods during meals and for between-meal snacks in the amount appropriate for the child's age.
- Inform the family about treatments and when they need to seek additional help.

Management Strategies for Infantile Colic (Petersen-Smith, 2004)

- Support parents and assure them the child is in good health.
- Reinforce parents' efforts to comfort the child.
- Instruct parents on strategies to calm infant (swaddling, decreasing environmental stimulation, rocking).
- Assess feeding techniques and instruct as needed.
- Provide an opportunity for parents to express frustrations

ADDITIONAL INFORMATION FOR THE CLINICAL SETTING

Preventing Spread of Rotavirus

Rotavirus	Incidence	Protecting Children	Dehydration Secondary to Gastroenteritis
Viral gastroenteritis causes approximately 80% of all cases of diarrhea in children younger than 1 year of age. Accounts for approximately one third of hospitalizations of children in industrialized countries. By 5 years of age, nearly every child will have had at least one episode of rotavirus-induced illness. Primary transmission of this virus is via the fecal-oral route. Virus is very hearty and stable on surfaces for long periods of time, increasing the risk for transmission through contaminated surfaces or food. The virus has been found in the respiratory tract of infected individuals, raising concern for transmission via infectious secretions.	Does not vary between industrialized and developing countries. Has not been shown to decrease with increased sanitation in developing nations. The incubation period for rotavirus is 1–3 days followed by fever, vomiting, diarrhea, and abdominal pain. Vomiting and diarrhea may be severe enough and require intervention to prevent dehydration. A primary factor in survival of rotaviral induced gastroenteritis is access to adequate medical care. Therapy primarily consists of oral rehydration.	The immunization schedule for ages 0–6 years of age now currently includes a recommendation for a three-dose series of the rotavirus vaccine (Rota). First dose is recommended between 6 and 12 weeks of age with the initial dose not to be started later than age 12 weeks (American Academy of Pediatrics, 2006).	Rotaviral gastroenteritis is self-limiting disease. Deaths due to dehydration. Early signs of dehydration require medical treatment: • Decreased number wet diapers • Sunken fontanel and eyes • Listlessness • Cool, pale skin Families should be given specific instructions regarding oral intake goals during treatment for rotavirus and instructed to return for follow up if a child is unable to meet the goals or the appearance of any of the above symptoms of dehydration.

Complementary Care for Diarrhea

- Products containing *Lactobacillus acidophilus*, such as yogurt, can be used to decrease the incidence of rotavirus diarrhea in infants 5–24 months of age (Blosser, 2004).
- *Lactobacillus* is a nonpathogenic bacterium that produces lactic acid from carbohydrates and is normally found in milk, feces of infants fed by bottle, and adults.
- The addition of *Lactobacillus acidophilus* to the diet changes the bacterial flora of the GI tract, hence treating the overgrowth of pathogenic or diarrhea-causing organisms in the GI tract.

Common Causes of Vomiting

Origin	Cause
Upper GI	Gastritis
	Esophagitis
	Pyloric stenosis
Small Intestine	Intestinal malrotation with volvulus
Colon	Hirschsprung's disease
	Intussusception
	Fecal impaction
Liver or Pancreas	Hepatobiliary dysfunction
Infections	Bacterial enteritis
	Otitis media
	Urinary track infection
	Viral gastroenteritis
	Hepatitis
	Sepsis
Neurological	Hydrocephalus
	Brain tumor
	Migraine headache
	Head trauma
	Congenital malformation
Other	Cow's milk protein allergy
	Maternal drug exposure and withdrawal
	Toxic ingestion
	Appendicitis
	Inborn error of metabolism
	Pneumonia
	Drug or alcohol ingestion
	Eating disorders
	Pregnancy

Short Bowel Syndrome

- The major symptoms of short bowel syndrome are diarrhea, malabsorption, malnutrition, and dehydration.
- Electrolyte imbalance is abnormal and usually secondary to diarrhea and malabsorption.

Hepatitis Viruses					
	HAV	**HBV**	**HCV**	**HDV**	**HEV**
Type of Virus	Enterovirus	Hepadnavirus	Flavivirus	Incomplete	Calicivirus
Transmission	Fecal–oral	Parenteral, sexual, vertical	Parenteral, sexual, vertical	Parenteral, sexual	Fecal–oral
Incubation Period	15–40 days	50–150 days	30–150 days	20–90 days	14–65 days
Diagnostic Tests	Anti-HAV IgM	HBsAg, anti-HBc IgM	Anti-HCV, PCR–RNA test	Anti-HDV	Anti-HEV
Mortality Rate	0.1–0.2%	0.5–2%	1–2%	2–20%	1–2% (20% in pregnant women)
Carrier State	No	Yes	Yes	Yes	No
Vaccine Available	Yes	Yes	No	Yes (HBV)	No
Treatment	None	Interferon-α, nucleoside analogues (lamivudine, tenofovir, adefovir, entecavir)	Interferon-α, (pegylated interferon in adults) plus ribavirin	Treatment for HBV	None

Source: Sokol & Narkewicz (2007).

Comparison of Hepatitis A (HAV), Hepatitis B (HBV), and Hepatitis C (HCV)

HAV	HBV	HCV
Usually rapid, acute	More insidious	Usually insidious
Common and early	Less frequent	Less frequent
Common	Mild to moderate	Mild to moderate
Common	Sometimes present	Mild to moderate
Rare	Common	Sometimes present
Rare	Common	Rare
Rare	Sometimes present	Sometimes present
Present	Present	Present

Sources: Diagneau (2007); Sokol & Narkewicz (2007).

Injuries Caused by Abdominal Trauma

Organ	Incidence and Description	Management
Abdomen	Approximately 8% of pediatric trauma Risk of blunt trauma injuries increased because of relative size and close proximity of organs Penetrating trauma accounts for <10% or pediatric abdominal trauma Gunshot wounds involve multiple organs in 80% of the cases	Serial examination is primary in decisions regarding surgical interventions Surgical intervention may be required if vital signs are persistently unstable along with aggressive fluid replacement. Laparoscopy may be indicated with peritoneal irritation and abdominal wall discoloration. CT is valuable for assessing intra-abdominal trauma.
Spleen	Most frequently injured abdominal organ in children Positive Kehr sign (pressure on the left upper quadrant eliciting left shoulder pain) related to diaphragmatic irritation from ruptured spleen Spleen injury suspected with left upper quadrant abrasions or tenderness Splenic injury may include capsular tear to a complete rupture	CT scan can be used to grade splenic injury. Treatment of choice is nonoperative management. Surgery is indicated for blood loss greater than 40 mL/kg or transfused blood in 24–36 hours or evidence of hemodynamic instability. With splenectomy penicillin prophylaxis is recommended *(continued)*

Injuries Caused by Abdominal Trauma (Continued)

Organ	Incidence and Description	Management
Liver	Accounts for 40% of all deaths associated with blunt abdominal trauma in children Right lobe injuries are more common Diagnosis based on Kehr sign (pressure on the right upper quadrant eliciting right shoulder pain) Severe hemorrhage is more common with injury to the liver than to other abdominal organs	Conservative management is recommended with ongoing monitoring of blood loss, hepatic function, and liver structure with serial CR scans or ultrasound. Operative management is reserved for life-threatening situations.
Pancreas and Duodenum	Less common in children than adults Seen in bicycle handlebar injuries, motor vehicle crashes, and nonaccidental trauma Diagnosis difficult unless obvious injury to overlying structures Diffuse abdominal tenderness, pain, and vomiting accompanied by elevation of amylase and lipase may be indicative of injury although often do not occur for several days after injury Duodenal injuries include hematomas and perforation Perforations are difficult to diagnose	Management includes nasogastric suction and parenteral nutrition. Nonoperative management is appropriate for contusions. Surgical interventions may be required with distal transection. Perforation is not always obvious on a CT scan.
Intestinal	Injury occurs less often than in solid intra-abdominal organs. Risk varies with the amount of intestinal contents, i.e., a full bowel is likely to shear more easily than an empty bowel. Lap belt or seatbelt in a motor vehicle crash results in a sudden deceleration and increase in intraluminal pressure and can lead to perforation.	Presence of a contusion over the seatbelt area and abdomen or back pain indicates a need to pursue the diagnosis of intestinal injury. Pneumoperitoneum in association with intestinal perforation occurs in about 20% of patients

Source: Marcdante (2006).

RESOURCES

American Academy of Pediatrics: http://www.aap.org

Celiac Sprue Association: http://www.csaceliacs.org

Crohn's and Colitis Foundation of America: http://ccfa.org

Food and Nutrition Information Center:
http://www.nal.usda.gov/fnic/

My Pyramid.gov: http://www.mypyramid.gov

United States Department of Agriculture Healthy Food
Guidelines: http://www.mypyramid.gov

REFERENCES

Bishop, W.P. (2006). The digestive system. In R.M. Kliegman, K.J. Marcdante, H.B. Jenson, & R.E. Behrman (Eds.). *Nelson essential of pediatrics* (5th ed., pp. 579–624). St. Louis: Elsevier,

Blosser, C.G. (2004). Complementary medicine. In C.E. Burns, A.M. Dunn, M.A. Brady, N.B. Starr, & C.G. Blosser (Eds.). *Pediatric primary care: A handbook for nurse practitioners* (3rd ed., pp. 1211–1248). St. Louis: Elsevier.

Burd, R.S., & Whalen, T.V. (2001). Evaluation of the child with suspected appendicitis. *Pediatric Annals, 30*(12), 721–725.

Daigneau, C.V. (2007). The child with gastrointestinal dysfunction. In M.J. Hockenberry & D. Wilson (Eds.). *Wong's nursing care of infants and children* (8th ed, pp. 1387–1435). St. Louis: Elsevier.

Deglin, J. & Vallerand, A. (2009). *Davis's drug guide for nurses* (11th ed.). Philadelphia: F.A. Davis.

Duderstadt, K.G. (2006). *Pediatric physical examination: An illustrated handbook*. St. Louis: Elsevier.

Letton, R.W. (2001). Pyloric stenosis. *Pediatric Annals, 3*(12), 745–750.

Marcdante, K.J. (2006). The acutely ill or injured child. In R.M. Kliegman, K.J. Marcdante, H.B. Jenson, & R.E. Behrman (Eds.). *Nelson essentials of pediatrics* (5th ed, pp. 179–216). St. Louis: Elsevier.

Mow, W. (2005). Disorders of the intestine. In L.M. Osborn, T.G. DeWitt, L.R. First, & J.A. Zenel (Eds.). *Pediatrics* (pp. 670–677). St. Louis: Elsevier.

Petersen-Smith, A.M. (2004). Gastrointestinal disorders. In C.E. Burns, A.M. Dunn, M.A. Brady, N.B. Starr, & C.G. Blosser (Eds.). *Pediatric primary care: A handbook for nurse practitioners* (3rd ed, pp. 839–884). St. Louis: Elsevier.

Potts, N. (2002). Gastrointestinal alterations. In N.L. Potts & B.L. Mandleco (Eds.). *Pediatric nursing: Caring for children and their families* (pp. 653–696). Clifton Park, NY: Delmar-Thomson Learning

Schnell, Z.B., Van Leeuwen, A.M., & Kranpitz, T.R. (2003). *Davis's comprehensive handbook of laboratory and diagnostic tests with nursing implications*. Philadelphia: F.A. Davis.

Sokol, R.J., & Narkewicz, M.R. (2007). Liver and pancreas. In W.W. Hay, M.J. Levin, J.M. Sondheimer, & R.R. Deterding (Eds.). *Current diagnosis & treatment in pediatrics* (18th ed, pp. 638–683). New York: Lange Medical Books/McGraw-Hill.

Venes, D. (Ed.). (2005). *Tabers cyclopedic medical dictionary*. Philadelphia: F.A. Davis.

Caring for the Child with an Immunological or Infectious Condition

KEY TERMS

allogeneic cell transplantation – Cell donation from a donor (family member) who has a compatible human leukocyte antigen

anaphylaxis – Immediate hypersensitivity reaction to an excessive release of chemical mediators affecting the entire body; a medical emergency

autoimmune disorder – Immune response against one of the body's own tissues or cells

autologous transplant – The child's own cells are taken, stored, and reinfused after the child has received chemotherapy

immune response – Defends the body against microorganisms, parasites, and foreign cells such as cancer cells and transplanted cells; key to a normal immune response is the body's ability to recognize foreign substances as non-self and then to mobilize defenses and attack the invaders

isogeneic transplantation – Cells are taken from an identical twin

pathogenicity – Percentage of children exposed to the pathogen who will eventually develop the disease

virulence – The severity of the health problems caused by the agent

FOCUSED ASSESSMENT

Anaphylaxis

Signs and symptoms of anaphylaxis develop suddenly and require prompt recognition and treatment.

- Wheezing
- Tachycardia
- Hypotension
- Cyanosis
- Alteration in level of consciousness
- Nasal congestion
- Facial edema
- Anxiety
- Hives
- Urticaria
- Nausea and vomiting
- Abdominal pain
- Laryngospasm
- A sense of impending doom
- Vascular collapse and cardiac arrest

Key Components of Physical Assessment for the Child with an Infectious Disease

Vital Signs
- Temperature (see Chapter 18, Expected Temperatures in Children)
- Heart rate
- Respiratory rate
- Blood pressure

Average Range for Pediatric Vital Signs

Age Group	Heart Rate	Respiration Rate	Blood Pressure Systolic	Blood Pressure Diastolic
Infant	80–150	25–55	65–100	45–65
Toddler	70–110	20–30	90–105	55–70
Preschooler	65–110	20–25	95–110	60–75
School-age	60–95	14–22	100–120	60–75
Adolescent	55–85	12–18	110–125	65–85

- Pain (the most commonly used pain scales are the numeric scale, the Wong Faces Scale, and the FLACC pain scale)

Respiratory Assessment

- Upper respiratory infection symptoms
- Breath sounds
- Work of breathing
- Pulse oximeter reading
- Skin/mucous membrane color
- Secretions; color, character, amount

Neurological Assessment

- Febrile seizures
- Early identification of neurological complications
- Level of consciousness (the pediatric Glasgcow Coma Scale consists of three components of assessment: eye opening, verbal response, and motor response)

Gastrointestinal Assessment

- Fluid intake
- Presence of vomiting or diarrhea

Skin

- Presence of rash, pruritus, lesions

CLINICAL ALERTS

Increased Risk for Infection

Something as simple and common as irritation from diaper rash, but also as a potential portal of entry for microorganisms.

Administration of Steroids

- Never stop steroids abruptly due to adrenal insufficiency (the greatest risks come from sudden withdrawal).
- Clinical manifestations of adrenal insufficiency include hypotension, weight loss, weakness, nausea, vomiting, anorexia, lethargy, confusion, and restlessness.
- Educate parents about the proper use of steroids; must be taken as directed.
- Slowly taper the use of steroids when it is time to discontinue use.

Systemic Lupus Erythematosus (SLE)

- Assess for signs and symptoms to ensure prompt recognition of an exacerbation (prevention is the most important component of nursing care).
- Emphasize the importance of rest and adequate nutrition to maximize immune system function.
- Facial rash, fatigue, and arthritic changes may put the child at risk depression and altered body image.
- Refer family to support group to help adjust to life with SLE.

Reye Syndrome Risk with Use of Aspirin

- Administration of salicylates (aspirin) to children with acute viral illness is linked to Reye syndrome.
- Educate parents regarding use of aspirin-free medications (Alka-Seltzer, Anacin, Ascriptin, Bayer Arthritis Pain and Aspirin preparations, Doan's, Dristan, Ecotrin, Excedrin, Kaopectate, Pamprin, Pepto-Bismol, Sine-Off Sinus Medicine, St. Joseph Adult Aspirin, Vanquish).
- The National Reye Syndrome Foundation can be accessed at www.reyessyndrome.org/

Preventing Cytomegalovirus (CMV) Infection in Immunocompromised Children

Cytomegalovirus (CMV) infection is a source of significant morbidity and mortality in immunocompromised children.

- Good hand washing is the best preventive measure.
- Disposable gloves should be worn when handling linen or underclothes soiled with feces or urine.
- CMV-negative blood should be provided to immunocompromised children.

Adverse Effects of Immunizations

- Local effects: Mild, occur most frequently. Symptoms include soreness, redness, and pain at the site of injection. Manage with heat or ice to the site.
- Systemic effects: Less frequent; fever and mild irritability. Manage the effects with acetaminophen (Children's Tylenol) administered before immunization; continuing every 4 hours as needed for 24 hours.

- Allergic reaction: Rare but serious. Seek immediate medical assistance if the child exhibits the following symptoms: high fever; altered mental status (excessive irritability, lethargy, nonresponsiveness, seizures); increased difficulty breathing; hoarseness or wheezing when breathing; hives, pale, cool skin.

Postexposure Treatment for Rabies

- Exercising caution with unknown animals is essential.
- Most exposures to rabies occur through bites of wild animals that allow contaminated saliva to enter the bite wound.
- If an animal has injured a child, the parents must contact their health care provider immediately!

Clusters of Human H5N1 Cases

- Clusters of human H5N1 cases ranging from 2 to 8 cases per cluster have been identified in most countries that have reported H5N1 cases.
- Nearly all of the cluster cases have occurred among blood relatives living in the same household.
- Most people in these clusters have been infected with H5N1 virus through direct contact with sick or dead poultry or wild birds.
- Limited human-to-human transmission of H5N1 virus cannot be excluded in some clusters.
- CDC Web site: http://www.cdc.gov/flu/avian/outbreaks/current.htm

DIAGNOSTIC TESTS

Human Immunodeficiency Virus (HIV) Testing

There are two primary methods for confirming the diagnosis of Human immunodeficiency virus (HIV):

- Enzyme-linked immunosorbent assay (ELISA): A test that identifies the presence of HIV antibodies and is performed within 48 hours after birth. The use of ELISA is ineffective in children younger than 18 months due to the presence of maternal antibodies.

- Polymerase chain reaction (PCR): A test that identifies the proviral DNA, specific to HIV. The PCR is more expensive but has greater sensitivity. PCR has a greater number of false-positive results.

Blood Culture

A simple blood culture can detect bacteria or fungi in the blood. To test for an infection in the blood:

- A phlebotomist will draw a sample of blood from a vein.
- In the laboratory, the blood sample will be mixed with substances that promote the growth of bacteria or fungi.
- In most cases, bacteria can be detected in the blood culture within 2 to 3 days. Some types of blood infections can take 10 days or longer and fungal infections in the blood can take up to 30 days for results.
- A normal blood culture (negative) result will report that no bacterium or fungus has been found in the blood.
- An abnormal result (positive) will report that a bacterium or fungus has been found in the blood.

Identification of an Infectious Disease

- Complete blood count (CBC) with differential
- Urinalysis (UA)
- Spinal fluid analysis
- Cultures from fluids, secretions, drainage
- Pulse oximetry
- Chest x-ray exam
- Computerized tomography (CT)

MEDICATIONS

Trimethoprim-Sulfamethoxazole (TMP-SMZ) (Bactrim or Septra) (trye-**meth**-oh-prim/sul-fa-meth-**ox**-a-zole)

Indications Prevention of *Pneumocystis carinii* pneumonia (PCP). Prevention of bacterial infections in an immunosuppressed child.

Actions The combination inhibits the metabolism of folic acid in bacteria at two different points.

Therapeutic Effects Bactericidal action against susceptible bacteria.

Pharmacokinetics
Absorption Well absorbed from the GI tract.

Contraindications and Precautions
Contraindicated in Hypersensitivity to sulfonamides or trimethoprim, megaloblastic anemia secondary to folate deficiency, severe renal impairment, and children <2 months of age.

Adverse Reactions and Side Effects Hepatic necrosis, nausea, vomiting, diarrhea, toxic epidermal necrolysis, Stevens-Johnson syndrome, erythema multiforme, rashes, agranulocytosis, aplastic anemia, and phlebitis with IV insertion.

Route and Dosage PCP prevention: **PO** (children): 75 mg/m^3 TMP/325 mg/m^3 SMZ q12hr on 3 consecutive days/week. Not to exceed 320 mg TMP/1600 mg/SMZ per day.

Nursing Implications
1. Assess the child for infection. Advise the family to notify the health care provider for any signs of infection.
2. Assess for allergy to sulfonamides.
3. Monitor lab values periodically throughout therapy. TMP-SMZ may produce elevated serum bilirubin, creatinine, and alkaline phosphatase.

Data from Deglin, J., & Vallerand, A. (2009). Davis's drug guide for nurses (11th ed.), pp. 1205–1207. Philadelphia: F.A. Davis.

Methylprednisolone (A-Methapred) (meth-ill-pred-**niss**-oh-lone)

Indications Anti-inflammatory or immunosuppressant agent

Actions Suppress inflammation and the normal immune response.

Therapeutic Effects Suppression of inflammation and modification of the normal immune response.

Pharmacokinetics
Absorption Well absorbed after oral administration.

Contraindications and Precautions
Contraindicated in Acute untreated infections.

Cautions Chronic use in children will result in decreased growth. During stress (surgery, infections) supplemental doses may be needed.

Adverse Reactions and Side Effects Peptic ulceration, anorexia, nausea, acne, decreased wound healing, hirsutism, petechiae and bruising, muscle wasting, osteoporosis, cushinoid appearance, and thromboembolism.

Route and Dosage PO (children): 0.417 mg/kg–1.67 mg/kg (12.5–50 mg/m²) per day in 3–4 divided doses. Rectal (children): 0.5–1 mg/kg (15–30 mg/m²) daily or every other day for at least 1 week. **IV, IM** (children): 139–835 mcg/kg (4.16–25 mg/m²) every 12–24 hours.

Nursing Implications

1. Assess for signs and symptoms of adrenal insufficiency (hypotension, weight loss, weakness, nausea, vomiting, anorexia, lethargy, confusion, restlessness).
2. Monitor fluid status, daily weights.
3. Monitor electrolytes and glucose levels.
4. Administer oral medications with food.
5. Instruct family regarding need to take medications as ordered due to risk of adrenal insufficiency with sudden withdraw of medication.
6. Instruct family regarding possibility of immunosuppression, need to avoid ill contacts and report possible infections to health care provider immediately.
7. Instruct family to inform health care provider promptly for severe abdominal pain, tarry stools, increased bruising, non healing sores, sudden weight gain, or behavior changes.
8. Immunizations should be discussed with health care provider on an individual basis.

Data from Deglin, J., & Vallerand, A. (2009). Davis's drug guide for nurses (11th ed.), pp. 350–367. Philadelphia: F.A. Davis.

Epinephrine (Adrenaline) (e-pi-**nef**-rin)

Indications IV: Management of severe allergic reactions

Actions Inhibits the release of mediators of immediate hypersensitivity reactions from mast cells.

Therapeutic Effects Maintenance of heart rate and blood pressure.

Pharmacokinetics
Absorption Well absorbed.

Contraindications and Precautions
Contraindicated in Hypersensitivity.

Adverse Reactions and Side Effects
CNS Nervousness, restlessness, tremor.
Cardiovascular Arrhythmias, hypertension, tachycardia.

Route and Dosage IV (severe anaphylaxis): 0.1–0.25 mg q5–15 minutes; may be followed by a 1–4 mcg/min continuous infusion (may be increased up to 1.5 mcg/kg per minute)

Nursing Implications
1. Assess volume status. Hypovolemia should be corrected prior to administration of IV epinephrine.
2. Monitor blood pressure, perfusion, ECG, respiratory rate, and urine output during administration.
3. Assess for hypersensitivity reaction: Rash, urticaria, swelling of face, lips, eyelids.
4. IV administration: Administer at a dilution of 1:10,000; this may be prepared through dilution of 1 mg of 1:1000 solution in at least 10 mL of 0.9% NaCl.

Administer each 1 mg of 1:10,000 solution over at least 1 minute.

Data from Deglin, J., & Vallerand, A. (2009). Davis's drug guide for nurses (11th ed.), pp. 480–484. Philadelphia: F.A. Davis.

Diphenhydramine (Benadryl) (dye-fen-**hye**-dra-meen)

Indications Relief of allergic symptoms caused by histamine release including: anaphylaxis, allergic rhinitis, allergic dermatoses. Relief of pruritis.

Actions Antagonizes the effects of histamine at H_1-receptor sites. Significant CNS depressant and anticholinergic properties.

Therapeutic Effects Decreased symptoms of histamine excess (sneezing, rhinorrhea, nasal and ocular pruritus, ocular tearing and redness, urticaria)

Pharmacokinetics
Absorption Well absorbed after oral or IM administration

Contraindications and Precautions
Contraindicated in Hypersensitivity.

Adverse Reactions and Side Effects Drowsiness, paradoxical excitation (more common in children). Anorexia, dry mouth.

Route and Dosage PO (children 6–12 years): 12.5–25 mg q4–6hr. **PO** (children 2–6 years): 6.25–12.5 mg q4–6hr. **IM/IV** (children): 1.25 mg/kg 4 times/day. Not to exceed 300 mg/day.

Nursing Implications
1. Provide child and family education regarding medication, caution not to exceed recommended dose.
2. Inform parents that medication may cause drowsiness or excitability in the child.
3. Provide education regarding common side effect of dry mouth. Management strategies include frequent mouth care and oral rinses.

Data from Deglin, J., & Vallerand, A. (2009). Davis's drug guide for nurses (11th ed.), pp. 424–426. Philadelphia: F.A. Davis.

Ganciclovir (Cytovene) (gan-**sye**-kloe-vir)

Indications Treatment of CMV retinitis in the immunocompromised child.
Prevention of CMV infection in the transplant child at risk

Actions CMV converts ganciclovir to its active form inside host cell, where it inhibits viral DNA polymerase.

Therapeutic Effects Antiviral effect directed against CMV-infected cells.

Pharmacokinetics
Absorption 5% to 9% absorbed with oral administration. IV administration results in complete bioavailability.

Contraindications and Precautions
Contraindicated in Hypersensitivity to ganciclovir or acyclovir

Adverse Reactions and Side Effects
Seizures, headache, malaise, drowsiness, ataxia
GI bleeding, nausea, vomiting, increased liver enzymes.
Neutropenia, thrombocytopenia, anemia.
Hypotension, hypertension
Renal toxicity

Route and Dosage Pediatric doses not established. IV (Adults): Induction 5 mg/kg q12hr for 14–21 days. Maintenance: 5 mg/kg per day or 6 mg/kg for 5 days/week; may increase to q12hr. PO (Adults): Maintenance: 1000 mg 3 times/day or 500 mg 6 times/day.

Nursing Implications
1. Pediatric dose not established.
2. Increased risk of bone marrow depression when used with antineoplastics or zidovudine
3. Assess the child during treatment for signs of infection, bleeding, or development of CMV retinitis.
4. Administer IV at slow rate, using in-line filter.
5. Advise the child/family to notify the health care provider for any signs of bleeding.

Data from Deglin, J., & Vallerand, A. (2009). Davis's drug guide for nurses (11th ed.), pp. 594–596. Philadelphia: F.A. Davis.

Amphotericin B (Amphocin) (am-foe-**ter**-i-sin)

Indications Treatment of active, progressive, potentially fatal fungal infections

Actions Binds to fungal cell membrane, allowing leakage of cellular contents

Therapeutic Effects Fungistatic action

Pharmacokinetics
Absorption Not absorbed orally.

Contraindications and Precautions
Contraindicated in Hypersensitivity

Adverse Reactions and Side Effects Headache, hypotension, diarrhea, nausea, vomiting, nephrotoxicity, hypokalemia, chills, fever, and hypersensitivity reactions

Route and Dosage Specific dosage and duration of therapy depend on infection being treated.
Amphotericin Deoxycholate IV (children): 0.25 mg/kg infused initially; increase by 0.25 mg/kg every other day to a maximum of 1 mg/kg per day.
Amphotericin B Cholesteryl Sulfate IV (children): 3–4 mg/kg per day
Amphotericin B Lipid Complex IV (children): 5 mg/kg per day.
Amphotericin B Liposome IV (children): 3–5 mg/kg q24hr

Nursing Implications

1. Premedication with antipyretics, corticosteroids, antihistamines, and antiemetics may reduce incidence of fever, chills, headache, nausea, or vomiting.
2. Monitor VS and above noted symptoms every 15–30 minutes during test dose and every 30 minutes for 2–4 hours after the test dose.
3. Monitor VS and above symptoms closely for first 1–2 hours of each subsequent dose.
4. Monitor for thrombophlebitis because the drug is highly irritating to tissues.
5. Monitor CBC and platelet counts weekly, BUN and serum creatinine every other day while increasing dose, then twice weekly. Monitor potassium and magnesium levels biweekly.
6. Ensure resuscitation equipment readily available before administration.

Data from Deglin, J., & Vallerand, A. (2009). Davis's drug guide for nurses (11th ed.), pp. 160–164. Philadelphia: F.A. Davis.

Vaccines

- Vaccine schedules may be obtained through the Centers for Disease Control and Prevention (CDC) Web site: http://www.cdc.gov/vaccines/recs/schedules/
- Vaccine Information Statements (in many languages) may be accessed at www.cdc.gov/nip or www.immunize.org

Type	Definition	Example
Inactivated	Disease-causing microbe is killed but is still capable of inducing the body to produce antibodies.	Inactivated poliovirus vaccine (IPV; injection)
Live (attenuated)	Disease-causing organism is not killed but under special conditions is designed to decrease virulence.	Measles vaccine (injection)
Toxoid	Inactivated form effective in producing an immune response geared toward a toxin-producing organism.	Tetanus toxoid (injection)

(continued)

Type	Definition	Example
Subunit	Portion of the virus or bacterium is used to produce the desired immunological response without the undesirable effects that are seen with some of the other surface antigens.	*Bordetella pertussis* vaccine included in the acellular DPT (injection)
Polysaccharide	Made from portions of the polysaccharides capsule and are effective in producing immunity in children older than the age of 2 years. At exposure the polysaccharide capsule does not elicit a T-cell response, the duration of immunity is variable and not life long.	Pneumovax (injection)
Conjugate	Links a recognizable antigen with the "hidden" bacterial antigen thereby enabling the immature immune system to identify the bacteria as non-self and respond.	*Haemophilus influenzae* type b (Hib; injection)
Recombinant	Inserts genes for production of the antigens desired into a low-virulent vector using genetic engineering.	Hepatitis B virus (HBV; injection)

TEACHING THE FAMILY

Anaphylaxis Reaction

- For children who have experienced an anaphylactic reaction the nurse must provide follow-up care to families to prevent recurrences.
- If the child has allergies that cannot be completely eliminated, a follow-up referral to an allergist for desensitization treatments or a self-administration epinephrine prescription, such as an EpiPen.
- It is important that parents are taught to recognize early indicators of anaphylaxis and are confident in their ability to act quickly on this assessment.

Immunizations

1. Discuss the immunization's purpose as well as the administration and potential side effects.
2. Give parents educational materials.
3. Tell parents about immunization clinics in nontraditional settings such as churches, synagogues, mosques, community centers, or shopping malls.
4. Provide opportunities and encourage parents to communicate their concerns about immunizations.
5. Encourage parents to investigate immunizations using reputable Web sites and other resources such as education pamphlets.
6. Assist the parents in understanding how to keep track of immunizations and when the next immunizations are due.
7. Assist parents in investigating funding resources for immunizations (this is a possible barrier to immunization for many families).

Use of Insect Repellants

Instruct parents to apply insect repellant to clothing and not to the child's skin to decrease the chance of systemic absorption of a potentially harmful substance.

Avian Flu Preparation

1. Discuss the differences between seasonal flu and pandemic flu.
2. Describe actions being taken by the health care community to monitor and prepare for the pandemic and encourage families to take an active role.
3. Assist families to establish their own plan for care in the event of a pandemic including:
   - Storage of a 2-week supply of food and water for the family
   - Maintenance of a supply of needed medications.
   - Maintenance of a supply of over-the-counter medications needed to treat symptoms of flu.
   - Establish a plan for family members living alone.
4. Encourage families to become involved with community groups to help prepare and plan for the pandemic.

5. Reinforce basic infection control techniques to limit the spread of influenza.
6. Provide families with links to CDC resources with preparation checklists. Encourage them to utilize the checklists to assist in preparation.

ADDITIONAL INFORMATION FOR THE CLINICAL SETTING

Complementary care: Nonpharmacological adjuncts to pain management:

- Guided imagery
- Hypnosis
- Prayer
- Meditation
- Music
- Aromatherapy
- Proper preparation (e.g., show diagrams, allow handling of equipment, introduce to child to personnel, visit special rooms where the child may go after the procedure)
- Distraction (e.g., blowing bubbles, singing songs, reading a book, playing with a favorite toy)
- Relaxation (guided imagery or hypnosis, easy-to-read relaxation books)

Systemic Lupus Erythematosus (SLE) Resources

The nurse can encourage an adolescent recently diagnosed with systemic lupus erythematosus (SLE) to contact a local support group. In addition, several good resources are available online through the organizations located at the following Web sites:

- Lupus Foundation of America
  http://www.lupus.org/
- National Institute of Arthritis and Musculoskeletal and Skin Disorders
  http://www.niams.nih.gov
- SLE Foundation, Inc.
  http://www.lupusny.org/
- Association of Rheumatology Health Professionals, American College of Rheumatology
  http://www.rheumatology.org/

- Arthritis Foundation
  http://www.arthritis.org/

Nursing Care for Anaphylaxis

- Perform cardiopulmonary resuscitation.
- Activate the emergency system.
- Ensure adequate airway: endotracheal intubation or oxygen.
- Administer epinephrine (adrenaline).
- Place a tourniquet proximal to the site of injection or insect sting.
- Keep the child lying flat, warm, and with feet slightly elevated.
- Administer corticosteroids and antihistamines.
- Determine the cause of the attack.

Communicable Diseases in Childhood

See Table 26–1 in Chapter 26 of Ward, S. & Hisley, S. (2009). *Maternal child nursing care: Optimizing outcomes for mothers, children & families.* Philadelphia: F.A. Davis.

Common Fungal Infections

Fungal Infection	Location	Treatment	Parent Information
Tinea Capitis (ringworm)	Begins as an infection of a single hair follicle but spreads rapidly in a circular pattern and produces a one inch in diameter lesion. The circular pattern becomes filled with dirty-appearing scales and the hairs involved break off.	Oral griseofulvin (Fulvicin)	1. Adolescents warned not to use alcohol due to tachycardia. 2. Children do not need to be kept home from school. 3. Family members must not share towels or combs.

(continued)

Common Fungal Infections (Continued)

Fungal Infection	Location	Treatment	Parent Information
Tinea Pedis (Athlete's Foot)	Skin lesions between the toes and on the plantar surface of the foot	Liquid preparations of clotrimazole (Lotrimin)	1. Antiseptic foot baths 2. Do not let others share personal items such as foot wear, towels, clothes, or sports equipment. 3. Wear thongs or swim shoes in public showers and stocking/shoes in locker rooms.
Tinea Cruris (jock itch)	Found on the inner aspects of thighs and scrotum	Liquid or powder preparations of clotrimazole (Lotrimin)	1. Shower or bathe frequently if necessary. 2. Dry scrotal area thoroughly when damp. 3. Wear cotton underwear 4. Do not let others share personal items such as foot wear, towels, clothes, or sports equipment.
Tinea Corporis (epidermal layer of the skin)	Fungal infection of the epidermal layer of the skin that has a circular lesion with a clear center and scaly inflammation	Topical clotrimazole (Lotrimin)	1. Do not let others share personal items such as foot wear, towels, clothes, or sports equipment.

The Role of the Nurse in Immunizations

The primary nursing goal is up-to-date immunizations for all children based on their particular health status. The pediatric nurse has several roles in the area of immunization:

- Address family concerns regarding immunizations.
- Organize and carry out vaccination programs and distributing accurate and timely information regarding childhood immunizations.

- Use the current immunization schedule and recognize that the complicated schedule may pose some challenges for parents.
- Ensure that the parent has a vaccine information sheet (VIS) that records the immunizations.
- Remind parents when the next immunizations are due.
- Stay abreast of current information and discuss the parents' concerns.
- Contact and immunize high-risk unimmunized children such as children who are homeless, immigrant, refugee, home schooled, frequently mobile, or who have chronic or life-threatening illnesses.
- Report adverse effects of the vaccine.

Legal Considerations in Immunization Education

The National Childhood Vaccine Injury Act of 1986 provides that parents or legal representatives of children receiving immunizations must be given a VIS developed by the Centers for Disease Control and Prevention (CDC) before immunization. The purpose of the VIS is to ensure uniform education regarding vaccines. The VIS must be used with the following vaccinations: DTaP, Td, MMR, polio, hepatitis B, Hib, varicella, and pneumococcal conjugate.

- Provide the parent or legal guardian with the appropriate VIS before immunization.
- Record on the medical record the date that the VIS was given, the date of publication for the VIS, the name, address, and title of the person giving the vaccine, the date of administration of vaccine, the manufacturer of the vaccine, and the vaccine lot number.
- The VIS must not be altered in any way.
- VIS forms (in many languages) may be accessed through the web at www.cdc.gov/nip or www.immunize.org
- Hardcopies may be ordered through the CDC website at www.cdc.gov/nip/publications
- Individual state health departments with camera-ready copies can be obtained.
- Additional resources and additional education provided to the parent must also be recorded.

Note: Additional VIS sheets are available for use with other common childhood vaccines.

Identifying Contraindications to Immunizations
Only one universal contraindication exists to all vaccines:

- Previous severe allergic reaction (anaphylaxis) to the vaccine or its component of vaccine.

Individual vaccines carry additional contraindications:

- DTaP: Progressive neurological disease, i.e., infantile spasms, encephalopathy
- MMR: Pregnancy, severe immunodeficiency

Circumstances requiring postponement of vaccine administration include:

- Moderate to severe illness.
- Administration of immunoglobulin within last 3 to 11 months (precise period depends on specific immunoglobulin).

Note: Individual vaccines may have additional contraindications and precautions. Safe administration of vaccines requires the nurse to screen for contraindications and precautions prior to administration.

RESOURCES

Lupus Foundation of America: http://www.lupus.org/

National Institute of Arthritis and Musculoskeletal and Skin Disorders: http://www.niams.nih.gov

SLE Foundation, Inc.: http://www.lupusny.org/

Association of Rheumatology Health Professionals, American College of Rheumatology: http://www.rheumatology.org/

Arthritis Foundation: http://www.arthritis.org/

Planning Checklists: http://www.pandemicflu.gov/plan/checklists.html

REFERENCE
Deglin, J., Vallerand, A. (2009). *Davis's drug guide for nurses* (11th ed.). Philadelphia: F.A. Davis.

Caring for the Child with a Cardiovascular Condition

KEY TERMS

cardiac output – Amount of blood discharged from the left or right ventricle per minute (Venes, 2005); the product of stroke volume (SV) and heart rate (HR)

stroke volume – Amount of blood ejected by the left ventricle with each heartbeat (Venes, 2005); the product of preload, after-load and contractility (inotropy).

FOCUSED ASSESSMENT

Syndromes Associated with Cardiac Disease

Syndrome/Disease/Chromosomal Aberrations	Cardiac Defect/Condition	Other Physical Findings
Down Syndrome	Atrioventricular canal defect (AVC), ventricular septal defect (VSD)	Down facies, developmental delay
Noonan Syndrome	Pulmonic valve stenosis, left ventricular hypertrophy (LVH)	Elfin facies, pectus deformity, joint laxity, undescended testes, spine abnormalities, hypotonia, seizures
Williams Syndrome	Supravalvular aortic stenosis, pulmonary artery (PA) stenosis	William's facies: small upturned nose, long philtrum (upper lip length), wide mouth, full lips, small chin, and puffiness around the eyes; hypercalcemia, dental abnormalities, renal problems, sensitive hearing, hypotonia, joint laxity, overly friendly personality
DiGeorge or Velo-cardio-facial Chromosome	Interrupted aortic arch, truncus arteriosus, ventricular septal defect (VSD), patent ductus arteriosus (PDA), tetralogy of Fallot (TOF)	Decreased immune response, low set ears, palate problems, hypoparathyroidism, hypocalcemia
Duchenne Muscular Dystrophy	Cardiomyopathy	Generalized weakness and muscle wasting first affecting the muscles of the hips, pelvic area, thighs, and shoulders; calves often enlarged
Marfan Syndrome	Aortic aneurysm, aortic and/or mitral regurgitation	Arms disproportionately long, tall and thin with laxity of joints, dislocation of lenses, spinal problems, stretch marks, hernia, pectus abnormalities, and restrictive lung disease

Syndrome	Cardiovascular Defects	Other Features
Trisomy 18	Ventricular septal defect (VSD), patent ductus arteriosus (PDA), pulmonic stenosis or pulmonic valve stenosis (PS or PVS)	Multiple joint contractures, spina bifida, hearing loss, radial aplasia (underdevelopment or missing radial bone of forearm), cleft lip, birth defects of the eye
Trisomy 13	Ventricular septal defect (VSD), patent ductus arteriosus (PDA), dextrocardia	Omphalocele, holoprosencephaly (an anatomic defect of the brain involving failure of the forebrain to divide properly), kidney defects, skin defects of the scalp
CHARGE	Tetralogy of Fallot (TOF), truncus arteriosus, vascular ring, interrupted aortic arch	Coloboma of the eye, *Heart defects*, *Atresia of the choanae*, *Retardation of Growth and development*, and *Ear abnormalities and deafness*
Fetal Alcohol Syndrome	Ventricular septal defect (VSD), patent ductus arteriosus (PDA), atrial septal defect (ASD), Tetralogy of Fallot (TOF)	Growth deficiencies, skeletal deformities, facial abnormalities, organ deformities: genital malformations; kidney and urinary defects, central nervous system handicaps
VATER (VACTERLS)	Ventricular septal defect (VSD)	*Vertebral anomalies, vascular anomalies, Anal atresia, Cardiac anomalies, Tracheoesophageal (T-E) fistula, Esophageal atresia, Renal anomalies, radial dysplasia, Limb anomalies, Single umbilical artery*
Turner Syndrome	Coarctation of the aorta (CoA), atrial septal defect (ASD), aortic stenosis or aortic valve stenosis (AS or AVS)	Kidney problems, high blood pressure, overweight, hearing difficulties, diabetes, cataracts, thyroid problems, lack of sexual development, a "webbed" neck, a low hairline at the back of the neck, drooping of the eyelids, dysmorphic, low-set ears, abnormal bone development, multiple moles

CLINICAL ALERTS

Renal Failure

Renal failure is considered when the output is less than 1 mL/kg per hour along with an elevation in serum creatinine and blood urea nitrogen.

- Monitor blood lab values for postoperative bleeding and post-pump electrolyte imbalances.
- Suction secretions.
- Maintain chest tubes that remove secretions and reexpand the lungs. Check drainage for quantity and color.

Postoperative Hemorrhage

Postoperative hemorrhage is considered when there is excessive chest tube drainage greater than 5–10 mL/kg in 1 hour or more than 3 mL/kg per hour in 3 consecutive hours.

- Assess for complications (e.g., cardiac, neurological, pulmonary, or hematological changes; infection; and delayed growth and development).
- Consider the child's level of development in order to provide developmentally appropriate care.
- Ensure rest, which is essential to promote healing and decrease the work load of the heart.
- Manage pain via comfort measures and the administration of medication.
- Group nursing care to avoid imposing unnecessary fatigue and weakness.
- Provide emotional support and information about home care.

Survival

- With any congenital defect, as long as there is mixing of oxygenated and deoxygenated blood, the child survives. A more definitive surgery such as a Fontan procedure is performed at a later date to correct the condition.

Tetralogy of Fallot

- The hallmark sign of Tetralogy of Fallot is cyanosis with crying or playing, which is relieved by squatting or drawing up the legs. These episodes are called "TET" spells: cyanotic events exacerbated by excitement and crying, then relieved by a decrease in pulmonary vascular resistance.

Kawasaki Disease

If the child has five out of six of the following signs, the diagnosis is Kawasaki disease:

- Persistent fever (5 days or more, spiking to 104°F [40°C])
- Skin rash
- Cervical lymphadenopathy, typically unilateral, greater than 1.5 mm in diameter
- Edema and erythema of hands and feet with eventual peeling of skin
- Irritation and inflammation of the mouth with "strawberry tongue," erythema, and cracking lips
- Conjunctivitis without exudate

Thrombus Formation

- Children with aneurysm formation as a result of Kawasaki disease require long-term follow-up for continued assessment related to other vascular changes such as stenosis or tortuosity (twisting) (AHA, 2004; Park, 2003).
- Occasionally, cardiac catheterization is indicated to diagnose aneurysm formation.
- Thrombotic agents such as streptokinase (Streptase), urokinase (Abbokinase), and alteplase (tPA or Activase) have been used with some success in thrombus formation.
- Long-term use of anticoagulants such as warfarin. (Coumadin) or clopidogrel (Plavix) may be used to prevent thrombus formation in the engorged or aneurysmal vessels.

Blood Pressure Post-Catheterization

- The child's blood pressure should remain within normal limits.
- Watch the pulse pressure (the difference between the systolic and diastolic BP; normal is <40 mm Hg).

Complications of Cardiac Transplantation

The four main complications of cardiac transplantation are:

- Rejection
- Infection
- Posttransplant lymphoproliferative disorder (PTLD)
- Transplant coronary artery disease (TCAD)

Postoperative Vital Signs

- Record vital signs every 15 minutes for the first few hours, then every 30 minutes, then once an hour until the child is stable.
- Adjust frequency based on stability of the patient.
- Document and report to the physician even the most subtle change in vital signs.

DIAGNOSTIC TESTS

Cholesterol Levels in Children			
	Desirable	Borderline	Associated with Higher Risk
Total Cholesterol	Less than 170 mg/dL	170–199	200 or more
LDL Cholesterol	Less than 110 mg/dL	110–129	130 or more

Tilt Test

The tilt test is used to diagnose neurally mediated syncope (NMS).

1. Place the child in a supine position on a table equipped with a foot board that may be tilted to an upright position between 45 to 90 degrees.
2. After a short time, tilt the table to a full 90-degree angle, standing the child upright.
3. If there is a remarkable drop in BP or HR and the child experiences syncope or presyncope, the tilt test is positive.
4. If the child does not exhibit any symptoms, lay the table flat again and administer isoproterenol (Isuprel) to stimulate a fast heart rate. Tilt the table again to elicit syncopal response or a drop in the blood pressure. If there is

no response in change in vital signs, the test is considered negative and other causative factors are evaluated.

Electrocardiogram

- An ECG or EKG is a graphic display of electrical activity produced by changes in the intracellular charge of the cardiac muscles.
- The components of an ECG or EKG are marked with the letters PQRST (Fig. 24-1)

Invasive Tests

Cardiac Catheterization
- Determines the pressures in heart and radiographic picture of heart anatomy.
- Interventional catheterization is a corrective procedure.
- Post-catheterization (monitor: pressure dressing in the groin, heart rate, respirations, and blood pressure).

Angiography
- Visualizes the structures and function of the ventricles, vessels, and valves; size and location of septal defects; directs medical treatment.

Biopsy
- Routine biopsies to assess for cardiac transplant rejection

Closure Devices
- Close simple intracardiac communications or shunts

Opening Devices
- Angioplasty or valvuloplasty
- Opens narrow vessels or valves

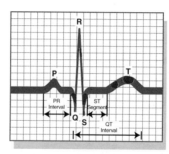

Figure 24-1 Components of electrocardiogram are PQRST.

Balloon Atrial Septostomy
- Emergent palliative procedure necessary to keep the child alive

Laboratory Values

- Lab values are unstable and require close monitoring.
- Electrolyte measurement (especially potassium) is the most critical lab test during the postoperative period because the cardiac bypass machine homolyses the cells, which creates a high concentration of extracellular potassium.
- Hemoglobin and hematocrit tests are required to check for bleeding and coagulation factors.
- Assess arterial blood gasses frequently to determine the concentrations of gases such as carbon dioxide and oxygen.

MEDICATIONS

Carvedilol (kar-**ve**-dil-ole)

Brand Name Coreg (co-rĕg)

Generic name Carvedilol

Classification(s) β-Adrenoreceptor blocker, α-adrenergic

Pregnancy Category C

Indications Coreg is indicated for the treatment of mild to severe heart failure of ischemic or cardiomyopathic origin.

Actions Beta blockade, slows tachycardia, vasodilation, decreases peripheral vascular resistance, decreases renal vascular resistance, reduces plasma renin levels, increases atrial natriuretic peptide levels

Therapeutic Effects Increase stroke volume, decrease blood pressure and improve renal flow, decrease heart rate.

Pharmacokinetics
Bioavailability 25–35%.
Onset of Effect 1–2 hours
Half-life 7–10 hours

Contraindications and Precautions Monitor for possible deterioration of CHF, liver injury, bronchospastic disease, thyrotoxicosis.

Adverse Reactions and Side Effects Chest pain, dizziness, hyperglycemia, bradycardia, nausea.

Route and Dosage
Oral: 0.07 mg/kg per dose
Maximum dose: 0.5 mg/kg
Once or twice daily dosing
Reduce dose for bradycardia <55 beats/min

Nursing Implications
1. Initiate with low dose and titrate up as tolerated.
2. Monitor blood pressure for 1 hour after initial dosing.
3. Monitor blood pressure, pulse and ECG frequently.
4. Take with food.

Data from Deglin, J., & Vallerand, A. (2009). Davis's drug guide for nurses (11th ed.), pp. 271–273. Philadelphia: F.A. Davis.

Idiopathic Primary Pulmonary Arterial Hypertension (IPAH)

- Prostacyclin (Flolan) dilates blood vessels and decreases pulmonary vascular resistance.
- Inhaled nitric oxide relaxes pulmonary (not systemic) vessels.
- Sildenafil (Revatio) decreases pulmonary artery pressures.
- Bosentan (Tracleer) blocks hormone that causes vasoconstriction.

ETHNOCULTURAL CONSIDERATIONS

Hypertension

- Hypertension has a higher incidence among black children than in other ethnic groups.
- Educate the child and family about the condition.
- Promote a reasonable sodium intake.
- Teach the family how to reduce the saturated fat and cholesterol in the child's diet.

TEACHING THE FAMILY

Hypercholesterolemia–Hyperlipidemia

- Treatment includes diet modification, exercise, and medication.
- Recommend balanced diet per day (less than 10% of total calories from saturated fatty acids, 30% or less total calories from fat, less than 300 mg of cholesterol).
- Pharmacological treatment is recommended for children over 10 years of age whose LDL is greater than 190 mg/dL.
- Recommend testing children 2 years old or older if the following factors apply:

At least one parent with high cholesterol (240 mg/dL or greater), family history of early heart disease such as a male parent or grandparent with Congenital Heart Disease (CHD) before age 55, or a female parent or grandparent with CHD before age 65, diabetes, obesity, immunosuppressant drug use (AHA, 2005).

Neurally Mediated Syncope (NMS)

- Inform the family of a teen of driving age who has syncope that he must be syncope free for 6 months in some states before he can drive again.

Pacemakers

- Permanent pacemakers may be placed in the abdomen in younger children and in the subclavicular area in older children.
- Pacemakers must be protected (consideration must be taken with children who are athletic).
- Pacemakers must be replaced every 5 to 10 years.
- Use of a pacemaker is controversial for vaso-vagal syncope.
- Pacemaker placement is not recommended for neutrally mediated syncope.

Caring for the Child with a Cardiac Condition

- A home health nurse may evaluate the child at intervals to see if help at home is needed and if a parent needs to take vital signs at night.

- The family must receive crucial information related to the timing and the routine of medication administration.
- Teach the family that one of the most important aspects of medication administration is proper dosing. Many medications are given in a liquid form. The medication dosing should always be in milliliters (mL) or cubic centimeters (cc) and not tsp or other household measures.
- Educate the family about the disease; there are many resources in print and on the Internet. Ensure that the most up-to-date information is provided.
- Educate the family that it is necessary for a team approach in treating the cardiac disease.

ADDITIONAL INFORMATION FOR THE CLINICAL SETTING

- The heart consists of four chambers, two reservoirs (atria) and two pumping chambers (ventricles; Fig. 24-2).
- There are four valves in the heart. Two are atrioventricular (AV) valves connecting the atria and ventricles (Fig. 24-3).
- There are major vessels that lead to and from the heart (Fig. 24-4).
- The vena cava carries the blood from body tissues to the right atrium.
- The superior vena cava lies above the heart and carries blood from the head, arms, and upper body.
- The inferior vena cava lies below the heart and carries blood from the legs, abdominal organs, and lower part of the body.

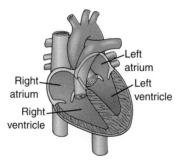

Figure 24-2 Chambers of the heart.

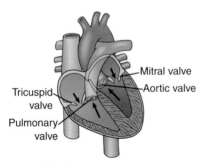

Figure 24-3 Valves of the heart.

- The pulmonary artery is the only named artery in the body that carries deoxygenated blood. It is called an artery because it carries blood away from the heart, but since it arises from the right ventricle, it carries deoxygenated blood. It carries this blood to the pulmonary capillary bed, where it interfaces with the alveoli in the lungs and "picks up" oxygen. From the lungs, the blood returns to the heart through the pulmonary veins into the left atrium (the only veins that carry oxygenated blood). The blood leaves the left ventricle through the aortic valve, through the aorta and out to the body.
- Venous system, venae cavae, right atrium tricuspid valve, right ventricle, pulmonic valve, pulmonary artery, and lungs pick up O_2. The pulmonary veins, left atrium, mitral valve, left ventricle, aortic valve, aorta, and arteriole system delivers O_2 via the blood to the cells of the body (Fig. 24-5).

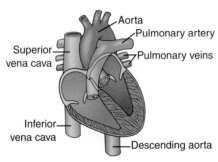

Figure 24-4 Vessels of the heart.

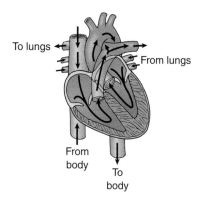

Figure 24-5 Normal blood flow.

- An atrial septal defect (ASD) results when the two septae fail to form properly (Fig. 24-6).
- A ventricular septal defect (VSD) is the most common congenital heart defect. The septum can have a single opening or be fraught with multiple defects (Fig. 24-7).

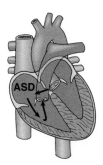

Figure 24-6 Atrial septal defect.

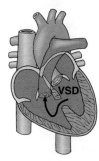

Figure 24-7 Ventricular septal defect.

- An atrioventricular canal defect (AVC) is somewhat of a combination of an ASD and VSD. However, it is much more than that, as it involves the valves. In its simplest definition, an AVC is a large hole in the center of the heart (Fig. 24-8).
- A patent ductus arteriosus is probably the simplest form of vessel defect. Remember that the ductus arteriosus is a normal structure during fetal life. In utero, the pulmonary resistance is high because the lungs are filled with fluid and not air. The blood is oxygenated through the placenta by the umbilical vein. Instead of the blood moving from the pulmonary artery (PA) to the lungs, the ductus is a pop-off valve for the large volume of fluid. As the blood flow follows the "path of least resistance," the blood moves through the ductus, into the aorta, and out to the body tissues. Directly after birth and the baby's first breaths, the pulmonary resistance starts to drop and the blood flows from the PA into the lungs. Since there is decreased flow through the PDA, the duct starts to close. Changes in prostaglandin level assist the closure as well. In 8 to 10% of the population, the PDA remains open (Fig. 24-9).
- Pulmonic stenosis or pulmonic valve stenosis (PS or PVS) is a malformation of the pulmonary artery or pulmonic valve. The narrowing of the valve causes an increased workload on the right ventricle which in turn leads to congestive heart failure (CHF) (Fig. 24–10).
- Pulmonary atresia is absence of the pulmonary valve, pulmonary artery, or both (Fig. 24-11).

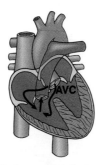

Figure 24-8 Atrioventricular canal defect.

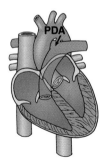

Figure 24-9 Patent ductus arteriosus.

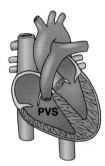

Figure 24-10 Pulmonary stenosis.

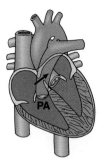

Figure 24-11 Pulmonary atresia.

- Aortic stenosis or aortic valve stenosis (AS or AVS) is a malformation and narrowing in the aorta or around the aortic valve. A narrowing in this area causes an increased workload on the left ventricle and eventually leads to hypertrophy (increase in size) and heart failure (Fig. 24-12).

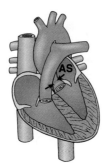

Figure 24-12 Aortic stenosis.

- Coarctation of the aorta (CoA) is a narrowing or stricture of the descending aorta distal to the carotid arteries. The coarctation is classified by its location: preductal, ductal, or postductal (Fig. 24-13).
- Tricuspid atresia (TA) occurs when there is an error of the formation of the tricuspid valve. As a single defect, this condition is incompatible with life, as no blood from the right atrium (RA) reaches the right ventricle (RV) and thus the right ventricular outflow tract (RVOT) leading to the PA and the lungs. For this reason, most children born with TA also have comorbidity with a septal defect such as ASD or VSD as well as a PDA. The deoxygenated blood must reach the pulmonary bed to sustain life (Fig. 24-14).
- Epstein's malformation occurs when the tricuspid valve is displaced into the right ventricle (Fig. 24-15).

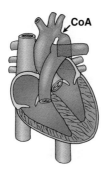

Figure 24-13 Coarctation of the aorta.

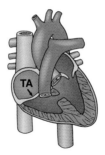

Figure 24-14 Tricuspid atresia.

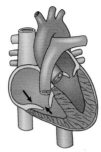

Figure 24-15 Epstein's malformation.

- Total anomalous pulmonary venous return (TAPVR) is a condition in which the pulmonary blood flow returns to the heart through the right atrium rather than the left (Fig. 24-16).
- Transposition of the great arteries or vessels (TGA or TGV) occurs in utero when the signals cross and instead of twisting there is simply a septation and the aorta arises from the right side of the heart and the pulmonary artery arises from the left (Fig. 24-17).
- In truncus arteriosus, the trunk has not twisted or septated. There are multiple variations of the condition, classed I to IV, but the general physiology is that the aorta and pulmonary arteries (PAs) are combined, with full mixing of blood. Sometimes the PAs arise from the aorta, either ascending or descending (Fig. 24-18).

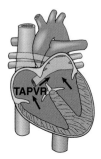

Figure 24-16 Total anomalous venous return.

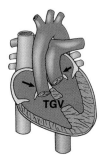

Figure 24-17 Transposition of the great vessels.

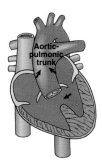

Figure 24-18 Truncus arteriosus.

- In tetralogy of Fallot, there are always four associated conditions: VSD, overriding aorta, hypertrophic RV, and pulmonary stenosis or atresia (Fig. 24-19).
- Hypoplastic left heart syndrome is a defect in which the left ventricle is extremely small or hypoplastic and unable to maintain an adequate cardiac output (Fig. 24-20).

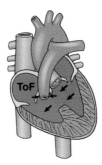

Figure 24-19 Tetralogy of Fallot.

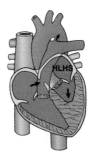

Figure 24-20 Hypoplastic left heart syndrome.

- Long Q-T syndrome (LQTS) is an electrophysiological condition predisposing the child to fatal arrhythmias such as ventricular tachycardia (VT), torsade de pointes, and ventricular fibrillation (Fig. 24-21).
- Narrow vessels or valves may be opened or dilated with a balloon angioplasty or valvuloplasty as an initial treatment or a stent may be placed in a vessel as a long-term treatment. This treatment is performed during a cardiac catheterization procedure. A special catheter with a balloon (similar to a Foley balloon) catheter is passed into the heart and into the narrow vessel. The balloon is then inflated, causing the stenotic area to expand (Fig. 24-22).

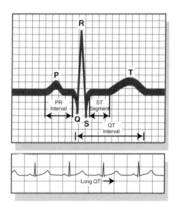

Figure 24-21 Long QT syndrome.

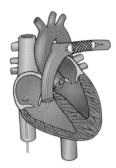

Figure 24-22 Balloon angioplasty with stent.

Postoperative Management

Provide immediate postoperative care in the intensive care unit:

- Record the vital signs frequently until the child is stable.
- Maintain "lines" (there may be several):
  - A peripheral IV line is used to administer fluid and medications.
  - A central venous pressure line (CVP) is inserted in a large vessel in the neck and is used to measure central venous pressure.
  - Intracardiac lines are inserted in the right atrium, left atrium, and pulmonary artery and are used to measure the pressures inside the cardiac chambers that provide essential information about cardiac output, blood volume, pulmonary pressures, ventricular function, and drug therapy response.

- Assess and maintain respiratory status. Respiratory assessment is done frequently.
- Provide oxygen via mechanical ventilation.
- Monitor fluid status. Accurately measure the intake and output of all fluids.
- Assess for signs and symptoms of infection.

A Way to Remember Cyanotic Defects

- All defects starting with a "T" are cyanotic defects.

Valve Replacement

- Replace every 5 years if originally replaced in infancy or childhood.
- If replaced in adolescence, replace approximately every 10 years.

Electrocardiogram

The abbreviations ECG/EKG are used interchangeably. (The K indicates the German spelling of cardiac.)

- An electrocardiogram (ECG) is a graphic display of electrical activity produced by changes in the intracellular charge of the cardiac muscles.
- An isoelectric line is the imaginary baseline of the ECG/EKG. One measurement in reading ECGs is how far the wave is from the baseline.
- A lead refers to the actual recording.
- The electrode is the device that is placed on the chest where the lead wire is attached.
- It typically takes two electrodes to make one lead.
- The electrical activity in the heart can then be graphed and evaluated.

Caring for the Child with a Cardiac Condition in a Clinic

- Monitor vital signs (heart rate, blood pressure, respiratory rate).
- Monitor the oxygen saturation of the patient's blood using a pulse oximeter (acceptable normal ranges are from 95 to 100% however, some children normally have a value as low as 85%. The nurse should confirm the range of normal oximeter readings with the practitioner).

- Review medications and discuss changes with the caregiver.
- Verify all medications and provide necessary instruction.
- Ensure that the family has enough medication refills. If there are any changes in medication or adjustments in dosages, document it in the child's record.
- Medications are frequently altered due to growth (weight) of the child.
- Laboratory tests may be required.
- Children requiring warfarin (Coumadin) to prevent thrombus must have the pro-time and international normalized ratio checked routinely. The ratio is checked frequently when this drug is first initiated, then every 4 weeks to 3 months after it is stabilized. Note any changes made to the dosage.
- Electrogram monitoring in the clinic usually includes a 12-lead ECG to identify potential or existing arrhythmias, chamber size, and strain on the heart muscle.
- Often the Holter monitor or event recorders are applied in the clinic.
- Other recording devices may be distributed to parents for home use (e.g., apnea monitors, pulse oximeters).

 Procedure 24-1 Taking a Blood Pressure Reading

Purpose

Taking the blood pressure is an indicator of the child's state of health. Blood pressure is the pressure of blood as it is forced against the arterial walls during a cardiac contraction.

Equipment

- Blood pressure cuff **(sphygmometer)** Stethoscope (Venes, 2005)

Steps

1. Measure the child's bare limb to determine the appropriate size cuff.
2. Have the child sit comfortably without dangling feet.
3. Encourage the child to be quiet and relaxed before taking the BP.
4. Apply the cuff to the arm.

Procedure 24-1 (Continued)

5. Palpate the brachial pulse just below and slightly medial to the antecubital area.

6. Rapidly inflate the cuff to about 30 mm Hg about the level at which the pulse disappears.

7. Slowly open the valve and watch the mercury drop.

8. Continue deflating the cuff, noting the point at which the pulse disappears or becomes muffled (fourth Korotkoff sound).

9. Document the procedure.

Clinical Alert Sometimes blood pressure is taken over clothing with the thought that children may become more afraid if asked to put on a gown. This practice will result in an inaccurate measurement of BP. In addition, the BP should not be taken in the same arm where an IV is placed.

Teach Parents

Teaching parents about the importance of taking the child's blood pressure as it is a physical sign concerning functions essential to life (Venes, 2005).

Subacute Bacterial Endocarditis (SBE)

- Subacute bacterial endocarditis (SBE) occurs subsequent to a bacterial infection or introduction of an infective agent into the child's blood stream.
- The infection may be caused by an invasive procedure such as surgery, urological procedures, or most often dental cleaning.
- Initially, vague symptoms may include a low-grade fever, malaise, loss of appetite, and muscle aches. A high fever, chills, sweating, stiff joints, or back pain can indicate that acute illness has occurred.
- As the condition worsens, symptoms of heart failure occur (Venes, 2005).
- Blood cultures to identify bacteria or fungi in the bloodstream may detect endocarditis.

The guidelines for administration and dosage of prophylactic antibiotics are determined by the American Dental Association

(ADA) and the American Heart Association (AHA). Guidelines for prescribing prophylaxis treatment were updated in April 2007:

- Patients with a prosthetic cardiac valve
- Patients who previously had endocarditis
- Patients with congenital heart disease only in the following categories:
  - Unrepaired cyanotic congenital heart disease, including those with palliative shunts and conduits
  - Completely repaired congenital heart disease with prosthetic material or device, whether placed by surgery or catheter intervention, during the first 6 months after the procedure
  - Repaired congenital heart disease with residual defects at the site or adjacent to the site of a prosthetic patch or prosthetic device (which inhibit endothelialization)
- Cardiac transplantation recipients with cardiac valvular disease
- If valve destruction occurs, the valve may need to be repaired or replaced

Sinus Arrhythmias

A normal irregular rhythm in which the rhythm varies with respiration is called sinus arrhythmia. Sinus arrhythmia has no adverse effect on the cardiac output.

- The heart rate increases with inspiration (Remember: "Inspiration" and "Increase" both start with an "I").
- The heart rate decreases with expiration.

Typical Post-Cardiac Catheterization Medical Orders

1. Admit to postsurgical observation unit.
2. Check vital signs (q15min × 4, then q1hr × 2, then q2hr × 2, then q4hr).
3. Check peripheral pulses with vital signs (especially on affected extremity).
4. Keep O_2 saturation above (95–100%) or _____.
5. Call house officer for HR > _____, BP > _____ (age and baseline dependent) and temperature >_____.
6. Give acetaminophen (Children's Tylenol) for pain (based on weight).

7. Keep the child flat in bed for 6 hours.
8. Check pressure dressing with Vital Signs for bleeding.
9. Call the medical doctor or house officer for complaints of abdominal pain or urine output. < _____ or no urine output.
10. Increase diet as tolerated.
11. Give _____antiemetic for nausea.

Note: The blank lines indicate the physician's particular medical order.

Administering Medication Properly

- It is crucial for the nurse to understand the desired and undesired effects of the child's medication.
- Before giving any medication, the nurse must check the proper dosage (with calculations) and route.
- At times, medications are given in very small amounts and an error in decimal placement can mean a fatal overdose or other detrimental effects.
- Be sure to use the 5 rights of medication administration.

Waking the Child during the Night for Vital Signs

- The best outcome for a child with a cardiac condition is proper healing along with adequate growth and development.
- Assess if the child needs to be awakened during the night for vital signs or can be allowed to sleep.

RESOURCES

American Heart Association: http://www.americanheart.org

Children's Heart Society: http://www.childrensheart.org

Congenital Heart Information Network: http://www.tchin.org

Cardiomyopathy: http://www.cardiomyopathy.org

Heart Rhythm Society: http://www.hrsonline.org

Kawasaki Disease: http://www.kdfoundation.org

Long QT Syndrome: http://www.long-qt-syndrome.com

March of Dimes: http://www.marchofdimes.com

Pectus: http://www.pectusinfo.com

Sudden Arrhythmia Death Syndrome (SADS) Foundation:
http://www.sads.org

REFERENCES

American Heart Association. (2004). Scientific statement: Diagnosis, treatment, and long-term management of Kawasaki disease. *Circulation, 110,* 2747–2771.

American Heart Association (AHA). (2005). Scientific Statement: Dietary recommendations for children and adolescents. *Circulation, 112,* 2061–2075.

Deglin, J., & Vallerand, A. (2009). *Davis's drug guide for nurses* (11th ed.). Philadelphia: F. A. Davis.

Park, M. (2003). *The pediatric cardiology handbook* (3rd ed). St. Louis: C.V. Mosby.

Venes, D. (Ed.). (2005). *Taber's cyclopedic medical dictionary* (20th ed.). Philadelphia: F.A. Davis.

Caring for the Child with an Endocrinological or Metabolic Condition

KEY TERMS

kussmaul breaths – Very deep and laborious breaths; in an attempt to correct metabolic acidosis, the respiratory system works hard to "blow off" excess carbon dioxide

FOCUSED ASSESSMENT

Proper Growth Assessment

- Plot the child's height and weight accurately at each outpatient visit on the appropriate growth chart.
- If the child is of short stature (below the 3rd or 5th percentile) and is not chartable on the usual chart or has Down syndrome, go to the Centers for Disease Control and Prevention (CDC) Web site to access the most appropriate chart, located at http://www.cdc.gov/nchs/about/major/nhanes/growthcharts/charts.htm.
- Be sure to use the same growth chart at each visit.
- Weigh an infant completely undressed (including diaper) and children in underwear only.

Signs and Symptoms of Diabetes Insipidus	
Infant	**Child**
Irritability	Excessive thirst (polydipsia)
Poor feeding (despite vigorous suck)	Excessive urine production (polyuria)
Failure to grow/thrive	Enuresis (nocturnal bed wetting)
Vomiting	
Constipation	
High fevers	

Signs and Symptoms of Acute Adrenocortical Insufficiency (Adrenal Crisis)

- Weakness, feeling tired, nausea, vomiting, loss of appetite, weight loss, low blood pressure, abdominal pain, fever, confusion, or coma

Assessing for Hyperreflexia of Muscles

- Tap on the facial nerve.
- Facial muscle spasm (Chvostek sign) confirms that the child has muscle pain, cramps, and probably twitches.
- These muscle manifestations may progress to numbness and tingling of the hands and feet as well as stiffness.
- Remember that infants and small children cannot express these manifestations and therefore may cry to communicate their pain.

Signs and Symptoms of Cushing's Syndrome

- Common signs and symptoms of Cushing's syndrome include weight gain, especially, pendulous abdomen; fatigue; muscle wasting and weakness, thin extremities; round "moon" face; facial flushing; fatty pad between shoulders (buffalo hump); and pink or purple stretch marks (striae) on abdominal skin, thighs, breasts, and arms.
- The child's skin is thin and fragile with little subcutaneous tissue, causing easy bruising; slow healing of cuts, insect bites, and infections due to a lessened inflammatory response.

- The child may exhibit depression, anxiety and irritability, euphoria, and frank psychoses; irregular or absent menstrual periods in females; and erectile dysfunction in adolescent males.
- Hyperglycemia may eventually lead to latent or overt diabetes, high blood pressure, or arteriosclerosis.
- Owing to the excess production of androgens, signs and symptoms related to secondary sexual characteristics can also be seen.

Signs and Symptoms of Diabetes Mellitus Type 1

- Excessive urination, in volume and frequency (polyuria)
- Loss of bladder control in children after they had already been trained, especially at night
- Excessive intake of water and/or food (polydipsia and/or polyphagia)
- Unintended weight loss over several days and tendency to be thin
- High glucose levels in the blood and urine (hyperglycemia and glycosuria)
- Nausea and vomiting, abdominal pain or discomfort
- Weakness and excessive fatigue
- Increased susceptibility to infection, especially urinary tract, respiratory, and skin infections
- Dehydration
- Blurred vision
- Irritability, restlessness, apathy

Signs and Symptoms of Diabetes Mellitus Type 2

- High blood glucose levels
- Sometimes mimic type 1 diabetes

Signs and Symptoms of Diabetic Ketoacidosis (DKA)

- Toddlers: Classic manifestations often absent
- Altered mental status, tachycardia, tachypnea, Kussmaul respirations, normal or low blood pressure, poor perfusion, lethargy and weakness, fever, acetone breath

CLINICAL ALERTS

Exogenous Hormones

- Alert parents of the dangers of hidden toxins in everyday products that can harm their children.
- Make parents aware of "endocrine disruptors".
- Refer parents to this Web site: http://www.mindfully.org/Pesticide/EDs-PWG-16jun01.htm.

Dehydration

- Dehydration can be seen in all cases, causing the infant/child to be irritable with many other manifestations: dry mucous membranes, decreased skin turgor (tenting of abdominal skin in infant), decreased tears when crying, sunken fontanel, and tachycardia.
- If dehydration is severe, the child's pulse may be thready and very rapid.
- Hypotension may be present and could lead to hypovolemic shock.

Hyponatremia

- Thoroughly and accurately track intake, output, and daily weights of the child.
- Hyponatremia (low serum sodium of less than 125 mEq/L) may cause seizures in the child with syndrome of inappropriate antidiuretic hormone secretion (SIADH).
- Keeping the serum sodium level as near as normal is the goal of treatment.

Thyroid Storm

- A rare and potentially fatal complication of hyperthyroidism
- Occurs in patients with untreated or partially treated thyrotoxicosis (a term often used interchangeably for hyperthyroidism) who experience a precipitating event such as surgery, infection, or trauma
- Must be recognized and treated on signs and symptoms alone, as laboratory confirmation often cannot be obtained in a timely manner

- Patients typically appear markedly hypermetabolic with high fevers, tachycardia, nausea and vomiting, tremulousness, agitation, and psychosis if untreated.
- Late in the progression of the disease (hyperthyroidism), patients may become stuporous or comatose with hypotension.

Symptoms of an Addisonian Crisis

- Sudden penetrating pain in the lower back, abdomen, or legs, severe vomiting and diarrhea, dehydration, low blood pressure, and a loss of consciousness
- If left untreated, a child with Addison's disease in crisis can die (NIH, 2004).

Cortisone Insufficiency

- Be aware of the signs and symptoms observed before an adrenal crisis (headache, dizziness, and nausea) or vomiting (stomachache) or wobbly knees.
- By the time the child exhibits extreme weakness and mental confusion, the adrenal crisis will be eminent.

Diabetic Ketoacidosis (DKA)

- Infection is the most frequent cause of DKA, particularly in known diabetics.
- Aggressive evaluation for infection is necessary.
- Empiric antibiotic therapy should strongly be considered until culture results return.
- Other patient-related issues may be the cause (noncompliance with insulin regimens, thelarche, adrenarche, menarche, caregiver's lack of competence, insulin pump failure).

DIAGNOSTIC TESTS

Diagnosis of Diabetes Insipidus

Water Deprivation Test

1. Monitor the patient's vital signs every hour if necessary and watch for fever and hypotension.

2. Collect urine and blood samples early in the day and test for osmolarity and electrolytes.
3. Deprive the child of water until significant dehydration occurs.
4. Weigh child every 2 hours until 2% to 5% of body weight is lost.
5. Monitor urine specific gravity hourly; stop when specific gravity is 1.014 or higher.
6. Complete test within 4 hours for an infant and 7 hours for a child.

Serum Levels

Diagnosis of diabetes insipidus is confirmed when the following values are found:

- High urine osmolarity (greater than 1200 Osmol/kg)
- High urine specific gravity (greater than 1.030)
- Low serum osmolarity (less than 275 mOsm/kg)
- Low serum sodium (less than 125 mEq/L)

Potassium Depletion

- Treatments for adrenal crisis cause potassium depletion; must closely watch the child's lab values.
- Watch for warning signs of hyperkalemia and hypokalemia (apnea, cardiac arrhythmias, paralysis, poor muscle control, weakness).

Hyperaldosteronism

- Blood chemistry studies indicate decreased potassium level, increased aldosterone level, and decreased renin activity.
- Urinalysis reveals an elevated aldosterone level.
- CAT scan of abdomen reveals an adrenal mass.
- EKG shows abnormalities.

Equivalent of A1C Level and Blood Glucose Level

Hemoglobin A1C Levels (mean %)		Mean Blood Glucose Level (mg/dL)
Normal	4	60
	4.5	
	5	90
	5.5	
	6	120
Slightly Elevated	6.5	
	7	150
	7.5	
	8	180
Elevated	8.5	
	9	210
	9.5	
	10	240
Severely Elevated	10.5	
	11	270
	11.5	
	12	300
	12.5	
	13	330
	13.5	
	14	360

Modified from the American Diabetes Association (2005). Standards of medical care in diabetes: Clinical practice recommendations. *Diabetes Care 28 (Suppl),* S4–S36.

Plasma Blood Glucose and Hemoglobin A1C Goals for Type 1 Diabetes by Age Group

Age Group (years)	Plasma Blood Glucose Goal Range (mg/dL)		Hemoglobin A1C (%)	Rationale
	Morning Before Meals	Bedtime/ Overnight		
Toddlers and Preschoolers (0–6 years)	100–180	110–200	< 8.5% (but > 7.5%)	High risk/ vulnerability to hypoglycemia
School-age (6–12 years)	90–180	100–180	< 8%	Risk of hypoglycemia and low risk of complications before puberty

(continued)

Plasma Blood Glucose and Hemoglobin A1C Goals for Type 1 Diabetes by Age Group (Continued)

Age Group (years)	Plasma Blood Glucose Goal Range (mg/dL)		Hemoglobin A1C (%)	Rationale
	Morning Before Meals	Bedtime/ Overnight		
Adolescents and Young Adults (13–19 years)	90–130	90–150	< 7.5%	Risk for severe hypoglycemia Developmental and psychological issues Lower goal of < 7.0% is reasonable if it can be achieved without excessive hypoglycemia

Modified from the American Diabetes Association (2007). Standards of medical care in diabetes – 2007. *Diabetes Care 30 (Suppl), S4–S41.*

MEDICATIONS

Desmopressin (DDAVP)

- Desmopressin (DDAVP) is a synthetic vasopressin analogue

Accurate Administration of Intranasal Medication Doses
- Instruct the child to blow his nose before medication is given.
- Administer intranasal DDAVP through a rhinal tube.
- Position the child on the side the medication is given to enhance absorption of the medication.
- Provide parents with clear instructions and refer them to the Family Resource Center Library (www.childrensmn.org) for patient family education materials.

Administration of Hormone Tablets

- Teach parents proper administration of the medication.
- Pills can be crushed in a spoon, dissolved with a small amount of water or other liquid immediately before

administration, and administered to the child with a syringe, dropper, or nipple.

- Toddlers can be allowed to readily chew the tablets (Postellon, 2006).
- Do not mix in a full bottle of formula (to avoid ruining the taste of the infant's sole source of nutrition).

Side Effects of Antithyroid Medications

Mild Effects	Severe Effects (can be *Fatal*)
Skin rash	Agranulocytosis (sore throat, high fever)
Mild leukopenia	Lupus-like syndrome
Loss of taste	Hepatitis
Arthralgia	Hepatic failure
Loss/abnormal hair pigmentation	Glomerulonephritis

Accurate Administration of Intravenous Calcium

- Check the IV site for accurate placement as infiltration of the intravenous calcium supplements cause extravasation and sloughing of the tissue around the site.
- Intravenous calcium supplements must be properly calculated, diluted, and administered strictly according to hospital's standards of care and protocols.

Steroid Administration

- Never stop steroid administration abruptly (can cause an adrenal crisis).
- Slowly wean according to the physician's orders.

Insulin Dosage and Frequency

- Dosage is based on the individual needs of the patient (common dosage for an adolescent is 1.0 to 1.7 units/kg per day; common dosage for a child is 0.75 to 1.0 units/kg per day).
- If treatment calls for two doses, usually 60% to 75% of the insulin is given before breakfast and the remainder is given with dinner.

Insulin Types and Peak Effects

Insulin Name	Insulin Type	Begins to Work	Peak Effect	Used Up
Humalog/ NovoLog	Short-acting	10–15 minutes	30–90 minutes	4 hours
Regular	Short-acting	30–60 minutes	2–4 hours	6–9 hours
NPH	Intermediate acting	1–2 hours	3–8 hours	12–15 hours
Ultralente	Intermediate acting	2–4 hours	6–14 hours	18 20 hours
Lantus	Long-acting	1–2 hours	2–22 hours	24 hours

Insulin "Cocktails"

Insulin Name	Insulin Type	Begins to Work	Peak Effect	Used Up
Lente	Premixed	1–2 hours	3–14 hours	18–20 hours
70/30 NPH/Regular	Premixed	30–60 minutes	3–8 hours	12–15 hours
75/25 NPH/Humalog	Premixed	10–15 minutes	30 minutes– 8 hours	12–15 hours

ETHNOCULTURAL CONSIDERATIONS

Shock in Dark-Complexioned Children

- When assessing for shock in children with a dark complexion look at the palms of the hands, feet, and lips to ascertain color changes.

Type 2 Diabetes

- Type 2 diabetes in children is often associated with ethnic background (African American, Hispanic, Asian, or American Indian), obesity (85% at diagnosis), and a family history of type 2 diabetes (74%–100%) as well as with insulin resistance.

TEACHING THE FAMILY

Hydrocortisone (A-Hydrocort) Administration

- Medication must be used as prescribed.
- Always have the injectable hydrocortisone available at home, school, and wherever the child travels.
- Keep an emergency kit on hand at all times with a cortisol supply. Administer to the child during acute illness, vomiting, diarrhea, or during stressful circumstances. When oral dose cannot be tolerated, injectable dose must be readily available.
- Administer the medication on time because this follows the child's body's normal cortisol release patterns (Wilson, 2006).

 Procedure 25-1 Teaching Parents How to Inject Insulin

Purpose

To teach parents how to inject insulin

Equipment

- Insulin bottle from refrigerator (remove up to one hour before injection to allow it to warm to room temperature)
- Appropriate syringe (U-30, U-50, or U-100)
- Alcohol wipes
- Container for the dirty, used syringe

Steps

1. Check the expiration date on the insulin bottle.
2. Wash hands.
3. Clean rubber stopper on insulin bottle with alcohol wipe.
4. Remove the syringe cap and pull air into the syringe line up the end of the black plunger to the exact amount the insulin dose will be.
5. Put the syringe needle through the bottle rubber top and push syringe plunger so that all the air goes from the syringe into the bottle.

(continued)

Procedure 25-1 (Continued)

6. Turn the insulin bottle upside down and pull the syringe plunger so that the insulin enters the syringe until the top of the black plunger exactly lines up with the dose of insulin to be given.

7. Remove every air bubble, always checking that the dose is exact.

8. Choose (or let the child choose) the site of the injection.

9. Clean the injection site with an alcohol swab.

10. Pinch up the skin slightly and gently, with the syringe at a 90-degree angle (perpendicular) to the skin, with a dart-like motion, insert the needle into the skin, release the skin.

11. Slowly inject the dose of insulin.

12. Discard the used syringe in a hard, rigid container with a tight-fitting lid.

13. Document the procedure.

Clinical Alert The nurse teaches the parents to evaluate the child for the signs and symptoms of either hypo- or hyperglycemia. In understandable terms explain these signs and symptoms to the parents so they can watch for them at home.

Hypoglycemia (LOW Blood Sugar)	Hyperglycemia (HIGH Blood Sugar)
Cold, pale skin (cold sweat)	Increased thirst, even if consuming a large amount of liquids
Shakiness/hand tremors	Loss of appetite, nausea/vomiting
Sudden hunger (crave salt/sweet)	Weakness, stomach pains/aches
Emotional outbursts (personality changes)	Heavy, labored breathing
Drowsiness/extremely tired	Fatigue, tired often sleepy
Pounding heartbeat/ palpitations	Large amounts of sugar in urine
Nervousness/dizziness	Ketones in urine
Anxiety/irritability	Frequent urination

Procedure 25-1 (Continued)

Headache, mental
    confusion, difficulty
    concentrating

Blurred/double vision

Numbness or tingling of
    lips/mouth
Poor coordination/
    staggering, unable to
    walk
Slurred or slow speech
Dilated, enlarged pupils
Fainting (needs emergency
    treatment *NOW*)

Teach Parents

If the child expresses that the injection is painful, the
following measures can be taken to decrease the pain:

Inject only room-temperature insulin.
Clear even the tiniest air bubbles from the syringe.
Allow the alcohol to dry completely.
Tell the child to relax muscles in the area of injection
    (the more tense the muscles during injection, the
    more painful the procedure).
Using the syringe like a dart, pierce the skin quickly.
Do not change the needle direction during insertion
    or withdrawal.
Never reuse needles/syringes.
Rotate sites with *each* injection (giving the insulin in
    the *same* place twice in one day can cause unneces-
    sary discomfort for the
    child and undue stress on
    the tissue).
Document exactly where
    each injection was given so
    as to avoid the same place
    more than once a day.
Create and keep a Diabetes
    Management Notebook
    with the plan and a place
    to record daily Blood

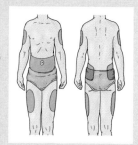

Sugar values as well as doses of insulin administered
including injection site.

Dealing with a Hypoglycemic Crises

- Recognize the signs of hypoglycemia (skin pale and sweaty, dizzy, shaky, tremors, confused, irritable, numb on lips or mouth, altered mental status).
- Check blood glucose level.
- If the blood glucose level is less than 70 mg/dL, rapidly give one of the following sources of carbohydrates (about 10–15 grams each), the right amount to treat hypoglycemia:
  - 1/2 to 3/4 cup of orange or grape juice (a juice box is good when you're away from home)
  - 2 glucose tablets or 2 doses of glucose gel
  - 2 to 4 pieces hard candy
  - 5 gumdrops
  - 1 to 2 tablespoons of honey
  - 1 small box of raisins
  - 6 oz. regular (not diet) soda (about half a can)
  - 2 tablespoons of cake icing
- Recheck blood glucose in 15 minutes, if reading is still below <70 mg/dL, then give another glass of juice, etc.
- Recheck blood glucose again after another 15 minutes.
- When blood glucose returns to at least 80 mg/dL, give a more substantial snack that is not sugar concentrated (i.e., cheese and crackers, bread and peanut butter) if the next meal is more than 30 minutes away or if a physical activity/exercise is planned.
- If the child is unconscious, give glucagon subcutaneously or intramuscularly (American Diabetes Association [ADA], 2007a).

Educating Different Groups on Diabetes

Content Topics	Parent	Child	Adolescent
Disease Process	Include type of diabetes, treatment options, and benefits of a healthy lifestyle.	Explain the disease simply. Begin to teach self-care. Include in treatment plan.	Talk to as an adult. Expect self-care, but with limitations.
Nutritional Guidelines	Address breastfeeding. Erratic eating habits How to read labels	Provide instruction on how to make appropriate food choices (restaurant). Discuss ways to change food behavior habits (fast food).	

Content Topics	Parent	Child	Adolescent
	Family goes grocery shopping. Controversy of artificial sweeteners	Provide guidelines for meal and snack planning. Address after-school and party eating habits. Discuss coordination of school, activities, and meals.	
Activities	Explain how activity and glucose level interact. Younger children have a high energy level. Incorporate walking into family outings.	Limit sitting in front of TV or computer. Play outside. Join a sport or activity. Walk to a friend's house if possible.	Explain how exercise increases glucose use. Decrease sedentary (computer) time. Exercise every day, not just on weekends. Increase time, amount, and frequency of activity.
Medications	Understand the medication to be given. Discuss dose, frequency, action, adverse reactions. Insulin storage, dose, administration technique if appropriate. Choose medication schedule to fit the family's lifestyle.	Needs supervision at all times. Plans medications around normal schedule. Provide for lunch time dose if needed (talk to school RN, teacher)	Educate on self-treatment Adapting to hectic high school schedule Treat to target blood glucose. Monitor patterns in blood glucose to improve control.
Complications Acute Chronic	Discuss signs/ symptoms of hypo/ hyperglycemia. Discuss DKA emergency procedures and when to go to the ER. Explain the risk of long-term uncontrolled diabetes and effect on neurological and vascular systems.	Begins to understand hyper/ hypoglycemia. Recognizes patterns. Links causes to high and low blood sugar. Understands consequences of actions.	Identify cause and effect of hyper/ hypoglycemia. Instruct on how to prevent high and low sugar levels. Discuss driving precautions. Explain effect of long-term, uncontrolled diabetes on neurological and vascular systems.

(continued)

Educating Different Groups on Diabetes (Continued)

Content Topics	Parent	Child	Adolescent
Outcome Criteria	Family lifestyle changes Discuss goals that can be met. Boost confidence in technical skills. Management of child during illness Understand blood glucose readings and hemoglobin A1C results.	Work toward independence. Learn technical skills; expect frustrations. Emotional immaturity	Goals should be realistic and attainable Problem solving each day How to manage heat, sun, dehydration
Psychosocial Adjustments	Avoid giving too much responsibility too soon. Identify friends at whose homes the child could spend the night. (friends know child's care routine.) Notify teachers, principal of child's health needs. Adaptation of family life to incorporate care without stress. Stress reduction Parental relief (who could stay overnight with family so parents can "get away")	Blood glucose testing before meals at friends, in restaurant, at school (in public) Learn weight control. Manage overnight stays. Promote healthy habits amid unhealthy environments.	Body image and weight concerns Puberty and effect of hormonal changes Learn to prevent complications. Prevent DKA. Modify high-risk behaviors. Diabetes and dating, sex, and conception Peer pressure Alcohol, tobacco, drugs

Source: Atkinson, A., & Radjenovic, D. (2006).

ADDITIONAL INFORMATION FOR THE CLINICAL SETTING

Weighing Children

Weigh an infant completely undressed (including diaper) and children in underwear only.

Daily Weights to Ensure Accurate Medication Doses

- Use metric system (kilograms) daily to ensure medication dosages are accurately calculated and administered.
- Recalculate medication dosages with every weight variance.
- Notify the physician if the dose ordered is inaccurate based on the current weight.

Helping Children Express Themselves About Growth Hormone Treatments

- Be honest about growth hormone treatments.
- Refer families to the Magic Foundation Web site (see Resources) for online videos.
- Help the child respond to the following questions:
  "How do you feel?"
  "What do you tell your friends about the GH medication?"
  "How have you changed since the GH treatments began?"
  "What advice do you have for other children beginning GH treatment?"

Action of Diuretics on the Kidney

Diuretics impede the sodium chloride reabsorption that occurs in the distal tubule of the kidney. This reduces the loss of free water and increases the concentration of the child's urine. Reduction in urine volume derives from a concomitant action on the proximal tubule, which causes reabsorption of sodium chloride from the glomerular filtrate, thus drawing additional water along. This results in both a smaller volume and a higher concentration of the urine (Chan & Roth, 2006).

Switching from Milk-Based Formula to Soy-Based Formula

- Soy-based formula may cause a decrease in absorption of levothyroxine (Synthroid).
- When an infant is switched from a milk-based formula to a soy-based formula, the dose of thyroid hormone may need to increase to maintain a euthyroid status (Postellon, 2006).

Proper Nutrition for Hypoparathyroidism

The following supplements have been used clinically and may be valuable adjuncts in the treatment of hypoparathyroidism:

- Calcium, if dietary intake is not adequate.
- Magnesium, which aids in the absorption of calcium; also, often low levels of magnesium are present in the case of hypoparathyroidism.
- Boron, which enhances the absorption of calcium.
- Vitamin K, produced by bacteria in the intestines or obtained through the diet (e.g., dark leafy greens) is important for the uptake of calcium by cells throughout the body.
- Foods rich in calcium include almonds, legumes, dark leafy greens, blackstrap molasses, oats, sardines, tahini, prunes, apricots, and sea vegetables.
- Calcium and vitamin D are thought to be best absorbed in an acidic environment (e.g., lemon juice may be added to salad to facilitate calcium absorption).
- Limit carbonated beverages, as they are high in phosphates and may reduce calcium absorption; dairy may diminish calcium absorption for similar reasons.
- Avoid caffeine (such as in coffee, black tea, colas, and chocolate); it can lead to calcium loss through the urine (A.D.A.M., 2006).

Adrenal Crisis

- Adrenal crisis is a life-threatening condition caused by the anterior pituitary gland not making enough adrenocorticotropic hormone (ACTH). Without ACTH, the adrenal gland cannot regulate bodily functions.
- Never stop steroids abruptly. Abrupt withdrawal can cause an adrenal crisis.
- Parents must seek emergency medical care immediately if there is suspicion of adrenal crisis.

Pheochromocytoma

- Perform frequent assessments.
- Never touch or manipulate an adrenal tumor. Palpation can cause further release of catecholamines, increasing the likelihood of a severe hypertensive crisis. This can cause potentially harmful tachyarrhythmias.

Clinical Comparison of Hypoglycemia and Hyperglycemia

Clinical Condition due to	Manifestations	Critical Nursing Actions
Hypoglycemia Too much insulin for amount of food eaten Injected insulin into muscle Too much activity for insulin dose Too much time between meals Too few carbohydrates eaten Illness or stress	Rapid onset Irritable Nervous Shaky feeling, tremors Difficult to concentrate Difficult to speak Behavior change Confused Repeats over and over Unconscious Seizure Tachycardia Shallow breathing Pale, sweaty Hungry Headache Dizzy Vision blurry or double Photophobic Numbness of mouth or lips	Give 15 grams of carbohydrates ($^1/_2$ glass orange juice). Recheck blood glucose in 15 minutes. If blood glucose level is <70 mg/dL give another 15 grams of carbohydrates. Recheck again in another 15 minutes. If unconscious, give IM glucagon.
Hyperglycemia Too little insulin for the food eaten Illness or stress Too many carbohydrates eaten Meals too close together Too many snacks Insulin given just under skin Too little activity	Gradual onset Lethargic Sleepy Slow response Confused Breathes deeply and rapidly Skin flushed and dry Mucous membranes dry Thirsty, hungry, dehydrated Weak, tired, headache Abdomen hurts Nausea and vomiting Vision blurry Shock	Give additional insulin at the usual injection time. Use sliding scale doses for specific level of blood glucose. Increase fluids. If ketone levels are elevated, give an extra insulin injection.

RESOURCES

Audio and visual injection techniques:
http://www.bddiabetes.com/us/main.aspx?cat=1&id=258

Growth charts: http://www.cdc.gov/growthcharts

Growth charts: www.growthcharts.com

Human Growth Foundation: http://www.hgfound.orgParenting:
http://www.primalspirit.com/ps3_1lyn-piluso.htm

Magic Foundation: http://www.magicfoundation.org/www

Short Stature Foundation:
http://www.kumc.edu/gec/support/dwarfism.html

REFERENCES

A.D.A.M. (2006). *Alternative medicine.* Retrieved from http://www.adam.com/ (Accessed July 15, 2008).

Atkinson, A., & Radjenovic, D. (2006). Meeting quality standards for self-management education in pediatric Type 2 diabetes. *Diabetes Care,* 40–46.

American Diabetes Association (ADA). (2007a). Nutrition recommendations and interventions for diabetes. *Diabetes Care,* S48–S65.

American Diabetes Association (ADA). (2007b). Standards of medical care in diabetes—2007. *Diabetes Care,* S4–S41.

Chan, J.C., & Roth, K.S. (2006, July 26). Diabetes insipidus. Retrieved from http://www.emedicine.com/ped/topic580.htm (Accessed November 20, 2008).

NIH Publication No. 04–3054 (2004, June). Addison's disease. Retrieved from http://www.endocrine.niddle.nih.gov/pubs/Addison/Addison.htm (Accessed April 13, 2009).

Postellon, D. (2006, August 23). EMedicine: Congenital hypothyroidism Retrieved from http://www.emedicine.com/ (Accessed November 20, 2008).

Wilson, T.A. (2006, November 17). EMedicine: Congenital adrenal hyperplasia. Retrieved from http://www.emedicine.com/ (Accessed November 20, 2008).

Caring for the Child with a Neurological or Sensory Condition

KEY TERMS

color blindness – An X-linked recessive inheritable color vision deficiency that causes loss of accurate color perception

encephalopathy – Generalized brain dysfunction marked by varying degrees of impairment of speech, cognition, orientation, and arousal, as well as trauma (Venes, 2005).

intracranial pressure (ICP) – Pressure of the cerebrospinal fluid in the subarachnoid space between the skull and the brain

meningocele – Protruding sac located on the cervical, thoracic, or lumbar spine at the level of the defect with a thin layer of muscle and skin usually covering the lesion

nystagmus – Rapid irregular involuntary eye movement caused by a disorder of the central nervous system which may be congenital or acquired

papilledema – Mass of blown-out blood vessels located around the optic nerve; an important sign of increased intracranial pressure (ICP)

strabismus – Condition of nonparallelism in the different fields of gaze causing visual lines to cross even when focused on the same object

tympanogram – Radiographic examination of the eustachian tubes and middle ear after introduction of a contrast medium (Venes, 2005).

FOCUSED ASSESSMENT

States of Consciousness Technique and Patient Response

State	Technique	Response
Alertness	Speak in a normal tone of voice.	Answers appropriately while opening his eyes and responding fully.
Lethargy	Speak in a loud voice.	Opens eyes, appears drowsy, answers questions appropriately but falls asleep easily.
Obtundation	Shake gently to arouse.	Opens eyes and looks at the stimuli, appears slightly confused; alertness and interest in surroundings decreased.
Stupor	Use a painful stimulus.	Responds only to painful stimuli; verbal responses slow or absent; ceases to respond to painful stimuli.
Coma	Apply repeated painful stimuli.	No response to internal or external stimuli, remains in unaroused state with eyes closed

Source: Bickley & Szilagi (2003).

Pediatric Glasgow Coma Scale (GCS)

- Monitor the child's neurological status by assessing his level of consciousness with the GCS (Fig. 26-1).

Pediatric Glasgow Coma Scale

Score for Infant/Nonverbal Child			Verbal Child	
Eye Opening	4	Spontaneously	Spontaneously	
	3	To speech	To verbal command	
	2	To pain	To pain	
	1	No response	No response	
Best Motor Response	6	Normal spontaneous movement	Obeys command	
	5	Withdraws to touch	Localizes pain	
	4	Withdraws to pain	Flexion withdrawal	
	3	Abnormal flexion	Abnormal flexion	
	2	Extension (decerebrate)	Extension (decerebrate)	
	1	No response	No response	
			2–5 years	>5 years
Best Verbal Response	5	Cries appropriately, coos	Appropriate words	Oriented
	4	Irritable crying	Inappropriate words	Confused
	3	Inappropriate screaming/ crying	Screams	Inappropriate
	2	Grunts	Grunts	Garbled
	1	No response	No response	No response

Adapted from Marcoux, K. (2005).

NEUROLOGICAL ASSESSMEMT

GLASGOW SCALE TOTAL

Pupils	Right	Size	
		Reaction	
	Left	Size	
		Reaction	
Eyes open	Spontaneously		4
	To speech		3
	To pain		2
	None		1
Best motor response	Obeys commands		6
	Localizes pain		5
	Flexion withdrawal		4
	Flexion abnormal		3
	Extension		2
	None		1

++ = Brisk
+ = Sluggish
— = No reaction
C = Eye closed by swelling

Usually record best arm or age-appropriate response

Best response to auditory and/or visual stimulus	>2 years		<2 years
	Orientation	5	5 Smiles, listens, follows
	Confused	4	4 Cries, consolable
	Inappropriate words	3	3 Inappropriale persistent cry
	Incomprehensible words	2	2 Agitated, restless
	None	1	1 No response
	Endotracheal tube or trach	T	
COMA SCALE TOTAL			

Hand Grip:
Equal
Unequal
R___L
Weakness

LOC:
Alert/oriented x4
Sleepy
Irritable
Comatose
Disoriented
Combative
Lethargic
Awake
Sleeping
Drowsy
Agitated

Muscle Tone:
Normal
Arching
Spastic
Flaccid Weak
Decorticate
Decerebrate
Other _____

Eye Movement:
Normal
Nystagmus
Strabismus
Other _____

Fontanel/Window:
Soft
Flat
Sunken
Tense
Bulging
Closed
Other _____

Mood/Affect:
Happy
Content
Quiet
Withdrawn
Sad
Flat
Hostile

Figure 26-1 Pediatric Glasgow Coma Scale.

Assigning a Numeric Value for Level of Response with Modified GCS

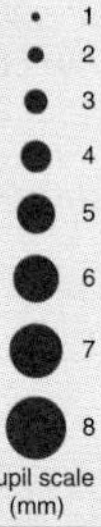

- Assign a value to each level of response (1–5); highest score is 15 (unaltered state of consciousness).
- 8 or below: Coma
- 3: Deep coma
- Coma scale scores may fluctuate if a change in neurological state occurs (e.g., cerebral ischemia, administration of paralytics and sedatives, regaining of consciousness).

Signs and Symptoms of Increased Intracranial Pressure in Infants	
Early Signs and Symptoms	**Late Signs and Symptoms**
Headache	Further decrease in level of consciousness (LOC)
Emesis	Bulging fontanels (infant)
Change in LOC	Decreasing spontaneous movements
Decrease in GCS score	Posturing
Irritability	Papilledema
Sunsetting eyes	Pupil dilation with decreased or no response to light
Decreased eye contact (infant)	Increased blood pressure
Pupil dysfunction	Irregular respirations
Cranial nerve dysfunction	Cushing's triad (late, ominous sign)
Seizures	

Adapted from Marcoux, K. (2005). Management of increased intracranial pressure in the ill child with an acute neurological injury. *AACN Advanced Critical Care, 16*(2), 212–231.

Assessing for Hypothermia

When using a hypothermia blanket, monitor the patient's temperature continuously to prevent hypothermia (a body temperature below 95°F or 35°C). Hypothermia causes shivering and an increase in ICP.

Kernig's Sign

Classic finding on examination for a child suspected of meningitis include a positive Kernig's or Brudzinski sign (Behrman, Kleigman, & Jenson, 2004).

- Place child in the supine position with hips flexed.
- When the lower leg is raised to straighten it, the child cries out or resists the leg extension.
- It is an abnormal finding if the child experiences pain behind the knee when it is fully extended.
- Bilateral increased resistance and pain upon extension of the knee is a positive Kernig sign and may indicate meningeal irritation.

Brudzinski Sign

- Lie the child flat.
- Attempt to raise the child's head toward her chest and place the chin on the chest.

- If there is pain or resistance, the child will immediately flex the hip and knee, which indicates meningeal inflammation may be present (Bickley & Szilagyi, 2003).

Reye Syndrome

There are several stages of Reye syndrome. The child may progress through all of the stages or stop at any stage if treatment is effective (McCance & Huether, 2002).

The Stages of Reye Syndrome

Stage I: Lethargy, vomiting, drowsiness, liver dysfunction

Stage II: Disorientation, combativeness, aggressiveness, delirium, hyperactive reflexes, hyperventilation, shallow breathing, stupor, liver dysfunction

Stage III: Obtundation, coma, decorticate posturing hyperventilation

Stage IV: Deepening coma, large fixed pupils, decerebrate posturing, loss of focular reflexes, liver dysfunction

Stage V: Loss of deep tendon reflexes, seizures, flaccidity, respiratory arrest, usually no liver dysfunction

Head Circumference Measurement	
Birth to 3 months (average head size at birth is 33–38 cm, 12–14 inches)	Head circumference increases 2 cm/month (0.75 inch)
4–6 months (average head size at 6 months is 43 cm, 17 inches)	Head circumference increases 1 cm/month (0.4 inch); average head size at 6 months is 43 cm (17 inches)
6–12 months (average head size at 1 year is 46 cm, 18 inches) By one year of age the child's head size has increased by 33%	Head circumference increases 0.5 cm/month (0.2 inch); average head size at 1 year is 46 cm (18 inches)

Near Drowning (Submersion Injuries)

- A submersion injury occurs when the child is submerged in water tries to breathe and aspirates water (wet drowning) or has a laryngospasm without aspiration (dry drowning).
- The most significant contributing factors to morbidity and mortality are hypoxemia with decreasing oxygen delivery to vital tissues.

- Central nervous system (CNS) damage may occur during the incident (primary injury) or may result from ongoing pulmonary injury, injury due to reperfusion, or multiorgan dysfunction (secondary injury).
- Early resuscitation is associated with an improved prognosis.
- Clinicians use an Orlowski scale to predict the likelihood of neurologically intact survival (Verive, 2006).

Orlowski Scale

Each item listed below is assigned one point. If a child has a score of 2 or less, there is a 90% likelihood of a complete recovery. If a child has a score of 3 or more, there is a 5% chance of survival (Verive, 2006).

- Three years of age or older
- Submersion time greater than 5 minutes
- No resuscitation efforts for more than 10 minutes after rescue
- Comatose on admission to the emergency room
- Arterial pH <7.10

Shaken Baby Syndrome

- Shaken baby syndrome results from major rotational forces and angular deceleration encountered when an infant is shaken forcefully (intentional or unintentional).
- Most victims are younger than 6 months of age and the source of the abuse is usually the father or a male acquaintance of the mother.
- The prognosis for an infant depends on the severity of the injury and response to medical therapy.
- A child may experience neuromotor impairment, visual impairment, and developmental delays.

Signs and Symptoms
- Seizure activity
- Apnea
- Bulging or full fontanelles
- Coma
- Hemorrhage
- Bradycardia
- Complete cardiovascular collapse

Symptoms Exhibited in Less Severe Shaken Baby Syndrome Cases

- Vomiting
- Hypothermia
- Poor feeding
- Failure to thrive
- Increased sleeping
- Lethargy
- Irritability
- Difficulty arousing
- The hallmark of shaken baby syndrome is an absence of external trauma to the head, face, and neck of an infant along with massive intracranial or intraocular pressure.

Hirschberg Asymmetrical Corneal Light Reflex Test

- Hold a penlight or flashlight in front of the child's face. Note the light reflection on the cornea in both eyes.
- Negative corneal light reflex exam (and normal muscle alignment) is when there is symmetrical placement on both eyes at the same time and in the same location on each eye.
- A positive asymmetrical corneal light reflex test (suggestive of strabismus) is when the light falls slightly medially to the center of the pupil on the iris. If this occurs, perform a cover test.

CLINICAL ALERTS

Monroe–Kellie Hypothesis

- The pressure–volume relationship between the blood, intracranial pressure (ICP), volume of cerebrospinal fluid (CSF), and brain tissue and cerebral perfusion pressure is the Monroe–Kellie hypothesis or Monroe–Kellie doctrine.
- This hypothesis states that if one of the components increases, the other components must compress (LeJune & Howard-Fain, 2002).
- The body tries to compensate by an increase in cerebrospinal fluid absorption, by a decrease in CSF production, by a reduction in blood volume or by a decrease in brain mass.
- When compression is exhausted, the intracranial pressure will rise.

- As a result of increased ICP, blood flow and oxygen delivery may be compromised.
- When blood flow and oxygen decrease, secondary brain injury occurs (Marcoux, 2005).

Patient Safety

When a child has increased ICP never place her head lower than her body. This position significantly increases the pressure more.

Seizure Precautions

- Maintain airway patency.
- Maintain a safe environment
- Do not place anything in the child's mouth during a seizure. A loose tooth may be aspirated or knocked out.
- Monitor oxygenation. Ensure the child's color remains pink; the pulse oximeter should read 95% or greater and the heart rate should be normal or slightly raised.
- Administer intravenous medications during a seizure slowly to reduce the risk of side effects such as respiratory or circulatory failure.
- Raise and pad the side rails of the crib or bed to protect the child from harm.
- Recommend that a helmet be worn to protect his head.
- Encourage the use of a medical identification bracelet at all times.

Cricoid Pressure

With neurological injuries apply cricoid pressure or empty the stomach contents with a nasogastric tube to avoid vomiting during intubation (Orlowski & Szpilman, 2001).

Autonomic Dysreflexia

- Autonomic dysreflexia is a stress syndrome caused by massive amounts of stimuli overloading the autonomic system, resulting in hyperactive sympathetic stimulation.
- Autonomic dysreflexia leads to extreme anxiety, headache, visual and auditory sensation changes, nausea, seizures, hypertension, peripheral vascular dilation or flushing, and bradycardia.

- Immediate management of hypertension and cardiac, and neurological complications is required.

DIAGNOSTIC TESTS

Determining Increased Intracranial Pressure (ICP)

- Magnetic resonance imaging (MRI) or computerized tomography (CT) is used to determine etiology and severity of increased ICP.
- Avoid computed tomography (CT) contrast in the presence of intracranial bleeding.
- Monitor ICP by inserting an intracranial catheter.

Brain Abscess

- Serum laboratory studies may be ordered (CBC, blood cultures, C-reactive protein).
- Usually moderate leukocytosis and elevated erythrocyte rate and C-reactive protein level occur.
- If the abscess is aspirated, culture the specimen to identify causative microorganism (Brook, 2004).

Hydrocephalus

- Use CT, MRI, and ultrasound to diagnose hydrocephalus.
- Cisternogram may be used to evaluate CSF flow dynamics in brain and spinal cord. This procedure reveals CSF concentration, leakage, obstruction, and pressure.

Audiologic Testing

One or several procedures may be used. The otoacoustic emissions test (OAE) and auditory brain stem evoked response (ABER) determine the degree of hearing loss.

MEDICATIONS

Phenytoin (Dilantin)

- Phenytoin (Dilantin) may cause gingival hyperplasia.
- The nurse observes for swelling and bleeding of the child's gums and provides good dental hygiene.

- Parents need to be taught the necessity of performing proper hygiene.

Mannitol (**man**-i-tol) (Osmitrol)

Classification(s) Osmotic Diuretic, Diagnostic Agent

Indications Reduction of intracranial pressure and treatment of cerebral edema

Action Increases the osmolarity of the glomerular filtrate, preventing the reabsorption of water and resulting in a loss of sodium chloride and water

Contraindications Use cautiously with dehydration, pulmonary congestion, renal disease and active intracranial bleeding (except during craniotomy)

Incompatibilities Do not add to blood products.

Adverse Reactions and Side Effects Seizures, hypotension, tachycardia, skin necrosis with infiltration, hyponatremia, diuresis, and urticaria

Route and Dosage Dosage for children <12 years of age not established

Nursing Implications
1. Do not administer electrolyte-free mannitol with blood products. If blood is administered, add at least 20 mEq of NaCl to each liter of mannitol.
2. Do not expose mannitol to low temperatures. If crystallization occurs, warm the bottle in a hot water bath and cool the medication to body temperature before administering.
3. Monitor serum electrolytes throughout therapy.

Data from Deglin, J., & Vallerand, A. (2009). Davis's drug guide for nurses (11th ed.), pp. 770–771. Philadelphia: F.A. Davis.

Seizure Medications

Type of Seizure	Medication	Dose Range	Adverse Reactions	Nursing Care
Partial Complex (Psychomotor)	Carbamazepine (Tegretol)	10–30 mg/kg per day in divided doses. Increase until best response is achieved.	Drowsiness, nausea, liver changes, increased appetite	Give with food but not milk.
	Valproic acid (Depakene)	0.1–0.2 mg/kg per day in two or three divided doses per day	Confusion, ataxia, nystagmus, nausea, gingival hyperplasia, bleeding disorders	Always give with food and monitor serum drug levels. Teach parents about oral hygiene and wear a medical alert tag. Teach parents to watch for adverse effects indicating toxicity.
	Phenytoin (Dilantin)	5 mg/kg per day in two to three divided doses	May cause dizziness, drowsiness, or physical incoordination. Avoid abrupt discontinuation of use. Daily multivitamin is recommended while on this medication.	Give with water, juice, or milk.
	Phenobarbital (Luminal)	Infants: 5–6 mg/kg per day in one or two divided doses		

Type of Seizure	Medication	Dose Range	Adverse Reactions	Nursing Care
	Fosphenytoin (Cerebyx)	Children 1–6 years: 6–8 mg/kg per day in one or two divided doses Loading dose of 10–20 mg/kg. Then 4–6 mg/kg per day		
Generalized Tonic–Clonic	Valproic acid (Depakene) and carba-mazepine (Tegretol) Phenytoin (Dilantin) Phenobarbital Ketogenic diet high in fat and low in protein and carbohydrates	May be an inexpensive medication. Causes a high level of ketones which decrease myoclonic or tonic–clonic seizure activity.	Monitor for sleepiness, hyperactivity, drowsiness, and school performance changes. Nausea, vomiting, headache, drowsiness, dizziness	This diet is hard to maintain for a long period of time because of the lack of food variety and difficulty of food preparation and parental involvement.
Absence (Petit Mal)	Ethosuximide (Zarontin) or Valproic acid	3–8 mg/kg per day		Avoid antacids.
Partial Simple	Topiramate (Topamax)	1–3 mg/kg per day	Weight loss, dizziness, diarrhea, cognitive dysfunction	Avoid antidepressants and antacids.

Community Education about DEET (N,N-diethyl-m-toluamide)

- Educate the community about DEET. Insect repellents containing DEET (N,N-diethyl-m-toluamide, also known as N,N-diethyl-3-methylbenzamide) with a concentration of 10% appear to be as safe as products with a concentration of 30% when used according to the directions on the product labels.
- The American Academy of Pediatrics recommends that repellents with DEET should not be used on infants younger than 2 months old.

Antimicrobial Therapy Used in Brain Abscesses

- Meningitis: Neonates: Cefotaxime+ampicillin; infants and children: ceftriaxone or cefotaxime+vancomycin
- Cyanotic congenital heart disease: Ampicillin+ chloramphenicol, or ceftriaxone+metronidazole, or ampicillin-sulbactam
- Otitis or sinusitis: Ampicillin+chloramphenicol, ceftriaxone+metronidazole or ampicillin-sulbactam
- Ventriculoperitoneal shunt or trauma: Vancomycin+antipseudomonal cephalosporin (i.e., cefepime or ceftazidime)
- Immunocompromised: Vancomycin+ceftazidime +metronidazole. If no response within 7 days, Amphotericin B should be added
- Endocarditis: prostatic valve: Vancomycin+gentamicin or ceftazidime; natural valve: ampicillin or an aminoglycoside or penicillin+ceftriaxone

Medications Containing Acetylsalicylic Acid		
Non-prescription	**Prescription**	**Topical**
Alka-Seltzer	Darvon	Acne cleaners
Excedrin	Norgesic	Acne creams
Pepto-Bismol	Robaxisal	Astringents
Anacin	Talwin	Facial masks
Kaopectate	Butalbital	Wart removers
Pamprin	Percodan	Dandruff shampoos
	Roxiprin	Muscle pain relief creams
	Lortab	Wintergreen scented oils
	Propoxyphene	Arthritis pain rubs
	Soma	Facial scrubs
		Sport strength sun block

ETHNOCULTURAL CONSIDERATIONS

Head Circumference in Infants of Asian Heritage

- Infants of Asian heritage generally have smaller head circumferences than Caucasian infants.
- When Asian infants are measured, the measurement obtained may indicate the infant is SGA; this may in fact not be true.
- The infant may be considered to be at risk for medical diseases and complications based on the data, which may be based on inaccurate conclusions.

TEACHING THE FAMILY

General Instructions

- Provide the family with specific instructions for care if the child will be cared for at home.
- Communicate information about bathing, feeding, medical equipment, tracheostomy suctioning, gastrostomy tubes, urinary catheterization, positioning, and range-of-motion exercises.
- Stress the importance of performing these procedures correctly.
- To validate parental understanding, require parents to demonstrate the tasks. Parents may appear reluctant and fearful.
- Remain supportive and patient as parents learn new skills.

Reye Syndrome

- Instruct parents not to administer any product containing acetylsalicylic acid (aspirin) to a child younger than the age of 19 because of the risk of Reye syndrome.

Ventricular Shunts

- Continuous monitoring and assessment is essential because hydrocephalus is a lifelong disorder.
- Recognize complications: Increased ICP and shunt malfunction (kinking, plugging within the ventricle from tissue, or exudate or obstruction at the distal end from thrombosis or displacement of tubing due to growth).
- Observe for signs of infection: Nausea and vomiting, headache, change in customary behavior, lethargy, unresponsiveness, elevated temperature.
- Instruct parents that the child cannot participate in contact sports.
- Emphasize the importance of safe transport and positioning during transport.

Language Disorder

- Encourage caregivers to help the children how to say speech sounds correctly, improve language comprehension, and develop conversational skills.

- Inform caregivers that the disorder may impact the child's educational and social interactions.
- Advise the family about how to find a speech pathologist in the community

ADDITIONAL INFORMATION FOR THE CLINICAL SETTING

Benefits of Massage

- Helps promote a sense of well-being and enhances self-esteem while benefiting the immune and circulatory systems.
- The resulting sense of well-being decreases the amounts of the circulating stress hormones cortisol and norepinephrine that may weaken the immune system.
- Decreased anxiety and tension allows people to feel more serene and enhances their ability to cope with life stressors.
- Different massage techniques have been integrated into various complementary therapies.
  - Gentle massage or stroking releases endorphins (the body's natural pain killers) and a feeling of comfort is experienced.
  - Stronger, more vigorous massage helps to stretch tense and uncomfortable muscles, leading to improved mobility and flexibility.
- Aids in relaxation by affecting the body system that controls blood pressure, digestion, and respiration.
- The stimulation of circulation improves the supply of oxygen and nutrients to the body's tissues and enhances skin tone.
- Stimulation of the lymphatic system improves the body's ability to eliminate lactic acid and other chemical wastes that cause muscle stiffness and pain (Woodham & Peters, 2006).

Cushing's Triad

- A child with significantly increased intracranial pressure may exhibit Cushing's triad. Symptoms of Cushing's triad

are hypertension (with widening pulse pressure), bradycardia, and an irregular respiratory pattern.
- Cushing's triad is usually indicative of impending herniation (the displacement of the foramen magnum) (Venes, 2005)

Intravenous Fluids

- Avoid hypotonic intravenous fluids (i.e., D5W) because they cross the blood–brain barrier, resulting in increased cerebral edema and ICP.

Intracranial Pressure Monitoring

- To monitor ICP accurately, a pressure line may be inserted. Several types of monitoring devices are available, including intracranial bolts, intraventricular catheters, and intraparenchymal fiber optic catheters.
- ICP monitoring is indicated for the child who has a Glasgow Coma Scale (GSC) score of less than 8, exhibits signs of increasing ICP, is status post major neurosurgical procedures, or has a high probability of having increased ICP.
- The best outcome for ICP monitoring is to maintain cerebral perfusion pressure between 50 and 70 mm Hg, maintain ICP at <20 mm Hg, and detect occurrences such as herniation or bleeding (Marcoux, 2005).

Signs and Symptoms of Seizures

Type of Seizures	Brain Location/Cause	Signs and Symptoms
Partial (focal)	Localized to one area	One area affected: Hands, lips, wrist, arms face. Impaired loss of consciousness at onset.
Partial Complex (psychomotor)	Temporal lobe	Loss of consciousness and loss of awareness or surrounding. Change in behavior: Lip smacking, picking, inappropriate mannerisms, confusion follows the seizure.

(continued)

Signs and Symptoms of Seizures (Continued)

Type of Seizures	Brain Location/Cause	Signs and Symptoms
Partial Simple		Lasts 5 minutes, child only remembers the aura. Automatisms are noted. No loss of consciousness or awareness. Motor signs are isolated to one area of the body and then spread to the rest of the body. May experience senses such as buzzing sounds, tingling, flashing lights, anxiety, fear or anger.
Generalized Tonic–Clonic	Genetic predisposition or brain injury secondary to anoxia.	Partial simple and complex seizures evolve to generalized seizures. Aura is experienced followed by loss of consciousness and tone. Patient falls to the floor with tonic clonic muscle contractions. Patient is postictal and confused after the seizure is over. Loss of urine may occur.
Atonic: Loss of muscle tone, drop attacks. Absence (petitmal) Tonic Myoclonic Clonic Myoclonic and Akinetic	Metabolic etiology	Sudden drop to the floor due to loss of motor muscle tone. Seen in children 2–4 years of age. No loss of consciousness but experiences loss of awareness. Nonconvulsive. Periods of staring or minor movements lasting seconds. May occur several times a day, interferes with learning and school work. Stiffening of the body that is sustained, involving all four extremities. Single or multiple jerks or flexion of limbs. Intermittent rhythmic jerking, one to three per second, may start in one body location and move or migrate to another location. Complete or total lack of movement

Source: Fox (2002).

Nursing Care for the Child Having a Seizure

1. Call for help (in a hospital setting use the designated emergency number; in the community setting, call 911).

2. Maintain safe environment and a patent airway. If the airway is occluded, open the airway with a jaw thrust maneuver. Administer oxygen if needed and available. Do not put anything in the mouth. If the situation warrants emergency medical care, qualified health care personnel can insert an appropriate sized oral airway.

3. Place the child on his side to prevent aspiration of secretions.

4. Loosen restrictive clothing to ensure adequate circulation to essential body organs.

5. Administer medications such as diazepam (Valium), lorazepam (Ativan), or fosphenytoin (Cerebryx) as ordered by the physician. An exception is in the neonate where these medications become toxic due to immature liver function.

6. Continue to monitor respiratory status and circulatory status throughout the seizure.

7. When the seizure is over, place the child in the recovery position or the left lateral recumbent position.

8. Inform the child that he or she has just had a seizure. Tell the family that the child may still be confused and disoriented for a short time.

9. Stay with the child (support is essential because a seizure can be frightening to both the child and family).

10. Document important details about the seizure (e.g., time and duration of seizure, antecedent activity or event, type or description of the seizure, assessment data, care measures provided such as positioning, oxygen, suctioning, mechanical ventilation or CPR, medication administration, physician notification or presence at the child's side, and response to seizure such as condition and disposition of the child after the seizure).

Complications from Encephalitis

- The complications may include motor or cognitive deficits, seizure disorders, hearing or vision loss, memory loss, and paralysis (Wisniewski, 2003).

- If a child has permanent or lingering problems, the treatment plan for them may be multidisciplinary.
- This multidisciplinary approach optimizes the child's recovery and maximizes skills necessary for life.

Liver Biopsy

- Monitor bleeding after a liver biopsy because child is predisposed to bleeding as the liver is highly vascular.
- After the biopsy, the physician places a dressing to splint the puncture site. Lie the child on the right side for 2 hours (Lewis et al., 2007).

Preventing Injury of the Sac (Spina Bifida)

- Use sterile technique to cover the defect as quickly as possible with a sterile, non-adherent dressing that is moistened with sterile saline to maintain moisture and prevent drying.
- Change dressing every 2 to 4 hours or as prescribed or when soiled.

Rectal Temperature

Do not obtain a rectal temperature of a child with spina bifida because rectal irritation and rectal prolapse may occur.

Ventricular Shunts

- A shunt may be placed to drain excessive intracranial CSF.
- Ventricular shunts have greatly improved the quality of life for children with hydrocephalus.
- A ventricular shunt consists of several parts including a proximal catheter that enters the lateral ventricle, a one-way valve that is set at a desired pressure to prevent CSF being drained too fast due to gravity, a small reservoir, and a distal catheter that terminates in the peritoneal cavity or alternate drainage site.
- The peritoneal cavity is the preferred site for placement of the distal catheter because of easy accessibility and decreased risk of complications.
- When the catheter is placed in the peritoneum, the shunt is called a ventriculoperitoneal shunt.

Measuring Head Circumference

 Procedure 26-1 Measuring Head Circumference

Purpose

Measuring head circumference is an important component of evaluation of a child's growth as well as his health status.

Equipment

- Flexible nonstretchable tape measure
- Child's chart

Steps

1. Obtain a flexible nonstretchable tape measure (preferably one in which one end inserts into the other end).

2. Allow the parent to hold the child in his or her arms or lap.

3. Remove braids, barrettes, or other hair decorations.

4. Place the tape measure over the most prominent part of the occiput (back of the head) and just above the supraorbital ridges (above the eyebrows).

5. Pull the tape measure snugly to compress the hair and underlying tissues.

6. Read the measurement to the nearest 0.1 cm or 1/8 inch.

7. Document the measurement on the chart.

Clinical Alert If an abnormal circumference is found based on the child's age, reposition the tape and measure the head circumference again. The new measurement should agree with the first measurement within 0.2 cm or 1/4 inch.

Teach Parents

To help ensure an accurate head circumference measurement, teach the parents how to hold the child firmly while offering verbal comfort and encouragement.

Intravenous Therapy

- If shunt surgery is anticipated, the nurse should not use scalp veins for intravenous therapy because the IV may be located near the surgical site.

Basal Skull Fracture

- Do not insert a nasogastric tube if a basal skull fracture is suspected because the tube may enter the brain through fracture.
- Insert an orogastric tube if needed (Brettler, 2004).

Common Acute Eye Disorders

Eye Disorder	Cause/Organism	Signs and Symptoms	Treatment
Conjunctivitis	An inflammation of the conjunctiva	Excessive tearing, erythematous, edema and with clear, watery, yellow or green drainage and eyelid crusting	Apply warm soaks to remove crusting, use good hand hygiene and apply cool compresses to edematous eyes.
Neonatal Conjunctivitis– Ophthalmia Neonatorium	Chemical irritation caused by maternal sexually transmitted diseases acquired at birth such as *Chlamydia, gonorrhea*, herpes.	Purulent drainage either white or yellowish.	Prophylactic antibiotic ointment is used in all neonates. Lack of treatment can cause eye damage.
Sty	A localized inflammatory swelling of one or more of the glands of the eyelid.	Painful, erythematous lesion on the lid margin. Slight edema, some lymph node tenderness or induration.	Apply warm moist compresses with an antibiotic ointment. Good hand hygiene is necessary.
Chalazion	Granuloma of the meibomian gland on the eyelid.	Hard, small nodule on either eye lid may be painful.	Apply warm moist compresses and massage, antibiotic ointment, may resolve the condition spontaneously.

Continued

Common Acute Eye Disorders (Continued)

Eye Disorder	Cause/Organism	Signs and Symptoms	Treatment
Blepharitis Marginalis	Staphylococcal infection of the lid margin.	Erythematous eyelid margin with crusted eye drainage.	Apply an antibiotic ointment to the lower affected eye lid. Apply warm moist compresses to remove crusting drainage.
Keratitis	Inflammation and infection of the corneal layers due to bacterial, viral, fungal, or foreign body infiltration.	Very painful, excessive tearing, photophobia, and erythema.	An ophthalmologist must examine the cornea to monitor or treat potential scarring and prevent loss of vision.
Periorbital Cellulitis	Inflammation of the subcutaneous tissues and skin about the eye may be bacterial or viral.	Edema, pain, erythema in the skin and orbital folds of the affected eye.	Use intravenous antibiotic therapy for 7 days.
Blocked Tear Duct (Dacryostenosis/ Dacryocystitis)	Obstruction of the nasolacrimal tear duct causing inflammation or cystitis.	Tearing, yellow drainage, crusting, small bump in the inner canthus of the affected eye. Usually unilateral, may be painful.	Apply warm compresses and gentle massage of the lacrimal sac with the forefinger milking any exudates toward the nose.

Chemical Burns

- Prompt assessment is essential.
- Monitor for signs of infection, hemorrhage, and increased intraocular pressure (IOP). Provide emotional and social support for the child and family.
- Follow-up care for evaluation of the cornea for scarring and IOP testing to determine post inflammatory response is necessary.
- Patching and administering eye medication may be required at home.
- School and normal activities are allowed after physician consultation.

Communicating with the Hearing Impaired Child

- Recognize behavioral cues suggestive of hearing loss.
- Obtain the child's attention before speaking.
- Face the child when speaking.
- Position yourself at the child's eye level.
- Speak slowly and loudly.
- Modify the environment; unnecessary noises should be reduced.
- Offer emotional support: a child with a hearing loss may face a potential stigma associated with his communication difficulty.

RESOURCES

American Academy of Pediatrics:
http://www.bt.cdc.gov/cdclinkdisclaimer.asp?a_gotolink=http://www.aap.org/family/wnv-jun03.htm

About Pediatrics.com:
http://pediatrics.about.com/cs/conditions/a/hydrocephalus_2.htm

About Pediatrics.com:
http://pediatrics.about.com/cs/conditions/a/hydrocephalus2.htm About Pediatrics.com

About Pediatrics.com:
http://pediatrics.about.com/cs/weeklyquestion/a/032002_ask.htm

American Foundation for the Blind Information Center:
http://www.afb.org

American Society for Deaf Children: http://www.deafchildren.org

American Speech-Language-Hearing Association:
http://www.asha.org

Alexander Graham Bell Association for the Deaf and Hard of Hearing: http://www.agbell.org

Colored blindness:
http://www.nlm.nih.gov/medlineplus/colorblindness.html

American Deafness and Rehabilitation Association:
http://www.adara.org

Centers for Disease Control and Prevention:
http://www.cdc.gov/ncbddd/autism/actearly

Epilepsy Foundation: http://www.epilepsyfoundation.org

Individuals with Disability Education Act of 2004 (IDEA): http://idea.ed.gov

March of Dimes: http://www.marchofdimes.com

Meningitis Foundation of America: http://www.musa.org

National Association of Neonatal Nurses: http://www.NANN.org

National Eye Institute: http://www.nei.nih.gov

National Headache Foundation: http://www.headaches.org

National Institute on Deafness and other Communication Disorders: http://www.nidcd.nih.gov/health/statistics/hearing.asa

Normal Growth of Young Children: http://pediatrics.about.com/cs/weeklyquestion/a/032002_ask.htm

National Institutes on Disability and Rehabilitation Research: http://www.ed.gov/about/contact/gen/index.htmo?src_1n

National Institute of Neurological Disorders and Stroke: http://www.ninds.nih.gov

National Reye's Syndrome, Inc.: http://www.reyessyndrome.org

National Spinal Cord Injury Association: http://www.spinalcord.org

Spina Bifida Association of America: http://www.sbaa.org

US Department of Health and Human Services: Health Resources and Services Administration Maternal and Child Health Bureau: http://depts.washington.edu/growth/module5/text/page5a.htm

REFERENCES

Behrman, R., Kleigman, R., & Jenson, H. (2004). *Nelson textbook of pediatrics* (16th ed.). Philadelphia: W.B. Saunders.

Bickley, L., & Szilagyi, P. (2003). *Bate's guide to physical examination and history taking* (8th ed.). Philadelphia: Lippincott Williams & Wilkins.

Brettler, S. (2004). Trauma nursing: Traumatic brain injury. Retrieved from http://www.rnweb.com/rnweb/article/articleDetail.jsp?id=110100 (Accessed July 22, 2008).

Brook, I. (2004). Microbiology and management of brain abscess in children. *Journal of Pediatric Neurology, 2*(3), 125–130.

Deglin, J., & Vallerand, A. (2009). *Davis's drug guide for nurses* (11th ed.). Philadelphia: F.A. Davis.

Fox, J.A. (2002). *Primary health care of infants, children and adolescents.* St Louis, MO: C.V. Mosby.

LeJune, M., & Howard-Fain, T. (2002). Caring for patients with increased intracranial pressure. *Nursing, 32*(11), 1–5.

Lewis, S., Heitkemper, M., Dirksen, S., O'Brien, P., & Bucher, L. (2007). *Medical-surgical nursing: Assessment and management of clinical problems.* St. Louis, MO: Mosby Elsevier.

Marcoux, K. (2005). Management of increased intracranial pressure in the ill child with an acute neurological injury. *AACN Advanced Critical Care, 16*(2), 212–231. Retrieved from http://www.nursingcenter.com/library/JournalArticle. asp? Article_ID=594176 (Accessed January 4, 2007).

McCance, K., & Huether, S. (2002). *Pathophysiology: The biologic basis for disease in adults and children* (4th ed.). St. Louis, MO: C.V. Mosby.

Orlowski, J.P., & Szpilman, D. (2001). Drowning: Rescue, resuscitation, and reanimation. *Pediatric Clinics of North America, 48*(3), 627–646.

Venes, D. (Ed.). (2005). *Taber's cyclopedic medical dictionary.* Philadelphia: F.A. Davis.

Verive, M. (2006). Near drowning. Retrieved from www.emedicine.com/ped/topic/2570.htm (Accessed November 23, 2008).

Wisniewski, A. (2003). Closing in on clues to encephalitis. *Nursing, 33*(4), 70–71.

Woodham, A., & Peters, D. (2006). Healing massage. *Saturday Evening Post,* May/June, 2006.

Caring for the Child with a Musculoskeletal Condition

KEY TERMS

cast syndrome – Results when a child is placed in a spica cast and a portion of the duodenum is compressed between the superior mesenteric artery and the aorta, causing vomiting, abdominal distention, and bowel obstruction

closed reduction – Treatment of bone fractures by placing the bones in their proper position without surgery (Venes, 2005)

compartment syndrome – Caused by an accumulation of fluid in the fascia; increases the pressure on the muscles, blood vessels, and nerve tissue that the fascia surrounds; too much pressure can cause tissue ischemia, nerve damage, and necrosis

open reduction – Treatment of bone fractures by the use of surgery to place the bones in their proper position (Venes, 2005)

FOCUSED ASSESSMENT

Performing the Neurovascular Assessment

Neurovascular status must be assessed carefully and every 1 to 2 hours for the first 48 hours and then every 4 hours after that if there is no compromise in circulation.

Pain
- Does the child complain of pain in the affected limb?
- Is it relieved by narcotic medication?

- Does it become worse when fingers or toes are flexed? If yes, notify the physician immediately (compartment syndrome).

Sensation
- Can the child feel touch on the extremity?
- Is two-point discrimination decreased? If yes, notify the physician immediately (compartment syndrome).

Motion
- Can the child move fingers or toes?
- Lack of movement may indicate nerve damage.

Temperature
- Does the affected limb feel warm?
- Does it feel cool? A cool extremity may change to feeling warm if a blanket is placed over it and the extremity is elevated. If the extremity is still cool after these interventions, there is poor circulation.

Capillary Refill Time (CRT)

Apply brief pressure to the nail bed and note how quickly pink color returns to the nail bed (normal, <3 seconds; circulation is poor if >3 seconds) (Fig. 27-1).

Color
- Note the color of the affected limb. Compare that color to the color of the unaffected limb. Pink is the norm.
- If the color is paler than in the unaffected limb, circulation is poor.

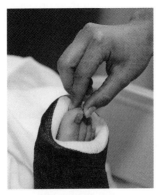

Figure 27-1 Assessing capillary refill time.

Pulses

- Check pulses distal to the injury or cast.
- If the pulse is difficult to locate, assess the area with a Doppler and mark the spot with an 'X'. If the cast covers the foot or hand, this may not be possible to assess.

Slipped Capital Femoral Epiphysis

Stage

- Preslip: The child complains of weakness in the leg. There is pain in knee or hip when standing or walking for long periods of time.
- Acute slip: The child falls and then reports hip pain.
- Chronic slip: The femoral head gradually slips off the femoral neck and then remodels for the incorrect position.
- Acute to chronic slip: Slow progressive slip that becomes more displaced.

Severity

- Grade I (preslip): Widening of the physis without any displacement of the epiphysis.
- Grade II (minimal slip): A one third displacement of the femoral head from the femoral neck.
- Grade III (moderate slip): More than one third but less than one half displacement of the femoral head from the femoral neck.
- Grade IV (severe slip): More than one half displacement of the femoral head from the femoral neck.

Classification of Fractures

- Classification of fractures is based on the location and description of the fracture.
- The location is where the fracture occurs along the shaft of the bone. Fractures are described in terms of the amount of injury.
- Closed fracture: No break in the skin.
- Open fracture: Bone has penetrated through the skin (type I, II, or III, based on the degree, severity of soft tissue damage, size of the wound, and amount of contamination), potential for infection is greatest with an open fracture.

Epiphyseal

- Type I: Separation of epiphysis; may be mistaken for a sprain; does not affect growth.
- Type II: Fracture separation of the epiphysis; circulation is intact; does not usually affect growth.
- Type III: Fracture through the epiphysis into the joint, does not usually affect growth if reduced properly.
- Type IV: Fracture through epiphysis into the joint and the metaphysis; open reduction and internal fixation necessary; can prevent growth disturbance.
- Type V: Rare occurrence; crush injury to epiphyseal plate; results in premature closure of epiphyseal plate and growth arrest.

Classification by Breaks

Transverse
Line crosses the shaft at a 90-degree angle.

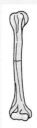

Spiral
A diagonal line coils around the bone.
Caused by a twisting force.

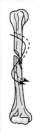

Oblique
A diagonal line across the bone.

Greenstick
Bone is bent, but not broken.
More common in children.

Comminuted
Three of more fractured fragments.

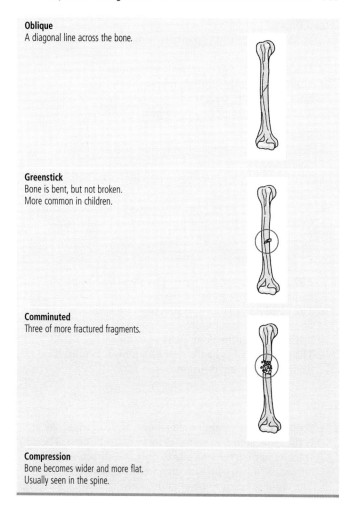

Compression
Bone becomes wider and more flat.
Usually seen in the spine.

Sprains

First Degree
- Mild; ligament is stretched and the affected joint is stable.
- Minimal pain, swelling, ecchymosis.
- Full range of motion and weight bearing.

Second Degree

- Moderate; ligament is partially torn and joint laxity is present.
- Moderate pain, swelling, and ecchymosis.
- Motion is slightly limited and painful.
- Mild joint laxity with tenderness over the joint.
- The patient may be unable to bear weight.

Third Degree

- Severe; ligament is completely torn and the joint is unstable.
- Significant swelling and severe ecchymosis occur within the first 30 minutes.
- Severe pain over the joint makes examination difficult.
- Cannot bear weight or otherwise use the extremity.

Gower Maneuver

- A child with muscular dystrophy uses the Gower maneuver to rise from the floor.
- The child moves to a kneeling position with hands on the floor to stabilize himself.
- With hands on the floor, he rises to his feet.
- The child uses his hands to walk up his legs until he reaches a standing position.

Scoliosis

- Scoliosis is a nonpainful lateral curvature of the spine and is the most common spinal deformity in children. The spine either curves laterally in only one direction ("C" curve) or in two opposite directions ("S" curve).
- The child is asked to bend at the waist with arms hanging loosely (Adam's position or bend over test) to determine scoliosis (Fig. 27-2).

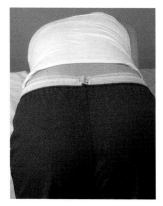

Figure 27-2 By doing the Adam's test or bend over test, scoliosis is obvious.

CLINICAL ALERTS

Complication of the Child with a Fracture: Compartment Syndrome

- Complications can occur when a child is immobilized in a cast. The major complication that can occur is compartment syndrome, which is caused by an accumulation of fluid in the fascia.
- The classic sign of compartment syndrome is unrelenting pain that is unrelieved by narcotics.
- Notify the physician immediately.
- The best treatment of compartment syndrome is prevention. Prevention is achieved by elevating the extremity to prevent excessive swelling and frequent neurovascular checks.

Osteomyelitis

- Osteomyelitis is an inflammation of bone and marrow, usually caused by infection.
- Acute osteomyelitis is a serious complication that may be caused by open fracture, penetration of the skin by a contaminated object, a septic joint, infected wound, bacterial infection from somewhere else in body (like

dental caries), blunt trauma, premature babies and infants with birth complications the first year of life.
- All types of osteomyelitis require immediate treatment (broad-spectrum antibiotics after blood cultures are drawn).
- Evaluate the child's response to the antibiotic therapy about 2 or 3 days after the initial dose.
- If the child demonstrates a response to the intravenous antibiotic therapy at this point, more blood cultures are drawn, intravenous antibiotics are stopped, and the child continues therapy on oral antibiotics for 4 to 8 weeks at home.
- If the child demonstrates poor response to the intravenous antibiotic therapy, antibiotic therapy is continued for a much longer time period.

Chronic Osteomyelitis

- Chronic osteomyelitis is uncommon and occurs when bone tissue dies as a result of the lost blood supply.
- Children with chronic osteomyelitis have had symptoms for longer than 3 weeks and there is a history of prior bone infection within weeks or months after surgery or trauma.
- The treatment for chronic osteomyelitis is prolonged, painful, and frustrating for the child and family. For the first few days of hospitalization, the affected limb is placed in a splint. Oral analgesics, including acetaminophen (Children's Tylenol), ibuprofen (Children's Motrin), or narcotic analgesics such as acetaminophen with codeine (Percocet) can be used to manage pain.
- Make the child as comfortable as possible.
- Monitor intravenous site for infiltration because the antibiotics used to treat osteomyelitis are caustic to the veins. A peripherally inserted central catheter (PICC) or tunneled central line is placed if intravenous therapy continues for more than 2 to 3 days.
- Use diversional activities while activity is limited.

DIAGNOSTIC TESTS

Orthopedic Imaging Tests

Diagnostic Imaging Test	Benefits	Limitations
Radiograph	Easily available Visualizes fractures well No sedation needed Inexpensive	Two-dimensional Does not visualize soft tissue such as cartilage. Patient must be positioned properly. Radiation exposure
Fluoroscopy	Guides many orthopedic procedures Can be used with contrast Real-time radiography Inexpensive	Radiation exposure
Arthrography	Provides visualization of joints Three-dimensional view	Risk of reaction to contrast Depends on the skill of the radiographer Radiation exposure
Computed Tomography (CT scan)	Cross-sectional view of anatomy More clear than radiographs Software programs can show reconstruction Can use contrast	Expensive May require sedation Risk of reaction to contrast
Bone Scan (nuclear medicine)	Excellent at finding changes in bone as a result of infection, trauma, or tumor	Takes 4 hours Not always available on emergency basis Cannot distinguish benign from malignant tumors Radiation exposure to entire body IV access required
Ultrasound	Easily available No radiation No sedation needed Good for visualizing soft tissue masses and cysts Painless Inexpensive	Limited use Depends on the skill of the radiographer
Magnetic Resonance Imaging (MRI)	Visualizes hard and soft tissue and bone marrow No radiation	Not readily available No metal Sedation may be needed Need experienced radiologist to read MRI

Blood and Body Fluid Analysis for the Child with Alterations in Musculoskeletal Conditions

Diagnostic Test	Function of the Test	Indications	Normal Values
Complete Blood Count (CBC)	Blood sample that evaluates many components.	Lower platelet count indicates a bleeding disorder. Greater WBC count indicates a bacterial infection or septic arthritis.	Platelets: 150,000– 400,000/µL WBCs: 4500– 10,000/µL
CBC Differential	Breaks down WBCs into various types (five total). Numbers indicate a percentage of total WBCs. Gives an indication of the type of infection.	↑Monocytes indicate a long-term infectious process. ↑Lymphocytes indicate an increase in viral illness. ↑Eosinophils indicate an allergic or parasitic condition. ↑Basophils indicate a chronic inflammatory condition. ↑Neutrophils (Polys) -Bands are immature neutrophils. -Segs are mature neutrophils. An increase in the band neutrophils suggest a severe bacterial infection such as sepsis.	0% for bands and 31%–57% for segs Presence of bands is highly indicative of a bacterial infection.

Diagnostic Test	Function of the Test	Indications	Normal Values
C-Reactive Protein (CRP)	Measures a protein in blood that is released when an infection is present.	>0.9 indicates an infection or septic arthritis.	<1.0 mg/dL
Calcium and Phosphate	Measures the amount of these minerals.	Low levels may indicate rickets.	Calcium: 8.5–11 mg/dL Phosphorus: 3.0–4.5 mg/dL
Rheumatoid Factor (Rh factor)	Measures the body's autoimmune response to an antigen.	If positive, may indicate juvenile arthritis. Not all children with juvenile arthritis have a positive Rh factor.	Negative
Erythrocyte Sedimentation Rate (ESR)	Measures the speed at which RBCs settle out in solution.	Elevated indicates septic arthritis; may also indicate infection.	0–10 mm/hr
Blood Cultures	Measures whether organisms grow out in the laboratory.	Can identify an organism causing infection; 40% of children with septic arthritis have a positive blood culture.	No growth
Bone Biopsies	Diagnose tumor or infection of the bone.	Osteomyelitis Bone tumor	Normal bone cells
Fluid Aspiration from Joints	Diagnose an infection of the joint or drain fluid from a joint to relieve pressure.	Drainage is purulent. Culture of fluid is positive.	Clear fluid No growth from culture

MEDICATIONS

Medications for Juvenile Arthritis (JA)

- Use approved nonsteroidal anti-inflammatory drugs (NSAIDs): Ibuprofen (Children's Advil), naproxen (Aleve), tolmetin (Tolectin), and choline magnesium trisalicylate (Trilisate), indomethacin (Indocin), and diclofenac (Cataflam). An NSAID is selected based on dosing schedule, patient preference, or medication taste because there is a lack of agreement on the best NSAID for patients with Juvenile Arthritis (JA).

- Common disease-modifying antirheumatic drugs (an agent that prevents or relieves rheumatism) (DMARDs): medications are methotrexate (Rheumatrex) (most commonly prescribed), cyclophosphamide (Cytoxan), sulfasalazine (Azulfidine) and infliximab (Remicade). It is effective in polyarticular JA and has been used for the past 10 years. The most common side effect of methotrexate (Rheumatrex) is gastrointestinal symptoms.

- New drugs potentially available for use with juvenile arthritis are leflunomide (Arava) and etanercept (Enbrel). Leflunomide is an immunosuppressant. Side effects are diarrhea, elevated liver enzymes, alopecia, and rash. It has been approved for use in patients with adult rheumatoid arthritis (RA), but has not yet been approved for use with children. There is a teratogenic potential that would be of concern with children, particularly adolescent girls. Etanercept (Enbrel) reduces the signs and symptoms of moderately severe to severe polyarticular juvenile arthritis. It is a potent inhibitor of tumor necrosis factor (TNF), which is a key proinflammatory cytokine found in the synovial tissue of patients with JA (Ilowite, 2002).

- Infliximab (Remicade) is another TNF-neutralizing agent. Efficacy data are limited for use of this medication.

- Prednisone (Deltasone) and other corticosteroids are very potent and should be administered at the lowest possible dose and for the shortest possible period of time. Side effects such as Cushing syndrome, osteoporosis, increased risk of infection, glucose intolerance, cataracts, and growth retardation can occur.

Neuromuscular Blocking Agent

When caring for a child treated with a neuromuscular blocking agent, remember:

- The child has total paralysis, including respiratory function.
- The child is not able to communicate.
- The child is anxious.
- The child is aware of all activity around him or her.

The nurse can:

- Anticipate the child's needs.
- Explain all procedures.
- Never leave the child alone.
- Reduce the child's anxiety (e.g., use a calm and reassuring manner, support her fear, encourage parents to stay with the child).
- Medicate with an anxiolytic (antianxiety agent).

Medications Used in Tetanus (Lockjaw)

Medications are used to alleviate the muscle spasms and seizures.

- Diazepam (Valium) is the drug of choice to control seizures.
- Lorazepam (Ativan) is an anticonvulsant. It may cause respiratory depression, especially when used in combination with other sedatives. Onset of action is 1 to 5 minutes intravenously, 30 to 60 minutes intramuscularly and 20 to 30 minutes orally, with a duration of action of 6 to 8 hours.
- Intrathecal baclofen (Lioresal) is a centrally reacting skeletal muscle relaxant. Avoid abrupt withdrawal. Administer oral doses with food or milk. Use with caution in children with a seizure disorder or impaired renal function (Robertson & Shilkofski, 2005).
- Dantrolene sodium (Dantrium) is a skeletal muscle relaxant. Use caution when administering to a child with cardiac or pulmonary impairment. Avoid unnecessary exposure to light. Do not allow it to extravasate into the surrounding tissue. Discontinue if benefits are not evident in 45 days (Robertson & Shilkofski, 2005).
- Midazolam (Versed) may be effective, but is contraindicated in patients with narrow-angle glaucoma and shock because

it causes respiratory depression, hypotension, and bradycardia. Cardiovascular monitoring is necessary. Reduce doses when given in combination with narcotics or in patients with respiratory compromise. Serum concentrations may be increased by cimetidine (Tagamet), erythromycin, itraconazole, ketoconazole, and protease inhibitors. Sedative effects may be antagonized by theophylline. The effects of the medication can be reversed with flumazenil (Romazicon) (Robertson & Shilkofski, 2005).

- Use neuromuscular blocking agents when the child is suffering severe unresponsive tetanus. The following are two nondepolarizing neuromuscular blocking agents:

Rocuronium (Zemuron) may cause hypertension, hypotension, tachycardia, and bronchospasm. There is a risk of increased neuromuscular blockade when administered in conjunction with aminoglycosides, clindamycin, tetracycline, magnesium sulfate, quinine, quinidine, succinylcholine, and inhalation anesthetics. There is a risk of a reduction in neuromuscular blocking effects when used in conjunction with carbamazepine, phenytoin, azathioprine, and theophylline. Peak effects occur in 0.5 to 1 minute. Duration is 30 to 40 minutes (Robertson & Shilkofski, 2005).

- Vecuronium bromide (Norcuron) may cause arrhythmias, rash, and bronchospasm. Use with caution in patients with renal or hepatic failure and neuromuscular disease. Infants from 7 weeks to 1 year of age are more sensitive to the medication and may have a longer recovery period. Children from 1 to 10 years may need higher and more frequent doses. Potency can be increased with administration of enflurane, isoflurane, aminoglycosides, magnesium salts, tetracyclines, bacitracin, and clindamycin. Neostigmine, pyridostigmine and edrophonium are antidotes. Onset is 1 to 3 minutes. Duration is 30-90 minutes (Robertson & Shilkofski, 2005).

ETHNOCULTURAL CONSIDERATIONS

Caring for a Hispanic Child

Hispanics have the following beliefs and they must be respected:

- "Mal ojo" or Evil Eye is an illness that affects a child when someone with special powers looks at or admires the child but does not touch the child. Touching a Hispanic child when making an admiring statement is important.

- Curanderos and curanderas treat a child through touch and prayer and have the child wear special amulets or charms to protect her.
- Saints help sick children and parents place holy pictures around the sick child.

TEACHING THE FAMILY

Instructions for Caregivers of a Child Who Is Casted for Clubfoot

- Call the physician if the child has a fever, infection, cast syndrome, or unrelieved pain.
- Take the child to the health care professional if the cast becomes loose, soft, or cracked.
- Perform good hygiene to prevent skin breakdown.
- Stimulate the child's development by reading and playing.
- Provide reassurance that when the cast is removed the child will quickly return to the expected developmental level.
- Encourage compliance with follow-up because there is potential for recurrence. Make first follow-up appointment with the parents for the child before the child is discharged.

Osteogenesis Imperfecta

Teach parents to:

- Watch for signs of a fracture (irritability, fever, refusal to eat).
- With an older child, watch for pain, swelling, and possible deformity at the site.

ADDITIONAL INFORMATION FOR THE CLINICAL SETTING

Preventing Cast Syndrome

- Reposition the child frequently.
- Encourage fluids and increased fiber in the child's diet.
- Cut a "belly hole" or a window to allow for abdominal expansion.

Procedure 27-1 Petaling a Cast

Purpose

The purpose of petaling a cast is to promote good hygiene by protecting the proximal edges of the long leg casts and the perineal area of the hip-spica casts from soiling.

Equipment

- Moleskin
- 1-inch waterproof adhesive tape
- Plastic bag to place adhesive tape on
- Scissors

Steps

1. Use scissors to cut 1-inch wide by 1 1/2 to 2 inches long strips of moleskin.

2. Use scissors to cut 1-inch wide strips of waterproof adhesive tape.

   The length of the waterproof adhesive tape should be about 1 1/2 to 2 inches long.

3. The edge on one end of both the moleskin and waterproof adhesive tape must be rounded.

4. Place strips of the 1-inch waterproof adhesive tape on the plastic bags.

5. Apply the first strip of waterproof adhesive tape to any edge of the cast that is likely to become soiled by urine or stool. Place the rounded ends of the moleskin and adhesive tape over the cast edge to the outside.

6. Tuck the straight (unrounded) end inside the cast.

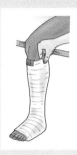

Procedure 27-1 (Continued)

7. With your forefinger, gently ensure that the inside end is flat and not sticking to the child's skin.

8. Repeat the procedure, overlapping each additional strip, until all rough edges are completely covered.

9. Begin the same procedure with the moleskin to edges of the cast that are not likely to become soiled by urine and stool.

10. Document the procedure.

Clinical Alert It is a good idea to petal the edges of the cast that are likely to be soiled by urine and feces on the first postoperative day and preferably before the Foley catheter is removed.

Teach Parents

The nurse can teach the parents that diapering needs to be modified. To achieve this, a small diaper or peripad is placed in the perineal area with all edges of the cast outside this small diaper. Then a larger diaper is placed outside the smaller diaper and taped in the normal fashion. The nurse needs to ensure that the perineal edges of the cast remain outside of the diaper.

Skin Traction

Skin traction is used for an extremity with a type of strapping material applied to the limb. It is used for short periods of time.

Russell's Traction

- Used when the child weighs more than 26.4 lbs. (12 kg).
- Most often used to stabilize femur fractures until a callus forms or with Legg–Calve–Perthes disease.
- The child lies supine with hip flexed and abducted.
- There are two lines of pull in Russell's traction and the hips need to remain in alignment (Fig. 27-3).
- Secure a trapeze on a cross-bar above the bed to assist with repositioning and maintaining upper body strength.
- A sling is placed under the knee. Assess placement of the sling frequently.
- Increase countertraction with the foot of the bed elevated and the head of the bed flat.

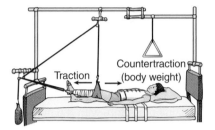

Figure 27-3 Russell's traction.

Skeletal Traction

Skeletal traction is used for long periods of time until the bone is ready for casting or open reduction (surgery to place the bones in their proper position).

- Crutchfield tongs: Used to treat cervical and thoracic fractures; tongs are placed into the skull (Fig. 27-4).
- 90/90 femoral traction: Most commonly used to treat femur fractures and complicated femur fractures (Fig. 27-5).
- Dunlop traction: Used to treat supracondylar fractures of humerus (Fig. 27-6).

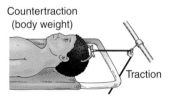

Figure 27-4 Crutchfield tongs.

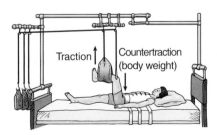

Figure 27-5 90/90 femoral traction.

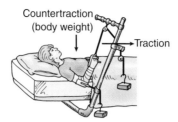

Figure 27-6 Dunlop traction.

Preventing Pneumonia

- Include assessment and methods to increase lung expansion.
- Initiate incentive spirometry in school-age and adolescent children.
- In younger children who cannot comprehend the concept of spirometry, encourage the same concept through other means (e.g., blowing bubbles or a party favor).

Talipes Equinovarus (Clubfoot)

When caring for an infant just delivered with clubfoot, the nurse can ask questions such as:

- "How are you feeling at this time?"
- "Do you know what this condition is called?"
- "Do you know anything about clubfoot?"
- "Can I stay with you to offer support while you hold the baby?"
- "After you rest we can talk more about the baby's condition."

Legg–Calve–Perthes Disease

There are four stages of Legg–Calve–Perthes Disease (LCPD):

- Aseptic necrosis (flattening of femoral head): Lasts several weeks, is characterized by synovitis and a decrease in ossification in the nucleus of the femoral head secondary to ischemia.
- Revascularization: Lasts 6 to 12 months, is characterized by increased joint space, increased cartilage thickness, and a decrease in size and density of femoral head.

- New bone formation: Lasts 1 to 2 years, is characterized by collapse and superolateral displaced head, and avascular bone is reabsorbed.
- Regenerative phase: Reconstitution of femoral head with remodeling and final healing.

Visiting Nurse's Responsibilities with a Child with Legg–Calve–Perthes Disease

- Assess the family's support systems in their own environment.
- Ensure that the family is able to provide the care needed.
- Ensure compliance with the use of the conservative devices.
- Ensure the non–weight-bearing status of the child.
- Assess the knowledge of the parents and child about ongoing care.
- Encourage the use of creative quiet activities and hobbies.
- Ask the family about follow-up care with the physician.

Caring for a Child with a Fracture in a Cast

- Elevate the casted extremity on pillows for at least the first 24 hours.
- Avoid indenting the cast.
- Observe the extremity for swelling and discoloration.
- Observe the extremity for sensation and movement.
- Call the health care professional if abnormalities are noted.
- Follow activity restrictions.
- Do not allow the affected limb to hang down for any length of time.
- Prevent the child from putting anything inside the cast.
- Keep a clear path for ambulation.
- Ensure the child uses crutches appropriately.
- Encourage rest.
- Encourage quiet activities.
- Instruct the child to move joints above and below cast.

Soft Tissue Injuries

Immediately after the initial injury, use the RICE acronym:

R: Rest the injured extremity prevents further injury and allows the ligament to heal.

I: Ice for the first 48 hours; keep ice packs in place for 15-minute intervals to decrease swelling.

C: Compression; apply an ace wrap or some other method to apply pressure to the affected joint to help reduce swelling of the joint.

E: Elevation and early motion of the affected joint; elevation reduces swelling and early motion of the affected joint helps keep the full range of motion of the joint.

Log Rolling

- Use log rolling to turn the child in Crutchfield tongs or after a spinal fusion.
- Two or more nurses turn the patient in complete unison.
- Turn head, shoulders, hips, and legs as one unit, keeping the back in a straight line (Fig. 27-7).

Tetanus (Lockjaw)

Signs and Symptoms

- Progressive stiffness and tenderness of the muscles in the neck and jaw
- Trismus (difficulty opening the mouth)
- Risus sardonicus (a peculiar grin)
- Opisthotonus posturing
- Laryngospasm of the respiratory muscles
- Tetanus prophylaxis through immunization is the key to preventing tetanus

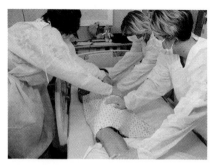

Figure 27-7 Logrolling technique.

Nursing Care
- Tetanus immune globulin (TIG) and antibiotics
- Closely monitored and respiratory support
- Fluids and electrolytes as well as caloric intake monitored
- Nasogastric (NG) feedings or Total Parental Nutrition (TPN)
- Endotracheal (ET) intubation (laryngospasms)
- Eliminate stimulation
- Frequent neurological assessments
- O_2 saturation and blood gases
- Oropharyngeal suctioning
- Medications
- Hydration and nutrition
- Collaboration

RESOURCES

Arthritis Foundation: http://www.arthritis.org

Muscular Dystrophy Association: http://www.mdausa.org

Osteogenesis Imperfecta Foundation: http://www.oif.org

REFERENCES

Ilowite, N. (2002). Current treatment of juvenile rheumatoid arthritis. *Pediatrics, 109*, 109–115.

Robertson, J., & Shilkofski, N. (2005). *Harriet Lane handbook: A manual for pediatric house officers,* 17th ed. St. Louis, MO: C.V. Mosby.

Venes, D. (Ed.). (2005). *Taber's cyclopedic medical dictionary* (20th ed.). Philadelphia: F.A. Davis.

Caring for the Child with an Integumentary Condition

KEY TERMS

dermis – Layer of skin containing the nerves, muscles, connective tissue, sebaceous and sweat glands, blood vessels, and lymph channels

epidermis – Layer of skin that serves as the outlet for the sweat glands and through which the hair follicles protrude

FOCUSED ASSESSMENT

Common Skin Lesions and Associated Conditions

Lesion Name	Description	Examples
Macule	Flat, circumscribed area that has color change and is <1 cm in diameter	Freckles Flat moles Petechiae Measles Scarlet fever
Papule	Raised, circumscribed area <1 cm diameter	Warts Moles Lichen planus Scabies
Patch	Macule that is flat, nonpalpable, of irregular shape, and >1 cm diameter	Port-wine stains Café-au-lait spots
Nodule	Raised, firm, circumscribed (deeper than a papule) 1–2 cm diameter	Lipomas Erythema nodosum
Tumor	Raised and solid. May be clear, deep in the dermis, <2 cm in diameter.	Lipoma Hemangiomas Neoplasms Benign tumors
Vesicle	Raised, circumscribed, superficial, filled with serous fluid, <1 cm in diameter	Varicella Herpes zoster (shingles)
Pustule	Raised, superficial-like vesicle, but fluid is purulent	Impetigo Acne

Lesion Name	Description	Examples
Bulla	Vesicle >1 cm in diameter	Blister
Wheal	Raised, irregular shape, cutaneous swelling, solid. Diameter is variable (usually transient)	Urticaria Insect bites Allergic reaction
Crust	Dried body fluid on the skin surface: serum, pus, or blood	Disease where the skin weeps: eczema, impetigo, seborrhea
Scales	Raised cluster of keratinized cells, irregular, diameter is variable, can be thick or thin, dry or oily	Seborrheic dermatitis Dry skin Skin flaking after allergic reaction
Lichenification	Rough, thickened epidermal area often in the flexor surface of extremity	Chronic dermatitis
Scar	Fibrous tissue, thin or thick, coloration may be lighter or darker than surrounding skin	Healing wound of any etiology
Keloid	Fibrous tissue (scar) of irregular shape, raised and grown beyond the boundary of the original wound	Postoperative wound healing (more common in persons of color)

(continued)

Common Skin Lesions and Associated Conditions (Continued)

Lesion Name	Description	Examples
Fissure	Linear crack in the epidermis may be deeper, moist or dry	Athlete's foot Cracks at the corner the mouth or anus
Erosion	Depressed, moist, loss of part of the epidermis	After rupture of vesicle or bulla, e.g., varicella
Ulcer	Concave, moist, loss of epidermis and dermis	Ulceration: stasis, decubitus

Adapted from Potter & Perry (2004).

Questions for Assessing Acne in an Adolescent

- When did your acne begin?
- What types of cleaning products, makeup, or moisturizers and hair care products are you currently using?
- Can you tell me what medications you are taking? Please include over-the-counter and natural products.
- What type of foods do you eat?
- Have you noticed any foods, activities, or environmental factors that affect your acne?
- Do you notice a change in your acne related to your menses? (female patients)
- What other dermatological problems have you had recently or in the past?
- Can you tell me how you feel about having acne?

Ringworm

The most common ringworm infections are as follows:

- Tinea capitis: Involves the hair of the scalp, usually seen in prepubertal children between the ages of 1 and 10 years.

- Tinea corporis: Involves the skin of the body, except the scalp, groin, hands, and feet; seen in children and adolescents.
- Tinea cruris: Known as "jock itch"; involves the inner thighs, inguinal creases, or perineal area (rare before adolescence).
- Tinea pedi: Athlete's foot, involves the kinesthetic webbed areas of the toes and feet; seen in children and adolescents.

Assessing for a Systemic Allergic Response

The nurse must recognize the key assessments in a systemic allergic response.

- Assess for edema or laryngospasms in the airway, which has the potential to cause blockage.
- Assess for cyanosis and listen for audible sounds of upper airway respiratory distress such as wheezing or stridor.
- Assess the vital signs, specifically hypotension.

Lyme Disease Presents in Three Stages

- In the first stage, days to weeks after the tick bite, the child has a mild local rash. The rash from Lyme disease may occur as a bull's-eye rash or as disseminated erythematous (red) rash and erythema migrans (bulls-eye rash) (CDC, 2005b).
- Other symptoms include headache, nuchal rigidity (stiff neck), and joint and muscle pain.
- In the second stage, the disease may last from a few days to up to 10 months after the tick bite. During stage 2, the infection spreads through the blood and the child may exhibit signs of arthritis (especially in the knees), arthralgia (muscle pain), cardiac dysrhythmias, lymphadenopathy, pericarditis, or meningoencephalitis.
- In the third stage, lasting from weeks to years after the tick bite (chronic stage), the child develops mild to severe arthritis. Neurological symptoms that occur in stage 3 include cranial nerve palsy, depression, meningitis, neuropathy, radiculopathy, and encephalopathy.

Questions for Gathering Important Information About Burns

- What was the offending agent?
- When did this burn occur?
- Who was present or witnessed the injury?
- What first aid was given?
- How did the burn feel when it first occurred?
- How does the burn feel now?
- Has the child had any like accidents or injuries before?
- What other medical history is important?

Classifying Hypothermia		
Classification	Body Temperature	Clinical Signs and Symptoms
Mild	90°–95°F (32.2°–35°C)	Shivering, rapid heart rate, rapid respiratory rate, vasoconstriction, increased urine output As temperature decreases, the child displays apathy, lethargy, and impaired judgment
Moderate	82.4°–90°F (28°–32.3°C)	Decreased heart rate, decreased respiratory rate, hypotension, loss of consciousness, decreased pupillary response
Severe	<82.4°F (<28°C)	Apnea, asystole, coma It may not be possible to readily differentiate between severe hypothermia and death

Source: McCullough, L., & Arora, S. (2004).

CLINICAL ALERTS

Group A *Streptococcus*

Group A *Streptococcus* can cause necrotizing fasciitis (flesh-eating bacteria). Be alert to the following clinical manifestations of necrotizing fasciitis:

- Bruising
- Crepitus
- Bullae filled with bluish/purple colored fluid over the induration (Lipsky, 2003).

Stevens–Johnson Syndrome (Erythema Multiforme)

Stevens-Johnson syndrome (also known as erythema multiforme) is a serious reaction that may be fatal (Knowles, Shapiro, & Shear, 2003; Venes, 2005).

- Stevens–Johnson syndrome is the leading cause of severe allergic response to a medication.
- This condition begins with a nonspecific upper respiratory system infection; however, the defining signs of this condition are bullae that appear on the lips, mouth, eyes, and genitalia, often in a target-like pattern.
- It is essential to eliminate the causative agent.
- Treat the skin lesions using aseptic technique along with an air- or fluid-filled bed, nutritional support, IV fluids, and pain management.
- Antibiotics can be given for secondary infections and an ophthalmologist should be contacted to assess for lesions in the eyes.
- As the fluid-filled lesions erupt and slough off internally and externally it is vital to ensure a patent airway. This may progress to the necessity of intubation and mechanical ventilation.
- As these lesions rupture large amounts of body surface area may become exposed. The child may experience large fluid losses and should be treated similarly to a burn patient.

A Severe Reaction to a Bite

A child who has had a severe reaction to bees or wasps should wear a medical alert bracelet or necklace and carry an EpiPen (epinephrine) or EpiPen Jr.

Material Safety Data Sheets

To protect personal and patient safety the nurse must:

- Know where to find material safety data sheets (MSDS) in your facility.
- Know your facility's special telephone hotline for MSDS information (usually in case of chemical exposure).
- Know the telephone number of the local poison control center, where you can receive accurate telephone advice and faxed information on management of spilled chemicals or ingested substances.

Hypothermia

- Hypothermia in children may have a metabolic or neurological etiology.
- The cause of hypothermia must be investigated when no environmental explanation is appropriate.
- Wet clothes increase the risk and should be removed as soon as possible and replaced with dry clothes.

DIAGNOSTIC TESTS

Monitoring Isotretinoin Therapy

- Approval for continued isotretinoin (Accutane) therapy depends on the patient's willingness to comply with pregnancy testing (girls) and blood testing of liver enzymes (both girls and boys).
- Liver enzymes must be tested once a month to ensure that liver damage is not occurring from the isotretinoin (Accutane).
- Teens are particularly difficult to manage because of their developmental age. They may feel invincible and may be less likely to comply with treatment unless they see a quick and direct improvement in their acne.

 Procedure 28-1 Obtaining a Fungal Culture

Purpose

To test for the presence of fungi and, if found, to identify the type.

Equipment

- Gloves
- Tongue blade
- Sterile cotton swab
- Sterile test tube

Steps

1. Explain the procedure to the child in age-appropriate terms.
2. Gather all supplies.
3. Using aseptic technique, place a sterile cotton swab against a plaque.
4. Vigorously rub the plaque with the cotton swab.

5. Place the swab into a covered, sterile test tube provided by the laboratory and place in a biohazard bag.

6. Have the specimen transported to the lab within 15–30 minutes to ensure accurate test results.

7. Monitor the child's oral mucosa for bleeding, which may result from attempting to remove the oral thrush (Elewski, 2002).

8. Explain to parents that final culture results will not be available for 48 to 72 hours, although preliminary results may be available sooner.

9. Document the procedure.

Clinical Alert The nurse must remember that attempting to remove the oral thrush can cause the lining of the oral mucosa to bleed.

Teach Parents

The final culture is not available for 48–72 hours; preliminary culture results may be available sooner.

Laboratory Results in Rocky Mountain Spotted Fever

Expect elevated white blood cells (WBCs), thrombocytopenia (low platelets), hyponatremia (decreased sodium in the blood), and elevated liver enzymes (CDC, 2005a). The child's WBCs will likely remain low in the early stage and rise to slightly abnormal in later stages.

WBCs: 5,000–10,000/mm³ (later stage: 10,000–12,000/mm³)
Platelets: 150,000–400,000/mm³ (thrombocytopenia: <150,000/mm³)
Sodium: 136–145 mEq/L (hyponatremia: <136 mEq/L)
Bilirubin (total): 0.3–1.0 mg/dL (hyperbilirubinemia: >1.0 mg/dL)
Urine testing may reveal red blood cells and protein (Gandhi, 2005).

MEDICATIONS

Tetracycline (Sumycin)

- Tetracycline (Sumycin) will autofluorescence in the presence of ultraviolet light, thus making the person noticeably "glow" in environments that are lit by black lights.

- Tetracycline (Sumycin) can also darken the teeth in children younger than the age of 8 years and should not be used in this age group.

Isotretinoin (Accutane)

- Isotretinoin (Accutane) causes severe birth defects.
- Women must not take this medication if there is any chance of becoming pregnant because of the risk of birth defects. It is important to discuss this with adolescents if pregnancy is a possibility.
- Pregnancy tests must be performed before treatment with this medication, monthly during treatment, and 1 month after the cessation of treatment.
- In addition, women must use two forms of birth control if considering this treatment.
- Visit iPLEDGE: Committed to Pregnancy Prevention program at http://www.ipledgeprogram.com/ to view the information appropriate for clients undergoing isotretinoin (Accutane) treatment.
- Other side effects include hypercholesteremia, drying of the mucous membranes, decrease in night vision, headaches, depression, and liver damage.

Benzathine Penicillin G (ben-za-theen pen-i-sill-in gee)
Bicillin L-A

Pregnancy Category B

Indications Treatment of a wide variety of infections: pharyngeal/tonsil/skin.
Prophylaxis for rheumatic fever

Actions Binds to bacterial cell wall, resulting in cell death.

Therapeutic Effects Bacteriostatic action against susceptible bacterial spectrum: Streptococci, staphylococci, and some gram-negative organisms

Pharmacokinetics
Absorption IM delayed and prolonged to sustain therapeutic blood levels.

Contraindications and Precautions Contraindicated in hypersensitivity

Adverse Reactions and Side Effects
Pain at injection site.

GI Diarrhea, epigastric distress, nausea/vomiting
Endocrine Rash
Respiratory Anaphylaxis

Route and Dosage
IM: Children >27 kg, 900–1.2 million units (single dose). **IM:** Children <27 kg, 300,000–600,000 units (single dose)

Nursing Implications
Assess for history of hypersensitivity.
Observe the patient for signs of anaphylaxis for a minimum of 15 minutes after injection.
Reconstitute with D_5W or 0.9% NaCl.
Administer deep into a well-developed muscle mass.

Data from Deglin, J., & Vallerand, A. (2009). Davis's drug guide for nurses (11th ed.), pp. 958–961. Philadelphia: F.A. Davis.

Ibuprofen (eye-byoo-**proe**-fen) Children's Advil/Motrin

Pregnancy Category B (first trimester)

Indications Mild to moderate pain. Inflammation

Actions Inhibits prostaglandin synthesis.

Therapeutic Effects Antipyretic, analgesic, nonsteroidal anti-inflammatory, antirheumatic

Pharmacokinetics
Absorption Well absorbed from the GI tract

Contraindications and Precautions Contraindicated in hypersensitivity. Cross-sensitivity with other nonsteroidal anti-inflammatory drugs (NSAIDs) and aspirin

Adverse Reactions and Side Effects Headache, constipation, nausea/vomiting

Route and Dosage
PO: Children 6 months–12 years: 20–40 mg/kg/day in 3–4 divided doses/day (every 6–8 hours).

Nursing Implications
Assess for history of sensitivity.
Assess pain and monitor temperature (if given as an antipyretic).
Ibuprofen may cause anticoagulation effects.

Data from Deglin, J., & Vallerand, A. (2009). Davis's drug guide for nurses (11th ed.), pp. 654–656. Philadelphia: F.A. Davis.

Topical Treatments

Classification	Names	Precautions
Anesthetics	Benzocaine (Americaine) Lidocaine and prilocaine (EMLA)	Allergy Do not use over wounds. Do not use over large areas; avoid the eyes.
Antibacterial	Bacitracin and polymyxin B (AK-Poly-Bac) Neomycin (Myciguent) Mupirocin (Bactroban)	Allergy Existing infection (for prevention of infection) Antibiotic resistance Use for only minor cuts/scrapes/burns.
Antifungal	Clotrimazole (Lotrimin) Ketoconazole (Nizoral) Miconazole (Aloe Vesta) Nystatin (Mycostatin)	Cautious use in nail and scalp infections
Anti-itch	Diphenhydramine (Benadryl)	Allergy Photosensitivity
Emollients	White petrolatum jelly Mineral oil Lanolin Glycerin	Allergy Choose fragrance-free products.
Steroids	Varying strengths Strongest: Group I: betamethasone (Diprolene) Group II: Desoximetasone (Decadron) Group III: Triamcinolone 0.5% (Kenalog) Group IV: Fluocinolone (Lidex) Group V: Hydrocortisone 0.2% (A-Hydrocort) Group VI: Desonide (Tridesilon) Group VII: Hydrocortisone 1% (A-Hydrocort)	Allergy Repeated use in the same area of the skin will cause thinning of the skin May inhibit the skin's ability to fight infection. Should be used in the lowest strength on the thin skin of the face and genitalia. Avoid the eye area: places the client at risk for glaucoma or cataract formation.

Data from Deglin, J., & Vallerand, A. (2009). *Davis's drug guide for nurses* (11th ed.). Philadelphia: F.A. Davis.

Topical Agents

- Topical agents that promote healing are frequently used for rashes: cow udder balm (bag balm), green tea extract, vitamin E preparations, aloe vera, milk, calamine, and colloidal oatmeal (Beltrani, 2002).

ETHNOCULTURAL CONSIDERATIONS

Vulnerable Populations

African Americans and Native Americans (CDC, 2006) and persons living in rural areas (Ahrens, 2001) are most vulnerable to fire-related injuries and death.

Pressure Ulcers

In children with dark pigmented skin, blanching may look red or purple.

TEACHING THE FAMILY

Impetigo

For a child with impetigo, teach the child and family the following:

- Wash your hands thoroughly and often.
- Do not scratch the lesions.

Cellulitis

- Teach the caregiver the following: Administer all antibiotics as ordered, even if the skin improves before completing the antibiotic course, because failure to finish the antibiotic may lead to recurrence of the infection.
- Use warm, moist packs to relieve discomfort as needed. Cool, moist packs are also acceptable if they relieve discomfort.
- Administer an analgesic, such as ibuprofen (Children's Advil) or acetaminophen (Children's Tylenol), if needed for comfort.
- If the infection is in a limb, elevate the limb to reduce swelling and increase comfort.
- Contact the physician if redness or edema worsens, if the child's pain increases, or if temperature remains above 101.5°F (38.6°C) for 48 hours after starting the antibiotic.

(Thomson Micromedex, 2006)

Herpes Simples Virus (HSV-1)

To decrease transmission of the virus and prevent future outbreaks, teach the child to do the following:

- Keep his hands away from his face.
- Wash his hands thoroughly. (To ensure that a young child washes for the proper amount of time, teach him to sing the alphabet song while washing.)
- Decrease stress.
- Avoid prolonged sun exposure.
- Use a moisturizing sunscreen on the lips during summer months.

(Hurtado, 2005)

Lice (Pediculosis)

Teach caregivers the following:

- To detect lice, examine the child's head under good lighting. Pay particular attention to areas behind the ears and at the nape of the neck.
- To treat lice, use an over-the-counter shampoo that contains permethrin (for an infant or young child) or lindane (for an older child).
- Wash the child's hair according to the instructions on the product.
- After shampoo is rinsed from the hair, remove nits by backcombing with a fine-tooth comb. Nits are easier to remove when the hair is damp.
- If the child cannot tolerate the medicated shampoo, an asphyxiant such as petrolatum or food oil (e.g., olive oil) may be used (Wiederkehr & Schwartz, 2003).
- Nits on eyelashes may be removed by applying petrolatum to the eyelashes twice daily for 8 days.
- Clean the home thoroughly (dust, vacuum, scrub), wash clothing and bedding, and wipe hats, bicycle helmet, and toys.
- If a soft or cloth toy is not washable, it must be placed in a sealed plastic bag away from family members' rooms for 14 days.
- All bed linens should be laundered in hot water and dried in a dryer.
- Pillows used by the child should be thrown away.
- Anti-lice spray can be used for furniture and other environmental objects that are not disposable.

- Hair-care items can be boiled (hot water above 140°F) or soaked in anti-lice shampoo and should never be shared.
- The child should stay home from school until lice-free, in keeping with the school's anti-lice policy. The child may need to be checked by the school nurse or day care provider before returning.
- The child should be rechecked for lice in 7 to 10 days if the itching resumes, if itching disrupts the child's sleep, or if the condition fails to clear after 1 week of treatment.
- More information is available from the National Pediculosis Association at http://www.headlice.org

Animal Bite Prevention

Teach children and families the following:

- Never leave a child alone with an animal.
- Never put your face close to an animal.
- Never tease or overexcite an animal.
- Avoid dogs and other animals that you do not know.
- Ask the owner's permission before touching or petting an animal.
- Play with animals only under adult supervision.
- Report strange animal behavior, even if you know the animal.
- Do not disturb animals that are eating, sleeping, or feeding their young.
- Spay or neuter pets to reduce aggression.
- Stay away from wild animals.
- Do not run away from an aggressive animal; instead, lie down in a ball, protect your face, and stay quiet.

(National Center for Injury Prevention and Control, 2008)

Burn Prevention

Teach parents the following:

- Set the home water heater no higher than 120°F to prevent scald injuries.
- When cooking, turn pot handles inward so children cannot reach them.
- Make sure electrical cords from cooking appliances are not dangling within the child's reach.

Managing Minor Burns

Teach parents and caregivers the following:

- Remove any clothing that is hot or has been in contact with an offending chemical.
- Cool a burn immediately using gauze or a clean cloth soaked in cool (54°F) saline solution or water.
- Do not put ice on a burn.
- Wash a wound with mild soap, and rinse well with water.
- Bacitracin (Baciguent) may be used topically to prevent infection. For moderate or major burns, the child will receive a different type of anti-infective and a tetanus booster.
- Cover the burn with gauze to prevent infection, decrease pain, and absorb drainage.
- Give acetaminophen (Children's Tylenol) or ibuprofen (Children's Advil) to decrease pain. If pain disrupts the child's sleep, play, or mood, give the medication on a schedule (Morgan, Bledsoe, & Barker, 2000).

Frostbite

Teach parents and caregivers the following:

- Place the child in a warm area, remove all wet and cold clothing, and replace with warm ones.
- If frostbite is in the hands or feet, they are immersed in warm tap water (100°F) for up to one half hour (McCullough & Arora, 2004).
- Check the water temperature frequently, as the body part cools the tub of water.
- Do not run warm water directly from the tap over the area, as tap water can change in temperature rapidly based on use by other household members. The water must also be monitored closely so a secondary burn does not occur in the process of rewarming.
- Do not rewarm the frozen part with massage or dry heat (McCullough & Arora, 2004).
- After rewarming is complete, the extremity is wrapped in a soft cloth and the child can be encouraged to rest.
- If no subsequent problems arise, the child can remove the soft cloth and return to inside activities.
- If parents suspect continued problems the heath care provider is called.

ADDITIONAL INFORMATION FOR THE CLINICAL SETTING

Infant Skin and Temperature

An infant's skin is very thin and contains very little subcutaneous fat. Temperature regulation becomes an important issue, as the infant tends to lose heat rapidly.

- Do not to leave an infant uncovered and exposed for a prolonged time.

Superficial Wound Management

- Superficial wounds are often closed with tissue adhesives (DERMABOND) that work like glue.

Cleansing an Adolescent's Face and Treating Acne

Follow these steps, giving the adolescent as much autonomy as possible in cleansing and treating the area:

1. Wash hands thoroughly.
2. Use a warm, moist cloth and antibacterial soap to soak and soften the crusting.
3. Gently wipe away as much crusting as possible.
4. Apply the prescribed topical antibiotic ointment using a cotton swab or a gloved finger.
5. Apply water-soluble moisturizer.
6. Wash hands thoroughly.

Family Compliance

- The best outcome for a child receiving an antibiotic is for the family to be adherent and administer the entire medication as prescribed.
- If the family has a history of nonadherence to a medical plan, or if the child cannot take the medication as prescribed, the nurse must notify the healthcare provider immediately. The healthcare provider may then choose to order a single dose of intramuscular penicillin instead of the oral medication.
- Using a topical anesthetic such as EMLA (lidocaine/prilocaine) at the injection site at least an hour before the injection can help decrease the pain.

Human Papillomavirus: Warts

Type of Wart	Treatment	Description
Common Wart (verruca vulgaris)	Topical keratolytic acids (OTC)	Applied by dropper or cotton swab. Place thick liquid directly on top of the wart, taking care to keep the highly acidic fluid off the surrounding skin. The wart will peel away in layers as the acid kills the superficial layers, one at a time.
	Liquid nitrogen cryosurgery	Application of liquid nitrogen to the wart by a practitioner is a common method of removal. It is mildly painful but efficient. The practitioner directs a narrow flow of liquid nitrogen to the wart, freezing and therefore killing the wart tissue.
Flat Wart (verruca plana)	Topical tretinoin cream (prescription)	Treatment is applied in a thin coating via a gloved finger.
Plantar Wart (verruca plantaris)	Topical keratolytic acids	Applied by dropper or cotton swab. Place thick liquid directly on top of the wart, taking care to keep the highly acidic fluid off the surrounding skin.
	Liquid nitrogen cryosurgery (with paring and topical chemodestruction to enhance effectiveness).	Application of liquid nitrogen to the wart by a practitioner is a common method of removal. It is mildly painful but efficient. The practitioner directs a narrow flow of liquid nitrogen to the wart, freezing and therefore killing the wart tissue.

Source: Krusinski, P.A., & Flowers, F.P. (2000).

How to Tell Oral Thrush from Formula or Breast Milk on the Tongue of the Infant

Gently scrape the white film on the infant's tongue with a tongue blade. If it comes off, it is formula or breast milk. If it does not come off, it is thrush.

Preventing Atopic Dermatitis Secondary Infection

- Use good hygiene.
- Follow prescribed treatment protocols.

- Maintain skin hydration.
- Assess rash frequently.

Removing a Tick

1. Clean the skin with a topical antiseptic.
2. Don gloves.
3. Using tweezers, grasp the tick firmly, as close to the skin as possible.
4. Pull the tick out with a firm, steady motion. Do not twist the tick.
5. Clean the skin again with a topical antiseptic.
6. Seal the tick in a bag, write the date on the bag, and place it in the freezer in case the tick needs to be tested for disease.

Classifying Burns

Determine the extent of the burn by calculating the total body surface area (TBSA). TBSA can be determined by using several methods:

- Lund and Browder Chart or the Burn Calculations Rule of 9's (Fig. 28-1)
- Categorized according to severity

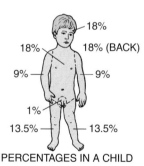

PERCENTAGES IN A CHILD

Figure 28-1 Rule of 9's.

Classification of Burn Severity		
Classification	Characteristics	Treatment
Mild	First or second degree, <10% body surface area (BSA) Third degree, <2% BSA No area of face, feet, hands, genitals burned	Can be treated on an outpatient basis.
Moderate	Second degree, 10%–20% BSA Third degree, <10% BSA	Can be treated in a burn unit or general hospital.
Severe	Second degree, >20% BSA Third degree, >10% BSA Burns on hands, feet, and genitals that may lead to functional impairment Smoke inhalation is present	Should be treated in a specialized burn center.

Sources: American Burn Association (2006); and Perry, C. (2003).

Criteria for Transfer to a Burn Center

- Partial-thickness burn over greater than 10% of body surface area (BSA)
- Burn involving face, hands, feet, or genitals
- Third-degree burn
- Electrical burn, including lightning injury
- Chemical burn
- Inhalation burn
- Burn injury in a person with a preexisting condition that could prolong the recovery period
- Burn injury in a person with coexisting trauma (e.g., fracture) when the burn poses a greater risk of morbidity or mortality than the trauma.
- The patient is a child in a facility without qualified personnel or equipment to care for a child.
- The patient needs special emotional, social, or long-term burn rehabilitation

(American Burn Association, 2006)

Overall Goals of Burn Treatment

The best outcome for a burned child considers the following interventions.

Burn Assessment

- The initial nursing assessment includes emergency care related to airway, breathing, and circulation (ABCs).
- After the ABCs are addressed and the child is being safely transported to an emergency room, the nurse or emergency medical technician (EMT) removes all clothing and jewelry to decrease continued burning at any site.
- Once the child is in a hospital, burn wounds are decontaminated and assessed for depth, surface area, and severity. The depth of the wounds is measured in millimeters or centimeters, circumference measurements are also necessary to provide a full clinical picture.
- The surface of the burn wound is assessed for color, blanching, desiccation (dryness), turgor/elasticity, blisters, or sloughed blisters.
- TBSA and all other skin assessments are taken into consideration to help classify the burn.

Fluid Resuscitation

- Children with burns greater than 15% of BSA require intravenous fluid resuscitation to maintain adequate perfusion.
- The IV fluid of choice is lactated Ringer's solution (Behrman, Kliegman, & Jenson, 2004).
- The Parkland formula is one means of determining the fluid needs of the child with a burn injury (Bollero et al., 2000). See page 568.
- Effectiveness of fluid resuscitation is monitored by adequate urine output. Normal urine output for children is 1 to 2 mL/kg per hour. If adequate urine output is not achieved, additional fluid resuscitation may be required.

Adequate Nutrition

- The caloric requirement for a patient with a >30% burn is 2000 to 2200 calories/day.
- In major burns enteral nutrition is necessary to keep up with the increased energy demand of the body, secondary to the stress response (Rimdeika et al., 2006).
- Enteral feeding is often initiated within 6 hours of the burn injury to support the child's increased needs.

Pain Management

- Initially morphine sulfate (Duramorph) is most commonly used for pain.

- The use of anxiolytics such as midazolam (Versed) or lorazepam (Ativan) is helpful
- Nonpharmacological interventions are also used

Meticulous Wound Care

- Wounds are initially decontaminated.
- Subsequent burn wound care includes cleansing the wound with a special solution or débridement.
- After cleansing, antibiotic ointment is applied and the wound is then re-dressed.
- Wounds can also be cleansed in a tub or a whirlpool, allowing the movement of the water to soften skin, and gently removing some loose dead skin.
- Escharotomy may be required if circulation or perfusion is impeded.
- Silvadene™ is the most commonly used burn cream to both prevent and treat burn infection.

Burn Recovery

- Burn injuries for children are managed by phases of recuperation as well as the type and severity of burns.
- The acute, or early phase, is from the time of the initial assault until wound closure.
- The second phase, recovery, is from the time of wound closure until scar maturation, which could be as long as 16 months (Selvaggi et al., 2005).
- For some children burn recovery may last a lifetime.

The Parkland Formula for Fluid Resuscitation

Fluid (milliliters) for first 24 hours: $4 \times$ patient's weight in kg $\times$ %TBSA

- Give half of the resulting IVF volume over the first 8 hours.
- Give the remaining half at an even rate over the next 16 hours.

Example: A child weighing 50 kg (110 lbs.) with a 20% TBSA burn
4 ml $\times$ 50 kg $\times$ 20% TBSA = 4000 mL.
First 8 hours, IVF = 2000 mL/8 hr = 250 mL/hr
Next 16 hours, IVF = 2000 mL/16 hr = 125 mL/hr
IVF = intravenous fluid; TBSA = total body surface area

(Behrman, Kliegman, & Jenson, 2004)

Using Distraction During Dressing Changes

- Use distraction techniques to reduce pain and anxiety based on the patient's age and developmental stage.
- Examples of distraction include singing, counting, watching television, focusing on a picture, talking about familiar events or places, playing a game, or blowing a pinwheel or bubbles.
- If the child is anxious or has severe pain, medication may be required before dressing changes.
- Praise the child when the dressing change is complete, focusing on all of the positive behaviors the child displayed.

Hypothermia

- Hypothermia is secondary to cold air exposure, wet clothes, and immersion in water.
- Hypothermia is a condition in which the child's core body temperature falls below 95°F (35°C).
- Hypothermia is a life-threatening emergency.

Types of Heat Loss	
Radiation	Heat loss from the head and areas with less subcutaneous fat and thin skin, e.g., prematurity of the newborn This is the most rapid method of heat loss and accounts for at least 50% of heat loss
Conduction	Transfer of heat away for the body by direct contact with a cooler surface, e.g., wet clothing or immersion
Convection	Transfer of heat away from the body by the movement of air over the skin surface, e.g., wind and drafts
Evaporation	Transfer of heat away from the body, e.g., skin moisture turned to vapor as it is dried by the movement of air
Respiration	Expiration of heat from the lungs, e.g., cold and windy weather

Pressure Ulcers

Pressure ulcers are the result of compression on one or more areas of the body for an extended period. Pressure ulcers occur when children and infants:

- Have decreased mobility.
- Have motor delays and cannot easily move their head or extremities.

- Have paralysis or other forms of limited mobility.
- Use mobility devices such as crutches, walkers, and wheelchairs.
- Have casts.
- Are malnourished.
- Have infections or anemia.
- Are bed bound for any period of time.
- Have decreased sensation to pressure or pain.

The four stages of ulcer formation can assist the nurse through skin assessment (Fig. 28-2).

Signs of Pressure Ulcer Formation

- The earliest sign of skin damage is a reddened area on the skin that does not disappear within 30 minutes of removing the cause of the pressure or irritant.
- The skin can appear to have an abrasion and look raw or rubbed.
- Further damage extends through the dermis forming the ulcer.

Nursing Care Related to Pressure Ulcer Formation

- Carefully inspect the child's skin at least three times a day, noting the color of the affected area, signs of infection, character of the skin lesion, wound edges, and drainage; measure the diameter; and determine the depth of the pressure ulcer.
- Address anemia by providing a diet high in iron.

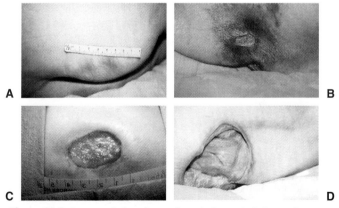

Figure 28-2 Stages of ulcer formation. *A.* Stage 1. *B.* Stage 2. *C.* Stage 3. *D.* Stage 4.

- Keep bed clothing straight and wrinkle-free to decrease areas of pressure.
- Use air, water, or gel mattresses and pads.
- Keep the child's skin both clean and dry.
- Keep the child off the affected area as much as possible.
- Stage 1 and 2 pressure ulcers are cleansed and allowed to dry.
- For stage 3: use hydrophilic gels or hydrocolloidal dressings for the ulcer.
- For stage 4 ulcers, surgical débridement and closure may be the treatment of choice.

Prevention of Pressure Ulcers

- Routinely move and shift the weight of the child off bony prominences on a regular basis.
- Move a child who is confined to bed at least every 2 hours.
- A child who is in a sitting position (e.g., in a wheelchair) should shift his weight every 15 minutes.
- If the child wears braces, inspect the skin for redness or irritation at least once a day. If any redness is noted, the nurse must not reapply the brace and notify the physician immediately.

RESOURCES

Braden Scale: http://www.bradenscale.com

iPLEDGE: Committed to Pregnancy Prevention: http://www.ipledgeprogram.com

National Pediculosis Association: http://www.headlice.org

Phoenix Society for Burn Survivors: http://www.phoenix-society.org

REFERENCES

Ahrens, M. (2001). The U.S. fire problem overview report: Leading causes and other patterns and trends [Electronic Version]. Quincy, MA: National Fire Protection Association.

American Burn Association (2006). National burn repository: 2005 report. Retrieved from http://www.ameriburn.org/NBR2005.pdf (Accessed July 27, 2008).

Behrman, R.E., Kliegman, R.M., & Jenson, H.B. (2004). *Nelson's textbook of pediatrics* (17th ed.). Philadelphia: W. B. Saunders.

Beltrani, V.S. (2002). An overview of chronic urticaria. *Clinical Reviews in Allergy and Immunology, 23*, 147–170.

Bollero, D., Stella, M., Calcagni, M., Guglielmotti, E., & Magliacani, G. (2000). Does inhalation injury really change fluid resuscitation needs? A retrospective analysis. *Annals of Burns and Fire Disasters. 13*, 198–200.

Centers for Disease Control and Prevention (CDC). (2005a, May). Rocky Mountain spotted fever. Retrieved from http://www.cdc.gov/ncidod/dvrd/rmsf/Epidemiology.htm (Accessed July 27, 2008).

Centers for Disease Control and Prevention (CDC). (2005b, October 7). Lyme disease prevention and control. Retrieved from http://www.cdc.gov/ncidod/dvbid/lyme/ld_prevent.htm (Accessed July 27, 2008).

Centers for Disease Control and Prevention (CDC). (2006, July 6). Mass casualties: Burns. Retrieved from http://www.bt.cdc.gov/masscasulties/burns.asp (Accessed July 27, 2008).

Deglin, J., & Vallerand, A. (2009). *Davis's drug guide for nurses.* (11th ed.). Philadelphia: F.A. Davis.

Elewski, B.E. (2002, January 24). Common fungal infections of the skin. Retrieved from http://merck.micromedex.com/index.asp?page=bpm_brief&article_id=CPM02DE405&hilight=candida|albicans (Accessed February 16, 2006).

Gandhi, M. (2005, June). Rocky mountain spotted fever. Retrieved from http://www.nlm.nih.gov/medlineplus/ency/article/000654.htm (Accessed July 27, 2008).

Hurtado, R. (2005). Herpes simplex. Retrieved from http://www.nlm.nih.gov/medlineplus/ency/article/001324.htm (Accessed July 28, 2008).

Knowles, S.R., Shapiro, L.E., & Shear, N.H. (2003, July). Cutaneous drug reactions. Retrieved from http://merck.micromedex.com/index.asp?page=bpm_brief&article_id=BPM01DE15&hilight=drug|reactions (Accessed February 27, 2006).

Krusinski, P.A., & Flowers, F.P. (2000, March). Common viral infection of the skin. Retrieved from http://merck.micromedex.com/index.asp?page=bpm_brief&article_id=CPM02DE404&hilight=herpesvirus (Accessed July 29, 2008).

Lipsky, B.A. (2003, July 1). Cellulitis, erysipelas, and necrotizing soft-tissue infections. Retrieved from http://merck.micromedex.com/index.asp?page=bpm_brief&article_id=BPM01ID08&hilight=cellulitis (Accessed February 25, 2006).

McCullough, L., & Arora, S. (2004). Diagnosis and treatment of hypothermia [Electronic Version]. *American Family Physician, 70*(12), 2325–2332.

Morgan, E.D., Bledsoe, S.C., & Barker, J. (2000). Ambulatory management of burns [Electronic Version]. *American Family Physician, 62*(9), 2015–2026.

National Center for Injury Prevention and Control. (2008). National dog bite prevention week. Retrieved from http://www.cdc.gov/ncipc/duip/biteprevention.htm (Accessed July 27, 2008).

Perry, C. (2003). Thermal injuries. In P.A. Maloney-Harmon & S.J. Czerwinski (Eds), *Nursing care of the pediatric trauma patient* (pp. 277–294). St. Louis, MO: W.B. Saunders.

Potter, P.A., & Perry, A.G. (2004). *Fundamentals of nursing* (6th ed.). St. Louis, MO: C. V. Mosby.

Rimdeika, R., Gudaviciene, D., Adamonis, K., Barauskas, G., Pavalkis, D., & Endzinas, Z. (2006). The effectiveness of caloric value of enteral nutrition in patients with major burns. *Burns: Journal of the International Society for Burn Injuries, 32*(1), 83–86.

Selvaggi, G., Monstrey, S., Van Landuyt, K., Hamdi, M., & Blondeel, P. (2005). Rehabilitation of burn injured patients following lightning and electrical trauma [Electronic Version]. *NeuroRehabilitation, 20*, 35–42.

Thomson Micromedex (2006). Micromedex healthcare series. Retrieved from http://www.thomsonhc.com/hcs/librarian/ND_PR/Main/SBK/2/PFPUI/LQ4m3Y21lSzztq/ND_PG/PRIH/CS/57CE9B/ND_T/HCS/ND_P/Main/DUPLICATIONSHIELDSYNC/85BB5A/ND_B/HCS/PFActionId/hcs.common.RetrieveDocumentCommon/DocId/1746/ContentSetId/31#pharmacokineticsSection (Accessed June 5, 2006).

Venes, D. (Ed.). (2005). *Taber's cyclopedic medical dictionary* (20th ed.). Philadelphia: F.A. Davis.

Wiederkehr, M., & Schwartz, R.A. (2003, October). Lice, scabies, and bedbugs. Retrieved from http://merck.micromedex.com/index.asp?page=bpm_brief&article_id=BPM01DE11&hilight=lice (Accessed March 18, 2006).

29

Caring for the Child with a Renal, Urinary Tract, or Reproductive Condition

KEY TERMS

urinary tract infection (UTI) – An acquired infection of the urinary system caused by bacteria, virus, or fungus (Hogan & White, 2003)

pyelonephritis – An infection in the renal pelvis that causes renal scarring and, with repeated infections, hypertension or end-stage renal disease

FOCUSED ASSESSMENT

Fluid Deficit

- A fluid deficit occurs when fluids are lost through diaphoresis, vomiting, diarrhea or hemorrhage.
- To determine normal values use calculation of daily maintenance fluid requirements. See page 581.

Fluid Deficit

Causes	Signs and Symptoms	Nursing Care
Diminished fluid intake	Dry skin	Determine the underlying
Diaphoresis	Sticky mucous membranes	cause.
Vomiting	Poor skin turgor	Replace fluids.
Diarrhea	Thirst	Replace electrolytes.
Nasogastric suction	Poor perfusion	Provide oral hydration.
Fever	Decreased urinary output	Provide IV hydration.
Hemorrhage	Weight loss	Measure intake and output.
	Fatigue	Monitor vital signs.
	Tachycardia	Monitor laboratory values.
	Tachypnea	
	Decreased blood pressure	
	High urine specific gravity	
	High hematocrit	

Fluid Excess

- A fluid overload occurs from conditions that create impaired fluid excretion, such as kidney disease or congestive heart failure. Fluid overload also can occur due to excessive administration of intravenous fluids (Venes, 2005).
- To determine normal values use calculation of daily maintenance fluid requirements. See page 581.

Fluid Excess

Causes	Signs and Symptoms	Nursing Care
Excessive oral/IV intake	Pulmonary edema	Determine the underlying
Hypotonic fluid overload	(crackles)	cause.
Kidney disease	Weight gain (fluid	Decrease fluid intake.
	retention)	Administer diuretics.
	Lethargy	Monitor vital signs.
	Decreased level of	Monitor laboratory values
	consciousness	(electrolytes).
	Slow, bounding pulse	
	Low urine specific gravity	
	Decreased hematocrit	

Vesicoureteral Reflux (VUR) and Urinary Tract Infection (UTI)

- Be aware that infants and small children cannot express urinary discomfort easily.
- Observe for discomfort during voiding or straining to void, dribbling of urine, and starting and stopping of the stream.
- Fever of unknown origin and irritability may suggest UTI, especially in nonverbal children.
- Take extreme care to obtain a reliable clean-catch urine specimen by helping older children collect the sample and properly handling a bagged specimen in younger children.
- Explain the urinary system to children old enough to understand it through the use of drawings, models, or dolls (Montagnino & Currier, 2005).

Hemolytic Uremic Syndrome

- Assess the child for abdominal symptoms, such as diffuse abdominal pain, intussusception (telescoping of the bowel), nausea, vomiting, diarrhea, and fever. These symptoms may occur up to 1 week after exposure to the *E. coli* O157.H7 toxin (Razzaq, 2006).
- Look for evidence of bleeding related to thrombocytopenia.
- Observe for petechiae, epistaxis (nosebleed), prolonged bleeding at venipuncture sites, and ecchymoses.
- Because of the increased risk for neurological sequelae, look for evidence of increased intracranial pressure (ICP), including altered level of consciousness and seizures.

Accurate Weight Measurement

- It is critical that children be weighed properly and their weights monitored carefully. An inaccurate weight recorded in a computer charting system can cause life-threatening harm for the patient.
- Weights are commonly ordered every 12–24 hours in children and must be done at the same time of day.

Glomerular Disease

Glomerular disease (glomerulonephritis) can be due to primary kidney disease or secondary multisystem diseases that cause damage to the glomerulus.

Poststreptococcal Glomerulonephritis

- A beta-hemolytic streptococcus is the cause of postinfectious glomerulonephritis.
- Gross hematuria, either tea- or coffee-colored urine, develops, accompanied at times by edema, which may be seen in the periorbital region (around the eye orbits).
- If the symptoms become more severe, the child may develop hypertension and headache.
- Severe disease causes significant proteinuria and possibly even ascites, due to fluid shifting (Lum, 2007).

Signs and Symptoms of Renal Trauma

- Localized flank tenderness
- Hematoma
- A palpable mass
- There also can be other symptoms related to abdominal injury such as tenderness, peritonitis, paralytic ileus, and resulting hypovolemic shock.

Signs and Symptoms of Acute Renal Failure

- Rash
- Bloody diarrhea
- Pallor
- Vomiting and diarrhea
- Abdominal pain
- Hemorrhage
- Shock
- Anuria or polyuria
- Other life-threatening signs and symptoms include gastrointestinal bleeding, hypertension, anemia, neurological symptoms, as well as the skin becoming ecchymotic.

History Information in Chronic Renal Failure

- Look for malaise, poor appetite, vomiting, bone pain, headache (if hypertensive), and polyuria.
- Listen for these problems in the patient's history: perinatal complications, oligohydramnios, recurrent UTIs, and enuresis.
- Stay alert for evidence of renal disease and hearing impairment in the patient's family history (Schwartz, 2005, p. 712).

Physical Examination Findings Correlated with Underlying Pathophysiological Mechanisms for Chronic Renal Failure

Organ System	Physical Findings	Correlation with Pathophysiological Mechanisms
Skeletal	Osteitis fibrosa (bone inflammation with fibrous degeneration) Bone demineralization (principally subperiosteal loss of cortical bone in the fibers, lateral ends of the clavicles, and lamina dura of the teeth) Spontaneous fractures, bone pain; osteomalacia (rickets or rachitic changes) with end-stage renal failure Edema Absent patella	Bone resorption associated with hyperparathyroidism, vitamin D deficiency, and demineralization Lowered calcium and raised phosphate levels
Cardiopulmonary	Hypertension, pericarditis with fever, chest pain, and pericardial friction rub, pulmonary edema, Kussmaul respirations Flow murmur Gallop Rub	Extracellular volume expansion as cause of hypertension Hypersecretion of renin also associated with hypertension Fluid overload associated with pulmonary edema and acidosis leading to Kussmaul respirations
Neurological	Encephalopathy (fatigue, loss of attention, difficulty problem solving) Peripheral neuropathy (pain and burning in the legs and feet, loss of vibration sense and deep tendon reflexes)	Uremic toxins associated with end-stage renal disease

Organ System	Physical Findings	Correlation with Pathophysiological Mechanisms
	Loss of motor coordination, twitching, fasciculations, stupor, and coma with advanced uremia Hypotonia Irritability	
Endocrine and Reproductive	Retarded growth in children (short stature) Osteomalacia High incidence of goiter Sexual dysfunction: menorrhagia, amenorrhea, infertility, and decreased libido in women; decreased testosterone levels, infertility, and decreased libido in men	Decreased growth hormone Elevated parathyroid hormone Decreased thyroid hormone Elevated hormones: luteinizing hormone (LH), follicle-stimulating hormone (FSH), prolactin, and LH-releasing hormone; decreased testosterone, estrogen, and progesterone
Hematological	Anemia, usually normochromic normocytic; platelet disorders with prolonged bleeding times (increase in bleeding gums)	Reduced erythropoietin secretion associated with loss of renal mass, leading to reduced red cell production in the bone marrow; uremic toxins associated with shortened red cell survival
Gastrointestinal	Anorexia, nausea, vomiting Mouth ulcers, stomatitis, ruinous breath (uremic fetor), hiccups, peptic ulcers, gastrointestinal bleeding, and pancreatitis associated with end-stage renal failure	Retention of urea, metabolic acids, and other metabolic waste products, including methylguanidine
Integumentary	Abnormal pigmentation and pruritus	Retention of urochromes, contributing to sallow, yellow color High plasma calcium levels associated with pruritus
Immunological	Increased risk of infection that can cause death Decreased response to vaccination	Suppression of cell-mediated immunity Reduction in number and function of lymphocytes Diminished phagocytosis. *(continued)*

		Correlation with Pathophysiological
Organ System	Physical Findings	Mechanisms
HEENT	Retinal changes Preauricular pits Hearing deficit	Uremic toxins
Abdomen	Palpable kidneys Suprapubic mass	

Physical Examination Findings Correlated with Underlying Pathophysiological Mechanisms for Chronic Renal Failure (Continued)

Varicocele

- Expect scrotal veins to distend when the patient stands and to decrease in visibility when the patient is supine.
- Look for accentuation of the veins with Valsalva maneuver.
- Be aware that testes are often smaller in varicocele.

Signs and Symptoms of Testicular Torsion

- The torsed testicle may be lying horizontally or appear higher in the scrotal sack than the opposite testicle.
- Although most commonly, the situation is unilateral, it may be bilateral. Scrotal edema is usually present within 12 hours.
- Especially in the neonate, the torsed testicle may feel quite hard.
- One way to differentiate the diagnosis of testicular torsion is to attempt to elicit the cremasteric reflex, which is normally absent on the torsion side.
- Prehn's sign, which is relief of pain from elevating the testicle, is also usually absent in torsion (Cole & Vogler, 2004).

CLINICAL ALERTS

Calculation of Daily Maintenance Fluid Requirements

Fluid balance means that the liquid in the body is regulated in such a way to maintain homeostasis (a state of equilibrium). The body's intake and output of fluid in a 24-hour period is approximately the same. Fluid balance is measured by daily discrepancies in body weight and by monitoring fluid intake and output. There are two methods of fluid maintenance:

- The surface area method is the most common and used for children >22 lbs. (10 kg): 1500 to 2000 mL/m² per day.

Daily Maintenance Fluid Requirements	
Child's Weight	**Daily Maintenance Fluid Requirement**
0–10 kg (0–22 lbs.)	100 mL/kg of body weight
11–20 kg (24.2–44 lbs.)	1000 mL + 50 mL/kg for each kg >10
>20 kg (>44 lbs.)	1500 mL + 20 mL/kg for each kg >20

Note: The method used to measure normal urinary output is 1–2 mL/kg per hour.

Types of Dehydration

Depending on the cause of the fluid loss, a child will lose water and electrolytes.

- *Isotonic* dehydration occurs when electrolyte and water deficits are present in balanced proportions (sodium and water are lost in equal amounts). Serum sodium remains in normal limits 130 to 150 mEq/L. This is the most common type of dehydration. Hypovolemic shock is the greatest concern.
- *Hypotonic* dehydration occurs when the electrolyte deficit exceeds the water deficit. Serum sodium concentration is <130 mEq/L. Physical signs are more severe with smaller fluid losses.
- *Hypertonic* dehydration is the most dangerous type and occurs when water loss is in excess of electrolyte loss. Sodium serum concentration is >150 mEq/L. Seizures are likely to occur.

Pathophysiology of Dehydration

Reasons for Dehydration
- Fever
- Vomiting
- Diarrhea
- Diaphoresis
- Hemorrhage
- Burns

- Trauma
- Diminished fluid intake

Possible Results of Dehydration
- Rapid and sudden extracellular fluid loss
  - Electrolyte imbalance
  - Intracellular fluid loss
  - Cellular dysfunction
- Hypovolemic shock (tachycardia, tachypnea, hypotension, cool, clammy, or cyanotic skin, decreased urine output)
  - Death

Sources of *E. coli* 0147.H7

- Undercooked ground beef is a primary source of *E. coli* 0147.H7, which can cause hemolytic uremic syndrome. Meat should be cooked until it reaches an internal temperature of 160°F and is no longer pink.
- *E. coli* outbreaks have originated in fast-food and other restaurants and have been linked to nonpasteurized cider, milk, juice, alfalfa sprouts, strawberries, and most recently, raw spinach.

Hematuria

- Hematuria usually is considered the cardinal marker of renal injury.
- Any degree of hematuria suggests underlying renal injury or anomaly.
- Hematuria out of proportion to the mechanisms of injury suggests a congenital anomaly or neoplasm.

Signs of Kidney Transplant Rejection

- Hypertension
- Decreased urinary output
- Fever
- Weight gain
- Edema
- Graft site pain
- Increasing BUN and creatinine levels

(Kenner et al., 2007).

DIAGNOSTIC TESTS

Sodium (Na⁺) Deficit (Hyponatremia; Serum Sodium Concentration <130 mEq/L)

Causes	Signs and Symptoms	Nursing Care
Decreased sodium intake	Dehydration	Determine the underlying cause.
Excessive sweating	Nausea	Administer IV fluids with the
Fever	Weakness	appropriate amount of
Malnutrition	Lethargy	sodium added.
Vomiting	Abdominal cramping	Monitor laboratory values
Diarrhea	Dizziness	(electrolytes).
Nasogastric suction	Weak pulse	
Diabetic ketoacidosis	Decreased blood pressure	
Kidney disease		

Sodium (Na⁺) Excess (Hypernatremia; Serum Sodium Concentration ≥150 mEq/L)

Causes	Signs and Symptoms	Nursing Care
Excessive salt intake	Oliguria	Determine the underlying cause.
Fever	Nausea	Monitor neurological status.
High insensible water loss	Vomiting	Monitor laboratory values
Diabetes insipidus	Muscle twitching	(electrolytes).
Hyperglycemia	Lethargy	
Kidney disease		

Potassium (K⁺) Deficit (Hypokalemia; Serum Potassium Concentration ≤3.5 mEq/L)

Causes	Signs and Symptoms	Nursing Care
Diuresis	Muscle weakness	Determine the underlying cause.
Starvation	Muscle cramping and	Monitor vital signs.
IV fluid without	stiffness	Offer high-potassium foods.
potassium added	Hypotension	Administer oral potassium
Diarrhea	Hyporeflexia	supplements (assess for
Vomiting	Cardiac arrhythmias	adequate output before
Nasogastric suction	(tachycardia or	administration).
Administration of	bradycardia)	Administer IV potassium
diuretics or corticosteroids	Fatigue	slowly.
Burns that are healing	Drowsiness	Obtain ECG (for IV potassium
Alkalosis		bolus).
		Monitor laboratory values
		(electrolytes).
		Evaluate acid–base status.

Potassium (K+) Excess (Hyperkalemia; Serum Potassium Concentration ≥5.5 mEq/L)

Causes	Signs and Symptoms	Nursing Care
Increased intake of potassium Severe dehydration Rapid administration of IV potassium chloride Potassium sparing diuretics Burns Kidney disease (failure) Adrenal insufficiency (Addison disease) Metabolic acidosis	Muscle twitching Muscle weakness Flaccid paralysis Hyperreflexia Oliguria Apnea (respiratory arrest) Bradycardia Ventricular fibrillation (cardiac arrest)	Determine the underlying cause. Monitor vital signs. Obtain ECG. Administer IV fluids as ordered. Administer IV insulin to facilitate potassium moving into cells (if ordered). Monitor laboratory values (electrolytes). Evaluate acid–base status.

Calcium (Ca²⁺) Deficit (Hypocalcemia; Serum Calcium Concentration <8.8 mEq/L)

Causes	Signs and Symptoms	Nursing Care
Inadequate dietary intake Vitamin D deficiency Feeding cow's milk to infants Advanced adrenal insufficiency	Tetany Convulsions Neuromuscular irritability Hypotension Tingling (nose, ears, toes and fingertips) Cardiac arrest	Determine the underlying cause. Administer oral calcium supplement as prescribed. Administer IV calcium slowly and monitor IV site (irritation). Monitor laboratory values (serum calcium and potassium levels).

Calcium (Ca²⁺) Excess (Hypercalcemia; Serum Calcium Concentration >10.8 mEq/L)

Causes	Signs and Symptoms	Nursing Care
Excessive vitamin D intake Acidosis Immobilization (prolonged periods of time) Increased bone catabolism Hyperthyroidism Kidney disease	Weakness Fatigue Constipation Anorexia Nausea Vomiting Thirst Bradycardia (cardiac arrest)	Determine the underlying cause. Obtain ECG. Monitor laboratory values (electrolytes).

Determining Problems with the Urinary Tract

- The renal ultrasound depicts the ureters but does not discern if there is an infection.
- A voiding cystourethrogram (VCUG) depicts urethral and bladder anatomy.
- An intravenous pyelogram (IVP) assists with identifying the size, shape, and position of the urinary system as well as elimination function by noting length of time for passage of contrast material through the kidneys.
- Nuclear cystography visualizes the bladder and is good for detecting VUR.
- Nuclear cortical scanning detects tubular damage and scarring

(Egland & Egland, 2006; Pagana & Pagana, 2003).

Voiding Cystourethrograms (VCUG)

Gradations of VUR are provided in the International Reflux Grading System, with a range from Grade I to Grade V (Fig. 29-1).

Grade I	Urine backs up into the ureter only, and the renal pelvis appears healthy, with sharp calyces.
Grade II	Urine backs up into the ureter, renal pelvis, and calyces. The renal pelvis appears healthy and has sharp calyces.
Grade III	Urine backs up into the ureter and collecting system. The ureter and pelvis appear mildly dilated, and the calyces are mildly blunted.
Grade IV	Urine backs up into the ureter and collecting system. The ureter and pelvis appear moderately dilated, and the calyces are moderately blunted.
Grade V	Urine backs up into the ureter and collecting system. The pelvis severely dilates, the ureter appears tortuous, and the calyces are severely blunted.

Source: Cendron & Benedict (2006, p. 1).

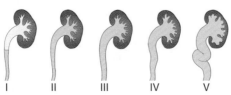

Figure 29-1 Gradations of VUR are found in the International Reflux Grading System, ranging from Grade I to Grade V.

Procedure 29-1 Urine Collection

Purpose

The purpose of collecting a urine specimen is to screen for early signs of disease

Equipment

Packaged urine culture set (usually contains three iodine or antiseptic towelettes and a sterile plastic collection container)

Steps

1. Wipe (or have the child wipe) the labia or penis with the three iodine or antiseptic solution towelettes. The customary procedure is to wipe the area three times.

   • In males, wipe the urethral tip three times in a circular fashion, once with each wipe.

   • In females, holding the labia open to expose the urethra, wipe the right side top to bottom and discard the wipe. Repeat on the left side, discarding the wipe. Finally, wipe top to bottom over the central area and the urethral meatus and discard that wipe.

2. Ask the child to start urinating into the toilet, bedpan, or urinal, and then to stop urinating.

3. Position the sterile urine container so that it catches about 3 to 4 ounces of "mid-stream" urine, which needs to be about 3–4 oz. of urine.

4. Remove the container and cap it, taking care not to contaminate the inner container with your gloved hands.

5. Allow the child to finish voiding into the toilet, bedpan, or urinal.

6. Do not keep the urine sample at room temperature any longer than 10 minutes, unless it is directly in transport to the laboratory. If the specimen cannot be sent to the laboratory immediately, it is necessary to refrigerate it in a plastic specimen bag.

7. Note the time and date of urine collection on the container label and in the patient's chart. The container label should also contain the patient's name and other identifying information, such as identification number.

Procedure 29-1 (Continued)

8. If the patient's parents will be responsible for collecting urine at home, instruct them in sterile collection and proper storage of the specimen.

9. Document the procedure.

Clinical Alert Do not keep a urine culture at room temperature any longer than 10 minutes, unless it is directly in transport to the laboratory. If the specimen cannot be sent to the laboratory immediately, it is necessary to refrigerate it in a plastic specimen bag to prevent the overgrowth of organisms that interfere with the interpretation of the culture and sensitivity to specific antibiotics. The specimen is plated on a nutrient medium and bacteria that are present are allowed to grow and then are counted. Usually, different antibiotic discs are placed on the inoculated medium to show which ones decrease the colony counts (sensitivity).

Teach Parents:

Parents may be responsible for collecting urine cultures of their children at home or in the medical office, so they must be instructed on the sterile techniques of handling the specimen. If the specimen is collected at home, it may need to be refrigerated before bringing it to the laboratory.

Urine Dipstick Test

To perform an accurate urine dipstick test, obtain proper quantities of urine to dip the sticks into, and then wait the appropriate amount of time to test each specimen (Fig. 29-2).

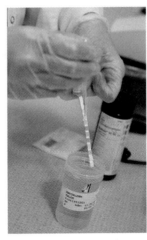

Figure 29-2 Nurses should be able to perform an accurate dipstick test.

Normal Urinalysis Values

Urinalysis Component	Normal Values
Appearance	Clear
Color	Amber yellow
Odor	Aromatic
pH	4.6–8.0 (average 6.0)
Osmolarity	50–1,400 mOsm/L
Protein	None or up to 8 mg/dL
	50–80 mg/24 hr (at rest)
	<250 mg/24 hr (exercise)
Specific gravity	Adult: 1.005–1.030 (usually 1.010–1.025)
	Elderly: values decrease with age
	Newborn: 1.001–1.020
Leukocyte esterase	Negative
Nitrites	Negative
Ketones	Negative
Crystals	Negative
Casts	None present
Glucose	Brand new specimen: Negative
	24-hour specimen: 50–300 mg/day or 0.3–1.7 mmol/day (SI units)
White blood cells (WBCs)	0–4 per low-power field
WBC casts	Negative
Red blood cells (RBCs)	Up to 2
RBC casts	None

Common Urinalysis Findings of Acute Renal Failure

Findings	Interpretation
Sediment	Intrinsic kidney failure
Color	"Dirty" brown: Intrinsic renal failure Reddish brown: Acute glomerulonephritis Bilious tinge: Mixed hepatic and renal failure
Proteinuria	Glomerulonephritis Interstitial nephritis Toxic and infectious causes
Casts	Red blood cells: Glomerulonephritis or vasculitis White blood cells: Interstitial nephritis Granular: Glomerulonephritis Uric acid crystals: Tumor lysis syndrome Calcium oxalate crystals: Ethylene glycol ingestion Acetaminophen (Tylenol) crystals: Acetaminophen toxicity acute

Renal Tubular Function

The fractional excretion of sodium (FE_{NA}) is an index of renal tubular function.

$$FE_{NA} = ([U_{NA}/P_{NA}]/Ucreat/Pcreat]) \times 100 \text{ (Schwartz, 2005, p. 711)}.$$

- An FE_{NA} greater than 2 is correlated with acute interstitial nephritis or acute tubular necrosis.
- An FE_{NA} less than 1 is correlated with hemolytic uremic syndrome, acute glomerulonephritis, or prerenal causes.

Laboratory Differential Diagnosis of Acute Renal Failure

	Prerenal		Intrarenal		Postrenal
	Child	Neonate	Child	Neonate	
Urine Na+ (mEq/L)	<20	<20–30	>40	>40	Variable, may be >40
FEna* (%) Should not be obtained after a diuretic is given as renders the test inaccurate	<1	<2–5	>2	>2.5	Variable, may be >2

(continued)

Laboratory Differential Diagnosis of Acute Renal Failure (Continued)					
	Prerenal		Intrarenal		Postrenal
	Child	Neonate	Child	Neonate	
Urine Osmolality (mOsmol/L)	>500	>300–500	>300	>300	Variable, may be <300
Serum BUN-to-Creatinine Ratio	>20	≥10	>10	>10	Variable, may be >20
Urinalysis	Normal		RBCs, WBCs, casts, proteinuria		Variable to normal, possible crystals
Comments	History: Diarrhea, vomiting, hemorrhage, diuretic Physical: Volume depletion		History: Hypotension, anoxia, exposure to nephrotoxins Physical: Hypertension, edema		History: Poor urine stream and output Physical: Flank mass, distended bladder

*Fractional excretion of sodium = [(urine sodium/plasma sodium) + (urine creatinine/plasma creatinine)] × 100.
RBCs, red blood cells; WBCs, white blood cells.
Source: Kliegman et al. (2006, p. 761).

Diagnostic Tools Determining Reason for Amenorrhea

- Genetic testing may be required to determine disorders such as Turner's syndrome.
- Pelvic ultrasound or transvaginal (ultrasound wand in the vaginal canal) is used to test for pregnancy, ovarian cysts, and other gynecological abnormalities. Patients normally are required to drink four 8-ounce glasses of water 1 hour before a pelvic ultrasound to elevate the bladder in order to view the pelvic organs.

Laboratory Tests for Amenorrhea	
Urine Pregnancy Test	Widely available over the counter, but more sensitive tests are available in clinical facilities.
Serum Pregnancy Test	Qualitative and quantitative tests show positive pregnancy and approximate duration of pregnancy, respectively. More accurate than urine pregnancy tests, and detect pregnancy earlier.

Thyroid-stimulating Hormone (TSH) Level	A general test for hypothyroidism and hyperthyroidism. May be accompanied by test of free thyroxine test to specify the disorder more clearly
Prolactin Level	Elevated in hyperprolactinemia, which may be seen with hypothyroidism or with a benign pituitary adenoma. Prolactin is a hormone produced in the pituitary gland and associated with breast-feeding.
Follicle-stimulating Hormone (FSH) Level	May be decreased in polycystic ovary syndrome (PCOS).
Luteinizing Hormone (LH) Level	May be increased in PCOS.
Testosterone Level	May be increased in PCOS, along with dehydroepiandrosterone (DHEA) level.

Tests for Testicular Torsion

- Doppler ultrasonography is the preferred diagnostic test and should be ordered immediately.
- The test can differentiate between ischemia; inflammation, such as that seen in orchitis (inflammation of a testis); and epididymitis (inflammation of the epididymis), often seen with gonorrhea.
- In possible false-negative results, a technetium scintigraphy test will show definitive testicular torsion (Ringdahl & Teague, 2006).
- The testicle may be enlarged and may have decreased or absent blood flow.

MEDICATIONS

Broad-Spectrum Antibiotics

- Stress to the parents the need for the child to complete the prescribed amount and to maintain adequate intake of fluids.
- For those children taking prophylactic low-dose antibiotics, taking the medication at night allows the drug more time in the bladder.
- Children who receive broad-spectrum antibiotics that are likely to alter GI and periurethral flora are at increased risk for UTI because these drugs disturb the natural defense against colonization by pathogenic bacteria (Hellerstein, 2007, p.4).

Common Anti-Infectives, Side Effects, and Nursing Interventions

Generic Drug Name Trade name	Side Effects	Nursing Interventions and Patient Teaching
Ampicillin (IV) *Marcillin*	Nausea, vomiting, diarrhea, Rash	Hold and notify MD if rash or diarrhea. With prolonged therapy periodically monitor renal, hepatic and hematological lab work.
Cefixime (PO) *Suprax*	Serious side effects: Stevens–Johnson syndrome, nephrotoxicity, blood dyscrasias Superinfections (can occur with any antibiotic)	Monitor BUN, serum creatinine, and input & output (I & O). Teach how to recognize superinfection, e.g., furry tongue, perineal itching. Tell the patient to take with yogurt/buttermilk to decrease superinfection by maintaining intestinal flora.
Cefotaxime (IV) *Claforan*	Mild diarrhea, mild abdominal cramping	Monitor fluid intake.
Ceftriaxone (IV) *Rocephin*	Serious side effect: Antibiotic-associated colitis manifested as severe abdominal pain, tenderness, fever, and diarrhea that is severe and watery	Assess bowel pattern or pain. Monitor I & O.
Cephalexin (PO) *Biocef, Keflex*	Serious side effects: Antibiotic-associated colitis and other superinfections, nephrotoxicity with preexisiting renal disease, angioedema, bronchospasm, and anaphylaxis (especially if allergies to penicillin or cephalosporins)	Monitor I & O for nephrotoxicity. Assess bowel activity, stool consistency, and increasing GI effects. Advise taking with food or milk if mild GI upset occurs. Assess mucous membranes and tongue for white patches.
Ciprofloxacin (PO) *Cipro*	Many IV incompatibilities Serious side effects: superinfection, nephrotoxicity, cardiac arrest, cerebral thrombosis Arthropathy may occur in children younger than 18 years.	Monitor I & O; assure that appropriate fluid intake maintained. Caution regarding sun exposure affecting eyes, skin.

Generic Drug Name Trade name	Side Effects	Nursing Interventions and Patient Teaching
		If patient wears contact lenses, remove if taking ophthalmic solution or ointment.
Gentamicin (IV) *Garamycin*	Serious side effects: Ototoxicity, nephrotoxicity	Monitor urinalysis. Therapeutic peak 5-10 mcg/mL and trough is 2 mcg/mL. The family should notify physician of any balance, hearing, urinary, or vision problems even after drug is completed.
Nitrofurantoin (PO) *Macrodantin, Furadantin*	Serious side effects: Stevens–Johnson syndrome, liver toxicity, peripheral neuropathy, impairment of pulmonary function	Monitor for peripheral neuropathy, e.g., numbness and/or tingling of extremities. Monitor for liver toxicity signs and symptoms. Monitor respiratory system and chest pain, cough, or difficulty with respirations.
Sulfamethoxazole/ Trimethoprim (PO) *Bactrim, Septra, Generic*	Serious side effects: Fatalities secondary to Stevens-Johnson syndrome, toxic epidermal necrolysis, fulminant hepatic necrosis and other blood dyscrasias, such as agranulocytosis, aplastic anemia	Contraindicated in children younger than 2 months of age; kernicterus may result if used with newborns. Monitor I & O; assess skin for pallor, purpura, and rash or overt signs of bleeding, swelling. Monitor hematology and liver and renal function lab results. Tell the family to report new symptoms, e.g., bruising, fever, sore throat, or other skin reactions.

Medications Used to Treat Complications of Acute Renal Failure

Medication	Action/Indication	Nursing Implications
Hyperkalemia		
Kayexalate	Exchanges sodium for potassium.	May require up to 4 hours to take effect.
Calcium gluconate 10%	Counteracts potassium-induced increased myocardial irritability.	Monitor for ECG changes. Intravenous infiltration may result in tissue necrosis.
Albuterol	Shifts potassium to the cells.	Give by inhalation.
Metabolic Acidosis		
Sodium bicarbonate or sodium citrate	Helps correct metabolic acidosis by exchanging hydrogen for potassium.	Do not mix with calcium. Complications include fluid overload, hypertension, and tetany.
Hypocalcemia		
Calcium gluconate 10%	Used in the presence of tetany; provides ionized calcium to restore nervous tissue function to control serum phosphorus.	Administer slowly to prevent bradycardia. Monitor for ECG changes.
Malignant Hypertension (B/P>95% for age)		
Sodium nitroprusside, nitroglycerin	Relaxes smooth muscle in peripheral arterioles.	Administer by continuous intravenous infusion; fall in blood pressure is seen within 10–20 minutes.

Medications Commonly Used for Children with Chronic Renal Failure

Medication	Action or Indication	Nursing Considerations
Vitamin and mineral supplement (Nephrocaps)	Adds vitamins and minerals missing from heavily restricted diet.	Only prescribed vitamins should be used; over-the-counter brands may contain elements that are harmful.
Phosphate binding agents: Calcium carbonate (Tums), calcium acetate (PhosLo), or sevelamer hydrochloride (Renagel)	Reduce absorption of phosphorus from the intestines.	Ensure that phosphate binding agent is aluminum free.

Medication	Action or Indication	Nursing Considerations
Calcitriol (Rocaltrol)	Replaces the calcitriol that kidneys are no longer producing to keep calcium balance normal.	Monitor serum calcium level. Ensure that calcium supplement is provided.
Epoetin alfa (Epogen, Procrit)	Stimulates bone marrow to produce red blood cells; treats anemia due to chronic renal failure (CRF).	Given by IV or subcutaneous injection. Monitor blood pressure as hypertension is an adverse effect. Monitor hematocrit and serum ferritin level according to facility guidelines.
Iron supplementation	Treats iron deficiency when epoetin alfa is prescribed.	May be administered orally or IV during hemodialysis.
Growth hormone (rhGH)	Used to stimulate growth in children with CRF.	Record accurate height measurements at regular intervals.
Antihypertensive agents: Angiotensin-converting enzyme (ACE) inhibitor (enalapril, lisinopril) Loop diuretics	Used with proteinuric kidney disease as it slows the progression to end-stage renal disease Used when volume overload is present.	Monitor renal function and electrolyte balance.

Medications Used for Enuresis

- Desmopressin (DDAVP) is a synthetic analogue of the antidiuretic hormone (ADH). This medication, administered orally or via a nasal spray, acts to lower nocturnal urinary production. The spray is given intranasally at doses of 1 to 40 mcg (1 to 4 sprays) each night, beginning with the lowest effective dose. If given orally, desmopressin (DDAVP) is available in 0.2 mg tablets given in dosages of 0.2 mg to 0.6 mg per night. Success rates range from 10% to 65%, but unfortunately, relapse rates are high, at 80%, when the drug is discontinued. Although there is a slight risk of water intoxication, the drug overall appears safe and efficacious (National Guidelines Clearinghouse, 2004).

- Imipramine (Tofranil) has been used for enuresis. Imipramine (Tofranil) may be used in a bedtime dose of 1 to 2.5 mg/kg with up to 60% effectiveness. As imipramine (Tofranil) is a tricyclic antidepressant, it is subject to risk of cardiac arrhythmia and therefore pretreatment EKG is required (National Guidelines Clearinghouse, 2004).

Topical Antifungal Medications for Candida vulvovaginalis

Medication	Pregnancy Category	Mechanism	Absorption	Use
Miconazole (Monistat products)	C	Damages fungal cell wall membrane, which causes nutrients to leak.	Small amount through the vagina	Apply topically, very sparingly, to external vagina once or twice daily in adolescents; may be applied with vaginal applicator in adolescents.
Nystatin (Mycostatin products)	B	Binds to sterols in fungal cell membrane, changing wall permeability	Not absorbed through mucous membranes, therefore safer for children	Gently massage cream or ointment into skin two to four times daily.
Clotrimazole (Lotrimin, Mycelex products)	B (topical)	Binds to phospholipids in cell membrane, causing cell wall permeability and loss of cell contents	Negligible through intact skin topically; 3% to 10% absorption when applied intravaginally	In children older than age 3, apply vaginal cream (Mycelex) 2% bid to external vagina. In children older than age 12 and adults, vaginal applicator may be used for cream.

Source: Taketomo, Hodding, & Kraus (2007).

ETHNOCULTURAL CONSIDERATIONS

Kidney Failure

"African Americans constitute about 32 percent of all patients treated for kidney failure in the United States, but only about 13 percent of the overall U.S. population. Anyone with high blood pressure, diabetes, or a family history of kidney disease is at risk and should have his or her kidney function tested" (Former U.S. Surgeon General Dr. Joycelyn Elders).

Enuresis

Toileting patterns and expectations vary among different cultural and ethnic groups. Enuresis may be considered more problematic for some people than for others, and expectations of bladder and bowel control vary among parents, teachers, health care professionals, and daycare providers.

TEACHING THE FAMILY

Arteriovenous (AV) Fistulas

- Teach the child (and family) with a new AV fistula to wash the access site with soap and water each day and always before dialysis.
- Instruct the child not to scratch the area or pick at scabs.
- Tell the child and family to check the area daily for signs of infection, including warmth and redness.
- Teach them to check for blood flow in the area daily by showing them the vibration (thrill) that should be present over the access site. Tell the child and family to notify a health care provider at the dialysis center if this vibration changes or stops.
- Urge the child to avoid traumatizing the arm with the access site, including by not wearing tight clothes or jewelry, carrying heavy objects, or sleeping on the arm.
- Instruct the child and family to remind all health care providers not to take blood or blood pressure measurements using that arm.
- Tell the child and family that needle sites should be rotated.
- Tell the child and family to apply gentle pressure to stop bleeding when the needle is removed. Also explain that gentle pressure should be applied if bleeding resumes later. A health care provider should be called if bleeding is excessive or does not stop within 30 minutes.

Vulvovaginitis

- Suggest tub baths with clear, warm water once to twice daily for 10 to 15 minutes, followed by washing with a bland soap such as unscented Dove, Basis, Aveeno, or Neutrogena. The soap should not be applied to the vulvar area, and the vulva should never be scrubbed.

- Discourage shampooing the hair in the bathtub to keep the vulva from being exposed to shampoo chemicals. Showering is a better option.
- Instruct the patient to gently pat the vulvar area dry after bathing.
- Sleeper pajamas are not recommended due to their occlusive nature.
- Underwear should be all cotton for greater ventilation, and they should be washed in mild, unscented detergent without bleach.
- Some health care providers recommend applying a small amount of A+D ointment, Vaseline, or Desitin ointment to protect the vulvar skin. Loose-fitting clothing is ideal, especially in warm weather.
- Persistent discharge is occasionally treated with certain oral or topical antibiotics.
- Pinworms may cause recurrent vulvovaginitis; it may be necessary to instruct parents to inspect their child's anal area at night with a flashlight or apply a small piece of cellophane tape over the anal area to catch the pinworms or their eggs (Emans, 2005).

Vaginal Candidiasis

Instruct the patient in the following:

- Wear cotton underwear to allow better ventilation.
- Avoid wearing wet clothing, such as bathing suits, for long periods.
- Avoid taking bubble baths and using perfumes or powder near the vaginal area.
- In menstruating females, avoid scented sanitary pads or tampons.
- Avoid excessive sugars and simple carbohydrates in the diet.
- Eat yogurt, which contains natural lactobacilli, to maintain normal bacterial balance in the GI tract, keeping yeast in check.

Causes of Secondary Amenorrhea

Review with the patient these possible causes of secondary amenorrhea:

- Pregnancy
- Corpus luteum cyst

- Lactation
- Menopause (premature or normal)
- Hypothyroidism or hyperthyroidism
- Chemotherapy
- Polycystic ovarian syndrome (PCOS)
- Diabetes mellitus
- Stress
- Excessive exercise
- Weight loss

(Herban, Hill, & Sullivan, 2004)

Cryptorchidism

- Teach patients and caregivers that human chorionic gonadotropin may cause penile growth, increased pigmentation, and pubic hair.
- Urge them to talk about any anxieties raised by the risk of testicular cancer and decreased fertility.

Gynecomastia

- Teach the patient and parents that gynecomastia is usually a temporary condition.
- If obesity is an issue, work with the patient and family members to establish an age-appropriate dietary plan. Referral to a nutritionist may be useful.
- Explain to the family and patient that certain blood tests may be used to eliminate any risk of pathological causes of the gynecomastia.
- Discuss ways the child can respond to hurtful comments from other children.

ADDITIONAL INFORMATION FOR THE CLINICAL SETTING

Fluid and Electrolyte Balance Nursing Interventions

- Obtain daily weights (same scale, same time and wearing the same clothing, infants are weighed naked and oftentimes older children only have on their underwear).
- Measure intake and output (weigh diapers to assess output). Assess hydration status which includes assessing for presence of tears, skin turgor, anterior fontanel (up to 18 months), sticky mucous membranes, sunken eyeballs,

urine and stool output, weight loss, tachycardia, tachypnea, decreased blood pressure, temperature and thirst.

- Laboratory tests include specific gravity, hematocrit, blood urea nitrogen (BUN), creatinine, Na^+, K^+, and Ca^{2+}.
- Assess type of acid–base disturbance (metabolic acidosis, metabolic alkalosis, or respiratory acidosis).
- Administer oral clear liquids as ordered (1 to 2 oz. every hour).
- Start an IV for fluid and electrolyte replacement as ordered.
- Before administering intravenous potassium (K^+), ensure the child has voided.
- Cleanse the perineal area and apply protective topical ointment.
- Encourage parents to be involved in the care of the child.
- Educate parents about signs and symptoms of dehydration, rehydration, and when to call the doctor.
- Encourage parents to be compliant with follow-up appointments.

Causes of UTI

- Bacterium, virus, or fungus
- Structural anomalies, catheterization, urinary tract instrumentation, and sexual activity (Lum, 2007; Wise & Cardinal-Busse, 2007).
- Boys are affected more than girls owing to a higher rate of congenital abnormalities (Lippincott Williams & Wilkins, 2004).
- Starting at 6 months, girls are at greater risk until school age and then again when they enter adolescence, owing to the proximity of the anus with fecal flora that are available to colonize easily within the urethra.
- Sexually active adolescent girls. The causative agent is *Chlamydia*.
- UTIs are also more common in uncircumcised males (Elder, 2004).
- Conditions associated with chronic perineal irritation such as poor hygiene, bubble baths, soaps, pinworms, or perineal trauma that experienced cyclists, dirt bikers, or equestrians may experience are important associations to consider in predisposing the individual to UTIs.

- Conditions such as constipation, neurogenic bladder, and voiding dysfunction, or a history of abnormal voiding patterns are potential underlying etiological factors.
- Fungus, particularly *Candida* (yeast) species in immunocompromised children (Kennedy, 2003).
- A child with a UTI may also have an anatomical abnormality called vesicoureteral

Hematuria

- The main sign of hematuria is blood in the urine.
- The color of the urine may be significant; tea-colored or brownish urine, especially if it contains protein and casts

Causes of Acute Renal Failure	
Prerenal, Hypovolemic, Hypotension	Dehydration Septic shock Heart failure Hemorrhage Burns Peritonitis Ascites Cirrhosis
Intrinsic, Intrarenal, Parenchymal	Acute tubular necrosis (nephrotoxins [drugs], reversible if caught early) Acute cortical necrosis (not reversible) Glomerulonephritis Interstitial nephritis Renal vein thrombosis Arterial thromboembolus (umbilical artery catheter) Disseminated intravascular coagulation Immune mediated (scleroderma) Hemoglobinuria, myoglobinuria (pigmented)
Postrenal (Obstruction)	Urethral obstruction (stricture, posterior urethral valves, diverticulum) Ureterocele Extrinsic tumor compressing bladder outlet Extrinsic urinary tract tumors Tumor lysis syndrome

Source: Kliegman et al. (2006, p. 760).

Signs and Symptoms of Electrolyte Imbalances in Acute Renal Failure

Electrolyte Imbalance	Clinical Manifestations	Clinical Treatment
Hyperkalemia (>6.0 mEq/L) Results from inability to adequately excrete potassium derived from diet and catabolized cells. In metabolic acidosis, there is also movement of potassium from intracellular fluid to extracellular fluid	Peaked T waves, widening of QRS on ECG Dysrhythmias: ventricular dysrhythmias, heart block, ventricular fibrillation, cardiac arrest Diarrhea Muscle weakness	Elimination of all intake of potassium (dietary, parenteral, or TPN) Administration of alkalinizing agents Kayexalate orally or in retention enema when K$^+$>7.0 mEq/L Other drugs may be ordered by physician, including calcium gluconate 10% solution, sodium bicarbonate, and regular insulin when K$^+$>7.0 mEq/L Dialysis if other methods to reduce the potassium level are ineffective
Hyponatremia In the acute oliguric phase, hyponatremia is related to the accumulation of fluid in excess of solute.	Change in level of consciousness Muscle cramps Anorexia Abdominal reflexes, depressed deep tendon reflexes Cheyne–Stokes respirations Seizures	Electrolyte replacement, sodium bicarbonate Dialysis to correct severe electrolyte disturbance
Hypocalcemia Phosphate retention (hyperphosphatemia) depresses the serum calcium concentration. Calcium is deposited in injured cells. Hyperkalemia and metabolic acidosis may mask the common clinical manifestations of severe hypocalcemia.	Muscle tingling Changes in muscle tone Seizures Muscle cramps and twitching Positive Chvostek sign (contraction of facial muscles after tapping facial nerve just anterior to parotid gland)	Calcium gluconate Low-phosphorus diet Phosphate binders, e.g., Tums tablets, calcium acetate and sevelamer. (Aluminum-based binders not utilized to prevent possible aluminum toxicity.) Calcium IV not given except for tetany to prevent calcium salt deposition into tissues) Dialysis to correct severe electrolyte disturbance

Complications of Acute Renal Failure

System	Complications
Metabolic	Hyperkalemia
	Metabolic acidosis
	Hyponatremia
	Hypocalcemia
	Hyperphosphatemia
	Hypermagnesemia
	Hyperuricemia
Cardiovascular	Pulmonary edema
	Arrhythmias
	Pericarditis
	Pericardial effusion
	Pulmonary embolism
	Hypertension
	Myocardial infarction
Gastrointestinal	Nausea
	Vomiting
	Malnutrition
	Gastrointestinal hemorrhage
Neurological	Neuromuscular irritability
	Asterixis (flapping tremor)
	Seizures
	Mental status change
Hematological	Anemia
	Bleeding
Infectious	Pneumonia
	Septicemia
	UTI
Other	Hiccups
	Increased parathyroid hormone level
	Low total triiodothyronine level
	Low thyroxine level
	Normal free thyroxine level

Four Stages of Chronic Renal Failure According to Glomerular Filtration Rate (GFR)

Percentage of Reduction of GFR	Stage of Renal Failure	GFR as Applied to Children Age 2 and Older*
35%–55% of normal	1. Reduced renal reserve	90 or higher
25%–35% of normal	2. Renal insufficiency	60–89
20%–25% of normal	3. Renal failure	30–59
<20% of normal	4. End-stage renal disease (ESRD)	15–29*

*If GFR <15, dialysis is needed.

Dialysis in Pediatric Nursing

Dialysis is a life-extending procedure for children with severe renal compromise. Dialysis may be done through the peritoneal wall (peritoneal dialysis) or through cleansing the blood by using a dialysis machine (hemodialysis).

Peritoneal Dialysis
- Utilizes the peritoneal membrane (abdominal lining) to filter blood and purify it.
- A dialysis solution composed of dextrose sugar and other minerals in water is inserted into the child's abdomen through an abdominal catheter.
- Through an osmotic process, the dialysis solution draws toxins, excess water, and waste chemicals from the blood into the dialysis solution.
- Then it is drained through an abdominal tube out of the abdomen. The amount of time the dialysis solution is in the abdomen is termed the dwell time, and the entire process of filling and emptying the abdomen is termed an exchange, which normally lasts 30 to 40 minutes.
- There are two essential types of peritoneal dialysis: continuous ambulatory peritoneal dialysis (CAPD) and continuous cycling peritoneal dialysis (CCPD).
- Nurses monitor the abdominal catheter sites for signs of infection or malfunctioning equipment and make certain that the returning dialysate solution remains clear.

Hemodialysis
- The child's blood is moved through a filter called a dialyzer, which is part of a complex machine.
- Extra water, extra salt, and toxic waste products are removed, while the blood pressure and electrolytes such as potassium, calcium, sodium, and bicarbonate are kept in balance.
- A special port is placed in the child, usually in the wrist, for vascular access. Through this port, the blood is removed through tubing into the dialyzer, cleansed, and then returned through a different set of tubes back to the child's body.
- Three types of ports are used: Arteriovenous (AV) fistulas, AV grafts, and venous catheters.
- It is imperative for pediatric nurses to teach the patient and parents or guardians how to keep the AV fistula, AV graft, or venous catheter safe and clean.

Dysfunctional Voiding

Dysfunctional elimination syndrome (DES), also called voiding dysfunction, is an abnormal but common pediatric elimination pattern associated with bladder and bowel withholding and incontinence. There are numerous types of voiding disorders:

- Urge incontinence
- Lazy bladder syndrome
- Giggle incontinence
- Bladder-sphincter dyssynergia
- Vaginal voiding

Alternative Treatments for Enuresis

- Hypnotherapy: Four to six sessions of hypnotherapy can train a child to awaken when his or her bladder feels full.
- Psychological evaluation: Although not every child with enuresis has psychological problems, there is an increased incidence of psychological issues in secondary enuresis, including parental divorce, school trauma, hospitalization, and sexual abuse (Practice Parameter for the Assessment and Treatment of Children and Adolescents With Enuresis http://www.aacap.org/galleries/PracticeParameters/ Enuresis.pdf).
  - Also, psychological counseling is vital. Associated psychological and educational problems include learning disabilities, attention–deficit/hyperactivity disorder (ADHD), low motivation, sensory problems, and family issues. Parents and other family members may need assistance in dealing with these issues.
- Acupressure or massage therapy: These may be useful in some cases of neurologically induced enuresis.
- Homeopathic remedies: These should be provided by a licensed homeopathic provider.
  - Promote adequate hydration by ensuring that the child is hydrated with 8 ounces of water with each meal and then encouraged to void every 2 hours.
- Behavioral management and biofeedback
  - Voiding charts and diaries may help in tracking behavior and recording successes.
  - Biofeedback training helps the patient gain control over bladder muscles and relaxes the external sphincter. Children wear electromyogram (EMG) patches near the perineum or abdomen to assist in training.

Exstrophy of the Bladder

- Exstrophy of the bladder is a congenital defect where the anterior surface of the bladder is open on the abdominal wall. The defect has a variety of degrees of severity.
- Ultrasound is the tool used to diagnose exstrophy of the bladder.
- Surgery is necessary within the first 48 hours of the infant's life.
- The area must be kept clean because urine on the skin can cause irritation.
- Diapers should be loose-fitted and changed frequently.
- The exposed bladder may be covered with Vaseline gauze (Stein, 2007).

Cryptorchidism

- Cryptorchidism is defined as absent, undescended, or ectopic testicles.
- Gentle compression of the inguinal canals should reveal a palpable nodule in undescended testicles (Fig. 29-3).
- The surgical repair is termed orchiopexy and is usually done between ages 1 and 2.
- Instruct the caregiver to have the child wear loose clothing to increase comfort; use appropriate analgesics as ordered, including acetaminophen (Children's Tylenol); observe for erythema, purulent discharge, fever, and increased pain at the incision site as potentially indicative of infection.
- Instruct the caregiver to change diapers more frequently and to avoid having the older child engage in any sports or straddle riding toys that might injure the surgical site (Kenner et al., 2007).

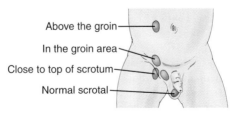

Above the groin

In the groin area

Close to top of scrotum

Normal scrotal

Figure 29-3 An undescended testis is palpable in various areas and needs to be surgically corrected.

Hypospadias and Epispadias

- Hypospadias and epispadias are genetic congenital conditions, which imply an abnormal positioning of the urethral meatus in boys.
- In hypospadias, the meatus is inferior to its usual position.
- In epispadias, the meatus is superior to its usual position and a surgical correction with possible penile urethral lengthening may be necessary (Montagnino & Currier, 2005).
- Recognize that parents of these children may be deficient in knowledge about the defects and their repair.
- Assess the parents' feelings about having a child with a congenital defect (Kenner et al., 2007).

Ambiguous Genitalia

- External reproductive organs that are not easily identified as male or female (Venes, 2005).
- The nurse may assist the patient's family by suggesting endocrinology and genetic referrals.
- Some patients with ambiguous genitalia become surgical candidates (Gray & Campbell, 2002).

RESOURCES

American Academy of Child and Adolescent Psychiatry: http://www.aacap.org

Bedwetting Store: http://www.bedwettingstore.com

National Guideline Clearinghouse: http://www.guideline.gov

National Kidney Foundation: http://www.kidney.org

REFERENCES

Cendron, M., & Benedict, J. (2006). Vesicoureteral reflux. Retrieved from http://www.emedicine.com/med/topic2838 (Accessed April 24, 2009).

Cole, F.L., & Volger, R. (2004). The acute, nontraumatic scrotum: Assessment, diagnosis, and management. *Journal of the American Academy of Nurse Practitioners, 16*(2), 50–56.

Davis' Drug Guide for Nurses (2009). Imipramine. Retrieved from http://www.drugguide.com/monograph_library/psychotropic_drugs/imipramine.htm (Accessed April 24, 2009).

Elder, J. (2004). Urinary tract infections. In R.E. Behrman, R.M. Kleigman, & H.B. Jenson. *Nelson's textbook of pediatrics* (17th ed., pp. 1785–1789). Philadelphia: W.B. Saunders.

Emans, S.J. (2005). Vulvovaginal problems in the prepubertal child. In S.J. Emans, M.R. Laufer, & D.P. Goldstein (Eds.). *Pediatric & adolescent gynecology* (5th ed.). Philadelphia: Lippincott Willliams & Wilkins.

Egland, A. & Egland T. (2006). Pediatrics, urinary tract infections and pyelonephritis. Retrieved from http://www.emedicine.com/emer/topic 769.htm (Accessed April 24, 2009).

Gray, M., & Campbell, F. (2002). Urinary system. In J.A. Fox (Ed.). *Primary health care of infants, children, & adolescents* (2nd ed., pp. 670–693). St. Louis, MO: Mosby.

Hellerstein, S. (2007). Urinary tract infection. Retrieved from http://www.emedicine.com/ped/topic2366.htm (Accessed April 24, 2009).

Herban Hill, N., & Sullivan, L.M. (2004). *Management guidelines for nurse practitioners working with children and adolescents* (2nd ed.). Philadelphia: F.A. Davis.

Hogan, M. & White, J. (2003). *Child health nursing: Reviews & rationales.* Upper Saddle River, NJ: PrenticeHall.

Kennedy, T. (2003). Urinary tract infection. In C. Rudolph & A. Rudolph (Eds.). *Rudolph's pediatrics* (21st ed., pp. 1667–1671). Chicago: McGraw-Hill.

Kenner, C., Moran, M., Zebold, K.F., Keating, B.J., & Amlung, S.R. (2007). Genitourinary alterations. In N.L. Potts & B.L. Mandleco (Eds.). *Pediatric nursing: Caring for children and their families* (2nd ed., pp. 623–659). Clifton Park, NY: Thompson Delmar.

Kliegman, R., Marcdante, K., Jenson, J. & Behrman, R. (2006). *Nelson essentials of pediatrics.* Philadelphia: Elsevier Saunders.

Lippincott Williams & Wilkins. (2004). *Straight A's in pediatric nursing.* Philadelphia: Lippincott Williams & Wilkins.

Lum, G.M. (2007). Kidney & urinary tract. In W.W. Hay, Jr., M.J. Levin, J.M. Sondheimer, & R. R. Deterding (Eds.). *Current pediatric diagnosis & treatment.* (18th ed). New York: Lange Medical Books/McGraw-Hill.

Montagnino, B., & Currier, H. (2005). The child with genitourinary dysfunction. In M.J. Hockenberry, D. Wilson, & M.L. Winkelstein (Eds.). *Wong's essentials of pediatric nursing* (7th ed., pp. 984–1010). St. Louis, MO: Mosby.

National Guideline Clearinghouse. (2004). Practice parameter for the assessment and treatment of children and adolescents with enuresis. Retrieved from http://www.guideline.gov (Accessed April 24, 2009).

Pagana, K., & Pagana, T. (2003). *Mosby's diagnostic and laboratory test reference.* Philadelphia: Mosby.

PDRhealth. (2007). Tofranil. Retrieved from http://www.pdrhealth.com/drug_info/rxdrugprofiles/drugs/tof1448.shtml (Accessed April 24, 2009).

Razzaq, S. (2006). Hemolytic uremic syndrome: An emerging risk. *American Family Physician, 74*(6), 991–996.

Ringdahl, E., & Teague, L. (2006). Testicular torsion. *American Family Physician, 74*(10), 1739–1744.

Schwartz, M.W. (2005). *The 5 minute pediatric consult.* Philadelphia: Lippincott Williams & Wilkins.

Stein, A.M. (Ed.). (2007). *Nursing review series: Pediatric nursing.* Clifton Park, NY: Thomson Delmar Learning.

Taketomo, C.K., Hodding, J.H., & Kraus, D.M. (2007). *Pediatric dosage handbook*. Hudson, OH: Lexi-Comp.

Venes, D. (Ed.). (2005). *Taber's cyclopedic medical dictionary* (20th ed.). Philadelphia: F.A. Davis.

Wise, B. & Cardinal-Busse, B. (2007). Common illness of the reproductive and urologic systems. In N. Ryan-Wenger (Ed.). *Core curriculum for primary care pediatric nurse practitioners*. St. Louis, MO: Mosby.

chapter

30

Caring for the Child with a Hematological Condition

KEY TERMS

allogeneic transplant – A transplant in which the recipient's human leukocyte antigens (HLA) are matched to a compatible donor, usually a sibling

autologous transplant – A transplant in which the ill child is her own donor of stem cells

febrile reaction – A fever greater than 1.8 degrees Fahrenheit from the baseline temperature

hemarthrosis – Bloody effusion within a joint and soft tissue bleeding (Sevier, 2005)

neutropenia – When an absolute neutrophil count is <1000/μL in infants <1 year of age and 1500/μL for those older than 1 year of age

pancytopenia – Reduction in all cellular elements of the blood caused by bone marrow hematopoiesis failure (Hillman, Ault, & Rinder, 2005)

plasmapheresis – Removal of plasma containing harmful components such as circulating complexes, antibodies (IgM, IgG), cholesterol

syngeneic transplant – A transplant in which the donor of the bone marrow is an identical sibling

FOCUSED ASSESSMENT

Anemia

Signs and Symptoms
- Mild anemia, may be asymptomatic and not diagnosed until blood tests are completed. Initial signs include fatigue, shortness of breath, headache, difficulty concentrating, dizziness, and pale skin.
- Moderate to severe anemia: Irritability, fatigue, delayed motor development, tachycardia, shortness of breath, decreased activity level, pale, listless, systolic heart murmur, hepatomegly, congestive heart failure.

Iron-Deficiency Anemia

Signs and Symptoms
- Asymptomatic (mild anemia)
- Decreased hemoglobin (Hgb) and hematocrit (Hct)
- Irritability, fatigue, delayed motor development, shortness of breath, decreased activity level, and pallor
- Remember that it is possible for an overweight child to be diagnosed with iron-deficiency anemia

Epistaxis

Signs and Symptoms
- Bleeding from the nose

Sickle Cell Disease (SCD)

Signs and Symptoms
- Result of vaso-occlusion
- Weakness
- Pallor
- Fatigue
- Tissue hypoxia
- Jaundice
- Pain

Beta-Thalassemia

Signs and Symptoms
- Enlarged liver and spleen
- Mild jaundice

- Growth retardation
- Moderate to severe anemia
- Bony deformities
- Increased susceptibility to infection

Hereditary Spherocytosis (HS)

Signs and Symptoms
- Hyperbilirubinemia
- Splenomegaly
- Negative Comb's test

Hemophilia

Signs and Symptoms
- Present with bleeding or known family history of bleeding disorders
- Hemarthrosis

von Willebrand's Disease

Signs and Symptoms
- Epistaxis
- Bleeding from the oral cavity
- Menorrhagia
- Easy bruising

Idiopathic (Immune) Thrombocytopenia Purpura (ITP)

Signs and Symptoms
- Detected after a recent viral infection
- Petechiae
- Bruising
- Mucocutaneous bleeding
- Epistaxis
- Menorrhagia (adolescent)

Disseminated Intravascular Coagulation (DIC)

Signs and Symptoms
- Excessive bleeding from orifices
- Petechia, purpura, and hypotension
- Multiorgan failure

Aplastic Anemia

Signs and Symptoms
- Pancytopenia
- Anemia, pallor, dizziness, and fatigue
- Petechia, epistaxis
- Increased susceptibility to infections and oral ulcerations

Neutropenia

- The nursing plan of care for children with neutropenia is based on the severity of neutropenia.
- Absolute neutrophil count (ANC) is a measure of the number of neutrophil granulocytes present in the blood.
- Calculation of the absolute neutrophil count (ANC) is the total number of white blood cells multiplied by the percentage of neutrophils (segs and bands). See page 647.
- The National Cancer Institute neutropenia grading system classifies slight neutropenia as grade 1 with ANC of less than 2000, minimal neutropenia grade 2 with ANC of <1500, and moderate neutropenia grade 3 with ANC less than 1000. The most severe neutropenia is grade 4 with an ANC of <500.

Signs and Symptoms
- Lymphadenopathy
- Organomegaly
- Pallor
- Bruising
- Petechia

Thrombosis

Risk Factors
- Prolonged immobility
- Disease states, obesity, medications, hereditary factors
- Major surgery or trauma

Signs and Symptoms
- Lungs: Shortness of breath, lightheaded, and increased heart rate
- Kidney: Blood in the urine
- Skin: Hemorrhagic spots
- Artery or extremity: Cold, pale, blue, and absent pulse

Complications
- Stroke
- Deep vein thrombosis
- Pulmonary emboli

CLINICAL ALERTS

Screening Guidelines

- According to the recommendations in the American Academy of Pediatrics screening guidelines, hemoglobin and hematocrit should be evaluated once during infancy (6–9 months of age), early childhood (1–5 years of age), late childhood (5–12 years of age), and adolescence (14–20 years of age).
- Identifies children who may benefit from treatment for anemia.

Iron-Deficiency Anemia

- Iron-deficiency anemia is defined as a microcytic, hypochromic anemia caused by an inadequate supply of iron (Nathan et al., 2003).
- Iron-deficiency anemia is more common in infants. Premature infants are at high risk due to their decreased fetal iron supply (Nathan et al., 2003).
- Be vigilant for overweight infants who may have iron deficiency anemia because of excessive milk ingestion, known as "milk baby." These infants will be chunky, pale, with a "porcelain like" appearance. Other clinical features of these "milk babies" include poor muscle development as well as being susceptible to infections.

A Child Who Is Asplenic

- Seek immediate medical attention if a child has a temperature greater than 101.5°F (38.6°C). The child needs blood cultures and broad-spectrum antibiotics to prevent sepsis.
- There is an inability to filter certain encapsulated bacteria, which causes a low-grade bacterial infection or serious sepsis.

- Ensure that parents know that is critical for children to receive the pneumococcal and *H. influenzae* type b vaccine and other routine vaccinations.

Accumulation of Iron (Hemosiderosis)

- Chronic blood transfusion therapy may cause iron to accumulate in tissues and organs that the body cannot eliminate. Treatment is necessary to prevent toxic levels of iron in the body, which may result in death.
- Chelating agents are used to remove iron from the body through excretion of urine and stool. The main chelating agent is deferoxamine B (Desferal) (Lo & Singer, 2002). This drug is rapidly excreted in the urine; therefore it must be administered intravenously or subcutaneously over 8 to 10 hours, usually at bedtime, at least 5 days a week.
- Teach parents and older children how to insert the butterfly catheter and administer the drug via an infusion pump at home without difficulty.
- Monitoring iron levels is indicated for patients on chelation therapy to evaluate compliance and effectiveness of treatment.
- Evaluate patients at risk for hemosiderosis for long-term complications. Complications that may occur are a result of iron deposits that may damage vital organs causing hearing loss, diabetes, organ failure, and ultimately death.

Administration of Intravenous Anti-D Antibody

- Is the newest treatment for acute ITP patients who are Rh+.
- Common side effects: Transient hemolytic anemia that often resolves as the IgG disperses, fever, chills, and headache after infusion.
- Closely monitor vital signs.

Intracranial Bleeding

- Intracranial bleeding is the most serious complication in idiopathic (immune) thrombocytopenia purpura (ITP).
- Alert caregivers to report any changes in level of consciousness or behavior, severe headaches, vision

616 ■ CLINICAL POCKET COMPANION

changes, ataxia, slurred speech, weakness or numbness, severe vomiting not associated with nausea.

Anaphylactic Reaction in Children Who Receive Antithymocyte Globulin (ATG)

- A severe anaphylactic reaction could occur (signs and symptoms include hypotension, tachycardia, shortness of breath, chest pain).
- Administer a test dose to check for allergic reaction, but be aware that an allergic reaction could occur beyond the test dose.
- If there is an allergic reaction, ATG may still be used following a desensitizing process and/or administration of pre-medications such as antihistamine and steroids.

Blood Transfusion Safety Measure

- To prevent a fatality, ensure a child receiving a transfusion is wearing a blood identification bracelet. The blood to be given must match identifying numbers on the bracelet.

The Administration Process for Blood Products

Pretransfusion

- Do not call for the product until it is needed.
- Verify the physician's orders including the appropriate product and volume to be infused. For packed red blood cell infusions appropriate volume is 10 to 13 mL/kg. Check with the institutional policies and procedures. The transfusion must be started within 30 minutes after the blood has left the blood bank.
- The maximum time for the infusion is 4 hours, which includes the first 30 minutes. Transfusion needs to start immediately due to the risk of bacterial contamination and cell lysis. Most blood banks will not accept blood back after 30 minutes.
- Follow institutional policy for obtaining, verifying, and transporting blood products obtained from the blood bank.
- Complete the appropriate forms and ensure accurate patient identification.
- Indicate product type and check for any special orders such as CMV safe, irradiated.

- Always check to see if any premedications were ordered before administration.
- Use PPE (personal protective equipment). Wear goggles and gloves.
- All blood products must be checked at the patient's bedside by two appropriate health care team members as per your institution's policy.
- Remember the two patient identifiers: Matching the numbers on the blood product and blood identification bracelet.

Initiation of the Transfusion

- Obtain baseline vital signs.
- Start the infusion slowly for the first 15 minutes.
- Designate a nurse to remain with the patient for the first 15 minutes of transfusion in the event of an adverse reaction.

During the Transfusion

- Do not infuse any other solutions simultaneously with blood through the same intravenous line; the only exception to this is normal saline (AABB Guidelines, 2004).
- Never add any medications to blood.
- Monitor vital signs per the institution's policy and procedures.
- All identification information that is attached to the blood product must remain attached until the transfusion is completed.
- Monitor for signs and symptoms of adverse reactions.

Posttransfusion

- Save the transfusion bag for at least 1 hour after the transfusion has ended.
- Complete the blood slip per the institution's policy.
- As per the American Association of Blood Bank (AABB). guidelines, include the following information on the child's medical record: Transfusion order, type of blood product, donor unit number, date and time of transfusion, pre and post vital signs, volume infused, required signatures, and any transfusion adverse events.
- Place the chart copy and blood bank copy of the blood slip in an appropriate area and keep on file as per policy and procedure.

Transfusion-Related Acute Lung Injury

- Transfusion-related acute lung injury (TRALI) occurs when there is an antigen–antibody reaction.
- The child who is experiencing TRALI may develop respiratory distress such as shortness of breath, hypoxia, hypotension, fever, and abnormal breath sounds.
- The reaction typically occurs within 1 to 2 hours after the transfusion has started and full-blown acute respiratory distress may occur within 6 hours (Knippen, 2006).
- Based on the severity of symptoms, respiratory support with a ventilator may be indicated. For mild cases of TRALI, supportive care is indicated.
- If this complication is suspected, it is reportable to the FDA (U.S. Food and Drug Administration, 2002).

DIAGNOSTIC TESTS

Hemoglobin and Hematocrit (Hgb & Hct)

- Complete blood count (CBC) and reticulocyte count are obtained to evaluate the hemoglobin and hematocrit.
- Anemia exists when the hemoglobin content is less than required to meet the oxygen demands of the body.
- Hemoglobin level is measured as the amount of hemoglobin per deciliter of whole blood. The average hemoglobin in the blood varies based on the age and gender of the individual. Normal Hemoglobin (Hgb; g/dL) lab values for children are:
  - Newborn: 12.7–18.6 g/dL
  - 2 Months: 9.0–14.0 g/dL
  - 2 Years: 10.5–12.7 g/dL
  - 6–12 Years: 11.2–14.8 g/dL
  - 12–18 Years: 10.7–15.7 g/dL
- The hematocrit is the percentage of whole blood that is composed of RBCs. The hematocrit measures both the number and size of the RBCs and is approximately three times greater than the hemoglobin value. The hematocrit indirectly measures the hemoglobin. The average hematocrit value is between 35% and 45% (Gilbert-Barness & Barness, 2003).

Complete Blood Count, Reticulocyte, and Peripheral Smear Lab Values for Children

- When evaluating for the presence of anemia, initial laboratory tests should include complete blood count (CBC) and a reticulocyte count. The CBC includes hemoglobin, hematocrit, red blood cell (RBC) indices, platelet count, white blood cell (WBC) count with a differential, and a peripheral smear to examine the morphology of the RBCs.
- For the patient with suspected anemia, the peripheral blood smear is imperative to confirm the appropriate diagnosis (Gilbert-Barness & Barness, 2003).

Normal Lab Values According to Age					
	Newborn	**2 Months**	**2 Years**	**6–12 Years**	**12–18 Years**
Red Blood Cell (RBC) Count	4.1–5.74	2.7–4.9	3.9–5.03	4.93–5.3	3.7–5.5
Hemoglobin (Hgb) (g/dL)	12.7–18.6	9.0–14.0	10.5–12.7	11.2–14.8	10.7–15.7
Hematocrit (Hct) (%)	37.4–56.1	28.0–42.0	31.7–37.7	34.0–43.9	33.0–46.2
White Blood Cell (WBC) Count	6.8–14.3	5.0–19.5	5.3–11.5	4.5–10.1	4.4–10.2
Platelets 10³/mm³(μL)	164–586	164–586	206–459	189–403	175–345

Normal White Blood Cell Differential Count According to Age

Age/White Blood Cell Component	Function	Newborn	2 Months	2 Years	6–12 Years	12–18 Years
Neutrophils (%)	Phagocytosis	19–49	15–35	13–33	32–54	34–64
Eosinophils (%)	Allergic reactions	0–4	0–3	0–3	0–3	0–3
Basophils (%)	Inflammatory reactions	0–1	0–1	0–1	0–1	0–1
Lymphocytes (%; B cells and T cells)	Humoral immunity (B cell) and cellular immunity (T cell)	38–46	42–72	46–76	27–57	25–45
Monocytes (%; macrophages)	Phagocytosis and antigen processing	0–9	0–6	0–5	0–5	0–5

Red Cell Lab Values for Children

Test	Reference Range	Comments
Mean Corpuscular Volume (MCV)	79–95 μm³	Average size of a single RBC, expressed as cubic microns (μm³)
Mean Corpuscular Hemoglobin (MCH)	25–33 pg/cell	Average weight of the Hgb within a RBC, expressed in picograms (pg)
Mean Cell Hemoglobin Concentration (MCHC)	31%–37% Hgb [g]/dl RBC	Average concentration of Hgb in each RBC
Reticulocyte Count	0.5%–1.5%	Measure of the production of mature RBCs by the bone marrow
Peripheral Smear	Size, shape, and structure of the RBCs, as well as an estimate of the amount of Hgb in the RBCs	Can indicate variations in size and shape of RBCs: microcytic, macrocytic, or normocytic

Evaluating a CBC

Blood Elements	Increase	Decrease
RBC (Hgb/Hct)	Polycythemia	Anemia
WBC	Leukocytosis	Leukopenia
Platelets	Thrombocytosis	Thrombocytopenia

Epistaxis Diagnostic Workup: Laboratory Tests to Diagnose Bleeding Disorder

Test	Range	Significance
Prothrombin Time (PT)	11–14 seconds	Measures the extrinsic pathway for bleeding, requires fibrinogen, prothrombin, and factors V, VII, and X. Prolonged times may indicate deficiencies of vitamin K liver factors, malabsorption, and liver disease.
Partial Thromboplastin Time (PTT)	25–38 seconds	Measures the intrinsic pathway for bleeding, requires factors V, VIII, IX, X, XI, and XII and fibrinogen and prothrombin. Prolonged times may indicate a bleeding disorder.

Source: Hillman, Ault, & Rinder (2005).

Further Testing for Infants Suspected of Having Sickle Cell Disease

- If sickle cell disease is suspected, infants will need further testing, such as a hemoglobin electrophoresis (Fixler & Styles, 2002).
- A hemoglobin electrophoresis is a more specific blood test that identifies sickle cell disease versus sickle cell trait in a child (Gilbert-Barness & Barness, 2003).

Procedure 30-1 Obtaining a Fecal Occult Blood Test Sample

Purpose
A fecal occult blood test (FOBT) is performed to detect hidden (occult) blood in the stool.

Equipment
- Hematest cards
- Gloves
- Sterile tongue blade
- Chemical reagent

Steps
1. Wash hands and don gloves.
2. Verify the identity of the patient.
3. Check the manufacturer's instructions for specific Hematest cards.
4. Keep the Hematest cards at room temperature.
5. Use a sterile tongue blade to remove a sample of stool from the diaper.
6. Place a smear of stool on both windows of the Hematest card as indicated on the instructions.
7. Cover the windows with the paper flaps and wait the correct amount of time before reading the results.
8. Apply the recommended drops of developing solution to the Hematest card.
9. Read the back flap of the sample card within the recommended time of application of developing solution.
10. The Hematest card should change color to indicate the test results.
11. Document the procedure.

Clinical Alert When the nurse records the results, it is important to notify the health care provider of any abnormal findings. In addition, the nurse should check the expiration date on the developing solution.

Teach Parents
It is important to teach the parents the rationale for the test.

Type and Screen and Type and Crossmatch

The best outcome exists for the child when the nurse understands the difference between the type and screen and type and crossmatch.

Type and Screen
- Obtained in anticipation that a child may need blood.
- ABO group and Rh type of patient identified.
- Does not remove blood from inventory.

Type and Crossmatch
- Obtained if almost certain the child will require blood.
- ABO/Rh compatible donor red cells combined.
- Crossmatch is good for 72 hours (Hillman et al., 2005).

Understanding Blood Type

- When the clinical criterion is met, the nurse may proceed and obtain the product to be infused from the institution's blood bank or pharmacy. Understand that blood type is essential information for the nurse.

Blood Type	Can GIVE to:	TAKE from:
A+	A+	A+, A–, O–
A–	A+, A–	A–, O–
B+	B+	B+, B–, O+, O–
B–	B+, B–	B–, O–
AB+	AB+	All types
AB–	AB–	A–, B–, AB–, O–
O+	A+, B+, AB+, O+	O+, O–
O–	All types	O–

MEDICATIONS

Ketorolac (Toradol)

Generic Name Ketorolac (Kee-**toe**-role-ak)

Pregnancy Category C (D if used in the 3rd trimester)

Indications Short-term (≤5 days) management of moderate to severe pain, including post operative pain.

Actions Inhibits prostaglandin synthesis by decreasing activity of the enzyme, cyclooxygenase, which results in a decrease of prostaglandin precursors.

Therapeutic Effects Pain relief

Pharmacokinetics
Oral Well absorbed; 100%
IM/IV Rapid and complete

Contraindications and Precautions
Contraindicated in Hypersensitivity to Toradol, aspirin, or other NSAIDs

Patients with peptic ulcer disease or anyone with bleeding tendencies

Adverse Reactions and Side Effects Dizziness, headache, rash, diarrhea, GI pain, bleeding, prolonged bleeding times, anaphylaxis, hypersensitivity reactions.

Route and Dosage Ketorolac injection is approved for use in pediatric patients only as a single IM or IV dose in children 2–16 years of age; the use of ketorolac injection in children <2 years of age, the use of multiple doses of the injection in children <16 years of age, and the use of the tablets in children <16 years of age are outside of product labeling; ophthalmic solutions are approved for use in children ≥3 years of age.

Single-dose treatment: Manufacturer's recommendations:
IM: 1 mg/kg as a single dose; maximum dose: 30 mg
IV: 0.5 mg/kg as a single dose; maximum dose: 15 mg

Nursing Implications
Teach the patient and parents medication administration.
Do not exceed 5 days of total use.
Avoid alcohol.
May cause drowsiness and impair the ability to perform activities requiring mental alertness.

Additional Information 30 mg of Toradol provides analgesia comparable to 12 mg of morphine or 100 mg of meperidine.

Data from Deglin, J., & Vallerand, A. (2009). Davis's drug guide for nurses (11th ed.), pp. 716–718. Philadelphia: F. A. Davis.

Pneumococcal and *Haemophilus influenzae* Type b (Hib) Vaccine

- Children with hereditary spherocytosis (HS) should receive the pneumococcal and *Haemophilus influenzae* type b (Hib) vaccine before the splenectomy to prevent life-threatening bacterial infections.
- Children should also be given prophylactic penicillin to prevent fatal infections.

Proper Replacement Factors

- Now recombinant factor products are the main treatment of hemophilia patients (Sevier, 2005).

Hematopoietic Growth Factors

- Hematopoietic growth factor is granulocyte colony stimulating factor (GCSF), also known as Neupogen.
- GCSF stimulates the WBC lines.
- Growth factors for the WBCs are given to prevent profound neutropenia and prevent the patient from being susceptible to life threatening infections.
- Given by subcutaneous injection once a day by child's caregiver.
- Possible side effects: Fever, bone pain, headache, local reaction at injection site.

ETHNOCULTURAL CONSIDERATIONS

Sickle Cell Disease

- Most prominent in children of African American or Mediterranean descent
- May also be seen in Hispanics, Caucasians, and Italians

Jehovah Witness

- It is against this faith to receive blood and blood products, including self-donation.
- All alternatives should be explored to respect these beliefs.
- If the child is in a life-threatening situation, the courts may be called in to make a decision.

TEACHING THE FAMILY

Nutritional Counseling for the Prevention of Iron-Deficiency Anemia

- Feed the infant breast milk or commercial infant formula for the first 12 months of life.
- Use iron-fortified cereal from 6 to 12 months of age.
- Do not feed the infant cow's milk before 12 months of age (for infants 12 months and older limit the amount of cow's milk to 18 to 24 ounces per day).
- Once solids are introduced, offering the bottle before the feeding helps prevent iron deficiency.
- It is important for adolescents on a vegetarian diet or weight reduction diet to understand proper dietary alternatives to prevent iron-deficiency anemia.
- Dietary alternatives such as red meats, beans, whole grains, nuts, and iron-fortified cereals are good sources of iron.

Education About Oral Iron

- Educating parents on the proper administration of oral iron is a vital nursing responsibility.
- The iron supplement needs to be taken between meals because absorption is improved in an acidic environment.
- Administering iron with a glass of orange juice may also enhance absorption.
- Iron supplements should not be taken with tea because they may adversely affect the absorption process.
- Inform parents that liquid iron preparations may stain teeth so it is important to administer the medication with a dropper or drink it through a straw. Encourage the child to rinse his or her mouth after taking this liquid medication.

- Make parents aware that iron can be constipating and it is necessary to increase the fiber and water intake to prevent this possible complication.
- Possible side effects of iron therapy include gastric upset, nausea, vomiting, and constipation. Black tarry stools are a common finding and are normal for children taking iron supplements.
- Encourage parents to keep no more than a 1-month supply in the home and to store it out of reach of small children because ingestion of excessive quantities may be toxic or even fatal.

Education About Sickle Cell Disease

- Ensure that families know signs and symptoms of sickle cell crisis so they can report them to health care provider.
- Educate the family about the goals of ongoing care including the prevention of complications such as infections, hypoxemia and vaso-occlusive crisis.
- Avoid strenuous activities that may precipitate hypoxia.
- Maintain rest and adequate hydration to avoid sickle cell crisis.
- Adhere to prophylactic penicillin as prescribed to prevent sepsis.
- Use supplemental folic acid to assist with red blood cell production.
- Instruct a patient who experiences a mild sickle cell crisis at home to stop what she is doing, rest, drink fluids, and take prescribed pain medication. If there is no improvement, tell her to seek help from health care provider or go to nearest emergency facility for treatment.
- Advise parents about genetic screening and counseling.

The Child with Hemophilia

- Instruct families on what signs and symptoms require prompt medical attention. Most importantly, any trauma to the head or a change in the level of consciousness is a medical emergency.
- Teach the family about the factor replacement products; including how to obtain the products.
- Teach parents how to administer prophylactic dose of factor replacement at home.

- Ensure that the family is aware that safety is of utmost importance. Injury prevention should be reviewed at all stages of development as risk factors change based on the child's age. Contact sports are highly discouraged. The child should be fitted for a safety helmet to prevent head injury when bike riding.
- Communicate to the family that an interdisciplinary team reviews home environmental factors that can affect the treatment plan.
- Inform the family that for children who have experienced bleeding into the joints, physical therapy may be necessary to preserve and maintain functional status.
- Encourage the child to wear a medical alert bracelet in the event that a medical emergency occurs outside the home.
- Reinforce to the family that genetic counseling is recommended because hemophilia is an inherited disorder (Lea & Williams, 2002).
- Collaboration with the social worker is essential to assist with insurance issues, obtaining medications and supplies, rehabilitation services, home nursing, and other concerns. The social worker is also available for emotional/ psychosocial support.
- Numerous resources are available at comprehensive hemophilia centers and also online by the National Hemophilia Foundation at www.hemophilia.org.

Diagnosing Idiopathic (Immune) Thrombocytopenia Purpura

- The following tests are required to confirm the diagnosis of ITP: CBC, peripheral smear examination, coagulation analysis, bone marrow aspirate if steroid therapy is implemented or to rule out an underlying malignancy.
- CBC usually shows isolated and severe thrombocytopenia, usually a platelet count of less than 20,000.
- Peripheral smear is often normal with the exception of thrombocytopenia with normal to large-sized platelets (Di Paola & Buchanan, 2002).

The Neutropenic Child

Teach families and children with neutropenia the following measures to reduce the incidence of infection:

- Always keep routine visits.
- Be aware of the signs and symptoms of infections such as fever (>101.5°F [38.6°C]).
- Avoid large crowds or anyone who may be sick with a cold, flu, etc.
- Keep the child's body clean by bathing every day, brushing teeth after meals and before bedtime.
- Avoid hot tubs.
- Always wash the child's hands before eating or touching the face, eyes, nose, mouth, etc.
- Avoid constipation and straining to have a bowel movement by drinking 2 quarts of fluid each day, exercising, and using a stool softener.
- Avoid putting anything in the child's rectum, including thermometers and suppositories.
- Avoid exposure to fresh flowers or live plants.
- Avoid exposure to stool droppings from pets and cleaning bird cages as well as cleaning cat litter boxes.
- Do not share bath towels or drinking glasses with others, including family members.
- Avoid eating the following items:
  - Raw milk or milk products; any milk product that has not been pasteurized, including cheese and yogurt made from unpasteurized milk
  - Raw or uncooked meat, fish, chicken, eggs, tofu
  - Any food that contains mold, for example, blue cheese
  - Raw honey (honey that has not been pasteurized)
  - Uncooked fresh fruit or vegetables
  - Any outdated foods or foods left at room temperature for more than 2 hours
- Adolescents should not use tampons, vaginal suppositories, or douche.
- Adolescents should avoid manicures, pedicures, acrylic nails, or nail tips.
- Adolescents should use an electric shaver instead of a razor.

ADDITIONAL INFORMATION FOR THE CLINICAL SETTING

Nursing Care for Iron-Deficiency Anemia

- Arrange for nutritional counseling and provide assistance in obtaining the recommended iron-fortified formula.
- Administer oral iron supplements.

Controlling Epistaxis (Nosebleeds)

1. Wear gloves and place child in a sitting position, leaning forward.
2. Apply direct pressure to anterior nasal septum for 10 to 15 minutes.
3. Remind the child to breathe through his mouth to avoid becoming anxious.
4. Apply ice to the nose area.
5. Monitor vital signs if there is a large amount of blood loss.
6. If severe nose bleeding persists beyond 10 to 15 minutes, begin nasal packing and apply topical adrenaline (epinephrine).
7. When infection is present, antibiotics may be ordered (Kucik & Clenney, 2005).
8. Keep child and family calm by providing support and reassurance.
9. Ensure family can demonstrate first aid measures necessary to control epistaxis.

Nonpharmacological Pain Interventions

- Distraction
- Guided imagery
- Relaxation techniques
- Music therapy
- Comfort care
- Cutaneous stimulation
- Play therapy

Idiopathic (Immune) Thrombocytopenia Purpura (ITP) Management

- Platelet count >20,000, asymptomatic; does not require treatment and platelet counts should be monitored.

- Platelet count <20,000, bruises, petechia, no bleeding; treat with steroid, immune gamma globulin (IVIG) or Anti-D antibody (WinRho).
- Platelet count <20,000, bleeding; hospitalization with close observation and a 2- to 3-day course of immune gamma globulin (IVIG).

Understand Institutional Guidelines Related to Intravenous Immune Gamma Globulin (IVIG)

- Understand that intravenous immune gamma globulin (IVIG) is a blood product and blood product consent may be necessary based on institutional guidelines.
- Administration of this product requires frequent measurement of vital signs to monitor for possible side effects.
- Side effects may include fever, chills, hypotension, nausea, and headache.
- It is important for the nurse to check product-specific information for administration guidelines (Di Paola & Buchanan, 2002).

Supportive Care for Patients with Aplastic Anemia

- Provide transfusions of red blood cells and platelets.
- Use transfusions cautiously to prevent development of antibodies and possible graft versus host disease.
- Antibiotics are given to treat infections but generally not recommended prophylactically.

Obtain Transfusion Consent

- Transfusion consent must be obtained before the transfusion of all blood products.
- Transfusion consent must include the description of the procedure for transfusion, risks/benefits, treatment alternatives, and appropriate signatures including the health care provider, signature of patient if 18 years or older, or signature of parent or other legal representative and witness (AABB, 2004).
- Provide the opportunity for the family to ask questions.
- The family has the right to revoke the consent if they wish.

Transfusion Products

Transfusion Product	Indications	Critical Nursing Actions
Red Blood Cells	Hemoglobin <8 grams on a stable patient with a chronic anemia Hypovolemia due to acute blood loss Evidence of impending heart failure secondary to severe anemia Patients on hypertransfusion regimen for sickle cell disease and history of: • Cerebral vascular accident • Splenic sequestration • Acute chest syndrome • Recurrent priapism • Preoperative preparation for surgery with general anesthesia • Hypoxia Children requiring increased oxygen carrying capacity (i.e., complex congenital heart, intracardiac shunting, severe pulmonary disease—acute respiratory distress syndrome [ARDS]): • Shock states (decreased blood pressure, increased peripheral vasoconstriction, pallor, cyanosis, diaphoresis, clamminess, mottled skin, increased oxygen requirement, decreased urinary output) • Cardiac failure • Respiratory failure requiring significant ventilatory support • Postoperative anemia	Observe for clinical signs and symptoms of anemia: Fatigue Syncope Pallor Tachycardia Diaphoretic Shortness of breath Inability to perform activities of daily living Don appropriate PPE (personal protective equipment) for all blood product transfusions. Monitor vital signs per hospital policy and procedure. Monitor hemoglobin and hematocrit Observe for adverse reactions. Store blood in a designated blood refrigerator. Generally 10-15 ml/kg of packed red blood cells are transfused (Khilnani, 2005).
Autologous Blood (Self-donated blood product)	For general scheduled surgical procedures in which there is clinical indications that a blood transfusion may be necessary during the intraoperative or postoperative period, the patient may elect to self-donate. Check with blood bank facilities for time criteria for this type of donation. For general surgical procedures, the recommended hemoglobin is 10 grams or greater and for ortho-pedic surgery, the recommendation is hemoglobin of 11.5 grams or greater.	Verify with the parent that self-donation has occurred. Patient identification and administration process is the same as with all other blood products.

Transfusion Product	Indications	Critical Nursing Actions
Whole Blood or Packed Red Blood Cells (PRBCs) Reconstituted with Fresh Frozen Plasma (FFP)	Hypovolemia due to acute blood loss non-responsive to crystalloids • Hct <35% • Hypovolemia due to acute massive blood loss (i.e., major trauma) • History of blood loss at delivery or large amount of blood drawn for lab studies (10% blood volume) • Cardiac patients Hct <40% (structural heart disease, cyanosis, or CHF) • Drop in Hgb to below 10 grams intraoperatively • Exchange transfusion	Same nursing actions applicable to red blood cell infusions In major trauma situations, may transfuse patient with O negative blood, the universal donor. Use blood warmer and rapid infuser if available.
Platelets	Platelet count <20,000 Active bleeding with symptoms of DIC or other significant coagulopathies Platelet count <50,000 with planned invasive procedure (i.e., surgical procedure, central line insertion, does not include drawing blood or intramuscular injection of intravenous catheter insertion) Prevention or treatment of bleeding due to thrombocytopenia (secondary to chemotherapy, radiation or bone marrow failure) Treatment of patients with severe thrombocytopenia secondary to increased platelet destruction or immune thrombocytopenia associated with complication of severe trauma Massive transfusion with platelet dilution.	Know normal platelet count (150,000 to 400,000). Obtain CBC. Assess bruising, petechiae, and bleeding.
Fresh Frozen Plasma (FFP)	Replacement for deficiency of factors II, V, VII, IX, X, XII, protein C, or protein S. Bleeding, invasive procedure, or surgery with documented plasma clotting protein deficiency (i.e., liver failure, DIC, or septic shock) Prolonged PT and/or PTT without bleeding.	Notify the blood bank to thaw FFP, product must be used within 6 hours of thawing. Don appropriate PPE for all blood product transfusions. Monitor vital signs per hospital policy and procedure.

(continued)

Transfusion Products (Continued)

Transfusion Product	Indications	Critical Nursing Actions
	Significant intraoperative bleeding (>10% blood volume/hr) in excess of normally anticipated blood loss that is at high risk of clotting-factor deficiency Massive transfusion Therapeutic plasma exchanges Warfarin anticoagulant overdose	Monitor coagulation studies. During FFP infusions, observe for adverse reactions.
Cryoprecipitate	Fibrinogen levels <150 mg/dL with active bleeding Bleeding or prophylaxis in von Willebrand's disease or in factor VIII (hemophilia A) deficiency unresponsive to or unsuitable for DDAVP or factor VII concentrates Replacement therapy, bleeding, or invasive procedure in patients with factor XIII deficiency Patients with active intraoperative hemorrhage in excess of normally anticipated blood loss that are at risk of clotting factor deficiency	Assess for signs and symptoms of bleeding. Don appropriate PPE (personal protective equipment) for all blood product transfusions. Monitor vital signs per hospital policy and procedure. Monitor coagulation studies. During cryoprecipitate infusions, observe for adverse reactions.
Granulocytes (White Cell Transfusion)	Bacterial or fungal sepsis (proven or strongly suspected) unresponsive to antimicrobial therapy Infection (proven or strongly suspected) unresponsive to antimicrobial therapy	Type and crossmatch required for all WBC transfusions. Premedications may be ordered, such as antihistamines or acetaminophen.
Factor VII	Factor VII deficiency Factor VIII inhibitors Factor IX inhibitors Idiopathic uncontrolled bleeding	Assess for signs and symptoms of bleeding. Don appropriate PPE for all blood products, even recombinant. Monitor coagulation studies. If undiluted, dilute vial with indicated amount of sterile water and administer intravenously as per manufacturer's guidelines.

Transfusion Product	Indications	Critical Nursing Actions
Factor VIII Concentrate	Hemophilia A (factor VIII deficiency). Patient with factor VIII inhibitors Patients with von Willebrand's disease	Assess for signs and symptoms of bleeding. Don appropriate PPE for all blood products. Monitor coagulation studies. Check product to see if refrigeration necessary. Record expiration date and lot number of product.
Factor IX Concentrate (Prothrombin Complex)	Hemophilia B Hemophilia A with factor VIII inhibitors Patients with congenital deficiency of prothrombin, factor VII, and factor X	Assess for signs and symptoms of bleeding. Don appropriate PPE for all blood products. Monitor coagulation studies. Record expiration date and lot number of product.
Intravenous Immunoglobulin (IVIG)	Congenital or acquired antibody deficiency Immunological disorders such as idiopathic thrombocytopenia (ITP), Kawasaki disease Posttransplant patients used prophylactically; newborns with severe bacterial infections	Don appropriate PPE (for all IVIG infusions). Monitor vital signs per hospital policy and procedure. Start infusion slowly and increase rate/titrate per physician orders. During IVIG infusion, observe for adverse reactions such as fever, chills, and headache. Product is obtained from the pharmacy. Record the expiration date and lot number of the product.

The Administration of Blood

- Strict observance to the institutional policy regarding the administration of blood products cannot be stressed enough.
- The accuracy of patient verification is a critical nursing action that can help prevent a transfusion reaction.

Transfusion Reactions

- Most transfusion reactions occur during the initiation of a transfusion, but a reaction can occur at any time during this process (AABB, 2004).

- These reactions can vary from a mild reaction, such as mild fever, to the most severe complication of death.
- Children who have received multiple transfusions are at higher risk for developing a transfusion reaction (Knippen, 2006).

Febrile Reaction

- The most common blood transfusion reaction is a nonhemolytic febrile reaction in which the child develops a fever >1.8°F from the baseline temperature.
- Occurs on initiation of the transfusion, but have been known to occur up to 12 hours posttransfusion.
- Signs and symptoms: Fever and chills, which then may progress to more serious complications such as tachycardia, tachypnea, and hypotension.
- Nursing care: Premedication with acetaminophen (Children's Tylenol) can sometimes prevent this type of reaction. Monitoring the child's temperature to recognize febrile reactions early and prevent progression. Stop the transfusion, monitor vital signs closely, and notify the physician.

Allergic Reaction

- A nonhemolytic reaction that occurs during a transfusion in which the child has had a previous exposure to a particular allergen in the blood product.
- Signs and symptoms: Rash, hives, pruritus, swelling of the lips, wheezing, and anxiety.
- Nursing care: Stop the transfusion immediately, monitor vital signs closely, and notify physician. The administration of an antihistamine such as diphenhydramine (Benadryl) resolves an allergic response.

Bacterial Contamination

- Occurs during the initiation of the infusion.
- Guidelines from the AABB (2004) require strict adherence to the completion of all transfusions in 4 hours or less to prevent this from happening.
- Signs and symptoms: Shaking chills, fever, vomiting, diffuse erythema, and the onset of hypotension that may progress to shock. In severe cases hemoglobinuria, actual renal failure, and DIC may develop.
- Nursing care: Stop the transfusion immediately, monitor vital signs closely, start a normal saline infusion, notify the physician, and prepare emergency care (support

oxygenation and ventilation, antibiotics, and vasopressors may be ordered). Nursing responsibilities also include obtaining blood samples for culture and sensitivity and sending the blood product with tubing to the blood bank also to be cultured.

Circulatory Overload

- This reaction is rare and occurs when the infusion is given too rapidly or an excessive quantity of blood is given.
- Signs and symptoms: Dry cough, dyspnea, rales, distended neck veins, hypertension/hypotension, bradycardia/tachycardia, clammy skin, and cyanosis of the extremities.
- Nursing care: Accurate verification of physician orders, double-checking the volume to be infused, and the use of an intravenous pump. If any of the signs and symptoms are identified, the nurse must immediately stop the transfusion, monitor vital signs closely, place the child upright with feet in a dependent position to increase venous resistance, notify physician, and prepare emergency care (support oxygenation and ventilation as well as diuretics may be ordered).

Acute Hemolytic Transfusion Reaction

- This reaction is rare but it is the most severe type of reaction. It occurs when the donor RBCs and the recipient plasma are incompatible, and there is an ABO mismatch. Acute hemolytic transfusion reactions occur upon initiation after exposure to a small amount of blood (Hillman et al., 2005).
- Signs and symptoms: Fever, shaking chills, pain at the intravenous site, tightness of the chest, difficulties breathing, impending sense of doom, pallor, jaundice, nausea/vomiting, red or black urine, flank pain, and progressive signs of shock such as tachycardia and hypotension.
- Nursing care: Stop the transfusion, monitor vital signs closely, start a normal saline infusion, verify patient identification, notify the physician, and prepare emergency care (support oxygenation and ventilation, antihistamines, fluids, diuretics, and vasopressors may be ordered). Other nursing responsibilities include obtaining blood and urine samples and sending them to the laboratory to analyze for the presence of hemoglobin, which indicates intravascular hemolysis. Insert a urinary catheter to monitor the child's output more accurately.

Complications of Apheresis

Complication	Critical Nursing Actions
Hypocalcemia	Obtain ionized calcium levels before treatment. Correct all abnormal levels before initiating treatment. For apheresis lasting longer than 1 hour in length, monitor ionized calcium levels every hour until the end of the procedure. Consider calcium drip if needed: • Calcium chloride: 20–25 mg/kg per dose used for acute hypocalcemia • Calcium gluconate: 100–500 mg/kg per day (Robertson & Shilkofski, 2005)
Hypotension	Hypotension may occur with onset of treatment. Be sure to have fluid readily available at bedside. Patients receiving inotropic support may need an increase in the rate of administration.
Risk for Bleeding	Prothrombin time (PT), partial thromboplastin time (PTT), fibrinogen level, platelet count, Hct, and activated clotting time (ACT) are measured before and after apheresis. Measure ACT at the bedside at regular intervals, and adjust citrate and/or heparin doses accordingly. Platelet or other blood products such as clotting factors may be required during the procedure.
Hypothermia	Hypothermia may result from the blood being circulated in the extracorporeal circuit outside the body. Use a blood warmer on the pheresis machine. Monitor frequent temperatures to avoid hypothermia. Assess the patient for other signs of hypothermia (e.g., bradycardia and shivering). Keep the child warm with blankets and/or an external warmer. Increase ambient room temperature.
Transfusion Reaction	Use leukodepleted blood. Monitor for transfusion reactions from the replacement products. Follow the transfusion reaction protocol if this occurs. Consider administration of an antihistamine for patients receiving multiple treatments.
Infection	Maintain strict sterile technique with all intravenous lines.
Air Embolism	Monitor tubing and connection sites. Check that all are secured properly.
Thrombus	Obtain platelet count before catheter placement and be aware when possible transfusion of platelets are necessary. Flush vigorously with adequate volumes of normal saline as per institution's policy.

RESOURCES

American Sickle Cell Anemia Association: http://www.ascaa.org

Aplastic Anemia and MDS International Foundation:
http://www.aamds.org

National Hemophilia Foundation: http://www.hemophilia.org

National Marrow Donor Program: http://www.marrow.org

Sickle Cell Anemia Association: http://www.sicklecelldisease.org

REFERENCES

American Association of Blood Banks (AABB) Guidelines. (2004). Bethesda, MD: AABB Press.

Deglin, J., & Vallerand, A. (2009). *Davis's drug guide for nurses* (11th ed.). Philadelphia: F.A. Davis.

Di Paola, J., & Buchanan, G.R. (2002). Immune thrombocytopenic purpura. *Pediatric Clinics of North America, 49,* 911–928.

FDA Patient safety news. October 2004.

Fixler, J., & Styles, L. (2002). Sickle cell disease. *Pediatric Clinics of North America, 49,* 1193–1210.

Gilbert-Barness, E., & Barness, L. (2003). *Clinical use of pediatric diagnostic tests.* Philadelphia: Lippincott Williams & Wilkins.

Hillman, R.S., Ault, K.A., & Rinder, H.M. (2005). *Hematology in clinical practice: a guide to diagnosis and management.* New York: McGraw-Hill.

Knippen, M. (2006). Transfusion-related acute lung injury. *AJN, 106*(6), 61–64.

Khilnani, P. (2005). *Practical approach to pediatric intensive care.* New York: Oxford University Press.

Kucik, C.J., & Clenney, T. (2005). Management of epistaxis. *American Family Physician. 71*(2), 305–311.

Lea, D., & Williams, J. (2002). Genetic testing and screening, use them as part of routine nursing practice. *American Journal of Nursing, 102*(7), 36–43.

Lo, L., & Singer, S. (2002). Thalassemia: Current approach to an old disease. *Pediatric Clinics of North America, 49,* 1165–1191.

Nathan, D.G., Orkin, S.H., Ginsburg, D., & Look, A.T. (2003). *Nathan and Oski's hematology of infancy and childhood* (6th ed.). Philadelphia: W.B. Saunders.

Robertson, J., & Shilkofski, N. (2005). *The Harriet Lane handbook* (17th ed.). Philadelphia: Elsevier Mosby.

Sevier, N. (2005). Inherited coagulation factor abnormalities: A pediatric review. *Journal of Pediatric Oncology Nursing, 22*(3), 137–144.

U.S. Food and Drug Administration. (2002). Current good manufacturing practice for blood and blood components: Adverse reaction file. Title 21 part 606.170(b).

Caring for the Child with Cancer

KEY TERMS

mucositis – A diffuse inflammation of the mucosa of the mouth, a change in the integrity of the mucous membranes characterized by soreness, redness, and swelling; lesions on the mucous membranes allow bacteria to attach themselves to the affected areas and are a source of localized and systemic infection

FOCUSED ASSESSMENT

Acute Lymphocytic Leukemia (ALL)

Signs and Symptoms
- Fever, fatigue, lethargy, anemia, pale skin, anorexia, bone or joint pain
- Increased white blood cell (WBC) count

Acute Myelogenous Leukemia (AML)

Signs and Symptoms
- Symptoms resembling the flu, anemia, pallor, fatigue, bone pain, fever, headache or dizziness, petechiae, easy bruising, nosebleeds, or bleeding gums
- Increased WBC count

Chronic Myelogenous Leukemia (CML)

Signs and Symptoms
- Fever, fatigue, weight loss, anorexia
- Increased WBC count and splenomegaly

Brain Tumors

Signs and Symptoms

- Depends on the tumor location, tumor type, and the age of the child
- Obstruction of cerebrospinal fluid (CSF) drainage leading to increased intracranial pressure (ICP)

Neurological Assessment

- Tumors of the brain or CNS are the second most common cancer in children after leukemia.
- Virtually all childhood brain tumors are primary tumors, meaning that they originate in the brain.

Performing the Neurological Exam

- The main focus of a physical assessment of a child with a brain tumor should be the neurological exam.
- A patient's baseline assessment is important to detect any subtle changes.
- The exam includes vital signs; pupil size, equality, and response to light; level of consciousness; strength and equality of grip of hands; and movement of the legs.
- Head circumference and the assessment of the anterior fontanel is also important in assessing an infant's intracranial pressure.
- Parents may first notice behavioral changes.
- The neurological exam can change rapidly.
- Timely responses to neurological changes are of vital importance for the child with a brain tumor.

Neuroblastoma

Signs and Symptoms

- Wide variety depending on site of primary tumor
- On palpation tumor crosses midline; hard painless mass in neck or abdomen

Wilms' Tumor (Nephroblastoma)

Signs and Symptoms

- Painless abdominal mass in one or both kidneys (seldom crosses midline)

Palpitation of the Abdomen in a Child with Wilms' Tumor
- Once a child has been diagnosed with Wilms' tumor, never palpate the abdomen or allow anyone else to do so.
- Palpating this kind of encapsulated tumor can cause it to rupture or lead to further metastasis.
- Place a warning sign on the child's hospital room door that says, "No abdominal palpation."

Rhabdomyosarcoma

Signs and Symptoms
- Depends on location of primary tumor and metastasis (head and neck, nasopharynx, genitourinary, extremities skeletal or smooth muscle perianal regions)

Retinoblastoma

Signs and Symptoms
- Leukocoria, strabismus, red painful eyes (blindness is a late sign)

Osteosarcoma

Signs and Symptoms
- Pain and swelling
- Limp
- Dull aching pain
- Palpation at site, tenderness, swelling, warmth, and erythema

Ewing's Sarcoma

Signs and Symptoms
- Pain or tenderness and swelling at the site of the tumor (chest wall tumor causes respiratory distress)

Hodgkin's Disease (HD)

Signs and Symptoms
- Painless, firm, cervical, or supraclavicular lymphadenopathy

Non-Hodgkin's Lymphoma (NHL)

Signs and Symptoms
- Pain or swelling (abdomen, chest and head/neck)

Liver Cancer

- Hepatoblastoma or Hepatocellular carcinoma

Signs and Symptoms
- The first sign is a mass in the abdomen (upper right side).
- Abdominal fullness, pain, vomiting, diarrhea, fever, abnormal weight loss, jaundice, or general itching

Medical Emergencies

Hemorrhagic Cystitis
Signs and Symptoms
- Bloody or painful urination

Tumor Lysis Syndrome
Signs and Symptoms
- Lethargy, nausea and vomiting, oliguria, flank pain, pruritus, tetany, and altered level of consciousness
- Renal failure can also occur.

Septic Shock
Signs and Symptoms
- Confusion, fever, tachypnea, decreased urinary output, and cold, clammy skin.
- Note: Decreased blood pressure is a late sign.
- Laboratory studies reveal acidosis and sometimes renal failure.

The Psychological Impact of Pediatric Cancer
Signs and Symptoms
- Shock, denial, confusion, fear, blame, and loss of control.

CLINICAL ALERTS

Brain Tumors

- First the tumor is staged.
- Tumor tissue is needed for the pathologist to determine the histological diagnosis so that proper treatment can be determined.

- Treatment may include surgical resection, radiation therapy, chemotherapy, or a combination of these.

Surgical Resection

- The extent of surgical resection (cutting off) of the tumor correlates with the prognosis.
- Radical resections are particularly important in children younger than 2 years of age because cranial radiation can be deferred in these patients.
- Because many brain tumors infiltrate into surrounding normal brain, complete resection often is not possible.

Discarding Chemotherapy Drugs

- When handling equipment or material that has contained chemotherapy drugs, discard it in a designated container that is properly labeled.
- Chemotherapy drugs are considered hazardous waste material.

Radiation

Radiation therapy is using ionizing radiation to break apart the bonds within a cell, damaging it and causing it to die. Address the radiation side effects:

- Nausea
- Alopecia
- Fatigue and malaise
- Low WBC count
- Skin desquamation
- Mucous membrane inflammation and irritation

Extravasation

- Chemotherapeutic drugs must be handled carefully to avoid extravasation (accidental leakage of drug into the subcutaneous tissues surrounding the injection site/IV site). This is caused by known vesicants or a chemotherapy agent that can produce a blister or tissue destruction.
- It is important to handle chemotherapy agents safely

- For central lines, it is important to make sure there is a blood return in the line to ensure patency before administering any chemotherapeutic agents by this route.
- Monitor closely the intravenous (IV) site.
- Before administering a known "vesicant," a chemotherapy agent that can result in tissue necroses and even potentially the loss of a limb, make sure the peripheral IV or central line is patent.
- It is important to flush the IV site and check a return blood flow.
- The nurse infusing these agents be specially trained and certified in the administration of chemotherapy agents. Through this training, the nurse learns that vigilant monitoring is paramount.

Medical Emergencies

Septic Shock
Septic shock response can occur immediately or up to 48 to 72 hours later.

Other Emergencies
- Superior vena cava syndrome: Obstruction or thrombus in the superior vena cava
- Superior mediastinum syndrome: Tracheal compression
- Pericardial effusion: Fluid in the pericardial cavity, between the visceral and the parietal pericardium. This condition may produce symptoms of cardiac tamponade, such as difficulty in breathing (Venes, 2005).
- Pleural effusion: Fluid in the thoracic cavity between the visceral and parietal pleura. It may be seen on a chest radiograph if the fluid exceeds 300 mL (Venes, 2005).
- Abdominal emergencies: Esophagitis, gastric hemorrhage, perirectal abscess, hemorrhagic pancreatitis, massive acute hepatomegaly, bowel obstruction.
- Neurological conditions: Stroke, seizure, spinal cord compression.
- Shock: Hypovolemic, cardiogenic, distributive.
- Hyperleukocytosis: WBC count >100,000 mm^3.

DIAGNOSTIC TESTS

Staging

- Staging describes the severity of the patient's cancer. It classifies tumors in relation to the degree of differentiation, possibility of responding to therapy, and prognosis (Venes, 2005).
- Stage 0 indicates early cancer that is present only in the layer of cells in which it began.
- Stages I, II, and III indicate more extensive disease, greater tumor size, and/or spread of the cancer to nearby lymph nodes or adjacent organs.
- Stage IV indicates that the cancer has spread to another organ(s).

Lumbar Puncture

- A lumbar puncture (LP), or "spinal tap," is the insertion of a needle into the subarachnoid space of the lumbar spinal cord to remove a sample of CSF to test for infection.
- Insert the needle with a stylet into the interspace between the third and fourth lumbar vertebrae under strict sterile technique (Fig. 31-1).
- It is used to introduce chemotherapeutic agents into the CSF space in cancer patients.

Neutropenia

- Neutropenic children have few WBCs and often do not show signs of infection, such as swelling, redness, or drainage.

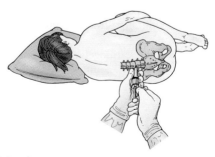

Figure 31-1 Lumbar puncture.

- The only sign may be fever.
- A fever in an oncology patient is 101.2°F (38.5°C) in a 24-hour period or 100.4°F (38.0°C) three times in a 24-hour period.
- A severe neutropenic patient has an absolute neutrophil count (ANC) of <500.
- An ANC of 500 to 1000 is considered moderately neutropenic
- ANC >1000 is considered mildly neutropenic.
- When a child undergoing chemotherapy develops a fever, it is considered an emergency.

Calculating the Absolute Neutrophil Count (ANC)
Formula:
ANC = (WBC × 10) × (Bands + Neutrophils)
Example: If WBC = 8.8, neutrophils = 82, bands = 5
            ANC = (8.8 × 10) × (82 + 5)
            ANC = (88) × (87)
            ANC = 7656

Liver Cancer

- Both hepatoblastoma and hepatocellular carcinoma can produce a protein called alpha-fetoprotein (AFP), which can be detected in the blood via a simple blood test.
- If AFP levels fall, it indicates that treatment is working. If AFP levels rise, it means the tumor is not responding.

Procedure 31-1 Checking Urine Specific Gravity

Purpose
The purpose of checking the specific gravity of urine is to measure the concentration of the particles in the urine.

Equipment
- Refractometer
- 3- or 5-mL syringe (needleless)

Steps
1. Have the child urinate into a urine collection receptacle.
2. Using a 3- or 5-mL syringe, draw up 0.5 mL of urine into the syringe

(continued)

Procedure 31-1 (Continued)

3. Place the syringe into a universal precaution container.

4. Take the urine specimen to the testing area.

5. Open the refractometer.

6. Place one drop of urine in the center of the square opening.

7. Close the lid.

8. Look through the focused eyepiece to see the horizontal line clearly.

9. Note where the blue horizontal line crosses the markings (see picture below).

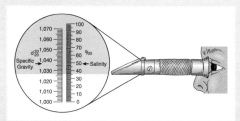

10. Document the procedure.

Clinical Alert If the institution does not have a refractometer, it is acceptable to use a urine dipstick, with the realization that this is not as detailed. The specific gravity markings on a urine dipstick are in increments of 0.005. On a refractometer, the markings are in increments of 0.001.

Teach Parents
The nurse can teach the parents about the purpose of a specific gravity measurement.

Checking Urine Specific Gravity

- Check urine specific gravity for patients receiving cytoxan, ifosfamide, cisplatin, high-dose carboplatin, high-dose methotrexate.
- Specific gravity must be less than or equal to 1.010 before the start of chemotherapy and then for at least 24 hours after its completion.

- If at any time the specific gravity rises above 1.010, the patient should receive a fluid bolus (extra fluid). DO NOT turn off the main IV. The bolus is in addition to the main intravenous fluid (IVF).
- If giving more than two or three fluid boluses, notify the oncologist on call.

Urine pH

- Monitor when the patient is receiving methotrexate (Amethopterin).
- Urine pH must be higher than 7.0 before starting methotrexate, and must be maintained at that level until the methotrexate serum blood level is <0.1 mg/dL.
- Before receiving high-dose methotrexate, patients are hydrated with IVF of D5$^1/_4$ with 40 mEq/L of $NaHCO_3$. The $NaHCO_3$ is needed to keep the urine alkalinized.

Bone Marrow Biopsy

Pretest

- Obtain a written, informed and signed consent for the procedure.
- Review the procedure with the child and parents. Explain that the child will receive topical anesthetic (EMLA) and/or pain medication before the procedure.
- If receiving conscious sedation, review the institution's policy on restriction of food and fluids.
- If parents choose to be present, explain how they might assist their child through diversionary activities, breathing techniques, and verbal support.

Intratest

- Depending on age, have the patient void before the procedure.
- Identify the patient.
- Take the patient to the treatment room.
- Assist the child to the desired position depending on the site to be used:
  - Proximal tibia (supine with pillow beneath knee)
  - Vertebral bodies (on side with head and knees tucked)
  - Posterior iliac crest (prone)
  - Anterior iliac crest or sternum (supine)
- Restrain as necessary with two adults.

- Record baseline vital signs and continue to monitor during procedure. If receiving conscious sedation, pulse and oxygen saturation monitoring are also necessary.

Posttest
- Apply pressure dressing if child's platelet count is 50,000 or less.
- Monitor vital signs and neurologic status for at least 1 hour or until child returns to a premedicated state.
- Observe site for bleeding, inflammation, or hematoma.
- Administer antiemetic and analgesic medications as needed.
- Instruct patient/family to report any redness, edema, bleeding, or pain at the site. Instruct patient/family to report chills or fever and to keep the site clean and change dressing as needed.

(Adapted from Van Leeuwen, A.M., Kranpitz, T.R., & Smith, L. (2006). *Davis's comprehensive handbook of laboratory and diagnostic tests with nursing implications.* Philadelphia: F.A. Davis, pp. 209–211.)

Bone Scan

Pretest
- Obtain a written, informed, and signed consent for the procedure.
- Explain the procedure to the child and family.
- Inform child and family that the technologist will administer an intravenous injection of an isotope and they will need to return 1 to 3 hours later for the scan.
- After the injection, encourage child to increase fluid intake and continue normal physical activity.

Intratest
- Confirm the child's identity.
- Ask the child to remove any jewelry, watches, and other metallic objects.
- Depending on the age of the child, ask the child to void.
- If the child is unable to lie still, sedation is necessary.
- Place the child supine with foam wedges to help maintain position and immobilization while multiple images are obtained.

Posttest

- If the child is sedated, monitor vital signs and neurologic status for at least 1 hour or until child returns to a premedicated state.
- Encourage increased fluid intake.
- Check the injection site for bleeding, redness, or hematoma (Van Leeuwen, 2006).

Lumbar Puncture

Pretest

- Obtain a written, informed, and signed consent for the procedure.
- Review the procedure with the child and parents. Explain that the child will receive topical anesthetic (EMLA) before the procedure.
- If parents choose to be present, explain how they might assist their child through diversionary activities, breathing techniques, and verbal support.

Intratest

- Confirm the child's identity.
- Take to treatment room.
- Obtain baseline vital signs and continue to monitor during procedure, particularly for signs of respiratory compromise due to positioning of the child. For infants, pulse and oxygen saturation monitoring may be required.
- Have emergency equipment readily available.
- Position and restrain the child in the knee chest position at the side of the examination table in order to best expose the L3–L4 site or the L4–L5 site. For older children the sitting position with neck and chest bent to the knees is an alternative.
- Instruct the child to breathe normally and to avoid unnecessary movement while vials of CSF are obtained.

Posttest

- Apply an adhesive dressing to the site.
- Observe site for bleeding, CSF leakage, or hematoma.
- Monitor vital signs and neurological status and compare to baseline values.

- The child should lie flat for at least 1 hour or according to the health care provider's instructions (Van Leeuwen, 2006).

Lymphangiogram

Pretest
- Obtain a written, informed, and signed consent for the procedure.
- Review the procedure with child and parents.
- Ask the child to remove any jewelry, watches, or other metallic objects before going to the radiology department.
- Ask the child and family if the child has an allergy to iodine or shellfish.

Intratest
- Confirm the child's identity.
- Have emergency equipment readily available.
- Obtain baseline vital signs and assess neurological status.
- Encourage the child to remain still throughout the procedure.
- Explain that a local anesthetic is injected before the injection of the contrast medium into the area between the first three toes of the foot or the web of skin between the fingers.
- Remind the child that he will need to inhale deeply and hold his breath while the x-ray images are taken.
- Monitor the child for complications related to the contrast medium (e.g., allergic reaction, anaphylaxis, bronchospasm).

Posttest
- Monitor vital signs and neurological status every 15 minutes and compare with baseline values.
- Observe the site for bleeding, inflammation, and hematoma and monitor for signs of infection.
- Observe for delayed allergic reaction or pulmonary embolus (shortness of breath, increased heart rate, pleuritic pain, hypotension, low-grade fever, and cyanosis) (Van Leeuwen, 2006).

MEDICATIONS

Chemotherapeutic Agents and Common Drugs Used with Cancer Patients

Agent	Indications	Route	Side Effects
Asparaginase (Elspar, Kidrolase) Classification: Antineoplastic Pharmacological action: Enzyme	Acute lymphoblastic leukemia (ALL)	IM, IV	Seizures, hyperglycemia Nausea/vomiting, rashes, coagulation abnormalities, hepatotoxic, pancreatitis, anaphylaxis (have emergency medications available)
Bleomycin (Blenoxane) Classification: Antineoplastic Pharmacological: Antitumor antibiotics	Hodgkin's disease Osteosarcoma Testicular embryonal cell carcinoma	IM, IV, SQ	Pulmonary fibrosis Pneumonitis, hypotension, nausea/vomiting, anorexia, hyperpigmentation, rashes, anaphylaxis (fever, chills)
Carboplatin **(Paraplatin, Paraplatin AQ)** Classification: Antineoplastic Pharmacological: Alkylating agent	Brain tumors Soft tissue sarcoma Osteosarcoma Retinoblastoma Neuroblastoma	IV	Ototoxicity, nausea/vomiting, constipation, diarrhea, stomatitis, renal and liver toxicity, hypocalcemia, hypokalemia, hyponatremia, hypomagnesemia Anaphylactic-like reactions

(continued)

Chemotherapeutic Agents and Common Drugs Used with Cancer Patients (Continued)

Agent	Indications	Route	Side Effects
Corticosteroid **(Dexamethasone, Decadron, Hydrocortisone, Prednisone)** Classification: Corticosteroid Pharmacological: Systemic corticosteroids, anti-inflammatory	ALL Non-Hodgkin's lymphoma HD Cerebral edema	PO, IV, IT	Immunosuppression Weight gain, hypertension, anorexia, nausea/vomiting, acne, delayed wound healing, hirsutism, petechiae, osteoporosis, - growth delay Cushinoid appearance
Cyclophosphamide **(Cytoxan, Neosar, Procytox)** Classification: Antineoplastic, Immunosuppressant Pharmacological: Alkylating agent	NHL HD ALL Neuroblastoma Wilms' tumor Bone and soft tissue sarcoma Retinoblastoma	PO, IV	Myelosuppression Nausea, vomiting, anorexia, diarrhea, pulmonary and myocardial fibrosis, hemorrhagic cystitis, leukopenia, hematuria, alopecia, sterility, SIADH May cause second neoplasm
Daunorubicin **(Daunomycin, Cerubidine)** Classification: Antineoplastic Pharmacological: Anthracyclines	ALL AML Osteosarcoma Soft tissue sarcoma	IV	Blistering, myelosuppression, cardiotoxic: arrhythmias, acute cardiac myopathy-delayed Nausea/vomiting, stomatitis, potentiation of radiation, alopecia, rash, hyperpigmentation of nails

Doxorubicin **(Adriamycin, Adria, DOX, Rubex)** Classification: Antineoplastic Pharmacological: Anthracyclines	ALL AML Osteosarcoma Soft tissue sarcoma Neuroblastoma	IV	Blistering, nausea/vomiting, stomatitis, esophagitis, diarrhea, red urine, anemia, hypersensitivity reaction, sterility. Cardiotoxic: arrhythmias, acute cardiomyopathy—delayed, potentiation of radiation, hyperpigmentation of nails, seizures, hypertension, edema, diarrhea, cough, shortness of breath, rash, thrombotic events
Epoetin/Erythropoietin **(Epogen, EPO, Procrit)** Classification: Biological Response Modifier Pharmacological: Hormone	Anemia	IV, SQ	Pulmonary edema, CHF, MI, hypotension, nausea/vomiting, anaphylaxis
Etoposide **(VP-16, VePesid)** Classification: Antineoplastic Pharmacological: Podophyllotoxin derivative	AML, ALL NHL HD Bone and soft tissue sarcoma Wilms' tumor Brain tumor Neuroblastoma Retinoblastoma	IV	Excessive leukocytosis, pain and redness at subcutaneous site.
Filgrastim (GCSF—granulocyte colony stimulating factor) **(Neupogen)** Classification: colony-stimulating factor Pharmacological: Hematopoietic progenitor mobilizer	Recovery drug for neutropenia	IV, SQ	Medullary bone pain

(continued)

Chemotherapeutic Agents and Common Drugs Used with Cancer Patients (Continued)

Agent	Indications	Route	Side Effects
Fluorouracil (5-FU, Adrucil) Classification: Antineoplastic Pharmacological: Antimetabolite	Brain tumors Germ cell tumors Osteosarcoma Soft tissue sarcoma NHL ALL	IV	Myelosuppression, nausea/vomiting (mild), mucositis (severe), hyperpigmentation of nails, nail loss, dermatitis, phototoxicity, myelosuppression, diarrhea, neurotoxicity (encephalopathy, hallucinations), hepatoxicity, hemorrhagic cystitis, alopecia, sterility, may cause second neoplasm
Ifosfamide (Ifex) Classification: Antineoplastic Pharmacological: Alkylating agent	Stops methotrexate from harming the cells when given in high doses	IV	Allergic reactions: rash, urticaria, wheezing
Leucovorin (Citrovorum factor, folinic acid, Wellcovorin) Classification: Antidote (for methotrexate), vitamins Pharmacological: Folic acid analog	Recovery drug to prevent hemorrhagic cystitis from ifosfamide and cyclophosphamide	IV, PO	*Dose dependent on methotrexate level *Given 24 hrs after first methotrexate level has begun
Mesna (Mesnex, Uromitexan) Classification: Antidote Pharmacological: Ifosfamide detoxifying agent	Prevention of ifosfamide-induced hemorrhagic cystitis	IV, PO, IM, IT	Dizziness, drowsiness, headache, anorexia, diarrhea, nausea/vomiting, unpleasant taste, flushing, flu-like symptoms

Methotrexate (MTX, Amethopterin) Classification: Antineoplastic Immunosuppressant Pharmacological: Antimetabolite	ALL Osteosarcoma NHL	IV	Myelosuppression, nausea/vomiting/stomatitis, alopecia, hepatotoxicity, neurotoxicity, photosensitivity, rash, pulmonary fibrosis, aplastic anemia
Ondansetron (Zofran) Classification: Antiemetic Pharmacological: 5-HT₃ antagonist	Prevention of nausea/vomiting association with chemotherapy	IV, PO	Headache, diarrhea, constipation, dry mouth, extrapyramidal reactions
PEG-L-asparaginase (pegaspargase) (Oncaspar) Classification: Antineoplastic Pharmacological: Enzymes	ALL HD	IM, IV	Seizures, pancreatitis, lip edema, headache, nausea/vomiting, diarrhea, DIC, hemolytic anemia, pancytopenia, chills, night sweats
Vincristine (Oncovorin, Vincasar PFS) Classification: Antineoplastic Pharmacological: Vinca alkaloids	Wilms' tumor Ewing's sarcoma Brain tumor	IV	Altered LOC, blistering, peripheral neuropathy, alopecia, constipation, SIADH, seizure, nausea/vomiting

IV = intravenous; IM = intramuscular; SQ = subcutaneous; PO = by mouth; IT = intrathecal.
Data from Deglin, J., & Vallerand, A. (2009). *Davis's drug guide for nurses* (11th ed.). Philadelphia: F.A. Davis.

Topical Anesthetics

- Use topical anesthetics when possible for procedure-related pain such as EMLA (Astra Zeneca) cream, which is a lidocaine/prilocaine 1:1 mixture.
- The nurse applies a thin coating of ointment to the projected insertion site(s) and covers the site(s) with a hydrocolloid dressing (such as DuoDERM).
- It is important to keep the cream on for at least 1 hour (sometimes longer) before the procedure (Bryant, 2003).

Common Antiemetics

Odansetron (Zofran)

- 0.15 mg/kg every 8 hours
- Duration
  - IV: 24 hours
  - PO: 8 hours
  - Not as effective as a prn
  - Not as effective if vomiting has begun
  - While the child is receiving chemotherapy, give 30 minutes before chemotherapy, then every 6 to 8 hours for 24 hours

Diphenhydramine (Benadryl)

- 1 mg/kg per dose every 6 hours
- PO/IV immediate onset
- Duration 4 to 7 hours
- Side effects: Sedation, dry mouth, blurred vision

Lorazepam (Ativan)

- IV: 0.4 mg/kg per dose every 6 hours
- IV duration: 4–6 hours
- Often used for anticipatory nausea/vomiting
- Side effects: Sedation, euphoria

Agents Known to Cause Extravasation

- TPN and other hyperosmolar fluids
- Dilantin
- Chemotherapeutic agents (doxorubicin, daunorubicin, mitomycin C, vincristine, vinblastine, VP-16, dacarbazine)

ETHNOCULTURAL CONSIDERATIONS

Caring for a Hispanic Child with Cancer

- Respect the family's values and incorporate their folk practices when possible.
- Provide written instruction for the child and parents in Spanish so they understand the plan of treatment.
- Do a thorough pain assessment and do not rely on verbal or observational cues, as Hispanics are known to be stoic and not express pain.
- Explore the parents' or caregivers' beliefs as well as the child's beliefs so that optimal pain control can be achieved.

TEACHING THE FAMILY

Suggestions for Nutrition

- Offer suggestions to the family to help the child maintain good nutrition.
- Encourage the family to plan a diet that includes foods from all four food groups.
- Refer to the nutritionist if necessary.

Nausea/Vomiting

- Offer plain, bland foods such as cereal, canned or fresh fruit, rice, pasta, toast, mashed potatoes, soup, crackers, or plain meat.
- Avoid spicy, heavy, or fatty foods.
- If food smells bother the child, choose cold or room-temperature foods; use a cup with a lid.
- Do not offer solid food and liquid at the same time, as this can induce nausea by making the child feel too full; give liquids 30 to 60 minutes after solid food.

Diarrhea

- Offer plenty of liquids.
- Suggest eating bananas, rice, applesauce, toast, and tea.
- Suggest cutting back on fiber in the diet.

Constipation

- Provide extra liquids; offer beverages that contain caffeine, like coffee, tea, and cola.
- Increase fiber in the diet.
- Encourage the child to increase activity level.

Poor Appetite

- Offer small amounts of food four or more times a day.
- Offer liquids between meals.
- Make every bite count by offering "power-packed foods."
- Start with small portions, and then gradually increase them.
- Allow the child to have foods and beverages that he or she especially likes.

Sore Throat and Mouth

- Offer soft foods such as pudding, Jell-O®, macaroni and cheese, applesauce, bananas, ice cream, Italian ice, popsicles.
- Avoid acidic foods like oranges and tomatoes, spicy foods, or foods that require a lot of chewing.
- Encourage good oral hygiene.

Heartburn or Reflux

- Do not give the child high-fat, spicy foods, caffeine, citrus juices, cinnamon, peppermint, or pepper.
- Keep the child upright for at least 1 hour after eating.

Difficulty Chewing or Swallowing/Dry Mouth

- Give the child soft, moist foods.
- Encourage sips of liquids while eating.
- Avoid hard foods that require a lot of chewing.
- Cut the food into small pieces.
- Use extra butter, sauces, or gravies.
- Offer hard candy to suck on.

Belching, Intestinal Gas, or Cramps

- Avoid gas-forming foods such as cabbage, broccoli, cauliflower, cucumbers, beans, and carbonated beverages.

- Encourage the child to eat or drink slowly.
- Do not allow the child to chew gum.

(Steen & Mirro, 2000).

Recognizing Signs and Symptoms of Infection

If any of these signs and symptoms or a combination of them occur, report them to the physician immediately.

- Fever
- Decrease in temperature
- Runny nose (or other respiratory illness)
- Sore throat
- Childhood disease such as chickenpox
- Lethargy
- Pale or ashen color
- Chills
- Diaphoresis
- Poor appetite
- Poor fluid intake
- Nausea, vomiting, or diarrhea
- Decreased urination
- Foul smelling urine, or pain or burning upon urination

ADDITIONAL INFORMATION FOR THE CLINICAL SETTING

Factors Predisposing to Childhood Leukemia	
Genetic Conditions	**Environmental Factors**
Down syndrome	Ionizing radiation
Fanconi syndrome	Drugs
Bloom syndrome	Alkylating agents
Shwachman syndrome	Nitrosourea
Klinefelter syndrome	Epipodophyllotoxin
Turner syndrome	Benzene exposure
Neurofibromatosis	Advanced maternal age
Li–Fraumeni syndrome	
Severe combined immune deficiency	

Visualization and Distraction

- Use visualization and distraction to help avoid anxiety before a procedure (e.g., imagine a trip to his favorite place).

- Have the child close his or her eyes while the nurse plays tour guide.
- Ask the child questions about the favorite place and encourage the child to be part of the story or trip.
- Use distraction depending on the child's developmental level (e.g., blowing bubbles, reading a story).

Bone Marrow Transplant

- This is the treatment option for children who have a second remission after relapse.
- The child is given high doses of chemotherapy and/or radiation to eradicate disease or cancer and then the patient is rescued with a source of stem cells that allows for recovery of healthy bone marrow.
- There are two basic types of bone marrow transplants: Autologous and allogeneic. In an autologous transplant, the patient's own peripheral blood or bone marrow is given back. An allogeneic transplant can be from a matched sibling, a relative, or an unrelated donor accessed through the National Marrow Donor Program.

When a Child Is Diagnosed with a Brain Tumor

- The family or the child does not understand the exact nature or future implications of a brain tumor.
- Treat the child as normally as possible.
- It is acceptable to communicate with the child and family while the child plays.
- Support the parents or caregivers and allow them time to "absorb" the diagnosis.

Things to say to the family:

- "It is important for you to verbalize and express your feelings."
- "You may find it helpful to talk with others who have had the same experience as you. I have contact information for a support group. Would you like me to make a call for you?"
- "I know this is a very difficult time for you. Let's take this a day at a time and make your child's daily routine as normal as possible.

Venous Access Devices

Name	Description	Advantage	Nursing Care
Central Implanted Ports such as **Infus-a-port, Mediport, Port-a-cath, or Norport**	A saucer-shaped plastic device with a self-sealing injection port that can be accessed from the top or side. Requires placement in operating room.	Decreased risk of infection Placed under the skin; reducing the chance of becoming dislodged or pulled out Limited noticeably (small bump under the skin) Patency is maintained by administering heparin after access Little maintenance or care: child can participate in regular activities	Cleanse skin with warm water and soap before use. Administer topical anesthetic such as EMLA (lidocaine and prilocaine) before accessing the port. Use a Huber needle to access the port. Observe the child during medication administration for dislodgment of the needle. When treatment complete the port must be surgically removed.
Central Groshong Catheter	A silicone, flexible and clear catheter. At the proximal end, there is a closed-tip two-way valve. Requires placement in operating room.	Easy for self-administered medications and fluids No heparin required No clamping needed due to two-way valve Minimal backflow Decrease possibility of air embolism	Weekly irrigation with normal saline Parents can learn catheter care (site must be kept clean and dry). Teaching includes: (1) strenuous activity and water sports are restricted and (2) safety as the catheter protrudes from body and may be pulled out. Offer support based on body image disturbance *(continued)*

Venous Access Device (Continued)			
Name	**Description**	**Advantage**	**Nursing Care**
Central Tunneled Catheter such as Broviac or Hickman	An open-ended silicone, flexible, radiopaque catheter. Requires placement in operating room	Easy for self-administered medications and fluids Decrease risk of infection	Daily heparin flushes Parents can learn catheter care (site must be kept clean and dry) When not in use must be clamped Teaching includes; (1) strenuous activity and water sports are restricted (2) safety as the catheter protrudes from body and may be pulled out
Peripherally Inserted Central Catheters	Catheter made of silastic or polyurethane material Single- or double-lumen available Inserted into antecubital fossa passing through the cephalic or basilic vein entering the superior vena cava	Does not require placement in operating room. Pediatric nurse practitioners can insert the line using a small lumen needle Decrease risk of infection	Flushed with saline using 5 to 10-mL syringe Not suitable for rapid fluid replacement (small lumen needle) Sometimes can be difficult to remove because of resistance

Insertion of Central Venous Catheters

- The insertion of central venous catheters is one of the most frequent surgical procedures performed (Fig. 31-2).
- Long-term central venous access devices make it safer to administer chemotherapy and total parenteral nutrition; also used to administer antibiotics and to obtain blood specimens (Alcoser & Rodgers, 2003).

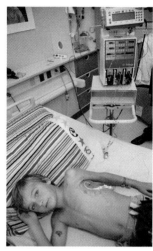

Figure 31-2 The insertion of a central venous catheter helps in administering chemotherapy and is one of the most frequent surgical procedures performed on children with cancer.

Nursing Care of Children with Cancer

- Children with cancer still want to be loved and treated like other children.
- Encourage these children to play and be involved in self-care activities as their condition allows.
- Encourage them to talk about their dreams, feelings, and fears.

Negative Effects of Chemotherapy

- Chemotherapy is toxic to the body because it kills not only cancer cells but healthy cells as well.
- As soon as chemotherapy is administered the nurse ensures that the child is also well hydrated so that the chemotherapeutic agent (or toxin) is flushed out of the system.
- Measure specific gravity of the urine to ensure proper hydration.
- The urine specific gravity should be 1.012 or below. If it rises above this, IV fluid boluses are required.

Loss of Hair (Alopecia)

- Explain that hair will probably start to fall out 10 days to 2 weeks after chemotherapy begins and that it may fall out in sections.

- Assure the child that once the chemotherapy has been completed, his or her hair will grow back.
- Emphasize that just because his or her hair falls out, it does not change the person the child is inside (just looks a little different for a short time).
- Suggest arranging for a first "cool hat" purchase before the child leaves the hospital.

Safe Handling of Chemotherapeutic Agents

- Use disposable gloves and gowns when handling or preparing chemotherapy medications to prevent contact with medication.
- Use aseptic technique when administering medications.
- Prepare drugs in a well ventilated room.
- Dispose all medications, contaminated needles, syringes, intravenous tubing, gloves, and gowns in an appropriate leak-proof, puncture-resistant container (Alcoser & Rodgers, 2003).

Neutropenic Patient Admitted to a Pediatric Unit

- Place the child in a private room by him- or herself for the best outcome.
- If a private room is not available, assigning the child to a room with a noninfectious child such as a fractured femur is acceptable.

Nutrition

- Maintain good nutrition.
- Assess for poor nutrition.
- Assess side effects of chemotherapy and recommend foods accordingly.
- Maintain the immune system.
- Try simple care measures first (enteral feedings or TPN may be the only option).
- Communicate to the parents that their child may eventually be able to eat independently again.

Infection

- Monitor for systemic and localized signs of infection every 2 to 4 hours.
- Take temperature every 4 hours.
- Report a single temperature >101.20°F (38.50°C) in a 24-hour period or 100.40°F (38.00°C) three times in a 24-hour period.
- Provide meticulous skin care and use good hand washing (instruct visitors).

- Use universal precautions and designated isolation precautions.
- Monitor and report lab values.
- Teach family about the principles of prophylactic antibiotics and signs and symptoms of infection.

Radiation Side Effects
- Nausea
- Alopecia
- Fatigue and malaise
- Low WBC count
- Skin desquamation
- Mucous membrane inflammation and irritation

Surgery
Surgery is used as an adjunct to both chemotherapy and radiation.

- It also has an important role in the diagnosis of a tumor via biopsy.

The biopsy is obtained through a fine-needle aspiration or an open biopsy procedure.

Pain Control
- Pain medications combined with adequate rest and sleep, massage, heat, distraction, and social support
- Topical anesthetics

Psychological Support
- Provide holistic nursing care.
- Encourage parents or another support person to stay with the child 24 hours a day.
- Involve the child-life specialist.
- Be present and listen.
- Provide family with community resources, reliable internet sources, or information about support groups.

Negative Effects of Chemotherapy
- Nausea and vomiting (administer antiemetics)
- Alopecia (address body image)
- Extravasation (prevent accidental leakage of drugs)
- Mucositis (keep oral cavity clean)
- Diarrhea (skin care, diet, and medication)
- Constipation (diet, activity, and medication)
- Anemia (signs and symptoms, diet, vitamin, RBC transfusion, administer hematopoietic growth factors)

- Thrombocytopenia (platelet transfusion)
- Neutropenia (assess fever, blood cultures, and administer antibiotics)

Medical Emergencies

Hemorrhagic Cystitis
- Maintain hydration.
- Test urine for blood, pH and specific gravity (see Procedure 31-1).
- If urine is positive for blood, notify the physician immediately.
- Monitor intake and output.
- Obtain daily BUN and creatinine levels.
- Administer MESNA (Mesnex, Uromitexan)

Tumor Lysis Syndrome
- Keep urine alkalinized.
- Maintain a low-phosphate diet.
- Administer allopurinol (Aloprim).
- Maintain adequate hydration.
- Monitor electrolytes.
- Obtain BUN and creatinine levels.
- Dialysis or exchange transfusions may be necessary.

Septic Shock
- When a neutropenic child is given antibiotics; take vital signs every 10 to 15 minutes during the antibiotic administration to recognize signs of septic shock.
- Administer large amounts of an isotonic fluid (normal saline).
- Check peripheral pulses and capillary refill to monitor perfusion.
- Use the ABCs and other emergent care measures:
  - Airway
  - Breathing
  - Circulation
  - Fluid resuscitation
  - Evaluation of etiology (CBC, electrolytes, DIC panel, blood cultures, liver and renal functions)
  - Blood products
  - Antibiotics
  - Vasopressors

Psychological Aspects
- Suggest support.
- Encourage adequate rest and nutrition for parents.
- Be honest.
- Use a multidisciplinary approach.
- Tailor information to developmental stage.
- Keep lines of communication open.
- Offer spiritual care.
- Help the child and his family express feelings.

Handling Siblings of an Ill Child

- While children with cancer are undergoing many stressful events, do not forget about their siblings (visiting a sick sibling is stressful for both sides).
- Help make the sibling's day special by telling her a story, or by giving her a sticker or a coloring book and crayons.
- Encourage the ill child to color a picture for his or her sibling and hang it in the room.
- A sincere demeanor and common pleasantries such as saying hello or calling the sibling by their name can make the visit special and less stressful.

RESOURCES

Association of Pediatric Hematology/Oncology Nurses:
http://www.apon.org

American Cancer Society (for children):
http://www.cancer.org/docroot/CRI/CRI_2_6x_Children_and_Cancer.asp

Candlelighters Childhood Cancer Foundation:
http://www.candlelighters.org

The Leukemia and Lymphoma Society: http://www.leukemia.org

REFERENCES

Alcoser, P., & Rodgers, C. (2003). Treatment strategies in childhood cancer. *Journal of Pediatric Nursing, 18*(2), 103–112.

Bryant, R. (2003). Managing side effects of childhood cancer treatments. *Journal of Pediatric Nursing, 18*(2), 113–125.

Deglin, J., & Vallerand, A. (2009). *Davis's drug guide for nurses* (11th ed.). Philadelphia: F.A. Davis.

Steen, G., & Mirro, M (2000). *Childhood cancer. A handbook from St. Jude Children's Research Hospital.* Cambridge, MA: Perseus.

Van Leeuwen, A.M., Kranpitz, T.R., & Smith, L. (2006). *Davis's comprehensive handbook of laboratory and diagnostic tests with nursing implications.* Philadelphia: F.A. Davis

Venes, D. (2005). *Taber's cyclopedic medical dictionary* (20th ed.). Philadelphia: F.A. Davis.

Caring for the Child with a Chronic Condition or the Dying Child

KEY TERMS

caregiver burden – Unrelenting pressure and anxiety in providing daily care to a child with disabilities while meeting other family needs; can be a major source of stress

chronic sorrow – Period of episodic grieving interspersed with periods of denial

end-of-life care – A holistic approach to care that includes physical, emotional, social, and spiritual interventions, and complementary care during the final 6 months of life

general growth failure – Growth that is slower than normal and the height and weight is in a lower percentile on the growth charts than those of children the same age

hospice care – A program that focuses on quality of life for dying persons; method of treating a serious illness when cure or meaningful improvement is no longer possible and end-of-life care describes a certain time frame where care is given during the final 6 months of life

palliative care – Type of care that the child receives at the end of life after it becomes obvious that no cure is possible; emphasizes physical, emotional, and spiritual care of the child and family

pathological grief – Deviation from a healthy or normal grief where intense grief feelings or a dysfunctional personality may easily bring about such behaviors as violence, addictions, or poor decision making

regression – An abnormal return to an earlier reaction, characterized by emotions or behaviors that are inappropriate for the current age and may include the loss of recently acquired skills (Venes, 2005)

respite care – Short-term care offered to families living with a child who has a chronic condition; the main goal is to provide temporary relief for family members from the burden and stress of sustained care giving (Venes, 2005)

technology dependent – Reliance on some type of medical device to compensate for the loss of normal use of a vital body function

FOCUSED ASSESSMENT

- Use either the numeric scale, the Wong faces scale, or the FLACC pain scale to determine a child's level of pain. See Chapter 18.

Impact of the Chronic Condition on the Infant

- Bonding process
- Pain
- Changes in diet and sleep may alter growth and development

Impact of the Chronic Condition on the Toddler

- Unable to achieve autonomy
- Pain, anxiety, and separation from parents
- Sensitive to bodily harm
- Hindered gross and fine motor development
- Stress and regression present

Impact of the Chronic Condition on the Preschooler

- Feels he or she is being punished for wrongdoing
- Reacts aggressively
- Regresses
- Withdraws from others
- Difficulty sleeping (fears falling asleep)

Impact of the Chronic Condition on the School-age Child

- Altered autonomy and peer relationships
- Interrupts independence
- Refuses to comply with treatments or to follow a special diet
- Cannot completely comprehend all information (reluctant to answer questions)
- May understand significance of illness and lifelong consequences

Impact of the Chronic Condition on the Adolescent

- There may be a dilemma where to place the adolescent; in a pediatric ward or on an adult floor?
- In spite of trying to achieve independence, dependence on caregivers may occur
- Lack of privacy
- Maladaptive coping behaviors
- Refuses treatments
- Easily overwhelmed and may show regression
- Worries about condition, self-esteem, identity, and family

Impact of the Chronic Condition on the Sibling

- May have decreased self-esteem
- May receive less attention and support from parents
- May have mood swings and lack understanding about the condition
- May display a negative attitude toward the ill sibling
- May have feelings of jealousy, embarrassment, resentment, loneliness, and isolation
- May think that he or she caused the condition or might acquire the condition too

Handling a Sibling Who Is Acting Out

Best outcome: The sibling has time to regain control and can express feelings. Some examples are below:

- "You seem very angry today." (reflection)
- "It is all right to be angry at your sister's condition and about the situation." (validating the sibling's feelings)

- "It must be difficult for you to have your sister in the hospital." (empathizing and understanding)
- The nurse can then help the sibling find a positive outlet for the anger such as art therapy (channeling).
- Encourage the sibling to tell an adult when the anger returns (providing an outlet).

Children Living with Chronic Conditions

Children living with a chronic condition experience one or more of these symptoms (Judson, 2004):

- Limitation in bodily functions appropriate for age and development
- Disfigurement
- Dependency on medical technology
- Dependency on medication or special diet to ensure normal functioning or control of the condition
- Ongoing need for medical care or related services compared to other children the same age
- Special ongoing treatments at home or at school

Emotional Responses to a Chronic Condition

- Disruption of family equilibrium
- Feelings of shock, chaos, anger, fear, disbelief, anxiety, pain, and stress ("emotional roller coaster")

Perceptions of Death

Infant
- Based on the degree of discomfort and the reactions of the parents and others in the environment

Toddler
- Has difficulty with separation from parents and/or disruption in routine

Preschooler
- Magical thinkers: Illness or injury may be viewed as punishment for bad behaviors
- Concrete thinkers: Death should not be described as "going to sleep."

School-age

- Understanding is not precise until the child can understand the concept of time
- After age 8 or 9 children understand the permanence of death.

Adolescent

- Adult level of understanding and fear of dependence on others
- Difficulty accepting death as reality and often think that death can be defied

Recognition of Physical Signs of Impending Death

- Loss of sensation
- Loss of the body's ability to maintain thermoregulation: skin may feel cool
- Loss of bowel and bladder function
- Loss of awareness or consciousness and slurring of speech
- Alteration in respiratory status
- Cheyne–Stokes respirations (a waxing and waning in the depth of respirations with regular periods of apnea)
- Noisy chest or respirations with the accumulation of fluid in the lungs or in the posterior pharynx
- Decreased, weak, or slow pulse rate and drop in blood pressure

Somatic Grief Response

- Somatic distress that includes feelings of tightness in the throat or chest, sighing
- Weakness or shortness of breath
- Preoccupation with the image of the deceased (e.g., hearing or seeing the person who died)
- Inability to focus on anything other than the loved one who died
- Emotionally distancing self from others
- Feelings of guilt
- Feeling responsible for the loved one's death
- Searching for what could have been done differently, thinking in terms of "if only I had done…"
- Hostile reactions that include feelings and expressions of anger
- Inability to complete daily tasks

Subtle Indicators of Grief

These subtle signs are warning signs and may not necessarily indicate a severe problem. It is the intensity and duration of these behaviors that are the deciding factors indicating the need for professional help.

- Absence of grief, such as showing little or no emotion
- Persistent blame or guilt
- Anxiety
- Aggressive and destructive outburst
- Depression and suicidal thoughts or actions
- Unwillingness to speak about the deceased
- Expressing only positive or only negative feelings about the deceased
- Prolonged dysfunction in school
- Always assuming a caregiver role
- Stealing or other illegal acts
- Signs of addictive behavior: drugs, food, certain activities

Paying Attention to Personal Needs

The nurse can pay attention to personal needs by asking:

- How do I feel?
- Am I comfortable caring for a child who is dying?
- Can I cope with the needs of the family as well?
- Am I becoming overwhelmed or attached when caring for this child and family?
- If the nurse feels uncomfortable with any of these questions, it is time for reflection and self-care.
- Determine if the situation becomes too great to bear.

CLINICAL ALERTS

Principles of Pain Medication Administration

- Administer pain medications orally for as long as possible.
- Alternative routes for pain medication administration include intravenous, subcutaneous, transcutaneous, transmucosal, rectal, nasal, epidural, and intrathecal.
- The enteral route (or through a gastrostomy tube) is the preferred route for children in the dying process.

- Adjuvants (drugs added to a prescription to hasten or increase the action of a principal ingredient in the medication) must be considered. They are medications not used as the principal pain medication but offer analgesia in certain situations, including anticonvulsants, antidepressants, or muscle relaxants (Hain et al., 2004).

MEDICATIONS

- Pain management includes medication and other traditional nursing comfort measures (e.g., clean sheets, good hygiene measures, oral care, and skin care).
- Answer questions about treatment, procedures, and medications honestly and at a level the child can understand.
- General growth failure means that the child grows more slowly than normal and that the height and weight are in a lower percentile on the growth charts than for children of the same age. It may result from the condition itself or from related treatments and medications.
- A large proportion of children taking herbal medications are also taking over-the-counter medications.

ETHNOCULTURAL CONSIDERATIONS

Cultural Practices

- The nurse must be knowledgeable about the cultural practices of the child and family.
- Include the right support person to facilitate the cultural care of the dying child.
- By including cultural rituals or customs, nursing care can provide comfort during the death process for the child and family.
- Special ceremonies or rites may be requested by the family and should be accommodated whenever possible.
- Other cultural care measures may include use of spiritual texts and symbols, using prayer or meditation, chanting, offering music, lighting a candle, listening in silence, being present in the moment, or including other methods of care as deemed appropriate by the culture.

Hispanic Culture and Grieving

- Hispanics are predominantly of the Roman Catholic faith tradition and have a close extended family network within the social structure. A child who dies is viewed as an angel who has returned to heaven. This belief brings comfort to the parents and the extended family, particularly the grandparents, and allows them to move on through the grieving process.
- To honor the deceased child, pictures are displayed in the home as a tribute, keeping the memory alive.
- Outward expressions of happiness (parties, celebrations, music in the house) are discouraged for usually a year.
- In some instances, the relatives wear black clothing to signify that they remember the loved one.
- If these traditions are not observed, there may be criticism from others and criticism is of the utmost concern to the family.

TEACHING THE FAMILY

The Sibling Needs to Say Good-Bye

- Visits from siblings are important and should be encouraged.
- Parents often try to protect the dying child by limiting visitation.
- Encourage siblings to write letters or draw pictures for the dying child as a way of saying good-bye.
- Siblings need to be included in the grieving process and to have the opportunity to say good-bye.
- The child who has been included in the death and mourning process with the family is able to let go in a healthy way (Kübler-Ross, 1983).

ADDITIONAL INFORMATION FOR THE CLINICAL SETTING

Other Terms Associated with a Chronic Condition

- Disability is similar to a chronic condition in that it also refers to the limitations that prevent or interfere with a child's ability to perform daily activities.

- Handicap is the inability to carry out tasks or access certain aspects of the environment due to one or more impairments. The terms "activity limitation" or "participation restriction" are preferred by many specialists in physical, occupational, and speech therapy as well as those in related fields (Venes, 2005).

Understanding the Type of Technological Equipment Required

Technology dependent children are grouped according to the type of equipment required. According to a United States Congress report, the groups are designated from the most complex equipment to the least complex equipment required:

- Group 1: Children who require a ventilator.
- Group 2: Children who require devices for total parenteral nutrition.
- Group 3: Children who have a daily dependence on some other device for respiratory or nutritional support (e.g., tracheostomy, oxygen support, tube feeding).
- Group 4: Children who require an apnea monitor, peritoneal dialysis, hemodialysis or other devices, such as catheters and colostomy bags.
- The infants and children who fall into groups 1 and 3 are further defined as needing high-technology care; medically fragile (Judson, 2004).

Impact of a Chronic Condition

- Creates a threat of the unknown, loss of control, and has long-term effects.
- Frequent hospitalizations or clinic visits may be needed.
- Disrupts normal home routines.
- Demands are placed on the caregiver.
- Parents may become controlling and overprotective.
- The child may have to cope with unfamiliar people, places, and medical treatments.
- The family may be overwhelmed and experience social, financial, and psychological strain.

Nursing Care of the Infant with a Chronic Condition

- Rock, hold, comfort, and use a soothing voice.
- Provide visual and auditory stimulation.

- Use group nursing care measures and protect nap time.
- Maintain the crib as a safe place.
- Encourage parents to hold the infant.
- Encourage siblings to visit.

Nursing Care of the Toddler with a Chronic Condition

- Maintain the bond between parents and child.
- Promote realistic developmental skills.
- Do not react negatively to regression.
- Praise the child for attempts at self-care.
- Instruct the parents on realistic methods of discipline.
- Manage pain.
- Maintain the home routine as much as possible.
- Allow the child to express his or her feelings through play.

Regression

- An abnormal return to an earlier reaction, characterized by emotions or behaviors that are inappropriate for the current age and may include the loss of recently acquired skills (Venes, 2005).
- Can be both physical and emotional.

Nursing Care of the Preschooler with a Chronic Condition

- Provide the opportunity to express fears and frustrations.
- Tell stories and read books.
- Allow the preschooler to use dramatic play.
- Ask the child-life specialist for assistance.
- Maintain a normal home schedule as much as possible and enforce consistent limits.
- Reassure the child that nothing he or she did caused the illness.
- Be honest when explaining and preparing the child for procedures.
- Understand the child's limited concept of time.

Nursing Care of the School-age Child with a Chronic Condition

- Maintain pain management.
- Reassure that personal behavior has not caused the illness.
- Answer questions at a level the child can understand.

- Use play as an outlet (unstructured).
- Include peers as much as possible.
- Communicate to family about nonverbal cues.
- Maintain open and honest dialogue.

Nursing Care of an Adolescent with a Chronic Condition

- Provide solitary time.
- Give realistic choices.
- Include the adolescent in medically related matters when possible.
- Use peer support and interaction.
- May expand networks to include support groups and community programming.

Nursing Care of a Sibling of a Child with a Chronic Condition

- Instruct parents to maintain familiar home routines as much as possible.
- Include the sibling in simple care.
- Provide information about the ill child.

Child Life Specialist

- Whenever a child is diagnosed with a chronic condition, it is important to involve the child life specialist.
- The child life specialist is an expert in child development and therapeutic play and can assist in diversion activities during procedures, arrange for therapeutic play, or simply let the child take time to play.

Caregiver Burden

- Caregiver burden, as described by Kuster et al. (2004), is the unrelenting pressure and anxiety in providing daily care to a child with disabilities while meeting other family needs and can be a major source of stress.

Respite Care

- Respite care is short-term care offered to families living with a child who has a chronic condition.

- The main goal of respite care is to provide relief for family members of the burden and stress of sustained care giving (Venes, 2005).
- Parents can also use respite care in situations in which someone besides them can accompany the child to a doctor's appointment.
- The availability of respite care varies in every community (Orloff et al., 2004).
- It is important to note that respite care is not always paid for by private insurance. Sometimes state agencies or national programs can reimburse the family for respite care.

Talking About the Chronic Condition

- When talking about the child's chronic condition with the family, the nurse must be sure to use the child's name and personalize the discussion.
- It is important that the nurse avoid labeling the child by, for example, saying "CF kids." Instead, the nurse can say, "Timmy will need ongoing care for his cystic fibrosis."
- This kind of communication places the emphasis on the child and not on the condition.
- It is also important to listen to the family so that home routines can be continued during hospitalization.

Establishing Trust with the Family

Godshall (2003) suggests that the nurse take the following actions when establishing trust:

- Consider the needs of the entire family; do not forget the siblings.
- Familiarize yourself with the child's condition and know about the disease process.
- Be open and honest.
- Show the family that the burden of care is understood. Burden of care includes the combination of physical, psychological, social, and financial burdens the family may face.
- Take time to listen to the child and to the caregiver.
- Include parents in the plan of care. Some parents like to participate in the child's care while the child is hospitalized. It is also important to maintain home rituals as much as possible while the child is hospitalized.

- Treat each child as an individual. It is essential that the nurse not label the child according to the disease process.
- Allow the child to make decisions about the care when possible. Decision making is especially important for the adolescent.
- Maintain confidentiality.
- Do not prematurely judge the parents. Some parents cannot stay with the child in the hospital because of personal needs and responsibilities.
- Arrange for continuity of nursing care.
- Assess the family's support systems and resources.

The Dying Child

Do Not Resuscitate

- A Do Not Resuscitate (DNR) request means withholding life-sustaining treatment and requires that no attempt be made to revive a child who has clinically died.
- Withholding life-sustaining medical treatment includes decisions to withhold, withdraw, or limit medical treatment.
- Some medical ethicists feel that there is no difference between withholding and withdrawing treatment if the treatment is no longer beneficial to the child. When making recommendations to withhold, withdraw, or limit medical treatment, the benefits of treatment must be weighed against the burden of continuing treatment for the child.
- A DNR order means that no lifesaving measures will be initiated in the event of cardiac or respiratory arrest.
- This decision also can mean removing medical equipment such as a ventilator or monitor, dialysis machine, feeding tube used for artificial nutrition, and intravenous fluids for hydration. Aggressive treatments such as chemotherapy or radiation therapy are also terminated.
- Wiegand (2006) states that the child and family participating in the process of withdrawal of life-sustaining therapy need consistency among health care providers and the delivery of consistent messages.
- All members of the interdisciplinary team need to communicate effectively with each other so that families receive ongoing and reliable information.

Before the Child Dies
- Complete the institution's checklist to ensure policies and procedures are followed.
- Contact the bereavement team.
- Create a file and include community resources.
- Make a follow-up ledger and phone call.

Facilitators and Barriers to Providing a "Good Death" Experience in the ICU	
Facilitators	**Barriers**
Make environment changes to facilitate dying with dignity.	Staffing patterns and nursing shortage
Communicate challenges.	Treatments based on medical regimens rather than on child and family needs
Manage pain and discomfort.	
Follow child's and family's wishes for end-of-life care.	
Promote early cessation of treatments if requested.	
Eliminate aggressive treatments, especially when the treatments are futile.	
Ensure effective communication among the total health care team.	

Source: Beckstrand, Callister, & Kirchoff (2006).

Care of the Dying Child
- Care of the dying child includes holistic nursing interventions that address the physical, emotional, and spiritual aspects:
  - Palliative care: Follows a medical model
  - Hospice care: Holistic approach; focuses on quality of life
  - End-of-life care: End of life is about 6 months away; the objective is peaceful death without pain
- Shift from the curative technological approach to providing care that enables the child to move toward death accessing own inner resources for healing.
- Help the child restore mental, physical, and spiritual balance to attain peace at the time of death.
- Be present.
- Use touch.
- Give the family choices.
- Assess the situation and determine the proper environment.

Complementary and Alternative Medicine

- Complementary and alternative medicine (CAM) has become increasingly popular in palliative care (e.g., relaxation, aromatherapy, acupuncture, or other therapies performed by a licensed practitioner). Other therapies, including dietary supplements and herbal remedies, are unregulated.
- The frequency and type of CAM are dependent on the child's condition and prognosis.
- Spiritual blessings and prayers may be beneficial to various types of chronic illnesses

Advantages of CAM

- Easy to understand
- Familiar methods
- Many are noninvasive
- Many have fewer side effects compared to medical treatments
- Help improve the overall quality of life
- Help maintain current state of health
- More holistic and in balance with nature (Suzuki, 2004)

Disadvantages of CAM

- Some treatments are complex
- They have not undergone adequate testing of effectiveness
- Many herbal preparations and remedies lack FDA approval
- Many are not covered by third-party reimbursement

The Hospice Approach

- Family-centered care is essential.
- A comprehensive, holistic approach can meet the child's physical, emotional, social, and spiritual needs.
- Effective symptom control and pain management are paramount.
- Care is provided by an interdisciplinary team.
- The child can be cared for at home or in a homelike environment.
- Coordination and continuity of care is a priority.
- In addition to regularly scheduled home care visits, services are available on a 24-hour, 7 days-a-week, on-call basis.
- The focus of care is on improving the quality of remaining life; that is, on palliative, not curative, measures.

- Bereavement follow-up services are offered to family members in the year after the death of the loved one (Lattanzi-Licht & Connor, 1995).

Children's Hospice International, 2005

- Children's Hospice International, 2005 states that it is important to give clear answers to children who are dying. Evasive answers may confuse the child.
- The child may be at a developmental level at which he or she may take conversations literally. When talking to the child, it is important to remember:
  - Do not tell the child that death is sleeping peacefully. The child may fear going to sleep.
  - Do not tell the child abstract concepts like, "It is God's will" or "You are such a good boy that God wants you to be with him." He or she may start to misbehave so as not to die.
  - Approach the child with compassion, honesty, support, and love (Children's Hospice International, 2005).

Critical Nursing Actions: Holistic Care for the Dying Child

Comfort Measures	Emotional Support	Spiritual Interventions	Complementary Care
Pain management Good hygiene Repositioning Nutrition and diet management Physical or occupational therapy Help the family create new rituals when the old ones no longer work due to the disease process.	Active listening and showing empathy Distraction Encourage positive coping. Encourage verbalization and ventilation of feelings. Psychotherapy referral Suggest support groups. Discuss topics about grief, loss, isolation, fear, guilt, and relationships. Discuss concerns about life after the child's death that relate to family, friends, and others.	Offering presence Meditation Music Prayer Read from spiritual text or poetry Allow for sacrament. Contact the family's religious or spiritual community. Discuss God/Higher Power or spiritual source.	Art therapy Energy-based therapy (healing touch, therapeutic touch, Reiki) Relaxation Guided imagery Acupuncture Reasonable exercise Aromatherapy

National Cancer Institute

- The National Cancer Institute (NCI) has resources available by calling the Cancer Information Service (CIS) Toll-free: 1-800-4-CANCER (1-800-422-6237) TTY (for deaf and hard of hearing callers): 1-800-332-8615.
- The NCI's Web sites are located at http://www.cancer. gov or http://www.cancer.gov/cancer_information/coping/ (click on the title under "End-of-Life Issues"). Cancer information specialists offer online assistance through the *LiveHelp* link on the NCI's Web site.

Fact Sheets

- The NCI fact sheet about hospice care includes contact information for hospice organizations.
- The NCI Advance Directives fact sheet discusses a patient's rights regarding medical treatment.
- The NCI fact sheet on Home Care for Cancer Patients provides information and resources related to home care services.
- The NCI booklet "Advanced Cancer: Living Each Day" provides support to cancer patients, families, and friends.

After the Child Dies

- Prepare the family about the child's appearance and description of the death.
- Offer the family the choice of seeing the child alone or with the nurse.

Handling the Child's Belongings

- Treat the child's belongings with respect and package in a special container instead of a plain plastic bag.
- Show sensitivity as these are the child's final possessions.

Grief

- Grief is a normal and appropriate emotional response to loss.
- Grief is unique to every individual and there is no timetable in which grief is complete.
- The stages of grief may come and go.
- Feelings of grief can return when least expected.
- Parents may not realize that grief begins the moment the child's diagnosis is communicated (Steen & Mirro, 2000).

Helping the Family Understand the Situation

- Listen empathetically and encourage the family to take the situation one day or one moment at a time.
- Help the family understand that there will be "good days" and inevitably "bad days."
- Give the family hope that over time the emotional pain may dissipate and that they can better come to terms with the experience of their child's death.

Coping Patterns

- Recognize exhibited coping patterns and find ways to support family:
  - Listen, sit silently, refer to pastoral care, offer spiritual care.
  - In case of destructive behavior to self or others call the physician or professional counselor.
  - Do not alter the coping pattern completely.

Pathological Grief

- Subtle indicators
- Suicidal or homicidal ideation
- Violent behavior
- Grief influenced by drugs and alcohol
- Extreme denial

Saying Good-bye

- Saying good-bye should not be rushed.
- Include siblings in the grieving process, encourage them to visit, and give them the opportunity to say good-bye.
- Call the child by his or her name.
- What to say to parents and family:
  - "I'm sorry"
  - "This must be terribly hard for you"
  - "Is there anyone I can call for you?"
  - "Would you like me to stay with you for a while?"

Caring for the Sibling of a Dying Child

- Listen and help the sibling express his or her feelings.
- Model to the family about how to acknowledge the sibling's presence during this difficult time (initiate a

simple conversation, turn on cartoons, offer a drink or snack, or show the sibling how to touch the dying child).

- Explain the situation to the sibling and relate appropriate information in terms understandable for the sibling's age.
- Help the sibling understand that he or she is not responsible for the death.
- Contact a child life specialist who can assist the sibling with art therapy.
- Encourage simple ways to be involved in the care such as making a final gift for the sibling to keep at the bedside.

RESOURCES

Compassionate Friends: http://www.compassionatefriends.org

National Cancer Institute: http://www.cancer.gov

End-of-Life Issues": http://www.cancer.gov/cancer_information/coping/

REFERENCES

Beckstrand, R.L., Callister, L.C., & Kirchhoff, K.T. (2006). Providing a "good death": Critical care nurses suggestions for improving end-life-care. *American Journal of Critical Care, 15*(1), 38–45.

Children's Hospice International (2005). Retrieved from http://www.chionline.org/resources (Accessed August 22, 2008).

Godshall, M. (2003). Caring for the families of chronically ill kids. *RN, 66*(2), 30–35.

Hain, R., Weinsten, S., Oleske, J., Orloff, S.F., & Cohen, S. (2004). Holistic management of symptoms. In B.S. Carter & M. Levetown (Eds.). *Palliative care for infants, children, and adolescents: A practical handbook* (pp. 163–195). Baltimore: The Johns Hopkins University Press.

Judson, L. (2004). Protective care: mothering a child dependent on parenteral nutrition. *Journal of Family Nursing, 10*(1), 93–120.

Kübler-Ross, E. (1983). *On children and death.* New York: Macmillan.

Kuster, P.A., Badr, L.K., Chang, B.L., Wuerker, A.K., & Benjamin, A.E. (2004). Factors influencing health promoting activities of mothers caring for ventilator assisted children. *Journal of Pediatric Nursing, 19*(4), 276–287.

Lattanzi-Licht, M., & Connor, S. (1995). Care of the dying: The hospice approach. In H. Wass & R.A. Neimeyer (Eds.). *Dying: Facing the facts.* Washington, DC: Taylor and Francis.

Orloff, S., Quance, K., Perszyk, S., Flowers, W., & Veale, E. (2004). Psychosocial and spiritual needs of the child and family. In K.M. Foley, B.S. Carter, & M. Levetown (Eds.). *Palliative care for infants, children, and adolescents* (pp. 141–162). Baltimore: The Johns Hopkins University Press.

Suzuki, N. (2004). Complementary and alternative medicine: A Japanese perspective. *Evidenced-based Complementary and Alternative Care, 1*(2), 113–118.

Steen, G., & Mirro, M. (2000). *Childhood cancer. A handbook from St. Jude Children's Research Hospital*. Cambridge, MA: Perseus.

Venes, D. (Ed.). (2005). *Tabers cyclopedic medical dictionary*. Philadelphia: F.A. Davis.

Wiegand, D. (2006). Withdrawal of life-sustaining therapy after sudden, unexpected life-threatening illness or injury: Interactions between patients' families, healthcare providers, and the healthcare system. *Journal of Critical Care, 15*(2), 178–187.

PHOTO AND ILLUSTRATION CREDITS

Chapter 1

First figure. Centers for Disease Control and Prevention, 2008.

Visual breast inspection. Dillon, P. (2007). *Nursing health assessment: A critical thinking, case studies approach* (2nd ed., p. 544). Philadelphia: F.A. Davis.

Arms raised overhead. Dillon, P. (2007). *Nursing health assessment: A critical thinking, case studies approach* (2nd ed., p. 544). Philadelphia: F.A. Davis.

Nipple assessment. Dillon, P. (2007). *Nursing health assessment: A critical thinking, case studies approach* (2nd ed., p. 550). Philadelphia: F.A. Davis.

Breast palpation. Dillon, P. (2007). *Nursing health assessment: A critical thinking, case studies approach* (2nd ed., p. 550). Philadelphia: F.A. Davis.

Testicular self-examination. Williams, L., & Hopper, P. (2007). *Understanding medical surgical nursing* (3rd ed., p. 896). Philadelphia: F.A. Davis.

Chapter 2

Figure 2-1 Dillon, P. (2007). *Nursing health assessment: A critical thinking, case studies approach* (2nd ed., p. 612). Philadelphia: F.A. Davis.

Figure 2-2 Scanlon, V., & Sanders, T. (2007). *Essentials of anatomy and physiology* (5th ed., p. 463). Philadelphia: F.A. Davis.

Figure 2-3 Scanlon, V., & Sanders, T. (2007). *Essentials of anatomy and physiology* (5th ed., p. 464). Philadelphia: F.A. Davis.

Figure 2-5 Dillon, P. (2007). *Nursing health assessment: A critical thinking, case studies approach* (2nd ed., p. 613). Philadelphia: F.A. Davis.

Figure 2-7 Scanlon, V., & Sanders, T. (2007). *Essentials of anatomy and physiology* (5th ed., p. 459). Philadelphia: F.A. Davis.

Chapter 6

Figure 6-1 Dillon, P. (2007). *Nursing health assessment: A critical thinking, case studies approach* (2nd ed., p. 836). Philadelphia: F.A. Davis.

Figure 6-2 Dillon, P. (2007). *Nursing health assessment: A critical thinking, case studies approach* (2nd ed., p. 837). Philadelphia: F.A. Davis.

Figure 6-3 Dillon, P. (2007). *Nursing health assessment: A critical thinking, case studies approach* (2nd ed., p. 838). Philadelphia: F.A. Davis.

Figure 6-4 Dillon, P. (2007). *Nursing health assessment: A critical thinking, case studies approach* (2nd ed., p. 838). Philadelphia: F.A. Davis.

Figure 6-5 Dillon, P. (2007). *Nursing health assessment: A critical thinking, case studies approach* (2nd ed., p. 838). Philadelphia: F.A. Davis.

Figure 6-6 Dillon, P. (2007). *Nursing health assessment: A critical thinking, case studies approach* (2nd ed., p. 838). Philadelphia: F.A. Davis.

Figure 6-7. Dillon, P. (2007). *Nursing health assessment: A critical thinking, case studies approach* (2nd ed., p. 838). Philadelphia: F.A. Davis.

Chapter 8

Figure 8-1 Holloway, B., Moredich, C., & Aduddell, K. (2006). *OB peds women's health notes: Nurse's clinical pocket guide,* p. 43, Philadelphia: F.A. Davis.

Figure 8-2 Holloway, B., Moredich, C., & Aduddell, K. (2006). *OB peds women's health notes: Nurse's clinical pocket guide,* p. 45, Philadelphia: F.A. Davis.

Figure 8-3 Dillon, P. (2007). *Nursing health assessment: A critical thinking, case studies approach* (2nd ed., p. 785). Philadelphia: F.A. Davis.

Chapter 9

Figure 9-8 Holloway, B., Moredich, C., & Aduddell, K. (2006). *OB peds women's health notes: Nurse's clinical pocket guide* (p. 53). Philadelphia: F.A. Davis.

Figure 9-11 Holloway, B., Moredich, C., & Aduddell, K. (2006). *OB peds women's health notes: Nurse's clinical pocket guide* (p. 55). Philadelphia: F.A. Davis.

Figure 9-12 Holloway, B., Moredich, C., & Aduddell, K. (2006). *OB peds women's health notes: Nurse's clinical pocket guide* (p. 56). Philadelphia: F.A. Davis.

Figure 9-13 Holloway, B., Moredich, C., & Aduddell, K. (2006). *OB peds women's health notes: Nurse's clinical pocket guide* (p. 57). Philadelphia: F.A. Davis.

Figure 9-14 Holloway, B., Moredich, C., & Aduddell, K. (2006). *OB peds women's health notes: Nurse's clinical pocket guide* (p. 59). Philadelphia: F.A. Davis.

Figure 9-15 Holloway, B., Moredich, C., & Aduddell, K. (2006). *OB peds women's health notes: Nurse's clinical pocket guide* (p. 60). Philadelphia: F.A. Davis.

Figure 9-16 Holloway, B., Moredich, C., & Aduddell, K. (2006). *OB peds women's health notes: Nurse's clinical pocket guide* (p. 60). Philadelphia: F.A. Davis.

Figure 9-17 Holloway, B., Moredich, C., & Aduddell, K. (2006). *OB peds women's health notes: Nurse's clinical pocket guide* (p. 60). Philadelphia: F.A. Davis.

Chapter 12

Figure 12-1 Holloway, B., Moredich, C., & Aduddell, K. (2006). *OB peds women's health notes: Nurse's clinical pocket guide* (p. 83). Philadelphia: F.A. Davis.

Figure 12-2 Dillon, P. (2007). *Nursing health assessment: A critical thinking, case studies approach* (2nd ed., p. 844). Philadelphia: F.A. Davis.

Chapter 13

Figure in Procedure 13-1. Holloway, B., Moredich, C., & Aduddell, K. (2006). *OB peds women's health notes: Nurse's clinical pocket guide* (p. 83). Philadelphia: F.A. Davis.

Chapter 15

Figure 15-1 Dillon, P. (2007). *Nursing health assessment: A critical thinking, case studies approach* (2nd ed., p. 857). Philadelphia: F.A. Davis.

Figure 15-2 Dillon, P. (2007). *Nursing health assessment: A critical thinking, case studies approach* (2nd ed., p. 856). Philadelphia: F.A. Davis.

Figure 15-3 Dillon, P. (2007). *Nursing health assessment: A critical thinking, case studies approach* (2nd ed., p. 856). Philadelphia: F.A. Davis.

Figure 15-4 Dillon, P. (2007). *Nursing health assessment: A critical thinking, case studies approach* (2nd ed., p. 857). Philadelphia: F.A. Davis.

Figure 15-5 Courtesy of Mead Johnson Nutritionals.

Procedure 15-2 Dillon, P. (2007). *Nursing health assessment: A critical thinking, case studies approach* (2nd ed., p. 857). Philadelphia: F.A. Davis.

Procedure 15-3, first photo. Dillon, P. (2007). *Nursing health assessment: A critical thinking, case studies approach* (2nd ed., p. 866). Philadelphia: F.A. Davis.

Procedure 15-3, second photo. Dillon, P. (2007). *Nursing health assessment: A critical thinking, case studies approach* (2nd ed., p. 866). Philadelphia: F.A. Davis.

Procedure 15-3, third photo. Dillon, P. (2007). *Nursing health assessment: A critical thinking, case studies approach* (2nd ed., p. 866). Philadelphia: F.A. Davis.

Palmar grasp. Dillon, P. (2007). *Nursing health assessment: A critical thinking, case studies approach* (2nd ed., p. 869). Philadelphia: F.A. Davis.

Toe or plantar grasp. Dillon, P. (2007). *Nursing health assessment: A critical thinking, case studies approach* (2nd ed., p. 869). Philadelphia: F.A. Davis.

Rooting and sucking reflexes. Dillon, P. (2007). *Nursing health assessment: A critical thinking, case studies approach* (2nd ed., p. 871). Philadelphia: F.A. Davis.

Extrusion reflex. Dillon, P. (2007). *Nursing health assessment: A critical thinking, case studies approach* (2nd ed., p. 871). Philadelphia: F.A. Davis.

Stepping reflex. Dillon, P. (2007). *Nursing health assessment: A critical thinking, case studies approach* (2nd ed., p. 870). Philadelphia: F.A. Davis.

Tonic neck or fencing reflex. Dillon, P. (2007). *Nursing health assessment: A critical thinking, case studies approach* (2nd ed., p. 868). Philadelphia: F.A. Davis.

Glabellar reflex. Dillon, P. (2007). *Nursing health assessment: A critical thinking, case studies approach* (2nd ed., p. 872). Philadelphia: F.A. Davis.

Babinski reflex. Dillon, P. (2007). *Nursing health assessment: A critical thinking, case studies approach* (2nd ed., p. 872). Philadelphia: F.A. Davis.

Moro reflex. Dillon, P. (2007). *Nursing health assessment: A critical thinking, case studies approach* (2nd ed., p. 868). Philadelphia: F.A. Davis.

Magnet reflex. Dillon, P. (2007). *Nursing health assessment: A critical thinking, case studies approach* (2nd ed., p. 873). Philadelphia: F.A. Davis.

Galant reflex. Dillon, P. (2007). *Nursing health assessment: A critical thinking, case studies approach* (2nd ed., p. 873). Philadelphia: F.A. Davis.

Crawling reflex. Dillon, P. (2007). *Nursing health assessment: A critical thinking, case studies approach* (2nd ed., p. 872). Philadelphia: F.A. Davis.

Crossed extension. Dillon, P. (2007). *Nursing health assessment: A critical thinking, case studies approach* (2nd ed., p. 872). Philadelphia: F.A. Davis.

Chapter 16

Figure 16-1 Stevens, B., Johnston, C., Petryshen, P., & Taddio, A. (1996). Premature infant pain profile: Development and initial validation. *Clinical Journal of Pain, 12*(1), 13–22.

Chapter 18

Figure 18-1 Dillon, P. (2007). *Nursing health assessment: A critical thinking, case studies approach* (2nd ed., p. 856). Philadelphia: F.A. Davis.

Figure 18-6B *Wong's essentials of pediatric nursing* (6th ed). St. Louis: Mosby. Copyright by Mosby, Inc. Reprinted with permission.

Figure 18-7 Wilkinson, J.M., & Van Leuven, K. (2007). *Fundamentals of nursing: Theory, concepts & application,* Vol. 2 (p. 254). Philadelphia: F.A. Davis.

Chapter 21

Heimlich maneuver, chest thrusts. Hopkins, T., & Myers, E. (2007). *Medical surgical notes* (2nd ed., p. 168). Philadelphia: F.A. Davis.

Heimlich maneuver, back blows. Hopkins, T., & Myers, E. (2007). *Medical surgical notes* (2nd ed., p. 168). Philadelphia: F.A. Davis.

Chapter 26

Figure 26-1 Teasdale, G., & Jennettt, B. (1974). Assessment of coma and impaired consciousness. A practical scale. *The Lancet, 13,*2(7872), 81–84.

Chapter 27

Figure 27-2 Dillon, P. (2007). *Nursing health assessment: A critical thinking, case studies approach* (2nd ed., p. 708). Philadelphia: F.A. Davis.

Assessment Tools: Transverse break. Williams, L., & Hopper, P. (2007). *Understanding medical surgical nursing* (3rd ed., p. 995). Philadelphia: F.A. Davis.

Assessment Tools: Spiral break. Williams, L., & Hopper, P. (2007). *Understanding medical surgical nursing* (3rd ed., p. 995). Philadelphia: F.A. Davis.

Assessment Tools: Oblique break. Williams, L., & Hopper, P. (2007). *Understanding medical surgical nursing* (3rd ed., p. 995). Philadelphia: F.A. Davis.

Assessment Tools: Greenstick break. Williams, L., & Hopper, P. (2007). *Understanding medical surgical nursing* (3rd ed., p. 995). Philadelphia: F.A. Davis.

Assessment Tools: Comminuted break. Williams, L., & Hopper, P. (2007). *Understanding medical surgical nursing* (3rd ed., p. 995). Philadelphia: F.A. Davis.

Chapter 28

Figure 28-1 Venes, D. (2005). *Taber's cyclopedic medical dictionary* (20th ed., p. 1931). Philadelphia: F.A. Davis.

Figure 28-2 Dillon, P. (2007). *Nursing health assessment: A critical thinking, case studies approach* (2nd ed., p. 239). Philadelphia: F.A. Davis.

Macules. Dillon, P. (2007). *Nursing health assessment: A critical thinking, case studies approach* (2nd ed., p. 231). Philadelphia: F.A. Davis.

Papule. Dillon, P. (2007). *Nursing health assessment: A critical thinking, case studies approach* (2nd ed., p. 233). Philadelphia: F.A. Davis.

Patches. Dillon, P. (2007). *Nursing health assessment: A critical thinking, case studies approach* (2nd ed., p. 233). Philadelphia: F.A. Davis.

Tumor. Dillon, P. (2007). *Nursing health assessment: A critical thinking, case studies approach* (2nd ed., p. 234). Philadelphia: F.A. Davis.

Vesicles. Courtesy of Centers for Disease Control and Prevention.

Pustules. Courtesy of Centers for Disease Control and Prevention.

Bullae. Courtesy of Centers for Disease Control and Prevention.

Wheals. Courtesy of Centers for Disease Control and Prevention.

Crust. Courtesy of Centers for Disease Control and Prevention.

Scales. Courtesy of Centers for Disease Control and Prevention.

Licherification. Courtesy of Centers for Disease Control and Prevention.

Keloids. Dillon, P. (2007). *Nursing health assessment: A critical thinking, case studies approach* (2nd ed., p. 237). Philadelphia: F.A. Davis.

Fissure. Dillon, P. (2007). *Nursing health assessment: A critical thinking, case studies approach* (2nd ed., p. 238). Philadelphia: F.A. Davis.

Ulcer. Dillon, P. (2007). *Nursing health assessment: A critical thinking, case studies approach* (2nd ed., p. 238). Philadelphia: F.A. Davis.

Index

Note: Page numbers followed by f refer to figures.

A

Abdomen
  acute, in neonate, 283
  assessment of, 339–400, 340f
    in appendicitis, 417–418
  auscultation of, 339
  in chronic renal failure, 580
  emergency conditions of, 645
  pain in, in children, 418
  palpation of, 339
  pediatric, 339–340, 340f
  preterm infant, 296–297
  quadrants of, 339, 340f
  trauma to, 431–432
Abdominal circumference, neonatal,
    272, 272f
Abducens nerve, 343
Abduction, of newborn, 219–220
ABO blood group, 623
ABO isoimmunization, 122
Abortion, 25
  spontaneous, 86, 91, 95
  therapeutic, 33–34
Abruptio placentae, 87, 92, 93–94, 93f
Abscess, brain, 507, 511
Absolute neutrophil count, 647
Abstinence, 25, 29
Abuse
  child, 384, 390, 393
  substance, 73–74, 122, 300,
    304–305, 385
Accessory nerve, 343
Acetaminophen
  for children, 353–356
  toxicity of, 356
Acetylsalicylic acid, 511. See also Aspirin
Acidosis, 402–403
  metabolic, neonatal, 295
  respiratory, neonatal, 295
Acne, 550
  isotretinoin monitoring in, 554
  treatment of, 563
Acoustic nerve, 343
Acoustic stimulation, fetal, 128
Acquired immunodeficiency syndrome
    in pregnancy, 111
  testing for, 438–439
Acrocyanosis, 251
  neonatal, 136, 280

Activity limitation, 679
Acupuncture/acupressure, 161
  in enuresis, 605
  in postpartum depression, 248
  in pregnancy, 84, 109
Acute hemolytic transfusion reaction,
    637
Acute lung injury, blood transfusion
    and, 618
Acute lymphocytic leukemia, 640
Acute myelogenous leukemia, 640
Adam's test, 530, 531f
Addisonian crisis, pediatric, 483
Adipose tissue, brown, 251
Adolescents, 6–7, 314. See also
    Children
  acne in, 550, 554, 563
  alcohol abuse evaluation for, 385
  amenorrhea in, 590–591, 598–599
  anorexia in, 386
  antidepressants in, 385–386
  chronic illness in, 673, 681
  communication with, 323
    about weight loss, 14
  death perceptions of, 675
  diabetes mellitus in, 492–494
  growth and development of, 322, 329
  health promotion screening for, 6–7
  informed consent process for,
    322–323
  obesity in, 389, 393
  pain management in, 369
  pregnancy in, 61, 122
  procedure preparation for, 361–362
  pubertal changes in, 18
  safety for, 7
  selective serotonin reuptake
    inhibitors in, 385–386
  substance abuse evaluation for, 385
  suicide by, 382–383
  syncope in, 462
  vital signs in, 333
  weight loss for, 14
Adrenal crisis, 480, 496
Adrenarche, 17, 18
Adrenocortical insufficiency, 436, 480,
    496
Afterpains (afterbirth pains), 202
Air embolism, apheresis-related, 638

Albumin
  in neonate, 261
  in pregnancy, 56
Albuterol, 405–406, 594
Alcohol use/abuse
  screening for, 8
  teratogenicity of, 45
Alertness, 500
Alkalosis, 402–403
  metabolic, neonatal, 295
  respiratory, neonatal, 295
Allen chart, 350, 350f
Allergic reaction
  diphenhydramine for, 442–443
  epinephrine for, 441–442
  immunization-related, 438
  systemic, 551
  transfusion-related, 636
Allogeneic cell transplantation, 434
Aloe vera, 357
Alopecia, chemotherapy-related,
  665–666
Alpha-fetoprotein, 63, 72, 647
Alpha-methyldopa, in pregnancy, 101
Ambiguous genitalia, 607
Ambulatory surgery center, 379
Amenorrhea, 63, 590–591, 598–599
Amniocentesis, 125–126
Amnioinfusion, 175, 187
Amnion, 41
Amniotic fluid
  assessment of, 148–149
  meconium-stained, 176, 189
  volume of, 127
Amniotic fluid embolism, 175, 197
Amniotic infection syndrome, 89
Amniotomy, 136, 179, 180f
  patient/family teaching for, 184
Amphetamines, teratogenicity of, 46
Amphotericin B, 444–445
Ampicillin, 592
Amylase
  in neonate, 261
  in pregnancy, 56
Analgesia, 161
  intrathecal, 162
  postpartal, 211
Anaphylaxis, 434, 435
  antithymocyte globulin and, 616
  epinephrine for, 441–442
  nursing care for, 449
  patient/family teaching for, 446
Androgen, reproductive system effects
  of, 34

Anemia, 611, 621
  aplastic, 613, 631
  iron-deficiency
    in children, 611, 614, 626–627,
      630
    in pregnancy, 81
  in pregnancy, 54, 82
Anesthesia, 161
  epidural, 162, 165, 167, 167f
  regional, 162, 167–171
Anesthetics, topical, 558, 658
  postpartum, 211
Aneurysm, in children, 457
Angel kiss, 267
Angiography, 459
Angioma, 51
Angioplasty, 459
Angiotensin-converting enzyme
  inhibitors, 595
Anorectal manometry, 422
Anorexia, 386
Anorexia nervosa, 78
Anthropometric measurements
  in children, 330–331
  in neonate, 271–272, 271f, 272f
Anti-D antibody, 615
Anti-itch agents, 558
Antianxiety drugs, 387
Antibiotics, 439–440
  in brain abscess, 511
  broad-spectrum, 591–593
  compliance with, 563
  in endocarditis prevention, 475–476
  in pregnancy, 120
  topical, 558
Anticoagulants
  in children, 457, 474
  patient/family teaching on, 247
Anticonvulsants, 388
  in eclampsia/preeclampsia, 99–101
Antidepressants, 387–388
  reproductive system effects of, 34
  suicide behavior and, 385–386
Antiemetics, 424, 425, 658
Antifungals, 596
  topical, 558
Antihypertensives, 595
  in pregnancy, 101–103
  reproductive system effects of, 34
Antipsychotics, 388
  reproductive system effects of, 35
Antiseizure medications, 507–508,
  509–510, 516
Antispasmodics, 424

Antithymocyte globulin, 616
Antithyroid medications, 487
Anus, 19f, 24f
Anxiety
  herbal remedies for, 10
  mindful breathing for, 391
  treatment of, 387
Aorta, 464f
  coarctation of, 468, 468f
Aortic stenosis, 467, 468f
Apgar Score, 136, 158
Apheresis, 638
Aplastic anemia, 613, 631
Apnea, 251
Appendicitis, 417–418, 419
Appetite, in cancer, 660
AquaMEPHYTON, 285–286
Aromatherapy, 161
  during labor, 173
  in postpartum depression, 248
  in pregnancy, 84
Arrhythmias, sinus, 476
Arterial blood gases, in children,
  402–403
Arteriovenous fistula, 597
Arthrography, 533
Asparaginase, 653
Aspiration, in preterm infant, 301
Aspirin
  patient/family teaching on, 247, 409
  prophylactic, 7
  Reye syndrome with, 437, 503, 512
Asplenia, in children, 614–615
Asthma, 398
  Action Plan for, 412, 415
  albuterol in, 405–406
  emergency treatment of, 414–415
  ethnocultural considerations in, 406
  peak flow meter for, 410–412
  persistent and intractable (status
    asthmaticus), 396
  resources on, 415
Athlete's foot, 450
Atopic dermatitis, 564–565
Atresia
  biliary, 416, 422
  esophageal, 407
  pulmonary, 466, 467f
  tracheoesophageal, 407
  tricuspid, 468, 469f
Atrial septal defect, 465, 465f
Atrial septum, neonatal, 255
Atrioventricular canal defect, 466, 466f

Attachment, infant-mother, 204,
  290–291, 316
Attachment therapy, 386
Attention-deficit/hyperactivity disor-
  der, 383, 386, 388
Audiologic testing, 507
Audiometry, 351
Autism A.L.A.R.M., 392–393
Autism spectrum disorder, 392–393
  resources on, 394
Autoimmune disorder, 434
Autologous epidural blood patch, 161,
  172
Autologous transplantation, 434
Autonomic dysreflexia, 506–507
Avian flu, 438, 447–448

B
Babinski reflex, 278, 315
Baby (maternal, postpartum) blues,
  203, 219
Bacitracin and polymyxin B, 558
Back pain, in pregnancy, 86
Baclofen, 537
Bacteriuria, asymptomatic, 89
Balloon angioplasty, 471, 472f
Balloon atrial septostomy, 460
Ballottement, 63
Band neutrophils, 534
Barbiturates, intrapartal, 166
Barium enema, 422
Barium swallow, 422
Barlow-Ortolani maneuver,
  275–276
Bartholin's glands, 19f
Basal body temperature, 25
Basal skull fracture, 519
Base excess, 402
Basophils
  cerebrospinal fluid, 352
  count of, 534, 620
  in neonate, 303
Bathing, neonatal, 288
Bee sting, 553
Behavior, neonatal, 260–261
Behavior assessment, for adolescents,
  6–7
Behavioral therapy, in enuresis, 605
Belching, cancer-related, 660–661
Bend over test, 530, 531f
Benzathine penicillin, 556–557
Benzocaine, 558

Benzodiazepines
  flumazenil reversal of, 164
  intrapartal, 164, 166
Beractant, 303–304
Beta blockers, reproductive system
  effects of, 35
Betamethasone
  for preterm infant, 263–264
  topical, 558
Bicarbonate
  in children, 402
  in neonate, 261
  in preterm infant, 295
Bilberry, 357
Biliary atresia, 416, 422
Bilirubin, 251
  neonatal, 256–258, 257f, 261, 300,
    300f
  in Rocky Mountain spotted fever,
    555
Binding-in, in pregnancy, 60
Biofeedback, 161
  in enuresis, 605
  in postpartum depression, 248
Biopsy
  bone, 535
  bone marrow, 649–650
  cardiac, 459
  endometrial, 27
  liver, 422, 517
  lung, 400–401
Bipolar disorder
  in children, 382
  resources on, 394
Birth. *See also* Labor
  assessment after. *See* Neonatal
    assessment
  Cesarean, 176
    anesthesia for, 168
    assessment after, 208
    infection with, 232–233
    vaginal birth after, 177
  documentation of, 290
  estimated date of, 63, 67–68
  forceps-assisted, 176, 191, 191f
  mother-infant bonding after, 204,
    290–291
  period after. *See* Postpartum period
    (puerperium)
  precipitate (precipitous), 185
  vacuum-assisted, 177, 192, 192f
Birth center, admission to, 144–145, 159
Birthmarks, 280

Bisacodyl, postpartal, 211
Bishop Score, 175, 180
Bites, 553
  prevention of, 561
  tick, 565
Bladder, postpartal assessment of, 204,
  208
Bleeding
  apheresis-related, 638
  intracranial, in children, 615–616
  post-tonsillectomy, 399
  in pregnancy, 91–95
Bleeding time, neonatal, 261
Bleomycin, 653
Blepharitis, 520
Blood, urinary, 582, 601
  in neonate, 262
Blood culture, 439, 535
Blood gases
  in at-risk neonate, 295
  in children, 402–403
  in neonate, 262, 295
Blood glucose, in preterm infant,
  306–307
Blood groups, 623
Blood patch, epidural, 161, 172
Blood pressure
  neonatal, 270
  pediatric, 333, 435, 457
  preterm infant, 309–310
  procedure for, 474–475
Blood transfusion
  acute hemolytic reaction with, 637
  acute lung injury with, 618
  administration of, 616–618, 635
  allergic reaction with, 636
  autologous blood for, 632
  bacterial contamination with,
    636–637
  circulatory overload with, 637
  consent for, 631
  cryoprecipitate for, 634
  documentation of, 617
  febrile reaction with, 636
  fresh frozen plasma for, 633–634
  initiation of, 617
  Jehovah's Witness and, 94–95,
    626
  packed red blood cells for, 633
  products for, 632–636
  reactions with, 635–636
  red blood cells for, 632
  safety for, 616

Blood transfusion (*Continued*)
  type and crossmatch for, 623
  verifications for, 616–617
  whole blood for, 633
Blood volume, in pregnancy, 54
Bloody show, 136
Blue nevus, 280
Blues, baby (maternal, postpartum), 203, 219
Body mass index, 78
  in children, 330–331, 349
Bone, biopsy of, 535
Bone marrow
  biopsy of, 649–650
  transplantation of, 662
Bone scan, 533, 650–651
Bony pelvis, 20, 21f
Bordetella pertussis vaccine, 446
Boron, in hypoparathyroidism, 496
Bowel, postpartal assessment of, 204
Bradycardia, fetal, 136
Brain abscess, 507, 511
Brain tumor, 641, 643–644, 662
Braxton Hicks sign, 63
Breast(s), 21
  development of, 341
  engorgement of, 202
  fibrocystic changes in, 13
  postpartal assessment of, 204
  postpartal infection of, 229, 229f, 236–237
  in pregnancy, 54
  self-examination of, 11–13
Breast cancer
  risk factors for, 9
  screening for, 7, 11
  self-examination for, 11–13
Breastfeeding
  discomfort with, 216
  electric milk expression and, 217
  infant readiness for, 209
  latch-on for, 202
  let-down reflex in, 202, 209
  manual milk expression and, 217
  milk storage with, 217
  neonatal jaundice with, 258
  nipple confusion and, 203, 217
Breath/breathing. *See also* Respiratory system
  Kussmaul, 479
  during labor, 173
  mindful, 391
  neonatal, 270, 287
  noisy, 347

  pediatric, 337, 347–348
  periodic, 252
  shortness of, in pregnancy, 85
Breath sounds, in children, 337, 347–348
Broad ligament, 20, 20f
Bromocriptine mesylate, in female infertility, 36
Bronchopulmonary dysplasia, 412–413
Bronchoscopy, 400
Broviac catheter, 664
Brown adipose tissue, 251
Brown nevus, 280
Brudzinski sign, 502–503
Bulbourethral gland, 24f
Bulimia nervosa, 78
Bulla, cutaneous, 549
BUN-to-creatinine ratio, 590
Burns, 552, 559
  assessment of, 567
  chemical, 520
  classification of, 565–566, 565f
  dressing change for, 569
  fluid resuscitation in, 567
  management of, 562
  nutrition in, 567
  pain management in, 567–568
  prevention of, 561
  recovery from, 568
  severity of, 566
  transfer for, 566
  treatment of, 566–568
  wound care in, 568
Butorphanol, 164–165

C
C-reactive protein, 535
Café-au-lait spots, 280
Caffeine, 496
  teratogenicity of, 45
CAGE questions, 385
Calcitriol, 595
Calcium
  deficit of, 584
  excess of, 584
  in hypoparathyroidism, 496
  intravenous, 487
  in neonate, 262
  in pregnancy, 56, 82
  serum, 535
Calcium gluconate, 594
Calories
  for children, 344
  in pregnancy, 82

Cancer, 640–670. *See also* Chronic illness; Dying child *and specific cancers*
  assessment in, 640–643
  bone marrow biopsy in, 649–650
  bone scan in, 650–651
  clinical alerts in, 643–645
  constipation in, 660
  diagnostic tests, 646–658, 646f
  diarrhea in, 659
  emergencies in, 643, 645, 668
  ethnocultural considerations in, 659
  gastrointestinal complications in, 660–661
  hemorrhagic cystitis in, 643, 668
  infection in, 661, 666–667
  lumbar puncture in, 646, 646f, 651–652
  lymphangiogram in, 652
  medications in, 653–658
  nausea/vomiting in, 659
  neutropenia in, 646–647, 666
  nursing care in, 665–669
  nutrition in, 659, 660, 666
  oral complications in, 660
  patient/family teaching in, 659–661
  psychological support in, 643, 667, 669
  resources on, 669, 687, 689
  septic shock in, 643, 645, 668
  sibling care in, 669
  staging of, 646
  treatments for, 643–645, 653–657, 661–668
  tumor lysis syndrome in, 643, 668
  urine specific gravity in, 647–649
  venous access devices for, 663–664
Candidiasis, vulvovaginal, 596, 598
Cannabis, in pregnancy, 74
Capillary refill time, 337, 526, 526f
Caput, 266
Caput succedaneum, 266
Car seat, 289
Carbamazepine, 509
Carboplatin, 653
Carboprost, in postpartal hemorrhage, 242
Cardiac arrest, in pregnancy, 97
Cardiac catheterization, 459
  medical orders after, 476–477
Cardiac output, 453
  pregnancy-related, 55, 124
Cardiopulmonary system, neonatal, 254–255, 254f

Cardiovascular system
  maternal, 54
  neonatal, 272
  pediatric, 330
    in acute kidney failure, 603
    assessment of, 330, 454–455
    in chronic renal failure, 578
    disorders of, 453–478. *See also specific conditions*
      clinical alerts for, 456–458
      clinical care for, 473–474
      diagnostic tests in, 458–460
      ethnocultural considerations in, 461
      home care for, 462–463
      laboratory values in, 460
      medications for, 460–461, 477
      patient/family teaching for, 462–463
      postoperative care for, 472–473
      resources on, 477
      syndromic, 454–455
      vital signs in, 477
Caregiver burden, 671, 681
Carvedilol, 460–461
Cast petaling, 540–541
Cast syndrome, 525
  prevention of, 539
Casts, urinary, 589
Cayenne pepper, 357
Cefixime, 592
Cefotaxime, 592
Ceftriaxone, 592
Celiac disease, 426
Cellulitis, 559
  periorbital, 520
Centigrade-Fahrenheit temperature conversion, 332
Central venous catheter, 663–664, 665f
Cephalexin, 592
Cephalhematoma, 266
Cephalic version, 177, 188, 188f
Cephalopelvic disproportion, 175–176
Cerebrospinal fluid
  analysis of, 352
  lumbar puncture for, 646, 646f, 651–652
Cerumen, cotton swabs for, 359
Cervical cancer, screening for, 8
Cervical cap, 30
Cervical mucus, 22
Cervical ripening agents, 182–183
  patient/family teaching for, 184–185

Cervix, 19f
  dilation of, 137, 138f
  effacement of, 137, 138f–139f
  intrapartal laceration of, 227
  in pregnancy, 54
  ripening of, 136, 182–183, 184–185
Cesarean birth, 176
  anesthesia for, 168
  assessment after, 208
  infection with, 232–233
  vaginal birth after, 177
Chadwick's sign, 51, 63
Chalazion, 519
Chamomile, 357
CHARGE association, 455
Chemical burns, 520
Chemotherapy, 653–657
  alopecia with, 665–666
  complications of, 665–667
  disposal of, 644
  extravasation with, 644–645, 658
  reproductive system effects of, 35
  safety for, 666
  venous access devices for, 663–664,
    665f
Chest
  neonatal, 272, 272f
  pediatric, 330, 336–337
  preterm infant, 296–298
Chest pain, in children, 348
Chest x-ray, in children, 400
Chewing, cancer-related difficulty
  with, 660
Cheyne-Stokes respirations, 675
Child abuse, 384, 390, 393
  resources on, 394
Child care, 289–290
Child life specialist, 681
Children, 2–6
  abdominal assessment in, 339–340,
    340f
  abdominal pain in, 418
  abdominal trauma in, 431–432
  acetaminophen for, 353–356
  acute kidney failure in, 589–590
  Addisonian crisis in, 483
  adrenal crisis in, 480, 496–497
  adrenocortical insufficiency in, 436,
    480, 496–497
  ambiguous genitalia in, 607
  ambulatory surgery center for, 379
  anaphylaxis in, 434, 435, 446–448,
    449, 616
  anorexia nervosa in, 386

anthropometric measurements for,
    330–331, 331f
  anti-D antibody in, 615
  antidepressants in, 385–386
  antithymocyte globulin in, 616
  anxiety in, 387
  aortic stenosis in, 467, 468f
  aplastic anemia in, 613, 631
  appendicitis in, 417–418, 419
  arteriovenous fistula in, 597
  asplenia in, 614–615
  asthma in, 396, 398, 406, 410–412,
    414–415
  atrial septal defect in, 465, 465f
  atrioventricular canal defect in, 466,
    466f
  attachment therapy and, 386
  attention-deficit/hyperactivity disor-
    der in, 383, 386, 388
  autism in, 392–393
  autonomic dysreflexia in, 506–507
  basal skull fracture in, 519
  bed confinement for, 363
  bee/wasp sting in, 553
  bipolar disorder in, 382, 387, 388
  bites in, 553, 561, 565
  bladder exstrophy in, 606
  blepharitis in, 520
  blood pressure in, 333, 457,
    474–475
  blood transfusion for. See Blood
    transfusion
  body mass index in, 330–331, 349
  brain abscess in, 507, 511
  brain tumor in, 641, 643–644, 662
  breath sounds in, 337, 347–348
  bronchopulmonary dysplasia in,
    412–413
  burns in, 552, 561, 562, 565–568,
    565f
  caloric requirements for, 344
  cancer in. See Cancer
  cardiac assessment in, 337–339,
    454–455
  cardiovascular assessment in, 330,
    454–455
  cardiovascular conditions in,
    453–478. See also specific
    conditions
  celiac disease in, 426
  cellulitis in, 559
  central venous line in, 420
  cerebrospinal fluid analysis in, 352
  chalazion in, 519

chemical burns in, 520
chest assessment in, 330, 336–337
child care for, 289–290
cholesterol in, 458, 462
chronic illness in. *See* Chronic illness
clinical alerts for, 347–349
clubfoot in, 539, 543
coarctation of aorta in, 468, 468f
communication with, 364–365
community health care for, 380
compartment syndrome in, 531
complete blood count in, 619, 621
congenital heart disease in, 465–471. *See also specific conditions*
conjunctivitis in, 519
constipation in, 420
cortisone insufficiency in, 483
cotton swabs for, 359
cranial nerve testing in, 343
cricoid pressure in, 506
critical care unit for, 379
cryptorchidism in, 599, 606, 606f
Cushing's syndrome, 480–481
Cushing's triad for, 514–515
cystic fibrosis in, 80, 401, 407–408, 413, 415
cytomegalovirus infection in, 437, 443–444
dehydration in, 482, 581–582
depression in, 385–386, 387–388
diabetes insipidus in, 480, 483–484
diabetes mellitus in, 489–494, 497–498
    type 1, 481, 485–486, 492–494
    type 2, 481, 488, 492–494
diabetic ketoacidosis in, 481, 483
diagnostic tests for, 349–352. *See also* Diagnostic tests
diarrhea in, 423, 429
differential white blood cell count in, 620
disability in, 359
disseminated intravascular coagulation in, 612
dying. *See* Dying child
dysfunctional voiding in, 605
ear assessment in, 335, 335f
emergency department care for, 379–380
encephalitis in, 516–517
endocrine assessment in, 330
enuresis in, 388, 595, 597, 605

epiglottitis in, 413–414
epispadias in, 607
epistaxis in, 611, 621, 630
Epstein's malformation in, 468, 469f
esophageal atresia in, 407
ethnocultural considerations for, 358–359. *See also* Ethnocultural considerations
Ewing's sarcoma in, 642
eye assessment in, 335, 350–351
eye conditions in, 519–520
failure to thrive in, 383
family medical history for, 325
fluid disorders in, 574–575, 581–582
fluid requirements for, 344–345
food jags in, 427
fracture in, 527–529, 531. *See also* Fracture
frostbite in, 562
gastrointestinal assessment in, 330
gastrointestinal conditions in, 416–433. *See also specific conditions*
gastrostomy tube for, 349
genitourinary assessment in, 330, 340–342
Glasgow Coma Scale for, 500–501
glomerulonephritis in, 577
group A *Streptococcus* infection in, 552
guided imagery for, 378
gynecomastia in, 599
head assessment in, 334, 334f
health assessment for, 330–333
health history for, 324–325
health insurance in, 362
hearing impairment in, 521
hearing screening in, 351–352
heart rate in, 333
heart sounds in, 338–339
heart transplantation in, 458
HEENT assessment in, 330
Heimlich maneuver for, 409–410
hematocrit in, 614, 618, 619
hematuria in, 582
hemoglobin in, 614, 618, 619
hemolytic uremic syndrome in, 576
hemophilia in, 612, 627–628
hemosiderosis in, 615
hepatitis in, 2, 286, 418, 430, 431
hepatoblastoma in, 643
hepatocellular carcinoma in, 643
herbal preparations for, 357, 362–363

Children (*Continued*)
hereditary spherocytosis in, 612, 625
herpes simplex virus infection in, 560
Hodgkin's disease in, 642
hospitalization for, 376–379
human papillomavirus infection in, 564
hydrocephalus in, 507
hyperaldosteronism in, 484
hypercholesterolemia-hyperlipidemia in, 462
hyperglycemia in, 490–491, 498
hyperreflexia in, 480
hypertrophic pyloric stenosis in, 420–421, 425–426
hypoglycemia in, 490–491, 492, 498
hyponatremia in, 482
hypoplastic left heart syndrome in, 470, 471f
hypospadias in, 607
hypothermia in, 552, 554, 569
idiopathic thrombocytopenic purpura in, 612, 615, 628, 630–631
immunization schedule for, 2. *See also* Immunization
impetigo in, 559
increased intracranial pressure in, 502, 506, 507, 514
informed consent for, 365
inguinal hernia in, 426–427
insulin for, 487–488, 489–491
intracranial bleeding in, 615–616
intussusception in, 417, 421
iron accumulation in, 615
iron-deficiency anemia in, 611, 614, 626–627, 630
irritable bowel syndrome in, 419, 427
Kawasaki disease in, 457
keratitis in, 520
kidney failure in, 456, 577–580
medications in, 594–595
kidney trauma in, 577
lactose intolerance in, 426
language disorder in, 512–513
lead exposure in, 359–360
Legg-Calve-Perthes disease in, 543–544
leukemia in, 640
lice in, 560–561
liver biopsy in, 517
liver cancer in, 647
long Q-T syndrome in, 471, 472f
Lyme disease in, 551

maltreatment of, 384, 390, 393, 394
massage for, 513
medications for, 353–358. *See also* Medications
meningitis in, 502–503
mindful breathing for, 391
mouth assessment in, 336
musculoskeletal assessment in, 330, 342
naloxone for, 349
near drowning in, 503–504
neck assessment in, 330, 334, 334f
nephroblastoma in, 641–642
neurally mediated syncope in, 462
neuroblastoma in, 641
neurological assessment in, 330, 342–343
neutropenia in, 613, 629, 646–647, 666
non-Hodgkin's lymphoma in, 643
nose assessment in, 336
nutrition for, 344–345, 363, 365–366
obesity in, 389, 393
observational impression of, 333
oro-/nasogastric tube for, 365–366
osteomyelitis in, 531–532
osteosarcoma in, 642
pacemaker in, 462
pain in, 345–346, 346f, 353–356, 367–369
pain scales for, 346–347, 346f
past medical history for, 325
patent ductus arteriosus in, 466, 467f
patient/family teaching for, 359–362. *See also* Patient/family teaching
periorbital cellulitis in, 520
peritonitis in, 419
pheochromocytoma in, 497
physical assessment in, 333–347
  abdominal, 339–340, 340f
  cardiac, 337–339
  chest, 336–337
  ears, 335, 335f
  eyes, 335
  general impression in, 333
  genitourinary, 340–342
  handwashing for, 349
  head, 334, 334f
  mouth, 336
  musculoskeletal, 342
  neck, 334, 334f
  neurological, 342–343
  nose, 336
  nutritional, 344–345

pain, 345–347, 346f
sinus, 336
skin, 333, 359
throat, 336
plan of care for, 372–373
platelets in, 619
postoperative hemorrhage in, 456
postoperative home care for,
374–375
posttraumatic stress disorder in,
381–382
posture of, 337
potassium depletion in, 484
pressure ulcers in, 569–571, 570f
privacy for, 316
probiotics in, 420
procedure preparation for, 360–362,
363–364. See also Procedure(s)
pulmonary atresia in, 466, 467f
pulmonic valve stenosis in, 466, 467f
pulses in, 337
rectal temperature in, 517
red blood cells in, 619, 620
reflexes in, 342–343
resiliency promotion for, 362
resources on, 370, 394
respiratory conditions in, 347–348,
396–415. See also specific
conditions
respiratory rate in, 333, 398, 435
restraints for, 367
retinoblastoma in, 642
review of systems for, 330
Reye syndrome in, 437, 503, 512
rhabdomyosarcoma in, 642
role modeling in, 378
rotavirus infection in, 428
safety for, 5, 348–349
scoliosis in, 530, 531f
seizures in, 506, 514–516
selective serotonin reuptake
inhibitors in, 385–386
shock in, 419, 488
short bowel syndrome in, 430
sickle cell disease in, 611, 621, 625,
627
sinus arrhythmias in, 476
sinus assessment in, 336
sinusitis in, 408
skin assessment in, 330, 333. See
also Skin
sleep disorders in, 385
sleep for, 4
slipped capital femoral epiphysis in,
527

social history for, 325
spina bifida in, 517
sprain in, 529–530
Stevens-Johnson syndrome in, 553
sty in, 519
subacute bacterial endocarditis in,
475–476
substance abuse by, 385
suicide assessment for, 382–383,
385–386
supraglottitis in, 413–414
syncope in, 458–459, 462
systemic allergic reaction in, 551
systemic lupus erythematosus in,
437
Tanner staging in, 341
tear duct blockage in, 520
temperature in, 331, 517
testicular torsion in, 580, 591
tetanus in, 537–538, 545–546
tetralogy of Fallot in, 456–457, 470,
471f
thalassemia in, 611–612
therapeutic play for, 377
throat assessment in, 336
thrombosis in, 457, 613–614
thyroid storm in, 482–483
tick in, 565
toilet training for, 391
total anomalous pulmonary venous
return in, 469, 470f
transposition of great arteries in,
469, 470f
tricuspid atresia in, 468, 469f
truncus arteriosus in, 469, 470f
twenty-four-hour observation unit
for, 379
ulcerative colitis in, 421
urinary tract infection in, 576,
600–601
varicocele in, 580
ventricular septal defect in, 465,
465f
ventricular shunt in, 512, 517
vesicoureteral reflux in, 576
violence by, 393
visual screening in, 350–351, 350f
vital signs in, 331–333
postoperative, 458
vomiting in, 419, 421, 425, 429
von Willebrand's disease in, 612
vulvovaginal candidiasis in, 596,
598
vulvovaginitis in, 597–598
warts in, 564

Children (*Continued*)
weight measurement in, 576
white blood cells in, 619, 620
Wilms' tumor in, 641–642
Chiropractic care, in pregnancy, 84
Chlamydia infection
in pregnancy, 110
screening for, 8
Chloride
in pregnancy, 56
sweat, 401
Cholasma, 51
Cholesterol
in children, 458, 462
screening for, 8, 10
Chorion, 41
Chorionic villi, 41
Chorionic villus sampling, 125
Chromosome, 41
Chronic illness. *See also* Cancer; Dying
child
in adolescent, 673, 681
caregiver burden in, 681
child life specialist in, 681
clinical alerts for, 676–677
discussion about, 682
ethnocultural considerations in,
677–678
family-nurse trust in, 682–683
focused assessment of, 672–676
impact of, 679
in infant, 672, 679–680
medications for, 677
nursing care in, 679–681
patient/family teaching about, 678
in preschooler, 672, 680
regression in, 680
respite care in, 681–682
in school-age child, 673, 680–681
sibling care and, 673, 681
technology for, 679
terms for, 678–679
in toddler, 672, 680
Chronic myelogenous leukemia, 640
Cigarette smoking
screening for, 8
teratogenicity of, 45
Ciprofloxacin, 592–593
Circulation, 464, 465f
neonatal, 254–255, 254f
Circulatory overload, transfusion-
related, 637
Circumcision, 266, 288
Citalopram, 387
Cleansing breath, 162

Climacteric, 1
Clinical alerts
abdominal pain, 418
abruptio placentae, 93–94
antidepressants, 385–386
appendicitis, 419
aspirin, 437
autonomic dysreflexia, 506–507
blood pressure, 475
brain tumor, 643–644
butorphanol, 164–165
cast petaling, 541
central venous line complications,
420
cervical laceration, 227
chemotherapy drug disposal, 644
compartment syndrome, 531
constipation, 420
cricoid pressure, 506
critical illness, 374
cytomegalovirus infection, 437
drug extravasation, 644–645
endometritis, 230–231
episiotomy-related hematoma, 210
fecal occult blood test, 622
fluid requirements, 580–581
flumazenil, 164
fourth-stage labor, 157
fractured clavicle, 301
gastrointestinal perforation, 419
gastrostomy tube, 349
handwashing, 349
head circumference, 518
human H5N1 virus, 438, 447–448
hyperglycemia, 490–491
hypoglycemia, 490–491
immunization, 437–438
infection risk, 349, 436
irritable bowel syndrome, 419
knee-chest position, 210
labor, 157, 164–166
labor-related cardiac output, 124
magnesium sulfate overdose, 99
maternal diabetes, 107
maternal hypotension, 165
microcephaly, 301
Monroe-Kellie hypothesis, 505–506
naloxone, 349
neonatal acute abdomen, 283
neonatal blood pressure, 301
neonatal ophthalmic emergency, 283
neonatal respiratory distress, 282
neonatal respiratory rate, 301
neonatal suctioning, 282
neonatal sun protection, 283

neonatal tachypnea, 282
newborn formula, 301
oro-/nasogastric tube, 366
osteomyelitis, 531–532
pain management, 676–677
patient safety, 506
peak flow meter, 411
peritonitis, 419
postpartal blood loss, 226–227
postpartal hematoma, 227–228, 228f
postpartal hemorrhage, 228–229
postpartal infection, 229–238, 229f
postpartal thrombophlebitis, 239–240
postpartal thrombosis, 239–240
postpartum depression, 240–241
pregnancy-related cardiopulmonary resuscitation, 97
pregnancy-related decreased cardiac output, 124
pregnancy-related hemodynamic changes, 124
pregnancy-related hemorrhage, 92
pregnancy-related seizure, 97–98
preterm labor, 107
probiotics, 420
rabies, 438
radiation therapy, 644
reflexes, 315–316
respiratory rate, 398
respiratory signals, 347–348
retractions, 398
Reye syndrome, 437
safety measures, 348–349
scrotal auscultation, 283
seizure precautions, 506
shock, 419
sitz bath, 215
spinal anesthesia, 165
steroid administration, 436
stool culture, 423–424
sudden infant death syndrome, 283
supine hypotension prevention, 61, 157
systemic lupus erythematosus, 437
urinary tract infection, 77
urine culture, 587
urine specific gravity, 648
uterine atony, 227
uterine palpation, 210
vaginal laceration, 227
vomiting, 419
Clitoris, 19f
Clomiphene citrate, in female infertility, 36

Clonus, in pregnancy, 104, 104f
Closed reduction, 525
Clothing, for neonate, 288
Clotrimazole, 596
Clubbing, in children, 348
Clubfoot, 539, 543
Coagulation factors, in pregnancy, 55
Coarctation of aorta, 468, 468f
Cocaine
    in pregnancy, 73
    teratogenicity of, 45
Coitus interruptus, 29
Cold stress
    in neonate, 256, 265
    in preterm infant, 294
Cold therapy, in labor pain, 174
Colic, 426, 427
Coloboma, 280
Colon cancer, screening for, 8
Color blindness, 351, 499
Colostrum, 51
Coma, 500
Comforting, in pain management, 368–369
Communication
    about chronic illness, 682
    nurse-adolescent, 323
        about weight loss, 14
    nurse-child, 364–365
        about growth hormone, 495
        about suicide, 383
        hearing impairment and, 521
    nurse-family
        about brain tumor, 662
        about dying child, 688
        about fetal anomaly, 49–50
        about perinatal loss, 95
    nurse-mother
        about dead newborn, 184, 200
        about infant clubfoot, 543
        about non-reassuring fetal heart rate, 186
    nurse-sibling, 673–674
    nurse–pregnant woman, 144, 159
Community settings, for child health care, 380
Compartment syndrome, 525
Complementary and alternative medicine/health care. *See also* Herbal preparations
    in diarrhea, 429
    for dying child, 685
    in menopause, 15
    in pain management, 448
    in pregnancy, 84, 108–109

Complete blood count, 534, 619, 621
Comprehensive health history, in child assessment, 325
Computed tomography, 400, 507, 533
Conditioned play audiometry, 351
Condom, 30
Conduction, heat, 255, 569
Condylomata acuminata, 89
Congestion, nasal, in pregnancy, 86
Conjunctivitis, 519
Consciousness
    Glasgow Coma Scale for, 500–501, 501f
    states of, 500
Constipation
    in cancer patient, 660
    in children, 416, 420, 424
    in pregnancy, 86
Contraception, 25, 28–34
    barrier, 29–30
    hormonal, 31–34
    implant, 32
    injection, 32
    intrauterine device for, 32–33
    medication-free, 29
    patch, 31–32
    patient/family teaching on, 28–34
Contraction stress test, fetal, 128
Convection, heat, 255, 569
Coombs test, 125
Coping patterns, 688
Corneal light reflex test, 350, 505
Corporal punishment, 318
Corpus luteum, 20f
Corticosteroids, 487, 536
    administration of, 436
    in cancer, 654
    clinical alert on, 436
    reproductive system effects of, 35
    side effects of, 424–425
    topical, 558
Cortisol, in pregnancy, 57
Cortisone insufficiency, pediatric, 483
Cotton swabs, for ear, 359
Coughing, 348
Couplet care, 202
Cover-uncover test, 350
Crack cocaine, teratogenicity of, 45
Crackles, 337, 348
CRAFFT questions, in substance abuse evaluation, 385
Cramps
    cancer-related, 660–661
    leg, in pregnancy, 85

Cranial nerves, 343
Crawling reflex, 279
Creatinine, in pregnancy, 56, 57
Creatinine clearance, in pregnancy, 57
Cricoid pressure, 506
Critical care unit, 379
Crohn's disease, 422
Crossed extension reflex, 280
Crust, cutaneous, 549
Crutchfield tongs, 542, 542f
Crying, neonatal, 261
Cryoprecipitate, 634
Cryopreservation, for infertility treatments, 40
Cryptorchidism, 599, 606, 606f
Culture
    blood, 439, 535
    fungal, 554–555
    sputum, 403
    stool, 423–424
    urine, 587
Cushing's syndrome, 480–481
Cushing's triad, 513–514
Cyclic vomiting, 421, 424
Cyclophosphamide, 654
Cystic fibrosis, 407–408
    nutrition in, 413
    resources on, 415
    respiratory function in, 413
    screening for, 80
    sweat chloride test of, 401
Cystitis, hemorrhagic, 643, 668
Cystogram, voiding, 422
Cytomegalovirus infection
    ganciclovir in, 443–444
    in immunocompromised children, 437
    in pregnancy, 49, 117

D
Dacryostenosis/dacryocystitis, 520
Dantrolene sodium, 537
Daunorubicin, 654
DDAVP, 486, 595
Death. See also Dying child
    perceptions of, 674–675
    signs of, 675
Decadron, in cancer, 654
Decidua, 51
Deep venous thrombosis
    Homans' sign in, 222
    postpartal, 239–240
DEET (N, N-diethyl-m-toluamide), 510

Dehydration, 581–582
  hypertonic, 581
  hypotonic, 581
  isotonic, 581
  pathophysiology of, 581–582
  pediatric, 482
Delivery. *See* Birth; Labor
Depression
  in children/adolescents, 385–386,
    387–388
  herbal remedies for, 10
  postpartum, 222, 240–241, 246, 248
  in pregnancy, 124
Dermatitis, atopic, 564–565
Dermis, 547
Desmopressin, 486, 595
Desonide, topical, 558
Desoximetasone, topical, 558
Despair, 372
Detachment, 372
Development. *See* Growth and
  development
Developmental psychopathology, 381
Dexamethasone
  in cancer, 654
  for preterm infant, 263–264
Dextroamphetamine, in pregnancy, 73
Diabetes insipidus, 480
  diagnosis of, 483–484
Diabetes mellitus
  gestational, 71, 86, 89, 106
  insulin in, 489–491
  patient/family teaching on, 492–494
  pediatric, 481, 488, 489–494,
    497–498
  postpartal complications in, 198
  pregestational, 90
  in pregnancy, 105–106, 107,
    109–110
  preterm birth and, 198
  type 1, 90
    blood glucose in, 485–486
    in children, 481
    in pregnancy, 105
  type 2, 90
    in children, 481, 488
    in pregnancy, 105
Diabetic ketoacidosis, 481, 483
Diagnostic tests. *See also* Procedure(s)
  A1C level, 485
  acoustic stimulation, 128
  albumin, 56
  alpha-fetoprotein, 72, 647
  amniocentesis, 125–126

amylase, 56
angiography, 459
anorectal manometry, 422
arthrography, 533
audiologic test, 507
barium enema, 422
blood culture, 535
blood gases, 402–403
blood glucose, 485–486
blood typing, 623
body mass index, 349
bone biopsy, 535
bone marrow biopsy, 649–650
bone scan, 533, 650–651
bronchoscopy, 400
C-reactive protein, 535
calcium, 56, 535, 584
cancer staging, 646
cardiac catheterization, 459
cerebrospinal fluid, 352
chest x-ray, 400
chloride, 56
cholesterol screening, 10, 458
chorionic villus sampling, 125
color blindness, 351
complete blood count, 534, 619–621
computed tomography, 400, 507,
  533
contraction stress test, 128
Coombs test, 125
corneal reflex, 350
cortisol, 57
cover-uncover test, 350
creatinine, 56, 57
creatinine clearance, 57
culture, 535
cystic fibrosis, 80
differential blood count, 534
Doppler ultrasonography, 127
electrocardiogram, 459, 459f
electronic fetal heart monitoring, 128
endocrine function, 27
endometrial biopsy, 27
erythrocyte sedimentation rate, 535
fetal, 125–128
fetal biophysical profile, 127
fibrinogen, 56
fluoroscopy, 533
follicle-stimulating hormone, 591
fungal culture, 554–555
gestational diabetes, 71
glucose, 56, 485–486
glucose-6-phosphate dehydrogenase
  deficiency, 80

Diagnostic tests (*Continued*)
  glucose challenge, 107
  glucose tolerance, 107–108
  group B *Streptococcus*, 71
  hearing, 351–352
  heart biopsy, 459
  hematocrit, 56, 71, 618, 619
  hemoglobin, 56, 71, 618, 619
  hemophilia, 80
  HIV testing, 438–439
  Hubner test, 27
  hysterosalpingography, 27
  hysteroscopy, 27
  infertility, 26–28
  intraesophageal pH, 422
  intravenous pyelogram, 422
  isotretinoin monitoring, 554
  joint aspiration, 535
  kick counts, 126
  Kleihauer-Betke test, 124
  laparoscopy, 27
  leukocytes, 56
  lipid screening, 10
  liver biopsy, 422
  lumbar puncture, 646, 646f, 651–652
  lung biopsy, 400–401
  luteinizing hormone, 591
  lymphangiogram, 652
  magnetic resonance imaging, 507, 533
  Meckel scan, 422
  neonatal, 261–262
  non-stress test, 128
  oral glucose tolerance, 107–108
  osmolarity, 484
  ovulation, 26–27
  pediatric, 349–352
    in cancer, 646–658, 646f
    in cardiovascular disorders, 458–460
    in endocrine system disorders, 483–486
    in gastrointestinal disorders, 420–424
    in genitourinary system disorders, 583–591, 585f, 588f
    in hematological system disorders, 618–623
    in immune system disorders, 438–439
    in musculoskeletal disorders, 533–535
    in neurological system disorders, 507
    in respiratory disorders, 400–403
    in skin disorders, 554–555
  percutaneous umbilical blood sampling, 125
  phosphate, 535
  platelets, 56
  postcoital test, 27
  potassium, 56, 484, 583–584
  pregnancy-related, 56–57, 66, 71–72, 79–80, 94, 107–108, 120, 124–128
  pregnancy test, 590
  prenatal, 66, 71–72, 79–80, 124–128
  preterm infant, 301–303
  prolactin, 57, 591
  protein, 56, 57
  pulmonary function tests, 401–402
  radiography, 421, 533
  red reflex, 351
  renal tubular function, 589–590
  Rh screening, 71
  rheumatoid factor, 535
  Rocky Mountain spotted fever, 555
  serum sodium, 484
  sickle cell disease, 79, 621
  sodium, 57, 583
  specific gravity, 484
  sputum culture, 403
  sweat chloride, 401
  Tay-Sachs disease, 79
  testosterone, 591
  thalassemia, 79
  thyroid hormones, 57
  thyroid-stimulating hormone, 591
  tilt test, 458–459
  triple test, 72
  tuberculin skin test, 403
  ultrasonography, 27, 71, 126, 421, 422, 533, 591
  urea nitrogen, 57
  uric acid, 57
  urinalysis, 586–588, 588f
  urinary tract imaging, 585, 585f
  urine chemistries, 57
  urine dipstick, 587, 588f, 589
  urine pH, 649
  urine specific gravity, 647–649
  vibroacoustic stimulation, 128
  visual acuity, 350, 350f
  voiding cystogram, 422
  voiding cystourethrogram, 585, 585f
  water deprivation test, 483–484
Dialysis, 604

Diapering, 288
  cast and, 541
Diaphragm, 29–30
Diarrhea
  in cancer patient, 659
  chronic, 423
  complementary care for, 429
Diastasis recti abdominis, 51
Diazepam, 537
Diet. *See* Nutrition
N, N-Diethyl-m-toluamide (DEET), 510
Diethylstilbestrol, 63
DiGeorge syndrome, 454
Digoxin, reproductive system effects of, 35
Dimenhydrinate, in pregnancy-related nausea and vomiting, 108
Dinoprostone, in labor, 182–183
Diphenhydramine, 442–443, 658
Diphtheria immunization, 2
Dipstick test, 587, 588f
Disability, 678
Discipline, 318
Disease-modifying antirheumatic drugs, 536
Disseminated intravascular coagulation, 89, 194–195
  pediatric, 612
  postpartal, 241
  pregnancy-related, 121
Distraction
  for discipline, 318
  for dressing change, 569
  for pain management, 368–369, 370
  for procedures, 661–662
Diuretics, renal effects of, 495
Do Not Resuscitate order, 683
Docusate sodium, postpartal, 210
Down syndrome, 71, 72, 454
Doxorubicin, 654
Dressing change, 569
Drowning, near, 503–504
Drug(s). *See also* Medications
  abuse of, 73–74, 122, 385
    neonatal abstinence syndrome and, 300, 304–305
  FDA pregnancy categories of, 46–47
  oral contraceptive interactions with, 28
  recreational use of, 73–74
  reproductive system effects of, 34–36
  teratogenicity of, 45–46

Dry mouth, cancer-related, 660
Duchenne muscular dystrophy, 454
Ductus arteriosus, 255
Ductus venosus, 254
Dunlop traction, 542, 543f
Duodenum, trauma to, 432
Dying child, 683–686. *See also* Cancer; Chronic illness
  care for, 676, 684–686
  complementary and alternative medicine for, 685
  coping patterns and, 688
  cultural practices and, 677
  Do Not Resuscitate order for, 683
  "good death" for, 684
  grief with, 687–688
  Hispanic culture and, 678
  holistic nursing care for, 686
  hospice care for, 685–686
  impending death signs in, 675
  National Cancer Institute resources for, 687
  resources on, 689
  saying good-bye to, 688
  sibling care and, 688–689
Dysfunctional voiding, 605
Dysmenorrhea, 1, 17
Dyspareunia, 25, 85
Dyspepsia, in pregnancy, 85
Dysplasia, 1
Dystocia, 176, 178–179
  pelvic, 176
  shoulder, 177, 192–193, 193f
  soft tissue, 177

E
Ears
  cotton swabs for, 359
  pediatric, 335, 335f
  in pregnancy, 55
Echinacea purpurea, 244–245, 357
Eclampsia, 96
  magnesium sulfate in, 99–101
  seizures in, 97–98
Ecstasy, in pregnancy, 73
Ectopic pregnancy, 89, 91
EDB (estimated date of birth), 63, 67–68
Edema, in pregnancy, 85
Effacement, 137
Effleurage, 162
Ejaculatory duct, 24f
Electrocardiogram, 459, 459f, 473, 474
  in long Q-T syndrome, 472f

Electronic fetal monitoring, 127–128, 152–156, 152f, 153f, 154f
Embolism, amniotic fluid, 175, 197
Embryo, 41. *See also* Fetus
  development of, 42–44
  drug effects on, 45–46
Emergency department, for children, 379–380
EMLA, 558, 563, 658
Emollients, 558
Emotional abuse, 384
Encephalitis, 516–517
Encephalopathy, 499
Encopresis, 381, 416
End-of-life care, 671
Endocrine system
  pediatric, 330
    assessment of, 479–481
    in chronic renal failure, 579
    disorders of, 479–499. *See also specific conditions*
      clinical alerts in, 482–483
      diagnostic tests in, 483–486
      ethnocultural considerations in, 488
      medications in, 486–488
      resources on, 498
  in pregnancy, 55
Endometriosis, 1
Endometritis, 222, 230–231
Endometrium, biopsy of, 27
Endotracheal tube, for neonate, 311–312
Enema, barium, 422
Engagement, fetal, 63
Engorgement, 202
Enuresis, 381, 388
  ethnocultural considerations in, 597
  psychological evaluation in, 605
  resource on, 607
  treatment of, 595, 605
Environment, in pain management, 368–369, 370
Enzyme-linked immunosorbent assay (ELISA) test, for HIV, 438
Eosinophils
  cerebrospinal fluid, 352
  count of, 534, 620
  in neonate, 303
Epidermis, 547
Epidural block, 162, 165, 167, 167f, 169, 170–171
  contraindications to, 170–171
  nursing actions after, 171

second stage labor and, 171
  shiver response with, 171
Epidural blood patch, 161, 172
Epiglottitis, 413–414
Epinephrine, 441–442
Epiphyseal fracture, 528
Episiotomy
  hematoma with, 210
  postpartal assessment of, 204
  postpartal care for, 208
Epispadias, 607
Epistaxis, 611, 621, 630
Epoetin, 655
Epoetin alfa, 595
Epstein's malformation, 468, 469f
Epstein's pearls, 280
Epulis gravidarum, 51
Equipment-dependent patient, 672, 679
Erosion, 550
Erythema multiforme, 553
Erythema toxicum, 266, 280
Erythroblastosis fetalis, 89
Erythrocyte(s), neonatal, 256
Erythrocyte sedimentation rate, 535
Erythromycin, 403–404
  in ophthalmia neonatorum, 284–285
  prokinetic effects of, 425
Erythropoietin, 655
Escherichia coli infection, 582
Escitalopram, 387
Esophageal atresia, 407
Estimated date of birth, 63, 67–68
Estrogen
  in pregnancy, 53
  reproductive system effects of, 35
  testing for, 27
Etanercept, 536
Ethnocultural considerations
  breast cancer screening, 11
  breastfeeding discomfort, 216
  burns, 559
  celiac disease, 426
  childhood obesity, 389
  colic, 426
  cultural models, 171
  cultural practices, 677
  culture understanding, 389
  customs and traditions, 287
  enuresis, 597
  genetic disease, 47
  gestational diabetes, 108
  head circumference, 511
  health care quality, 183–184

Hispanic child with cancer, 659
Hispanic culture, 538–539
hypertrophic pyloric stenosis, 425–426
infant attachment, 316
infant feeding, 6
infertility care, 34
Jehovah's Witness, 626
kidney failure, 596
labor, 159
labor pain, 172
labor-related communications, 183–184
lactose intolerance, 426
lead exposure, 359
neonatal jaundice, 264
neonatal weights, 305
pediatric hypertension, 461
perinatal death, 184
postpartal period, 215–216
pregnancy, 57
pregnancy health promotion, 81–82
pregnancy-related bleeding, 94–95
pregnancy-related hypertension, 75
pregnancy-related skin changes, 215
prenatal assessment, 75
pressure ulcers, 559
preterm labor and birth, 183, 305
puberty, 316
RhoGAM administration, 132
sexual history, 34
shock, 488
sickle cell disease, 625
skin assessment, 359
stereotyping and, 171, 358
type 2 diabetes mellitus, 488
Ethosuximide, 510
Etoposide, 655
Evaporation, 255, 569
Ewing's sarcoma, 642
Exercise
    in gestational diabetes mellitus, 109
    in postpartum depression, 248
    in pregnancy, 84
Expiratory reserve volume, 401
External otitis media, 408–409
Extracorporeal membrane oxygenation, for preterm infant, 308
Extrusion reflex, 277
Eye(s)
    neonatal, 90, 267, 283, 284–285
    pediatric, 335, 350–351, 350f
        disorders of, 519–520
    in pregnancy, 55

F
Faces pain scale, 346f
Facial nerve, 343
Factor IX, transfusion of, 635
Factor VII, transfusion of, 634
Factor VIII, transfusion of, 635
Failure to thrive, 383
Fallopian tubes, 19f
Fallot, tetralogy of, 267–268, 456–457, 470, 471f
Family, 372–380. See also Patient/family teaching
    care compliance of, 563
    child's hospitalization and, 376–379
    community health care settings for, 380
    coordinated care for, 375–376
    critical illness and, 374
    follow-up care teaching for, 375
    health screening for, 373
    home care teaching for, 374–375
    infant bonding with, 290–291
    medical home for, 375–376
    plan of care for, 372–373
    resources for, 380
    spiritual care for, 363
    teaching tips for, 374
Family medical history, in child assessment, 325
Fatigue, in pregnancy, 83–84, 85
Febrile reaction, 610
    with blood transfusion, 636
Fecal occult blood test, 622
Feeding, infant, 2–3, 6
Femoral traction, 542, 542f
Fencing reflex, 278
Fennel, 357
Fentanyl citrate, in labor pain, 168
Fern test, 148–149
Ferning, 17
Ferrous sulfate, 81
Fertility awareness contraception, 29
Fetal alcohol syndrome, 455
Fetal biophysical profile, 127–128
Fetal heart rate, 63, 68, 68f, 128
    acceleration of, 136, 153f
    auscultation for, 145–146
    baseline, 136
    bradycardiac, 136, 156
    deceleration of, 137
    early deceleration of, 154f
    electronic monitoring of, 152–156
        accelerated rate on, 153f
        early decelerated rate on, 154f

Fetal heart rate (Continued)
   external monitor for, 152f
   internal monitor for, 152f
   interpretation of, 155–156
   late decelerated rate on, 154f
   normal rate on, 153f
   variable decelerated rate on, 154f
  late deceleration of, 154f
  long-term variability in, 137, 138
  monitoring of, 128, 137
  non-reassuring, 185–186
  normal, 153f
  resources on, 160
  short-term variability in, 137, 138
  tachycardiac, 137, 156
  variability in, 138
  variable deceleration of, 154f
Fetal lie, 63
Fetus, 41. See also Labor; Neonate
  alcohol effects on, 45
  amphetamine effects on, 46
  anomalies in, 49–50
  antepartum assessment of, 68–69,
   70f, 124–128. See also Prenatal
   assessment
   acoustic stimulation/vibroacoustic
    stimulation test in, 128
   amniocentesis in, 125–126
   auscultation in, 68, 68f
   biophysical profile in, 127–128
   chorionic villus sampling in, 125
   contraction stress test in, 128
   Doppler ultrasonography in, 127
   electronic monitoring in,
    145–146, 152–156, 152f, 153f,
    154f. See also Fetal heart rate
   kick counts in, 126
   Leopold maneuver in, 68, 68f, 69f
   non-stress test in, 128
   percutaneous umbilical blood
    sampling in, 125
   ultrasonography in, 126
   umbilical velocimetry in, 127
  attitude of, 136, 140f
  caffeine effects on, 45
  cephalopelvic disproportion of,
   175–176
  cocaine effects on, 45
  compromise of, 86–87
  cranial molding in, 137
  crowning of, 136
  development of, 42–44
  drug effects on, 45–46
  engagement of, 63

  erythrocytes in, 256
  external cephalic version of, 188,
   188f
  head of, 139f–140f
  heart rate of. See Fetal heart rate
  lead effects on, 46
  lie of, 63, 140f
  macrosomic, 86
  malpresentation of, 137
  marijuana effects on, 46
  opiate effects on, 45
  position of, 64, 137, 142f–143f,
   159–160
  presentation of, 64, 68, 70f
   breech, 136, 141f, 142f, 189
   cephalic, 136, 141f, 142f–143f
   shoulder, 141f
  radiation effects on, 46
  resources on, 50
  resuscitation of, 176, 186
  sedative effects on, 45
  station of, 137
  teratogen effects on, 45–47
  tobacco effects on, 45
  vitamin effects on, 45
Fever, with blood transfusion, 636
Feverfew, 357
Fibrinogen, in pregnancy, 56
Fibrocystic changes, in breasts, 13
Filgrastim, 655
Fingers, pregnancy-related numbness
  and tingling of, 85
First Signs program, 392–393
Fissure, 550
Fistula, arteriovenous, 597
FLACC pain scale, 347
Flatulence, in pregnancy, 85
Fluid(s)
  for children, 344–345
  deficit of, 574–575, 581–582
  excess of, 575
  requirements for, 580–581
Fluid therapy
  in burns, 567
  nursing interventions for, 599–600
  Parkland formula for, 568
  precautions for, 514, 519
Flumazenil, 164
Fluocinolone, 558
Fluoroscopy, 533
Fluorouracil, 656
Fluoxetine, 387
Fluvoxamine, 387
Folic acid, in pregnancy, 82

Follicle-stimulating hormone, 591
Follicle-stimulating syndrome, 27
Fontan procedure, 456
Fontanels, 137, 139f–140f, 334, 334f
Food(s). *See also* Nutrition
  E. coli in, 582
  in hypoparathyroidism, 496
  solid, for infant, 3, 316–317
Food jags, 427
Foramen ovale, 255
Forced inspiratory volume, 402
Forced vital capacity, 402
Forceps-assisted birth, 176, 191, 191f
Formula, infant, 218, 301, 496
Fosphenytoin, 510
Fracture
  casting for, 539, 540–541, 544
  classification of, 527–529
  closed, 527
  closed reduction of, 525
  comminuted, 529
  compartment syndrome with, 531
  compression, 529
  epiphyseal, 528
  greenstick, 529
  oblique, 529
  open, 527
  open reduction of, 525
  skull, 519
  spiral, 528
  transverse, 528
Fresh frozen plasma, 633–634
Friedman curve, 151f
Frostbite, 562
Functional residual capacity, 402
Fundal massage, 224–226
Fundus, uterine, 64, 65, 66f, 86
Fungal infection, 449–450
  amphotericin B in, 444–445
  culture in, 554–555
  topical agents in, 558
Furosemide, in pregnancy, 102

G
Galant reflex, 279
Gamete intrafallopian transfer, 39
Ganciclovir, 443–444
Gas, cancer-related, 660–661
Gastroenteritis, rotaviral, 428
Gastroesophageal reflux, 424
  cancer-related, 660
Gastrointestinal system
  neonatal, 259, 273

  pediatric, 330
    in acute kidney failure, 603
    assessment of, 417–418
    in chronic renal failure, 579
    disorders of, 416–433. *See also*
      specific disorders
      clinical alerts in, 418–420
      diagnostic tests in, 420–424
      ethnocultural considerations in,
        425–426
      medications for, 424–425
      patient/family teaching in,
        426–432
      resources on, 432
  in pregnancy, 55
Gastrostomy tube, 349
Gavage feedings, for infant, 366–367
General growth failure, 671, 677
Genetic disorders
  chromosomal, 50
  ethnocultural considerations in, 47
  in pregnancy, 79–80
Genetics, 41
Genitalia
  external, 18–19, 19f
  internal, 19–20, 19f, 20f
Genitourinary system
  neonatal, 273
  pediatric, 330, 340, 341. *See also*
    specific genitourinary conditions
    assessment of, 574–580
    clinical alerts on, 580–582
    diagnostic tests in, 583–591, 585f,
      588f
    ethnocultural considerations in,
      596–597
    medications for, 591–596
    patient/family teaching for,
      597–599
    resources on, 607
  in pregnancy, 55
  preterm infant, 296–297
Gentamicin, 593
German measles, in pregnancy,
  115–116
Gestation, 41. *See also* Pregnancy
  multiple, 197
Gestational age, 269, 274–275, 275f
  average for, 294
  birth weight and, 294
  large for, 294
  small for, 294
  viability and, 293–294

Gestational diabetes mellitus, 89, 106
    diet and exercise in, 109
    ethnocultural considerations in, 108
    insulin therapy in, 109–110
Gestational trophoblastic disease, 91
Ginger, in pregnancy-related nausea
    and vomiting, 108–109
Gingiva, 336
Glabellar reflex, 278
Glasgow Coma Scale, 500–501
Glomerular filtration rate, in chronic
    kidney failure, 603
Glomerulonephritis, 577
Glossopharyngeal nerve, 343
Gloves, 349
Glucose
    blood, 485–486, 492
        in neonate, 265
        in pregnancy, 56, 107–108
    cerebrospinal fluid, 352
        in neonate, 262
    urinary, 588
        in neonate, 262
Glucose-6-phosphate dehydrogenase
    deficiency, 264
    screening for, 80
Glucose challenge test, in pregnancy,
    107
Glucose tolerance test, in pregnancy,
    107–108
Gonad, 17
Gonadotropin-releasing hormone
    agonists, in female infertility, 37
Gonadotropin-releasing hormone
    antagonists, in female infertility, 37
Gonorrhea
    in pregnancy, 110
    screening for, 8
Good death, 684
Goodell sign, 51, 64
Gower maneuver, 530
Graafian follicle, 17
Granulocyte colony stimulating factor,
    655
Granulocyte transfusion, 634
Grasping reflex, 277, 315
Gravidity, 64
Great arteries, transposition of, 469,
    470f
Grief, 675, 687–688. *See also* Dying
    child
    Hispanic culture and, 678
    pathological, 671, 688

    somatic manifestations of, 675
    subtle manifestations of, 676
Groshong catheter, 663
Group A *Streptococcus,* 552
Group B *Streptococcus,* prenatal screen-
    ing for, 71, 110
Growth
    assessment of, 479
    failure of, 671, 677
    resources on, 499
Growth and development, 314–315
    adolescent, 316, 322–323, 329
    anticipatory guidance for, 317
    clinical alerts for, 315–316
    communication and, 364–365
    discipline and, 318
    ethnocultural considerations in, 316
    infant, 316–317, 318–320, 326–327
    informed consent and, 322–323
    milestones in, 326–329
    newborn, 318–319, 326
    parent inquires about, 317
    parental concerns about, 317
    patient/family teaching for, 316–318
    preschooler, 321, 328
    preterm infant, 310–311
    privacy considerations in, 316
    procedure preparation and,
        360–362, 363–365
    reflexes in, 315
    resources on, 323
    school-age child, 321–322, 329
    toddler, 320–321, 328
Growth factors, hematopoietic, 625
Growth hormone, 495, 595
Grunting, 347
Guided imagery, 378
Gums, pregnancy-related hyperplasia
    and bleeding of, 85
Gynecomastia, 599

H

H_1-receptor antagonists, intrapartal, 166
Haemophilus influenzae type b
    immunization, 2, 446, 625
Handicap, 679
Handwashing, 349
Head
    circumference of, 271, 271f, 331,
        331f, 503, 511, 518
    neonatal, 272
    pediatric, 334, 334f
    preterm infant, 296–297

Headache, postdural puncture, 162, 166
Health care provider, 376
Health history, pediatric, 324–325
Health insurance, for children, 362
Health promotion. *See also* Patient/family teaching
  adolescent, 6–7
  adult, 7–8
  ethnocultural considerations in, 81–82
  older adults, 15–16
  perimenopausal women, 15
  pregnancy, 82–87
Health screening, 372, 373
Health surveillance, 372, 373
Hearing
  impairment of, 521
  testing of, 351–352, 507
Heart
  anatomy of, 463, 463f, 464f
  chambers of, 463, 463f
  congenital disorders of, 465–472. *See also specific disorders*
  oxytocin effects on, 131
  in pregnancy, 54
  in preterm infant, 296–298
  prostaglandin effects on, 131
  terbutaline effects on, 131
  transplantation of, 458
  valves of, 463, 464f
Heart rate
  fetal. *See* Fetal heart rate
  pediatric, 333, 435
  preterm infant, 296
Heart sounds, pediatric, 338–339
Heartburn, cancer-related, 660
Heat loss, 569
  in neonate, 255–256
Heat therapy, in labor pain, 174
Heel-drop Jarring test, 417
Hegar sign, 64
Heimlich maneuver, 409–410
HELLP syndrome, 96
Hemangioma, strawberry, 267
Hemarthrosis, 610
Hematocrit
  neonatal, 262
  pediatric, 614, 618, 619
  in pregnancy, 56, 71
  preterm infant, 302
Hematological system, pediatric, 610–639. *See also specific conditions*
  in acute kidney failure, 603

  assessment of, 611–614
  in chronic renal failure, 579
  clinical alerts for, 614–618
  diagnostic tests for, 618–623
  medications for, 624–625
  patient/family teaching for, 626–629
  resources on, 639
Hematoma
  episiotomy-related, 210
  postpartal, 222
  vaginal, 227, 228f
  vulvar, 227, 228f
Hematopoietic growth factors, 625
Hematuria, 262, 582, 601
Hemodialysis, 604
Hemoglobin, 256
  glycosylated, 89
  neonatal, 262
  pediatric, 614, 618, 619
  in pregnancy, 56, 71
  preterm infant, 302
Hemoglobin A1C, 485–486
Hemoglobin F, 256
Hemolytic disease of newborn, 122
Hemolytic uremic syndrome, 576
Hemophilia, 612, 625
  patient/family teaching in, 627–628
  screening for, 80
Hemorrhage
  intrapartal, 194–197
  postoperative, in children, 456
  postpartal, 222, 223–224, 228–229, 242–243
    nursing actions for, 248
  pregnancy-related, 91–95, 93f
    diagnostic tests in, 94
    ethnocultural considerations in, 94–95
    identification of, 92
Hemorrhagic cystitis, 643, 668
Hemorrhoids, postpartal, 211
Hemosiderosis, 615
Hepatitis A virus infection, 418, 430, 431
  immunization against, 2
  in pregnancy, 48
Hepatitis B virus infection, 418, 430, 431
  immunization against, 2, 286, 446
  in pregnancy, 48, 113–114
Hepatitis C virus infection, 418, 430, 431
Hepatitis D virus infection, 430
Hepatitis E virus infection, 430

Hepatoblastoma, 643, 647
Hepatocellular carcinoma, 643, 647
Herbal preparations
  in children, 357, 362–363
  in labor, 187
  in menopausal symptom treatment, 15
  pregnancy-related contraindications to, 38
  screening for, 10
  topical, 558
Hernia, inguinal, 426–427
Heroin, in pregnancy, 74
Herpes simplex virus infection
  in children, 560
  in pregnancy, 49, 118–119
Hickman catheter, 664
Hip, developmental dysplasia of, 266
Hirschberg asymmetrical corneal light reflex test, 505
Hoarseness, 348
Hodgkin's disease, 642
Holding therapy, 386
Homans' sign, 89–90, 204, 222
Home care
  for cardiovascular disorders, 462–463
  patient/family teaching for, 512
  postoperative, 374–375
Hormones, exogenous, 482
Hospice, 671, 685–686
Hospitalization, for child, 376–379
Huhner test, 27
Human chorionic gonadotropin (hCG), 64, 72
  in female infertility, 37
Human immunodeficiency virus (HIV) infection
  in pregnancy, 111
  testing for, 438–439
Human papillomavirus (HPV) infection, 564
  in pregnancy, 111
Humor, in postpartum depression, 248
Hydatidiform mole, 86, 90, 91
Hydralazine, in pregnancy, 103
Hydramnios, 86, 90
Hydrocephalus
  diagnosis of, 507
  ventricular shunt for, 512, 517
Hydrochloride, in labor pain, 168
Hydrochlorothiazide, in pregnancy, 102

Hydrocortisone
  in cancer, 654
  topical, 558
Hydromorphone, in labor pain, 168
Hydrops fetalis, 90
Hydrotherapy, 162
Hymen, 19f
Hyperaldosteronism, 484
Hyperbilirubinemia, 251
Hypercholesterolemia-hyperlipidemia, 462
Hyperemesis gravidarum, 86, 107
Hyperglycemia
  pediatric, 490–491, 497
  preterm infant, 301–302
Hyperkalemia, 594
  in acute renal failure, 602
Hyperleukocytosis, 645
Hyperprolactinemia, 1
Hyperreflexia, assessment of, 480
Hypertension
  pediatric, 461
  pregnancy-related, 75, 95–105. See also Eclampsia; Preeclampsia
    antihypertensives in, 101–103
    chronic, 95
    gestational, 95
    patient/family teaching for, 103
  screening for, 8
Hyperthyroidism, 482–483
  in pregnancy, 106
Hypertrophic pyloric stenosis, 420–421, 425–426
Hyperventilation
  during labor, 173–174
  in pregnancy, 85
Hypnosis, in postpartum depression, 248
Hypnotherapy, 162
  in enuresis, 605
Hypocalcemia
  in acute renal failure, 602
  apheresis-related, 638
Hypoglossal nerve, 343
Hypoglycemia
  neonatal, 256, 261
  pediatric, 490–491, 492, 497
  preterm infant, 301–302, 306–307
Hyponatremia
  in acute renal failure, 602
  pediatric, 482
Hypoparathyroidism, nutrition in, 496
Hypopigmentation, 280
Hypoplastic left heart syndrome, 470, 471f

Hypospadias, 266, 607
Hypotension
    apheresis-related, 638
    maternal, 52, 61, 62f, 85, 157, 165
Hypothermia, 554, 569
    apheresis-related, 638
    classification of, 552
    monitoring of, 502
Hypothyroidism, in pregnancy, 106
Hysterosalpingography, 25, 27
Hysteroscopy, in female infertility, 27

I

Ibuprofen, 358, 557
    postpartal, 211
Icteric discoloration, 251
Idiopathic primary pulmonary arterial
    hypertension, 461
Idiopathic thrombocytopenia purpura,
    612, 615, 628, 630–631
Ifosfamide, 656
Illotycin, in ophthalmia neonatorum,
    284–285
Imipramine, 596
Immune globulin
    intravenous, 631, 635
    Rh (RhoGAM), 65, 129–131, 132
Immune response, 434
Immune system
    maternal, 55
    neonatal, 259
    pediatric
        assessment of, 435–436
        in chronic renal failure, 579
        disorders of, 434–452. See also
            specific conditions
            clinical alerts in, 436–438
            diagnostic tests in, 438–439
            medications for, 439–446
            patient/family teaching for, 446
            resources on, 452
Immunity, 251
    acquired, 251
    active, 251
    natural, 251
    passive, 251–252
Immunization, 445–446
    adverse effects of, 437–438
    contraindications to, 452
    legal considerations in, 451–452
    nursing role in, 450–451
    patient/family teaching on, 447
    in pregnancy, 120

resources on, 445
    schedule for, 2
Immunoglobulins, in neonate, 262
Imperforate anus, 266
Impetigo, 559
Implant contraception, 32
Implantable port, 663
In vitro fertilization, 39
Incubator, weaning from, 306
Infant, 2–6, 314. See also Children;
    Neonate; Preterm infant
    car seat for, 289
    child care for, 289–290
    chronic illness in, 672, 679–680
    clubfoot in, 539, 543
    colic in, 426, 427
    cryptorchidism in, 599
    death perceptions of, 674
    DEET contraindication in, 510
    diabetes insipidus in, 480
    feeding of, 2–3, 6
    gavage feedings for, 366–367
    growth and development of,
        318–319, 326–327
    Heimlich maneuver for, 410
    immunization schedule for, 2
    increased intracranial pressure in,
        502
    nutrition for, 2–3, 218, 316–317,
        366–367
    pain management in, 368
    plagiocephaly prevention for, 4–5
    preterm, 50
    procedure preparation for, 360
    respiratory assessment in, 412–413
    safety for, 5
    shaken baby syndrome in, 504–505
    sickle cell disease in, 621
    skin of, 563
    sleep for, 4
    solid foods for, 3, 316–317
    teething in, 3–4
    temperament of, 319–320
    temperature in, 563
    thrush in, 564
    vital signs in, 333
Infection
    neonatal, 259, 309
    pediatric, 449–450
        in acute kidney failure, 603
        apheresis-related, 638
        assessment of, 435–436
        with blood transfusion, 636–637
        bone, 531–532

Infection (*Continued*)
    cancer-related, 661, 666–667
    E. coli, 582
    fungal, 444–445, 449–450
    medications for, 439–440
    risk for, 349, 436
    tests for, 439
    urinary tract, 576, 600–601
    postpartal, 229–238, 229f, 241
    patient/family teaching for, 246–247
    vertical transmission of, 90–91
Infertility, 25
    female
        advanced reproductive technologies for, 39–40
        diagnostic tests in, 26–28
        sexual history for, 34
        treatment of, 36–37
    male, diagnostic tests in, 28
Infliximab, 536
Influenza
    avian, 438, 447–448
    immunization against, 2, 8
    oseltamivir for, 404–405
Informed consent, 324, 365
    for adolescent, 322–323
Inguinal hernia, 426–427
Insect repellant, 447, 510
Insomnia, in pregnancy, 86
Inspiratory capacity, 401
Inspiratory reserve volume, 401
Insulin, 487–488, 489–491
    in pregnancy-related diabetes mellitus, 109–110
Insurance, for children, 362
Intimate partner violence, 66, 123
Intracranial bleeding, in children, 615–616
Intracranial pressure, 499
    hypothermia effect on, 502
    increase in, 506
        body position and, 506
        diagnosis of, 502, 507
        mannitol for, 508
    monitoring of, 514
    Monroe-Kellie hypothesis of, 505–506
Intracytoplasmic sperm injection, 39
Intraesophageal pH, 422
Intrathecal analgesia, 162
Intrauterine device, 25, 32–33
Intrauterine growth restriction, 78, 86
Intrauterine insemination, 39
Intrauterine resuscitation, 176, 186

Intravenous immune globulin, 631, 635
Intravenous pyelogram, 422, 585
Intubation, cricoid pressure in, 506
Intussusception, 416, 417, 421
Iron
    in neonate, 262
    in pregnancy, 54, 82, 83
    supplemental, 595, 626–627
    tissue accumulation of, 615
Iron-deficiency anemia, 630
    in children, 614, 626–627
    in pregnancy, 54, 81
Irritable bowel syndrome, 416, 419, 424, 427
Isogeneic transplantation, 434
Isoimmunization, 90
    ABO, 122
    Rh, 122, 129–131
Isotretinoin, 556

J
Jaundice, 252
    neonatal, 258, 264, 281, 300, 300f
        caring for, 307–308
Jehovah's Witness, 94–95, 132, 626
Jock itch, 450
Joint aspiration, 535
Juvenile arthritis, 536, 546

K
Kangaroo care, 252
Karyotype, 41
Kawasaki disease, 457
Keloid, 549
Keratitis, 520
Kernicterus, 90, 252
Kernig's sign, 502
Ketoacidosis, diabetic, 481, 483
Ketogenic diet, 510
Ketorolac, 624–625
Kick counts, 126
Kidney
    diuretic effects on, 495
    neonatal, 259
    transplantation of, 582
    trauma to, 577
Kidney failure
    acute, 577, 589–590
        causes of, 601
        complications of, 603
        electrolyte imbalances in, 602
        medications in, 594

chronic, 578–580
dialysis in, 604
medications in, 594–595
stages of, 603
clinical alert on, 456
ethnocultural considerations in, 596
Kleihauer-Betke test, 124
Klinefelter syndrome, 50
Kussmaul breaths, 479

L

Labetalol, in pregnancy, 102, 103
Labia majora, 19f
Labia minora, 19f
Labor. *See also* Birth; Pregnancy
active phase of, 136
amnioinfusion in, 187
amniotic fluid embolism during, 197
amniotomy in, 175, 179, 180f, 184
aromatherapy during, 173
assessment during, 144–149, 163–164
amniotic fluid identification in, 148–149
electronic fetal monitoring in, 152–156, 152f, 153f, 154f. *See also* Fetal heart rate
fetal heart tone auscultation in, 145–146
for pain, 163
vaginal examination in, 146–148
augmentation of, 175
Bishop Score in, 175, 180
bleeding during, 194–197
breathing patterns in, 173
breech presentation with, 189
cervical ripening agents for, 182–183, 184–185
clinical alerts for, 157, 164–166
closed-glottis pushing in, 156
comfort during, 172
communication during, 183
contractions in, 177–178, 178f
dystocia with, 176, 177, 178–179, 192–193, 193f
effective pushing in, 156
ethnocultural considerations in, 159, 183–184
external cephalic version during, 188, 188f
false, 137, 144
first stage of, 137, 150–151

five P's of, 138–143, 138f–139f, 140f, 141f, 142f–143f
forceps-assisted, 191, 191f
fourth stage of, 156–157
Friedman curve for, 151f
hemorrhage during, 194–197
herbal induction of, 187
hospital/birth center admission for, 144–145, 159
hypertonic contractions in, 176, 177, 178, 178f, 183
hyperventilation during, 173–174
hypotonic contractions in, 176, 177, 178, 178f
induction of, 176
latent phase of, 137
maternal hypotension during, 165
in multiple gestation, 197
nonherbal induction of, 187
nurse communications about, 144, 173
open-glottis pushing in, 156
oxytocin in, 157–158, 180–182
pain during, 163–164
anxiety–tissue anoxia–pain connection in, 163
cold application for, 174
combined spinal-epidural anesthesia for, 169
epidural anesthesia for, 169, 170–171
ethnocultural considerations in, 172
during first stage, 167
heat application for, 174
nonpharmacological measures for, 164
opioids for, 167–168
perineal anesthesia infiltration for, 169
pharmacological measures for, 166–171
pudendal nerve block for, 169
regional blocks for, 169
during second stage, 167–168, 167f
spinal anesthesia for, 169, 170–171
with vaginal birth, 168
passage/passenger relationship in, 142, 142f–143f
passageway of, 139
passenger in, 139, 139f–140f, 141f
patient/family teaching for, 172, 184–185

Labor (*Continued*)
  placental variations in, 194
  powers of, 138–139, 138f–139f
  precipitate (precipitous), 177
  in preeclampsia, 198–200
  preterm, 183, 184
  prostaglandin E$_1$ in, 182
  prostaglandin E$_2$ in, 182–183
  psychosocial influences in, 143
  pushing in, 156
  resources on, 134, 160, 174
  second stage of, 137, 150–151
  shoulder dystocia with, 192–193, 193f
  spinal anesthesia for, 165
  station of, 142, 142f
  third stage of, 137, 156–157
  transition phase of, 138
  trial of, 177, 185
  umbilical cord prolapse during,
      189–190, 190f
  umbilical cord variations in, 194
  uterine contractions in, 138–139,
      177–181, 178f, 183
  uterine rupture with, 193
  vacuum-assisted, 192, 192f
Lactational amenorrhea method, for
    contraception, 29
Lactobacillus, 420, 429
Lactogenesis, 202
Lactose intolerance, 416, 426
Language disorder, 512–513
Laparoscopy, in female infertility, 27
Large intestine, trauma to, 432
LARRY acronym, 223
Last menstrual period, 64
Latch-on, 202
Laxatives, 424
Lead
  exposure to, 359–360
  teratogenicity of, 46
Leflunomide, 536
Let-down reflex, in breast feeding, 209
Legg-Calve-Perthes disease, 543–544
Legs, postpartal assessment of, 204
Leiomyoma, 1
Leopold maneuvers, 64, 68, 68f, 69f
Lethargy, 500
Leucovorin, 656
Leukemia, 640, 661
Leukocytes, in pregnancy, 56
Leukocytosis, 621
Leukopenia, 621
Leukorrhea, 51
  in pregnancy, 86

Lice, 560–561
Lichenification, 549
Licorice, 357
Lidocaine, topical, postpartum, 211
Ligamentum arteriosum, 255
Ligamentum teres, 254
Ligamentum venosum, 254
Light therapy, in pregnancy, 84
Linea alba, 52
Linea nigra, 52
Lipoproteins
  high-density, 10
  low-density, 10
Lips, 336
Lithium carbonate, 387, 388
  reproductive system effects of, 36
Liver
  biopsy of, 422, 517
  cancer of, 643, 647
  neonatal, 256–258
  trauma to, 432
LMP (last menstrual period), 64
Lochia alba, 202, 204, 206, 206f
Lochia rubra, 137, 202, 204, 206,
    206f
Lochia serosa, 203, 204, 206, 206f
Lockjaw (tetanus), 537–538,
    545–546
Logrolling, 545, 545f
Long Q-T syndrome, 471, 472f
Lorazepam, 537, 658
Lumbar puncture, 646, 646f,
    651–652
  headache after, 162, 166
Lung(s)
  biopsy of, in children, 400–401
  function tests in, 401–402
  neonatal, 253–254, 254f
    betamethasone for, 263–264
    dexamethasone for, 263–264
  transfusion-related injury to, 618
Lung sounds, pediatric, 337
Luteinizing hormone, 591
  in pregnancy, 54
  testing for, 27
Lyme disease, 551
Lymph nodes, of head and neck, 334,
    334f
Lymphangiogram, 652
Lymphocytes
  cerebrospinal fluid, 352
  count of, 534, 620
  in neonate, 303

M

Macrosomia, 176
Macule, 548
Magnesium, in hypoparathyroidism, 496
Magnesium sulfate
overdose of, 99
in pregnancy, 99–101
in preterm labor, 107
Magnet reflex, 279
Magnetic resonance imaging
in children, 507, 533
postpartal, 222
Mannitol, 508
Manometry, anorectal, 422
Marfan syndrome, 454
Marijuana
in pregnancy, 74
teratogenicity of, 46
Massage, 513
fundal, 224–226
in postpartum depression, 248
in pregnancy, 84
Mastitis, 222, 229, 229f, 236–237
Material safety data sheets, 553
MDMA (methylenedioxymethamphetamine), in pregnancy, 73–74
Mean arterial pressure, 52
Mean cell hemoglobin concentration, 620
Mean corpuscular hemoglobin, 620
Mean corpuscular volume, 620
Measles immunization, 2, 445
Mechanical ventilation, 399
in neonate, 311–312
Meckel scan, 422
Meconium, 176
in amniotic fluid, 189
Meconium aspiration syndrome, 189
Medical home, 375–376
Medications
acetaminophen, 353–356
acetylsalicylic acid in, 511
albuterol, 405–406, 594
alpha-methyldopa, 101
amphotericin B, 444–445
ampicillin, 592
antibiotics, 120, 511, 591–593
anticancer, 653–657
antiemetics, 424, 425, 658
antifungal, 596
antihypertensive agents, 595
antiseizure, 507–508, 509–510
antispasmodics, 424

antithyroid, 487
AquaMEPHYTON, 285–286
asparaginase, 653
baclofen, 537
benzathine penicillin, 556–557
beractant, 303–304
betamethasone, 263–264
bisacodyl, 211
bleomycin, 653
breastfeeding and, 212
broad-spectrum antibiotics, 591–593
calcitriol, 595
calcium, 487
calcium gluconate, 594
calcium nitroprusside, 594
carbamazepine, 509
carboplastin, 653
carboprost, 242
carvedilol, 460–461
cefixime, 592
cefotaxime, 592
ceftriaxone, 592
cephalexin, 592
chronic illness, 677
ciprofloxacin, 592–593
clotrimazole, 596
corticosteroids, 424–425, 487, 536, 654
cyclophosphamide, 654
dantrolene sodium, 537
daunorubicin, 654
DEET, 510
desmopressin, 486, 595
dexamethasone, 263–264
dimenhydrinate, 108
dinoprostone, 182–183
diphenhydramine, 442–443, 658
disease-modifying antirheumatic drugs, 536
docusate sodium, 210
doxorubicin, 654
echinacea purpurea, 244–245
epinephrine, 441–442
epoetin, 655
epoetin alfa, 595
erythromycin, 284–285, 403–404
erythropoietin, 655
etanercept, 536
ethosuximide, 510
etoposide, 655
extravasation of, 658
ferrous sulfate, 81
filgrastim, 655
fluorouracil, 656

Medications (*Continued*)
  fosphenytoin, 510
  furosemide, 102
  ganciclovir, 443–444
  gentamicin, 593
  growth hormone, 595
  hematopoietic growth factors, 625
  hepatitis B vaccine, 286
  herbal preparations, 10
  hormone tables, 486–487
  hydralazine, 103
  hydrochlorothiazide, 102
  hydrocortisone, 489
  ibuprofen, 211, 358, 557
  ifosfamide, 656
  imipramine, 596
  infliximab, 536
  insulin, 487–488
  intrapartal analgesia, 166–171, 167f
  iron supplementation, 595
  isotretinoin, 556
  for juvenile arthritis, 536
  kayexalate, 594
  ketorolac, 624–625
  labetalol, 102, 103
  laxatives, 424
  leflunomide, 536
  leucovorin, 656
  lidocaine, 211
  lorazepam, 537, 658
  magnesium sulfate, 99–101
  mannitol, 508
  mephyton, 285–286
  mesna, 656
  methotrexate, 657
  methylergonovine, 212–213, 242
  methylprednisolone, 440–441
  metoclopramide, 108
  miconazole, 596
  midazolam, 537–538
  misoprostol, 182, 243
  morphine sulfate, 358
  naloxone, 305, 349
  neuromuscular blocking agents, 537
  nifedipine, 102, 103
  nitrofurantoin, 593
  nitroglycerin, 594
  nonsteroidal anti-inflammatory
    drugs, 536
  nystatin, 596
  ondansetron, 657, 658
  opioids, 168, 211
  oral contraceptive effectiveness
    and, 28
  oseltamivir, 404–405
  oxytocin, 157–158, 181–182, 242
  PEG-L-asparaginase, 657
  phenobarbital, 509
  phenytoin, 507–508, 509, 510
  phosphate-binding agents, 594
  phytonadione, 285–286
  postpartal, 242–243
  prednisone, 536
  prokinetics, 424
  promethazine, 108
  prostaglandins, 182–183, 243
  proton pump inhibitors, 424
  pyridoxine, 108
  Rho(D) immune globulin, 129–131,
    132
  rocuronium, 538
  screening for, 10
  selective serotonin reuptake
    inhibitors, 596
  sodium bicarbonate, 594
  sodium citrate, 594
  sodium nitroprusside, 103
  stool softener, 210–211
  for tetanus, 537–538
  tetracycline, 555
  topical agents, 558
  topical anesthetics, 658
  topiramate, 510
  trimethoprim-sulfamethoxazole,
    439–440, 593
  valproate, 387
  valproic acid, 509, 510
  vecuronium, 538
  vincristine, 657
  vitamin K, 285–286
  warfarin, 245–246
  witch hazel, 211
Meditation, in postpartum depression,
  248
Melanosis, pustular, 281
Membranes
  artificial rupture of, 175, 179, 180f,
    184
  premature rupture of, 86, 90, 121
  preterm premature rupture of, 90
  preterm rupture of, 90
  spontaneous rupture of, 177
Menarche, 17, 18
Meningitis
  Brudzinski sign in, 502–503
  Kernig's sign in, 502
Meningocele, 266, 499
Meningococcal immunization, 2

Menopause, 1, 22
    symptom treatment in, 15
Menorrhagia, 25
Menstrual cycle, 21–23, 22f, 23f
Mental status, in children, 342
Meperidine hydrochloride, in labor
    pain, 168
Mephyton, for neonate, 285–286
Mesna, 656
Metabolic screening, neonatal,
    283–284
Methamphetamines, in pregnancy, 73
Methotrexate, 657
Methyldopa, in pregnancy, 101
Methylenedioxymethamphetamine, in
    pregnancy, 73–74
Methylergonovine, postpartal,
    212–213, 242
Methylprednisolone, 440–441
Metoclopramide, in pregnancy-related
    nausea and vomiting, 108
Miconazole, 596
Microcephaly, 267
Midazolam, 537–538
Migraine, 425
Milia, 281
Mindful breathing, 391
Minerals, in renal failure, 594
Mini pill contraception, 32
Misoprostol
    in labor, 182
    in postpartal hemorrhage, 243
Mittelschmerz, 1, 17
Molding, cranial, 267
Mongolian spots, 281
Monocytes
    count of, 534, 620
    in neonate, 303
Monosomy X, 50
Monroe-Kellie hypothesis, 505–506
Montgomery tubercles (glands), 52
Mood, postpartal, 219
Mood stabilizers, 387, 388
Morning after pill, 32
Moro reflex, 279, 315
Morphine sulfate, 358
Mother-baby care (couplet care),
    202
Motion, extremity, 526
Mouth
    cancer-related disorders of, 660
    dry, 660
    pediatric, 336
Mucositis, 640

Multigravida, 64
Multipara, 64
Multiple gestation, 86, 121
Mumps immunization, 2
Mupirocin, 558
Muscular dystrophy, 546
    Gower maneuver in, 530
Musculoskeletal system
    neonatal, 273
    pediatric, 330, 342
        assessment of, 525–531
        in chronic renal failure, 578
        disorders of, 525–546. *See also*
            specific conditions
        capillary refill time in, 526,
            526f
        clinical alerts for, 531–532
        diagnostic tests for, 533–535
        ethnocultural considerations in,
            538–539
        medications for, 536–538
        neurovascular assessment in,
            525–526
        patient/family teaching for, 539
        pulses in, 527
        resources on, 546
    in pregnancy, 56
    preterm infant, 296–297
Mutation, 41
Myelomeningocele, 267

N
Naegele's rule, 64, 67–68
Naloxone, 349
    during labor, 171
Nasal congestion, in pregnancy, 86
Nasal flaring, 347
Nasogastric tube, for children,
    365–366
National Cancer Institute, 687–688
Natural family planning, 29
Nature, 314
Nausea
    in cancer patient, 659
    in pregnancy, 85, 86, 108
Near drowning, 503–504
Neck, pediatric, 334, 334f
Necrotizing enterocolitis, 267
    for preterm infant, 308–309
Necrotizing fasciitis, 552
Neglect, 384
Neomycin, 558
Neonatal abstinence syndrome, 300,
    304–305

Neonatal assessment, 268–282
abdominal circumference measurement in, 272, 272f
in at-risk neonate, 293–300
Barlow-Ortolani maneuver in, 275–276
body measurements in, 271–272, 271f, 272f
cardiovascular system, 272, 293
chest circumference measurement in, 272, 272f
clinical alerts in, 282–283
diagnostic tests in, 283–284
gastrointestinal, 273
genitourinary, 273
gestational age, 274–275, 275f, 293–294
head, 272
head circumference measurement in, 271, 271f
immediate, 268–269
later, 270–282
length measurement in, 273–274
medications in, 284–286
metabolic screening in, 283–284
musculoskeletal, 273
neurological, 273, 293
oral and nasal suctioning for, 268–269
patient/family teaching in, 287–290
reflexes in, 277–280. See also Reflex(es)
resources on, 291–292
respiratory system, 272, 293
skin, 280–282
temperature in, 270
vital signs in, 270
weight measurement in, 271, 271f
Neonatal intensive care unit, 305–306, 311
Neonate, 314. See also Neonatal assessment
abdominal circumference in, 272, 272f
abduction prevention for, 219–220
acrocyanosis in, 136, 280
acute abdomen in, 283
albumin in, 261
amylase in, 261
Apgar Score for, 158
AquaMEPHYTON for, 285–286
assessment of. See Neonatal assessment
Barlow-Ortolani maneuver for, 275–276

bathing of, 288
behavioral states of, 260–261
betamethasone for, 263–264
bicarbonate in, 261
bilirubin in, 256–258, 257f, 261, 300, 300f
bleeding time in, 261
blood gases in, 262, 295
blood glucose in, 262, 265
blood pressure in, 270, 309–310
blood values for, 261–262
blood volume in, 256
breathing by, 270, 287
calcium in, 261
chest circumference in, 272, 272f
circumcision of, 288
cleft lip and palate in, 305
clothing for, 288
cold stress in, 256, 265
death of, 184, 200
dexamethasone for, 263–264
diagnostic tests for, 261–262
diapering of, 288
documentation for, 290
endotracheal tube in, 311–312
erythrocytes in, 256
erythromycin for, 284–285
gastrointestinal system of, 259, 273
genitourinary system of, 273
gestational age of, 274–275, 275f
viability and, 293–294
glucose in, 262, 265
growth and development of, 318–319, 326
head circumference in, 271, 271f, 331, 331f
heat loss in, 255–256
hematocrit in, 262
hemoglobin in, 256, 262
hemolytic disease of, 122
hepatitis B vaccine for, 286
high-risk. See Preterm infant
hypoglycemia in, 256, 261
immune system of, 259
immunoglobulins in, 262
infection in, 90–91, 259, 309
intrapartal suctioning in, 189
iron in, 262
jaundice in, 258, 264, 281, 300, 300f, 307–308
kidney of, 259
laboratory values for, 261–262
length of, 273–274

liver of, 256–258
lung sounds in, 253
lungs of, 253–254, 254f
maternal bonding with, 204, 290–291
mechanical ventilation in, 311–312
medications for, 263–264
musculoskeletal system of, 273
neurological system of, 273
nourishment promotion for, 209, 218
ophthalmic disorders in, 267, 283, 284–285
oral and nasal suctioning for, 268–269
pain in, 294
penile care for, 288
pH in, 262, 295
physiological transition of, 251–265
    cardiopulmonary, 254–255, 254f, 293
    gastrointestinal, 259
    genitourinary, 259
    hematopoietic, 256
    hepatic, 256–258, 257f
    immunological, 259
    in non-hospital setting, 264–265
    psychosocial, 260–261
    respiratory, 252–253, 253f, 293
    thermogenic, 255–256
phytonadione for, 284–285
platelets in, 256, 262, 302
pulse in, 269, 270
reactivity-inactivity in, 260
red blood cell count in, 262
red blood cell enzyme defects in, 264
red reflex in, 283
resources on, 291–292
respiratory distress in, 282
respiratory rate in, 269, 270
scrotal auscultation in, 283
sepsis in, 309
sibling adjustment to, 218
skin of, 280–281
    color of, 269, 281–282
sleep in, 260–261
suctioning of, 268–269, 282, 287
sudden death of, 283
sun protection for, 283
tachypnea in, 282
temperature in, 255–256, 269, 270, 294
urinary values for, 262

vital signs in, 270
weight gain in, 209
weight of, 271, 271f, 282, 294
white blood cells in, 262, 303
withdrawal syndrome in, 300, 304–305
Nephroblastoma, 641–642
Nerve block, for labor, 167–171
Nettle, 357
Neural tube defect, 42, 71, 72
Neurally mediated syncope, 462
Neuroblastoma, 641
Neurological examination, in brain tumor, 641
Neurological system
    neonatal, 273
    pediatric, 330, 342–343
        in acute kidney failure, 603
        assessment of, 436
        cancer-related disorders of, 645
        in chronic renal failure, 578–579
        disorders of, 499–523. See also specific conditions
            clinical alerts in, 505–507
            diagnostic tests in, 507
            ethnocultural considerations in, 511
            focused assessment of, 500–505
            medications for, 507–511
            patient/family teaching in, 512–513
            resources on, 521–522
        in pregnancy, 54
        preterm infant, 296–298
Neuromuscular blocking agents, 537, 538
Neutral thermal environment, 252
Neutropenia, 610, 646–647, 666
    in children, 613, 629
Neutrophils
    in cancer, 646–647
    cerebrospinal fluid, 352
    count of, 534, 620
Nevus, 267, 280
Nevus flammeus, 267, 281
Nevus vasculosus, 267, 281
Newborn. See Neonate; Preterm infant
Nifedipine, in pregnancy, 102, 103
Nipple, inspection and palpation of, 12
Nipple confusion, 203
Nissen fundoplication, 416
Nitrazine tape test, 148–149
Nitrofurantoin, 593
Nitroglycerin, 594

Nocturia, in pregnancy, 85
Nodule, 548
Non-Hodgkin's lymphoma, 643
Non-stress test, fetal, 128
Nonshivering thermogenesis, 252
Nonsteroidal anti-inflammatory drugs, 536
  postpartal, 211
Noonan syndrome, 454
Nose
  pediatric, 336
  in pregnancy, 55
Nosebleed, 611, 621, 630
Nuchal cord, 176
Nuclear cortical scanning, 585
Nuclear cystography, 585
Nulligravida, 64
Nullipara, 64
Nurture, 314
Nutrition
  in burns, 567
  in cancer patient, 659, 666
  in cystic fibrosis, 413
  in gestational diabetes mellitus, 109
  in hypoparathyroidism, 496
  infant, 2–3, 209, 217, 218, 316–317, 366–367
  in iron-deficiency anemia, 626
  pediatric, 344–345, 363, 365–366
  in pregnancy, 82–83
Nystagmus, 499
Nystatin, 596

O

Obesity
  childhood, 389, 393
  pregnancy and, 123
Obesogenic role, 381
Obtundation, 500
Obturator sign, 418
Occult blood test, 622
Oculomotor nerve, 343
Old Cat, for child's health history, 324
Older adults, health promotion for, 15–16
Olfactory nerve, 343
Oligohydramnios, 176
Omphalitis, 267, 416
Ondansetron, 657, 658
Oocyte, 17
Oogenesis, 17
Open reduction, 525
Operculum, 52

Ophthalmia neonatorum, 90, 267, 284–285, 519
Opioids
  in labor pain, 167–168
  postpartal, 211
  teratogenicity of, 45
Optic nerve, 343
Oral contraceptives, 31
  drug interactions with, 28
Orlowski scale, 504
Orogastric tube, for children, 365–366
Oseltamivir, 404–405
Osmolality, urinary, 590
Osmolarity, urinary, 588
Osteogenesis imperfecta, 539, 546
Osteomyelitis, 531–532
Osteoporosis
  risk factors for, 9
  treatment of, 15
Osteosarcoma, 642
Otitis media, prevention of, 408–409
Ova, stool culture for, 423–424
Ovary (ovaries), 19f, 54
Ovulation, testing for, 26–27
Oxycodone and acetaminophen, postpartal, 211
Oxytocin, 180–182
  complications of, 187
  contraindications to, 181
  in labor, 157–158
  in postpartal hemorrhage, 242
  precautions for, 181
  in pregnancy, 53, 131

P

Pacemaker, in children, 462
Pa_{CO_2}
  neonatal, 262
  pediatric, 402
  preterm infant, 295
Pain
  abdominal, 418
  acute, 324, 345, 346
  burn-related, 567–568
  cancer-related, 667
  chronic, 324, 345, 346
  extremity, 525–526
  injection, 563
  labor. *See* Labor, pain during
  pediatric, 345–347, 346f, 353–356, 367–369, 418, 630
  postpartal, 211, 216–217
  in preterm infant, 294, 295f
  referred, 162

somatic, 162
visceral, 162
Pain management
in cancer, 667
for children, 353–356, 367–369, 630
complementary care in, 448, 630
in labor. *See* Labor, pain during
postpartal, 211, 216–217
Pain scales, 346–347, 346f
Palliative care, 671
Palmar erythema, 52
Palmar grasp reflex, 277, 315
Pancreas
in pregnancy, 56
trauma to, 432
Pancytopenia, 610
Pao_2
neonatal, 262
pediatric, 403
preterm infant, 295
Papilledema, 499
Papilloma, periauricular, 281
Papule, 548
Parasites, stool culture for, 423–424
Parathyroid gland, in pregnancy, 55
Parenting, 389–391
Parenting techniques, 389–391. *See
also* Family; Patient/family teaching
Parity, 64
Parkland formula, 568
Paroxetine, 387
Partial thromboplastin time, 621
Participation restriction, 679
Parturition, 203. *See also* Birth; Labor
Past medical history, in child assess-
ment, 325
Patch, cutaneous, 548
Patch contraception, 31–32
Patent ductus arteriosus, 466, 467f
Pathogenicity, 434
Pathological grief, 671, 688
Patient/family teaching
adolescent health promotion, 7
adolescent safety, 7
amniotomy, 184
anaphylaxis, 446
animal bite prevention, 561
anticoagulants, 247
arteriovenous fistula, 597
aspirin, 247, 409
avian flu, 447–448
birthing center, 159
breast milk expression, 217
breast milk storage, 217

burn management, 562
burn prevention, 561
cancer-related constipation, 660
cancer-related diarrhea, 659
cancer-related gastrointestinal
complications, 660–661
cancer-related heartburn/reflux, 660
cancer-related infection, 661
cancer-related nausea/vomiting, 659
cancer-related nutrition, 659
cancer-related oral complications,
660
cancer-related poor appetite, 660
car seat use, 289
cellulitis, 559
cervical ripening agents, 184–185
child care arrangements, 289–290
child with disability, 359
cleft lip and palate, 305
clubfoot, 539
complementary care, 84
contraception, 28–34
cotton swab use, 359
cryptorchidism, 599
cystic fibrosis, 407–408
diabetes mellitus, 492–494
education-related empowerment,
47–48
esophageal atresia, 407
external otitis media prevention,
408–409
family tips for, 374
follow-up care, 375
frostbite, 562
gynecomastia, 599
Heimlich maneuver, 409–410
hemophilia, 627–628
herpes simplex virus, 560
home care, 512
hydrocortisone administration, 489
hypercholesterolemia-
hyperlipidemia, 462
idiopathic thrombocytopenic
purpura, 628
immunization, 447
impetigo, 559
infant feeding, 2–3, 316–317
infant formula, 218
infant safety, 5
infant sleep, 4
infant teething, 3–4
inguinal hernia, 426–427
insect repellant, 447
insulin administration, 491

Patient/family teaching (*Continued*)
  iron-deficiency anemia, 626–627
  iron supplements, 626–627
  labor, 172, 184–185
  language disorder, 512–513
  lead exposure, 359–360
  lice, 560–561
  maltreatment prevention, 390
  neonatal breathing difficulties, 287
  neonatal bulb suctioning, 287
  neonatal intensive care unit,
    305–306, 311
  neurally mediated syncope, 462
  neutropenia, 629
  nipple confusion, 217
  osteogenesis imperfecta, 539
  pacemaker, 462
  parenting techniques, 389–391
  peak flow meter, 410–412
  pediatric safety, 5
  perineal care, 216
  plagiocephaly prevention, 4–5
  post-tonsillectomy discharge, 408
  postpartal analgesia, 216–217
  postpartal bleeding, 247
  postpartal discharge, 220
  postpartal period, 216–219
  pregnancy, 47–50, 58–59
  pregnancy health promotion, 82–87
  pregnancy-related discomforts,
    85–86
  pregnancy-related exercise, 84
  pregnancy-related fatigue, 83–84
  pregnancy-related herbal contraindi-
    cations, 38
  pregnancy-related hypertension, 103
  pregnancy-related nausea and vomit-
    ing, 108–109
  pregnancy-related nutrition, 82–83
  prenatal, 75
  preterm labor, 184
  puerperal infection, 246–247
  Reye syndrome, 512
  salicylates, 409
  sibling of dying child, 678
  sickle cell disease, 627
  sinusitis prevention, 408
  sleep hygiene, 390–391
  stool culture, 424
  teething, 3–4
  toilet training, 391
  TORCH infections, 48–49
  tracheoesophageal atresia, 407
  umbilical cord care, 287–288
    uncircumcised penis care, 288
    ventricular shunt, 512
    vulvovaginitis, 597–598
Peak flow meter, 410–411
Pectus carinatum, 336
Pectus excavatum, 336
Pediculosis, 560–561
PEG-L-asparaginase, 657
Pelvic dystocia, 176
Penis, 24f
  care for, 288
Percutaneous umbilical blood sam-
    pling, 125
Perforation, gastrointestinal, 419
Periauricular papilloma, 281
Pericardial effusion, 645
Perimenopause, 1, 22
  health promotion counseling for, 15
Perineum, 19f
  anesthetic infiltration of, 169
  postpartal assessment of, 207
  postpartal care for, 213–215, 216
  postpartal infection of, 232–233
Periodic breathing, 252
Peripheral blood smear, 620
Peripherally inserted central catheter,
    664
Peritoneal dialysis, 604
Peritonitis, 419
Personality, infant, 319–320
Pertussis immunization, 2
pH
  intraesophageal, 422
  neonatal, 262, 295
  pediatric, 402
  preterm infant, 295
  urinary, 588, 649
    neonatal, 262
Phenobarbital, 509, 510
Phenylketonuria, 262
Phenytoin, 507–508, 509, 510
Pheochromocytoma, 497
Phosphate, serum, 535
Phosphate-binding agents, 594
Phytonadione, for neonate, 285–286
Pica, 78, 82
Piskacek sign, 64
Placenta
  battledore, 194
  circumvallate, 194
  succenturiate, 194
Placenta accreta, 194
Placenta increta, 194
Placenta percreta, 194

Placenta previa, 87, 92, 93f
Placental abruption, 87, 92, 93–94, 93f
Plagiocephaly, prevention of, 4–5
Plantar grasp reflex, 277, 315
Plasmapheresis, 610
Platelet(s)
  in children, 619
  count of, 534
  in idiopathic thrombocytopenic
    purpura, 630–631
  in neonate, 256, 262, 302
  in pregnancy, 56
  in Rocky Mountain spotted fever,
    555
  transfusion of, 633
Play, therapeutic, 377
Plethora, 267, 281
Pleural effusion, 645
Pneumococcal immunization, 8, 625
Pneumonia, prevention of, 543
Pneumovax, 446
Poisoning, acetaminophen, 356
Poliovirus immunization, 2, 445
Polycythemia, 252, 621
Polyhydramnios, 90
Polymerase chain reaction (PCR) test,
  for HIV, 439
Port wine stain, 267
Postcoital test, 27
Postdate pregnancy, 176
Postdural puncture headache, 162, 166
Postpartum blues, 203, 219
Postpartum depression, 222, 240–241
Postpartum period (puerperium), 203
  aspirin avoidance during, 247
  assessment in, 204–208, 205f,
    223–226
  bladder care in, 208
  bleeding in, 223–224, 226–227,
    228–229, 242–243
    nursing actions for, 248
    patient/family teaching for, 247
  blood loss measurement in, 223
  breastfeeding during. See
    Breastfeeding
  cervical laceration, 227
  depression in, 240–241, 246, 248
  diabetes and, 198
  diagnostic tests in, 241
  discharge teaching for, 220
  disseminated intravascular coagula-
    tion in, 241
  endometritis in, 230–231
  episiotomy care in, 208, 210

ethnocultural considerations in,
    215–216
  fundal massage in, 224–226
  hematoma in, 227–228, 228f
  hemorrhoid care in, 211
  infant abduction prevention during,
    219–220
  infant nourishment in, 209, 217,
    218
  infection in, 229–238, 229f, 241
    diagnostic tests for, 241
    endometrial, 230–231
    mammary, 236–237
    patient/family teaching for,
      246–247
    pelvic, 238
    urinary tract, 234–235
    wound, 232–233
  knee-chest position avoidance in,
    210
  lochia assessment in, 206, 206f
  mastitis in, 229, 229f, 236–237
  maternal mood changes in, 219
  medications in, 210–211, 242–243,
    247
  methylergonovine in, 212–213
  mother-infant attachment in, 209
  nonsteroidal anti-inflammatory
    drugs in, 211
  opioid analgesics in, 211
  pain relief in, 211, 216–217
  patient/family teaching in, 216–219,
    246–247
  perineal assessment and care in,
    207, 213–215, 216
  psychosocial complications in,
    240–241, 246
  resources on, 221, 249
  septic pelvic thrombophlebitis in,
    238
  sibling adjustment during, 218
  sitz bath in, 213–215
  skin changes in, 215
  stool softener in, 210–211
  thrombophlebitis in, 238, 239–240
  thrombosis in, 239–240
  topical anesthetic in, 211
  urinary tract infection in, 234–235
  uterine assessment in, 204–206,
    205f
  uterine atony in, 224–226, 227
  vaginal laceration, 227
  vital signs in, 203, 226–227
  voiding assessment in, 208

Postpartum psychosis, 223, 240–241
Poststreptococcal glomerulonephritis, 577
Postterm pregnancy, 177
Posttraumatic stress disorder, in children, 381–382
Posture, of child, 337
Potassium
  deficiency of, 484, 583
  excess of, 584
  in pregnancy, 56
Prednisone, 536
  in cancer, 654
Preeclampsia, 86, 95
  assessment for, 96–97
  blood pressure in, 198
  cardiovascular assessment for, 96–97
  central nervous system assessment for, 97
  fetal status in, 200
  hepatic assessment for, 97
  intrapartal nursing care in, 198–200
  magnesium sulfate in, 99–101
  medication administration in, 198
  neurologic examination in, 199
  psychological examination in, 199
  pulmonary examination in, 199
  renal assessment for, 97
  renal balance in, 198–199
  risk factors for, 96
  seizures in, 97–98, 199
  SPASMS mnemonic in, 104–105
Pregestational diabetes mellitus, 90
Pregnancy. *See also* Prenatal assessment
  ABO isoimmunization in, 122
  abruptio placentae in, 87, 92, 93–94, 93f
  acceptance of, 60
  acceptance of child in, 60
  adolescent, 61, 122
  after age 35, 123
  anemia in, 82
  antibiotics in, 120
  antihypertensives in, 101–103
  back pain in, 86
  bedrest in, 122
  binding-in in, 60
  bleeding during, 91–95, 93f
  blood volume changes in, 54
  breast changes in, 54
  cardiac output in, 55, 124
  cardiopulmonary resuscitation in, 97
  cardiovascular system changes in, 54

  cervical changes in, 54
  Chlamydia infection in, 110
  clonus in, 104, 104f
  clotting factors in, 55
  complementary care in, 84, 108–109
  complications of, 89–135
    bleeding, 91–95, 93f
    endocrine, 105–110
    genetic disease and, 79–80
    hypertensive, 95–105
    infectious, 110–120
  constipation in, 86
  cytomegalovirus infection in, 49, 117
  danger signs in, 58, 86–87
  depression in, 124
  diabetes mellitus in, 105–106
    diet and exercise for, 109
    insulin therapy for, 109–110
    preterm labor and, 107
  diagnostic tests in, 56–57, 66, 71–72, 79–80, 94, 107–108, 120, 124–125
  discomforts of, 85–86
  disseminated intravascular coagulation in, 121
  drug effects during, 45–48
  dyspareunia in, 85
  dyspepsia in, 85
  ectopic, 89, 91
  edema in, 85
  endocrine system changes in, 55–56
  estrogen effects in, 53
  ethnocultural considerations in, 57, 75, 81–82, 94–95, 215
  exercise in, 84
  eye changes in, 55
  fatigue in, 83–84, 85
  ferrous sulfate in, 81
  finger numbness and tingling in, 85
  first trimester, 70
    danger signs in, 86
    discomforts of, 85
  flatulence in, 85
  gastrointestinal tract changes in, 55
  genetic screening in, 79–80
  gestational diabetes mellitus in, 89, 106, 108, 109–110
  glucose challenge test in, 107
  glucose tolerance test in, 107–108
  gonorrhea in, 110
  group B *Streptococcus* in, 71, 110
  gum disorders in, 85
  health promotion for, 78–88

ferrous sulfate in, 81
genetic screening in, 79–80
heart changes in, 54
hemodynamic changes in, 124
hepatitis B virus infection in, 49, 113–114
herpes simplex virus infection, 49, 118–119
hormones in, 53
human immunodeficiency virus infection in, 111
human papillomavirus infection in, 111
hypertension in, 95–105. *See also* Eclampsia; Preeclampsia
hyperthyroidism in, 106
hyperventilation in, 85
hypothyroidism in, 106
immune system changes in, 55
immunizations in, 120
infection in, 110–120
insomnia in, 86
integumentary system changes in, 54
intimate partner violence and, 66, 123
iron-deficiency anemia in, 54, 81
iron in, 54, 82, 83
isotretinoin contraindication in, 556
leg cramps in, 85
leukorrhea in, 86
loss of, 91, 95, 184
magnesium sulfate in, 99–101
maternal tasks of, 60–61
molar, 86, 90, 91
multiple gestation in, 86, 121
musculoskeletal system changes in, 56
nasal congestion in, 86
nausea and vomiting in, 85, 86
medications for, 108
patient/family teaching for, 108–109
neurological system changes in, 54
nocturia in, 85
non-nutritive substances in, 82
nose changes in, 55
nursing-care goals for, 75
nutrition in, 82–83
obesity and, 123
in older gravida, 123
ovarian changes in, 54
oxytocin in, 53, 131
pancreas changes in, 56

parathyroid changes in, 55
patient/family teaching for, 47–50, 58–59, 75, 82–87
physiological adaptations in, 52–56, 53f, 58
pica in, 82
placenta previa in, 92, 93f
placental abruption in, 92, 93f
postdate, 176
postterm, 177
preeclampsia in. *See* Preeclampsia
progesterone effects in, 53
prolactin effects in, 53
prostaglandin in, 53, 131
psychiatric complications of, 122
psychosocial adaptations in, 59
ptyalism in, 86
pyelonephritis in, 110
recreational drug use in, 122
reflexes in, 104, 104f
relationship reordering in, 60
relaxin effects in, 53
resources on, 87, 134
respiratory system changes in, 55
Rh isoimmunization in, 122
Rho(D) immune globulin in, 129–131, 132
rubella infection in, 48–49, 115–116
safe passage in, 60
second trimester, 70
danger signs in, 86
discomforts of, 85
seizure in, 97–98
shortness of breath in, 85
sickle cell disease and, 121
skin changes in, 54, 215
substance abuse during, 73–74, 122
supine hypotension syndrome in, 52, 61, 61f, 85, 157
syphilis in, 111
teratogen exposure in, 45–46
terbutaline in, 131
tests for, 590
thalassemia and, 122
third trimester, 71
danger signs in, 86–87
discomforts of, 85–86
throat changes in, 55
thromboembolism in, 121, 123
thyroid changes in, 55
tocolytic agents in, 131–132
TORCH infections during, 48–49, 112–119
toxoplasmosis in, 48, 112–113

Pregnancy (Continued)
trauma in, 133–134
tuberculosis in, 111
urinary frequency in, 85
urinary system changes in, 55
urinary tract infection in, 77, 86,
110, 120
urine sample in, 76–77
uterine growth in, 53f, 54, 65, 66f
vaginal changes in, 54
varicosities in, 85
vitamin B_{12} deficiency in, 83
vitamin D deficiency in, 81
vitamins in, 82
vomiting in, 86, 107
medications for, 108
patient/family teaching for,
108–109
vulvar changes in, 54
weight gain in, 83, 87
Premature Infant Pain Profile, 294,
295f
Prenatal assessment, 63–77
alpha-fetoprotein screening in, 72
estimated date of birth in, 67–68
ethnocultural considerations in, 75
fetal heart tones in, 68, 68f
fetal presentation in, 68, 70f
first trimester, 70
after first visit, 68–69, 68f, 69f, 70f
first visit for, 65–68
gestational diabetes screening in, 71
goals of, 75
group B Streptococcus screening in,
71, 110
health history in, 65
hemoglobin/hematocrit in, 71
hypertension in, 75
intimate partner violence screening
in, 66
Leopold maneuvers in, 68–69, 68f,
69f
patient/family teaching in, 75
physical examination in, 65, 66f
pregnancy history in, 67
pregnancy signs in, 67
recreational drug use screening in,
73–74
Rh screening in, 71
screening/diagnostic tests in, 66,
71–72, 79–80, 124–128
second trimester, 70
teratogen exposure in, 45–46
third trimester, 71

triple test in, 72
ultrasonography in, 71
urine sample for, 76–77
Prenatal care, 42–44. See also Prenatal
assessment
after first visit, 68–69, 68f, 69f, 70f
first visit for, 42, 65–68
Prenatal diagnosis, 71, 124–128
Preschoolers, 314. See also Children
chronic illness in, 672, 680
death perceptions of, 674
growth and development of, 321,
328
pain management in, 368
procedure preparation for, 360–361
sleep for, 4
vital signs in, 333
Pressure ulcers, 569–571, 570f
Preterm birth, 183
in diabetes mellitus, 198
Preterm infant, 50. See also Neonate
abdominal assessment in, 296–297
aspiration in, 301
assessment of, 293–300
betamethasone for, 263–264
bilirubin in, 300, 300f
blood gases in, 295
blood glucose in, 301–302
blood pressure in, 301, 309–310
cardiac assessment in, 296–298
chest assessment in, 296–298
circulation of, 293
clavicular fracture in, 301
clinical alerts for, 301
cold stress in, 294
developmental care for, 310–311
dexamethasone for, 263–264
diagnostic tests for, 301–303
endotracheal tube for, 311–312
ethnocultural considerations for,
305
extracorporeal membrane oxygenation for, 308
fractured clavicle in, 301
genitourinary assessment in,
296–297
head assessment in, 296–297
hematocrit in, 302
hemoglobin in, 302
hyperglycemia in, 301–302
hypoglycemia in, 301–302, 306–307
incubator weaning for, 306
intensive care unit for, 305–306, 311
jaundice in, 300, 300f, 307–308

lung maturity in, 293
mechanical ventilation for, 312
medications for, 303–305
microcephaly in, 301
musculoskeletal assessment in, 296–297
necrotizing enterocolitis in, 308–309
neurological system in, 293, 296–298
nutrition for, 301
pain in, 294, 295f
patient/family teaching for, 305–306
pH in, 295
radiology in, 302
red blood cells in, 302
resources on, 312–313
respiratory distress syndrome in, 302
respiratory rate in, 301, 307
retinopathy in, 308
skin assessment in, 296–299
S.T.A.B.L.E. program for, 311
surfactant therapy for, 303–304
tachypnea in, 307
temperature in, 294
transport team for, 311
weight of, 305
white blood cells in, 303
withdrawal syndrome in, 300, 304–305
Preterm labor, 86, 121
clinical alert on, 107
patient/family teaching for, 184
risk factors for, 133
tocolytic therapy in, 131–132
Primigravida, 64
Privacy, for children, 316
Privilege withholding, for discipline, 318
Probiotics, 417
Procedure(s)
amniotic fluid assessment, 148–149
Barlow-Ortolani maneuver, 275–276
cast petaling, 540–541
fecal occult blood test, 622
fetal heart tone auscultation, 145–146
fundal massage, 224–226
fungal culture, 554–555
head circumference measurement, 518
insulin injection, 489–491
intrapartal vaginal examination, 146–148
mid-stream urine sample, 76–77

newborn blood pressure, 309–310
newborn length, 273–274
newborn suctioning, 268–269
oro-nasogastric tube, 365–366
preparation for, 363–364
adolescent, 361–362
consent in, 365
infant, 360
preschooler, 360–361
school-age child, 361
toddler, 360
sitz bath, 213–215
spinal anesthesia, 170
stool culture, 423–424
urine collection, 586–587
urine specific gravity, 647–648
Progesterone
in female infertility, 37
in pregnancy, 53
testing for, 27
Progestins, reproductive system effects of, 35
Prokinetics, 424, 425
Prolactin, 53, 57, 591
Promethazine, in pregnancy-related nausea and vomiting, 108
Propoxyphene napsylate and acetaminophen, postpartal, 211
Prostaglandin, 1
in pregnancy, 53, 131
Prostaglandin E$_1$, in labor, 182
Prostaglandin E$_2$, in labor, 182–183
Prostate gland, 24f
Protein
cerebrospinal fluid, 352
in pregnancy, 56, 82
urinary, 588, 589
in neonate, 262
in pregnancy, 57
Protest, 372
Prothrombin complex transfusion, 635
Prothrombin time, 621
Proton pump inhibitors, 424
Pruritus gravidarum, 52
Pseudocyesis, 64
Psoas sign, 418
Psychological/psychosocial factors
in cancer, 643, 667, 669
in enuresis, 605
in labor, 143
in neonatal physiological transition, 260–261
in postpartal period, 240–241, 246
in pregnancy, 59

Psychopathology, developmental, 381
Psychosis, postpartal, 223, 240–241
Ptyalism, 52
  in pregnancy, 86
Puberty, 17, 18
  ethnocultural considerations in, 316
Pubic hair, 341
Pudendal nerve block, 169
Puerperium. *See* Postpartum period
  (puerperium)
Pulmonary artery, 464, 464f
Pulmonary atresia, 466, 467f
Pulmonary function testing
  in children, 401–402
  peak flow meter for, 410–412
Pulmonary vein, 464, 464f
Pulmonic stenosis, 466
Pulmonic valve stenosis, 466, 467f
Pulses
  in musculoskeletal injury, 527
  neonatal, 269, 270
  pediatric, 337
Pushing, in labor, 156
Pustule, 548
Pyelogram, intravenous, 422
Pyelonephritis, 574
Pyloric stenosis, hypertrophic,
  420–421, 425–426
Pyridoxine, in pregnancy-related
  nausea and vomiting, 108
Pyruvate kinase deficiency, 264

Q
Quickening, 64

R
Rabies, 438
RADAR, for intimate partner violence
  screening, 66
Radiation, heat, 255, 569
Radiation therapy, 644, 667
  teratogenicity of, 46
Radiography, 533
Radiology, in preterm infant, 302
Radionuclide scan, 422
Rage reduction therapy, 386
Rebirth therapy, 386
Rebound tenderness, 417
Red blood cells
  neonatal, 262
  pediatric, 619, 620
  preterm infant, 302
  urinary, 588, 590

Red reflex, 283, 351
Referred pain, 162
Reflex(es)
  Babinski, 278, 315
  in children, 342–343
  corneal, 350, 505
  crawling, 279
  crossed extension, 280
  extrusion, 277
  fencing, 278
  Galant, 279
  glabellar, 278
  grasping, 315
  magnet, 279
  Moro, 279, 315
  neonatal, 277–280
  palmar grasp, 277, 315
  plantar grasp, 277, 315
  in preeclampsia, 199
  in pregnancy, 104, 104f
  red, 283, 351
  rooting, 277, 315
  stepping, 278
  sucking, 277, 315
  toe grasp, 277
  tonic neck, 278
  trunk incurvation, 279
Reflexology, in pregnancy, 84
Regression, 672, 680
Relaxation exercise, in pregnancy, 84
Relaxin, in pregnancy, 53
Renal failure, in children, 456
Renal tubular function, 589
Reproductive health history, 26
Reproductive system
  in chronic renal failure, 579
  female, 18–23, 19f, 20f
    drug effects on, 34–36
    external structures of, 18–19, 19f
    focused assessment of, 18
    health history for, 26
    internal structures of, 19–20, 19f,
      20f
    menstrual cycle and, 21–23, 22f, 23f
  male, 23–24, 24f
Residual volume, 402
Resiliency, in children, 362
Respiration
  Cheyne-Stokes, 675
  heat loss with, 569
  pediatric, 347–348
Respiratory distress
  neonatal, 282
  pediatric, 337

Respiratory distress syndrome, 252
  in preterm infant, 302
Respiratory rate
  neonatal, 269, 270, 301
  pediatric, 333, 398, 435
  in preeclampsia, 199
  preterm infant, 297–298, 307
Respiratory syncytial virus infection,
  414
Respiratory system
  infant, 412–413
  maternal, 55
  neonatal, 253–254, 254f, 272
  pediatric, 396–415
    assessment of, 396, 397, 412–413,
      436
    in cystic fibrosis, 413
    disorders of. *See also specific*
      conditions
    clinical alerts in, 398–399
    diagnostic tests in, 400–403
    emergency, 397, 413–415
    ethnocultural considerations in,
      406
    maternal obstetric history and,
      398–399
    medications for, 403–406
    patient/family teaching in,
      407–412
    resources on, 415
    suctioning and, 399
  preterm infant, 296–298
Respite care, 672, 681
Restraints, for children, 367
Reticulocyte count, 620
  in preterm infant, 302
Retinitis, cytomegalovirus, 443–444
Retinoblastoma, 642
Retinopathy of prematurity, 308
Retractions, 336, 396
Reye syndrome, 437, 503
  patient/family teaching on, 512
Rh factor, 65, 122
  screening for, 71
Rh immune globulin (RhoGAM), 65,
  129–131, 132
Rh isoimmunization, 122, 129–131
Rhabdomyosarcoma, 642
Rheumatoid factor, 535
Rhonchi, 337, 348
RICE acronym, 544–545
Ringworm, 449, 550–551
Rinne test, 352
Rocky Mountain spotted fever, 555

Role modeling, for children, 378
Romberg test, 342
Rooting reflex, 277, 315
Rotavirus infection, 428
  immunization against, 2
Round ligament, 20, 20f
Rovsing sign, 418
Rubella
  immunization against, 2
  in pregnancy, 48–49, 115–116
Rule of 9's, 565, 565f
Russell's traction, 541, 542f

S
Safety
  for adolescents, 6
  for chemotherapy, 666
  in increased intracranial pressure,
    506
  for infants and children, 5, 348
  material safety data sheets for, 553
St. John's wort, 357
  in postpartum depression, 248
Salicylates, patient/family teaching for,
  409
Salpingectomy, 90
Salpingostomy, 90
Scales, cutaneous, 549
Scar, 549
School-age children, 314. *See also*
  Children
  chronic illness in, 673, 680–681
  death perceptions of, 675
  growth and development of,
    321–322, 329
  pain management in, 368–369
  procedure preparation for, 361
  vital signs in, 333
Scoliosis, 530, 531f
Screening. *See also* Diagnostic tests
  adolescent health promotion, 6–7
  alcohol use/abuse, 8
  alpha-fetoprotein, 72
  aspirin prophylaxis, 7
  breast cancer, 7, 11
  cervical cancer, 8
  Chlamydia infection, 8
  cholesterol, 8, 10
  cigarette smoking, 8
  colon cancer, 8
  cystic fibrosis, 80
  genetic, in pregnancy, 79–80
  gestational diabetes, 71

Screening (*Continued*)
glucose-6-phosphate dehydrogenase deficiency, 80
gonorrhea, 8
group B *Streptococcus,* 71, 110
hearing, 351–352
hemophilia, 80
herbal preparations, 10
hypertension, 8
intimate partner violence, 66
lipoprotein, 10
medication, 10
metabolic, neonatal, 283–284
prenatal, 66, 71–72, 79–80
recreational drug use, 73–74
Rh, 71
sickle cell disease, 79
Tay-Sachs disease, 79
testicular cancer, 13–14
thalassemia, 79
triglycerides, 10
vision, 8
Scrotum, 24f
auscultation of, 283
Sedatives
intrapartal, 164, 166
teratogenicity of, 45
Segmented neutrophils, 534
Seizures
medications for, 509–510
nursing care for, 516
precautions for, 506
in preeclampsia, 199
in pregnancy, 97–98
signs and symptoms of, 514–515
Selective serotonin reuptake inhibitors, 387
female reproductive system effects of, 34
suicide behavior and, 385–386
Semen analysis, 28
Seminal vesicle, 24f
Sensation, extremity, 526
Separation, child-parent, 372, 376–378
Sepsis, neonatal, 309
Septic shock, 668
Sertraline, 387
Sex chromosomes, 17
disorders of, 50
Sexual abuse, 384
Sexual history, 34
Shaken baby syndrome, 504–505
Shiver response, with epidural block, 171

Shock, 419
in children, 488
septic, 643, 645, 668
Short bowel syndrome, 422, 430
Shoulder dystocia, 177, 192–193, 193f
Siblings
acting out by, 673–674
of cancer patient, 669
of chronically ill child, 673, 681
of dying child, 678, 688–689
new baby adjustment of, 218
Sickle cell disease
in children, 611, 621
ethnocultural considerations in, 625
patient/family teaching in, 627
pregnancy and, 121
resources on, 639
screening for, 79
Simian crease, 267
Sinus arrhythmias, 476
Sinuses, pediatric, 336
Sinusitis, 408
Sitz bath, 203, 213–215
Skeletal traction, 542, 542f, 543f
Skene's ducts, 19f
Skin
color of, 281–282, 333, 338, 348, 359
infant, 563
layers of, 547
lesions of
in children, 548–552
in neonate, 280–281
neonatal, 280–282
pediatric, 547–573
acne of, 550, 563
assessment of, 330, 333, 548–552
in chronic renal failure, 579
clinical alerts in, 552–554
color changes in, 348
diagnostic tests in, 554–555
ethnocultural considerations in, 559
fungal infection of, 449–450
lesions of, 548–552. *See also specific conditions*
medications in, 555–558
patient/family teaching in, 559–562
resources on, 571
ringworm of, 550–551
wound management for, 563
in pregnancy, 54, 215
preterm infant, 296–299
Skin traction, 541, 542f

Skull, plagiocephaly prevention for, 4–5
Skull fracture, basal, 519
Sleep
  hygiene for, 390–391
  neonatal, 4, 260–261
  pediatric, 4
    disorders of, 385
Slipped capital femoral epiphysis, 527
Small for gestational age, 78
Snoring, 347
Social history, in child assessment, 325
SODA, for child's health history, 325
Sodium
  deficit of, 583
  excess of, 583
  fractional excretion of, 589
  in pregnancy, 57
  in Rocky Mountain spotted fever, 555
  urinary, 589
Sodium bicarbonate, 594
Sodium citrate, 594
Sodium nitroprusside, 594
  in pregnancy, 103
Sore throat, in cancer patient, 660
Sorrow, chronic, 671
Soy-based formula, 496
SPASMS mnemonic, 104–105
Specific gravity, urinary, 588, 647–649
  in neonate, 262
Sperm
  analysis of, 28
  intracytoplasmic injection of, 39
Spermicides, 30
Spherocytosis, hereditary, 612
Spina bifida, 517
Spinal block, 167, 167f, 169
  administration of, 170
  complications of, 165, 166
  contraindications to, 170–171
  headache after, 166
  hypotension with, 165
Spinal-epidural anesthesia, 169
Spinal tap, 646, 646f, 651–652
Spinnbarkheit, 18
Spiritual care, for parents, 363
Spironolactone, female reproductive system effects of, 36
Spleen
  absence of, 614–615
  trauma to, 431
Sponge, contraceptive, 30
Sprain, 529–530

Sputum culture, 403
S.T.A.B.L.E. program, 311
Status asthmaticus, 396
Stepping reflex, 278
Stereotyping, 358
Sterility, 26
Sterilization, 33
Stevens-Johnson syndrome, 553
Stimulants, 388
Stool culture, 423–424
Stool softener, postpartal, 210–211
Stork bite, 267
Strabismus, 499
Strawberry hemangioma, 267
Strength, assessment of, 342
Streptococcus, group B, prenatal screening for, 71, 110
Stretch marks, 52
Striae gravidarum, 52
Stridor, 348
Stroke volume, 453
Stupor, 500
Sturge-Weber syndrome, 281
Sty, 519
Subacute bacterial endocarditis, 475–476
Subinvolution, 203
Submersion injury, 503–504
Substance abuse
  maternal, 73–74, 122
  neonatal abstinence syndrome and, 300, 304–305
  pediatric, 385
Sucking reflex, 277, 315
Suctioning
  neonatal, 189, 268–269, 282, 287
  postoperative, 399
  preoperative, 399
Sudden infant death syndrome, 283
Sufentanil citrate, in labor pain, 168
Suicide, 382–383, 385–386, 388
Sulfamethoxazole/trimethoprim, 593
Sun protection, for neonate, 283
Superior mediastinum syndrome, 645
Superior vena cava syndrome, 645
Supine hypotension syndrome, 52, 61, 61f, 85, 157
Supraglottitis, 413–414
Surfactant, 252
  synthetic, 303–304
Surgery, in cancer, 667
Swallowing, cancer-related difficulty with, 660
Sweat chloride test, 401

Sympathetic blockade, 162
Syncope, 462
    tilt test in, 458–459
Syphilis, in pregnancy, 111
Systemic lupus erythematosus
    clinical alert on, 437
    resources on, 448–449, 452

T

Tachycardia, fetal, 137
Tachypnea, neonatal, 282, 307
Tachysystole, 137
Talipes equinovarus, 539, 543
Tamoxifen, female reproductive system
    effects of, 35
Tanner stage, 340, 341
Tantrums, 320–321
Tay-Sachs disease, screening for, 79
Tea tree oil, 357
Tear duct blockage, 520
Technology-dependent patient, 672,
    679
Teething, 3–4
Telangiectasia, 267
Telangiectatic nevus, 267, 281
Temperament, infant, 319–320
Temperature
    Centigrade-Fahrenheit conversion
        for, 332
    extremity, 526
    infant, 563
    neonatal, 270
    pediatric, 331, 517
    preterm infant, 294
Teratogen, 42
Terbutaline
    in pregnancy, 131
    in preterm labor, 107
Testicular torsion, 580, 591
Testis (testes), 24f
    self-examination of, 13–14
Testosterone, 24, 591
TET spells, 457
Tetanus, 537–538, 545–546
    immunization against, 2, 545
Tetanus toxoid, 445
Tetracycline, 555
Tetralogy of Fallot, 267–268, 456–457,
    470, 471f
Thalassemia
    in children, 611–612
    pregnancy effects of, 122
    screening for, 79
Thelarche, 18

Theoretical effectiveness, 26
Therapeutic play, 372, 377
Thermogenesis, 252
    nonshivering, 252
Throat
    pediatric, 336
    in pregnancy, 55
    sore, in cancer patient, 660
Thrombocytopenia, 621
Thrombocytopenia purpura, idio-
    pathic, 612, 615, 628, 630–631
Thrombocytosis, 621
Thromboembolism, in pregnancy, 121,
    123
Thrombophlebitis, postpartal, 223,
    239–240
    septic, 238
Thrombosis
    apheresis-related, 638
    in children, 457, 613–614
    postpartal, 223, 239–240
Thrush, 564
Thyroid gland, in pregnancy, 55
Thyroid hormone
    in pregnancy, 57
    reproductive system effects of, 36
Thyroid-stimulating hormone, 591
Thyroid storm, pediatric, 482–483
Thyrotoxicosis, 90
Thyroxin (T_4), in pregnancy, 57
Tick bite, 565
Tidal volume, 401
Tilt test, 458–459
Time-out, for discipline, 318
Tinea capitis, 449, 550
Tinea corporis, 450, 551
Tinea cruris, 450, 551
Tinea pedis, 450, 551
Tissue adhesives, 563
Tocolysis, 90
    contraindications to, 132
    nursing care for, 131–132
Toddlers, 314. See also Children
    chronic illness in, 672, 680
    death perceptions of, 674
    growth and development of,
        320–321
    procedure preparation for, 360
    sleep for, 4
    vital signs in, 333
Toe grasp reflex, 277
Toilet training, 391
Tonic neck reflex, 278
Tonsillectomy

bleeding after, 399
  patient/family teaching for, 408
Topical agents/medications, 558
Topiramate, 510
TORCH infections, 48–49, 112–119
Torticollis, 281
Total anomalous pulmonary venous return, 469, 470f
Total lung capacity, 402
Toxic shock syndrome, 26
Toxoplasmosis, in pregnancy, 48, 112–113
Tracheoesophageal atresia, 407
Traction
  skeletal, 542, 542f, 543f
  skin, 541, 542f
Transcutaneous electrical nerve stimulation, 162
Transfusion-related acute lung injury, 618
Transplantation
  allogeneic, 610
  autologous, 610
  syngeneic, 610
Transposition of great arteries, 469
Trauma
  abdominal, 431–432
  infant, 504–505
  in pregnancy, 133–134
Triamcinolone, topical, 558
Tricuspid atresia, 468, 469f
Tricyclic antidepressants, female reproductive system effects of, 34
Trigeminal nerve, 343
Triglycerides, screening for, 10
Triiodothyronine (T_3), in pregnancy, 57
Trimethoprim-sulfamethoxazole, 439–440, 593
Triple test, in prenatal assessment, 72
Tripod position, 414
Trisomy, 42
Trisomy 13, 455
Trisomy 18, 455
Trisomy XXY, 50
Trochlear nerve, 343
Truncus arteriosus, 469, 470f
Trunk incurvation reflex, 279
Trust, nurse-family, 682–683
L-Tryptophan, female reproductive system effects of, 36
Tubal embryo transfer, 39
Tubal ligation, 25
Tuberculin skin test, 403

Tuberculosis, in pregnancy, 111
Tumor. *See* Cancer *and specific tumors*
Tumor lysis syndrome, 643, 668
Tuning fork testing, 351–352
Turner syndrome, 50, 455
Twenty-four-hour observation unit, 379
Twins, 197
  dizygotic, 41
  monozygotic, 41
Tympanic membrane, 335, 335f
  rupture of, 399
Tympanogram, 499
Tympanometry, 351

U
Ulcer, 550
  pressure, 569–571, 570f
Ulcerative colitis, 421, 422
Ultrasound, 533
  fetal, 126, 127
  for ovulation, 27
  in pediatric gastrointestinal disorders, 421, 422
  prenatal, 71
  renal, 585
  in testicular torsion, 591
Umbilical artery, 255
Umbilical cord
  care of, 287–288
  percutaneous blood sampling of, 125
  prolapse of, 189–190, 190f
  variations in, 194
  velamentous insertion of, 194
Umbilical vein, 254
Umbilical velocimetry, 127
Urea nitrogen, in pregnancy, 57
Uric acid, in pregnancy, 57
Urinalysis, 586–588, 588f
  in acute kidney failure, 589
  in neonate, 262
  in Rocky Mountain spotted fever, 555
Urinary frequency, in pregnancy, 85
Urinary output, 345
Urinary tract infection, 574, 576, 600–601
  postpartal, 234–235
  during pregnancy, 77, 86, 120
Urine
  blood in, 262, 582, 601
  collection of, 586–587

Urine *(Continued)*
  mid-stream sample of, 76–77
  pH of, 649
  specific gravity of, 647–649
User effectiveness, 26
Uterine, postpartum assessment of,
    205f
Uteroplacental insufficiency, 138
Uterus
  anatomy of, 19f, 20, 20f
  atony of, 224–226, 227
  contractions of, 138–139, 177–178,
      178f, 183
  fundus of, 64
  hypertonic contractions of, 176,
      177, 178, 178f
  hypotonic contractions of, 176, 177,
      178, 178f, 183
  involution of, 137, 202, 204–206,
      205f
  labor-related contractions of,
      138–139
  massage of, 224–226
  postpartal assessment of, 204–206,
      205f
  pregnancy-related growth in, 53f,
      54, 65, 66f
  rupture of, 193
  subinvolution of, 203

V

Vaccine, 445–446. *See also*
    Immunization
Vaccine information sheet, 451–452
Vacuum-assisted birth, 177, 192, 192f
Vagina, 19f
  hematoma of, 227, 228f
  intrapartal examination of, 146–148
  intrapartal laceration of, 227
  in pregnancy, 54
Vaginal bleeding, in pregnancy, 86, 87
Vaginal ring, 32
Vaginitis, in pregnancy, 86
Vagus nerve, 343
Valerian, 357
Valproate, 387, 388
Valproic acid, 509, 510
Valvuloplasty, 459
Varicella immunization, 2
Varicocele, 580
Varicosities, in pregnancy, 85
Vasa previa, 194
Vasectomy, 26

VATER (VACTERLS) association, 455
Vecuronium, 538
Velo-cardio-facial syndrome, 454
Vena cava, 463, 464f
Vena caval syndrome, 52, 61, 61f
Venous access devices, 663–664, 665f
Venous system, 464, 465f
Ventricular septal defect, 465, 465f
Ventricular shunt, 512, 517
Verbal reprimand, for discipline, 318
Verruca plana, 564
Verruca plantaris, 564
Verruca vulgaris, 564
Version, fetal, 177
Vesicle, cutaneous, 548
Vesicoureteral reflux, 576
Vibroacoustic stimulation, fetal, 128
Vincristine, 657
Violence, youth, 393
Viral gastroenteritis, 428
Virulence, 434
Vision screening, 8, 350–351, 350f
Visual acuity, 350, 350f
Visualization, for procedures, 661–662
Vital capacity, 402
Vital signs
  in intrapartal hemorrhage, 195
  neonatal, 270
  pediatric, 331–333, 435
    night-time waking for, 477
    postoperative, 458
    postpartal, 203, 226–227
Vitamin A, teratogenicity of, 45
Vitamin B_{12} deficiency, in pregnancy,
    83
Vitamin C, in pregnancy, 82
Vitamin D
  deficiency of
    in pregnancy, 81
    teratogenicity of, 45
  in hypoparathyroidism, 496
  in pregnancy, 82
Vitamin E, teratogenicity of, 45
Vitamin K
  in hypoparathyroidism, 496
  for neonate, 285–286
Vitamins, in renal failure, 594
Voiding, dysfunctional, 605
Voiding cystogram, 422
Voiding cystourethrogram, 585, 585f
Vomiting
  pediatric
    in cancer, 659

causes of, 429
cyclic, 421
medications for, 425
in pregnancy, 85, 86, 107, 108
Von Willebrand's disease, 612
Vulva
hematoma of, 227, 228f
in pregnancy, 54
Vulvovaginitis
candidial, 596, 598
patient/family teaching on, 597–598

W
Warfarin, 245–246
Warts, 564
genital, 89
Wasp sting, 553
Water, insensible loss of, 252
Water deprivation test, 483–484
Water intake, in pregnancy, 82
Weber test, 351
Weight
maternal, 83, 87
neonatal, 209, 271, 271f, 282, 294
pediatric, 345, 495
for drug dose, 495
measurement of, 576
Wharton's jelly, 268
Wheal, 549

Wheezing, 337, 348
White blood cells
cerebrospinal fluid, 352
complete count of, 534
differential, 303, 534, 620
neonatal, 262, 303
pediatric, 619
preterm infant, 303
in Rocky Mountain spotted fever, 555
urinary, 588, 590
in neonate, 262
Williams syndrome, 454
Wilms' tumor, 641–642
Witch hazel, postpartal, 211
Withdrawal syndrome, in neonate, 300, 304–305
Wong-Baker faces pain scale, 346f
Wristbands, in pregnancy-related nausea and vomiting, 109

Y
Youth violence, 393
resources on, 394

Z
Zygote, 26
Zygote intrafallopian transfer, 39